Leininger's Transcultural Nursing

Concepts, Theories, Research & Practice

Fourth Edition

Marilyn R. McFarland, PhD, RN, FNP-BC, CTN-A
Professor
School of Nursing
University of Michigan-Flint

Hiba B. Wehbe-Alamah, PhD, RN, FNP-BC, CTN-A
Professor
School of Nursing
University of Michigan-Flint

Mc
Graw
Hill
Education

New York   Chicago   San Francisco   Athens   London   Madrid   Mexico City
Milan   New Delhi   Singapore   Sydney   Toronto

Leininger's Transcultural Nursing: Concepts, Theories, Research & Practice, Fourth Edition

1 2 3 4 5 6 7 8 9   LCR   23 22 21 20 19 18

ISBN 978-0-07-184113-9
MHID 0-07-184113-X

Notice

Medicine is an ever-changing science. As new research and clinical experience broaden our knowledge, changes in treatment and drug therapy are required. The authors and the publisher of this work have checked with sources believed to be reliable in their efforts to provide information that is complete and generally in accord with the standards accepted at the time of publication. However, in view of the possibility of human error or changes in medical sciences, neither the authors nor the publisher nor any other party who has been involved in the preparation or publication of this work warrants that the information contained herein is in every respect accurate or complete, and they disclaim all responsibility for any errors or omissions or for the results obtained from use of the information contained in this work. Readers are encouraged to confirm the information contained herein with other sources. For example and in particular, readers are advised to check the product information sheet included in the package of each drug they plan to administer to be certain that the information contained in this work is accurate and that changes have not been made in the recommended dose or in the contraindications for administration. This recommendation is of particular importance in connection with new or infrequently used drugs.

This book was set in Minion pro by Cenveo® Publisher Services.
The editors were Susan Barnes and Christina M. Thomas.
The production supervisor was Rick Ruzycka.
Project management was provided by Neha Bhargava, Cenveo Publisher Services.
The cover designer was Randomatrix.

This book is printed on acid-free paper.

Library of Congress Cataloging-in-Publication Data

Names: McFarland, Marilyn R., author. | Wehbe-Alamah, Hiba B., author. |
    Preceded by (work): Leininger, Madeleine M. Transcultural nursing.
Title: Leininger's transcultural nursing : concepts, theories, research, &
    practice / Marilyn R. McFarland, Hiba B. Wehbe-Alamah.
Other titles: Transcultural nursing
Description: Fourth edition. | New York : McGraw-Hill Education, [2018] |
    Preceded by Transcultural nursing / Madeleine Leininger, Marilyn R.
    McFarland. 3rd ed. c2002. | Includes bibliographical references and index.
Identifiers: LCCN 2016035145| ISBN 9780071841139 (pbk. : alk. paper) | ISBN
    007184113X (pbk. : alk. paper)
Subjects: | MESH: Transcultural Nursing | Culturally Competent Care |
    Philosophy, Nursing
Classification: LCC RT86.54 | NLM WY 107 | DDC 610.73—dc23 LC record available at https://lccn.loc.gov/2016035145

About the Authors

Marilyn R. McFarland, PhD, RN, FNP-BC, CTN-A is a Professor in the School of Nursing at the University of Michigan-Flint. Dr. McFarland earned her PhD in Nursing with a focus in Transcultural Nursing from Wayne State University, Detroit, Michigan; Master of Science in Nursing from Wayne State with a major in Medical Surgical nursing and minors in Teaching in Nursing, Gerontological Nursing, and Transcultural Nursing; and Bachelor of Science in Nursing also from Wayne State. Her family nurse practitioner certificate was earned from Saginaw Valley State University in 2005.

As a Certified Transcultural Nurse and as a Transcultural Nursing Author and Scholar, Dr. McFarland has been nationally and internationally recognized for her contributions to transcultural nursing by the Transcultural Nursing Society having received their 1993 Leininger Award for Excellence in Transcultural Nursing. She was also the 1994 Recipient of the Leininger Transcultural Nursing Award for Excellence and Creative Leadership in Transcultural Nursing and Human Care from Wayne State University, College of Nursing. In addition to individually publishing numerous book chapters and articles, Dr. McFarland co-authored two texts with Dr. Madeleine Leininger: *Culture Care Diversity and Universality: A Worldwide Nursing Theory* (2006) and *Transcultural Nursing: Concepts, Theories, Research, & Practice* (2002), which was the recipient of the 2003 American Journal of Nursing's Book of the Year Award. Published in 2015, she co-authored the third edition of *Leininger's Culture Care Diversity and Universality: A Worldwide Nursing Theory* with Dr. Hiba Wehbe-Alamah.

Dr. McFarland is a past editor of the Journal of the Transcultural Nursing; past chair of the Transcultural Nursing Certification Commission whose members developed a revised certification examination process under her guidance; and past member of the TCNS Board as well as serving on numerous Society committees. With Dr. Leininger, Dr. McFarland co-presented the 2011 Keynote Address at the 37th Annual TCNS International Conference in Las Vegas, Nevada. She is also a member of the National Organization of Nurse Practitioner Faculties; Michigan Council of Nurse Practitioners; American Nurses' Association; the Michigan Nurses' Association; and ANA-Michigan (formerly RN-AIM). As a career-long member of Sigma Theta Tau International, she is active in the local Pi Delta chapter based at UM-Flint.

Dr. McFarland has taught at the undergraduate level in the areas of gerontology, fundamentals of nursing, and health assessment. She currently teaches nursing at the graduate level with focus on transcultural health care, advanced practice nursing role development, and graduate translational research. She has served on many doctoral nursing dissertation committees nationally as well as on master's theses committees statewide and currently supervises numerous graduate-level translational research projects. Her clinical practice is focused on diverse and underserved clients in pediatric private practice and in caring for underserved women at a local health department family planning clinic.

As a leader in transcultural nursing, Dr. McFarland has studied, practiced, consulted, and lectured throughout the United States and in various parts of Europe, Kenya, Taiwan, and Australia. She has conducted transcultural research studies focused on Polish, Anglo-American, African-American, Mexican-American, and German-American elders, using Leininger's Theory of Culture Care Diversity and Universality as well as co-participating in a metasynthesis of culture care theory research studies guided by the Theory of Culture Care Diversity and Universality. Along with Dr. Wehbe-Alamah and Dr. Margaret Andrews, Dr. McFarland is currently planning to conduct an ethnohistorical study of key transcultural scholars and their contributions to the discipline. Her scholarly interests include the Scholarship of Teaching and Learning (SOTL); the translation of evidenced-based research into clinical practice; and the integration of transcultural nursing theory into nurse practitioner practice across the lifespan and in diverse settings.

Hiba B. Wehbe-Alamah, PhD, RN, FNP-BC, CTN-A is a Professor in the School of Nursing at the University of Michigan-Flint. Dr. Wehbe-Alamah earned her PhD degree and post Master's certificate in Transcultural Nursing from Duquesne University in Pittsburgh, Pennsylvania; Master of Science in Nursing (Family Nurse Practitioner) and Bachelor of Science in Nursing from Saginaw Valley State University, University Center, Michigan. She holds an advanced-level certification in transcultural nursing and was inducted as a Transcultural Nursing Scholar in 2011 by the Transcultural Nursing Society. She is the recipient of numerous awards including the University of Michigan-Flint Scholarly or Creative Achievement Award (2017), Teaching of Excellence Award (2016), and Provost Innovative Teaching Prize (2015); the Transcultural Nursing Society Madeleine M. Leininger Award (2015); and the National American Arab Nurses' Association Angel of Mercy Award (2014).

As a member of the Transcultural Nursing Society, National American Arab Nurses Association, National Organization of Nurse Practitioner Faculties, Michigan Council of Nurse Practitioners, American Nurses Association, Michigan Nurses Association, American Academy of Nurse Practitioners, and Sigma Theta Tau International, Dr. Wehbe-Alamah is nationally and internationally known for her contributions to Transcultural Nursing and Health Care. She has presented, guest-lectured, and published in the United States, Australia, Europe, Asia, and the Middle East, and played a key role in providing cultural competence educational training to registered nurses, advanced practice nurses, nursing faculty, nursing students, and diverse health care providers in 45 states and the District of Columbia as part of a 3-year federally funded Nurse Education, Practice, and Retention grant project entitled *Developing Nurses' Cultural Competencies: Evidence-based and Best Practices.*

Dr. Wehbe-Alamah led an interdisciplinary project involving faculty and students from Nursing, Computer Science, and Art departments at the University of Michigan-Flint to create the first prototype for a transcultural computer-based simulation game. As a member of the Transcultural Nursing Society Certification Commission, she co-developed an international online certification exam for advanced transcultural nurses and contributed test questions to the basic transcultural nursing certification exam for registered nurses. In addition, she teaches and advises nursing students at the undergraduate, master's, and doctoral levels in courses focused on women's health and transcultural health care. She chairs many doctoral translational research projects and is a member of numerous doctoral dissertation committees. Her clinical practice centers on women's health and the underinsured at a local community health department. Dr. Wehbe-Alamah's scholarly and research interests include obesity; women's health; mental health; primary care; creative teaching methodologies; computer simulation games; technology use in the academic setting; Asian, African-American, and Middle-Eastern health and well-being; health disparities; cultural healers and generic/folk beliefs and practices; and promoting cultural competence for diverse health care providers, nursing students, practicing nurses, and nursing faculty.

Contents

Color insert appears between pages 18 and 19

Contributors

Margaret M. Andrews, PhD, RN, CTN-A, FAAN
Interim Dean and Professor of Nursing
School of Nursing
University of Michigan-Flint
Flint, Michigan
USA

Lenny Chiang-Hanisko, PhD, RN
Associate Professor
Florida Atlantic University
Christine E. Lynn College of Nursing
Boca Raton, Florida
USA

Marilyn K. Eipperle, MSN, RN, FNP-BC, CTN-A
Lecturer II
School of Nursing
The University of Michigan-Flint
Flint, Michigan
USA

Pamela Embler, PhD, RN
Clinical Assistant Professor of Nursing
University of Tennessee
College of Nursing
Knoxville, Tennessee
USA

Valera A. Hascup, PhD, MSN, RN, CCES
Assistant Professor
Saint Peter's University
Jersey City, New Jersey
USA

Ann O. Hubbert, PhD, RN, CTN-A
Director and Professor, School of Nursing
College of Health Sciences
Boise State University
Boise, Idaho
USA

Robert H. Kelch, DNP, RN, FNP-BC
Family Nurse Practitioner
Health Delivery, Inc.
Saginaw, Michigan
USA

Janee F. Koc, MSN, RN, FNP-BC
Family Nurse Practitioner
Triumph Cancer Center
Flint, Michigan
USA

Rebecca C. Lee, PhD, RN, PHCNS-BC, CTN-A
Associate Professor
University of Cincinnati, College of Nursing
Cincinnati, Ohio
USA

Mary Brigid Martin, PhD, RN-BC, FNP, CTN-A
Faculty, Graduate Nursing
Keiser University
Fort Lauderdale, Florida
USA

Joanna M. Maxwell (Basuray), PhD, RN
Professor of Nursing
Towson University
Towson, Maryland
USA

Marilyn R. McFarland, PhD, RN, FNP-BC, CTN-A
Professor
School of Nursing
University of Michigan-Flint
Flint, Michigan
USA

Sandra J. Mixer, PhD, RN, CTN-A
Associate Professor of Nursing
University of Tennessee, College of Nursing
Knoxville, Tennessee
USA

R. Amadea Morningstar, BS, MA, RPE, RYT
Director, Ayurveda Polarity Therapy and
Yoga Institute
Santa Fe, New Mexico
USA

Edith J. Morris, PhD, RN, PPCNP-BC
Research Associate
Cincinnati Children's Hospital Medical Center
Cincinnati, Ohio
USA

Margaret A. Murray-Wright, MSN, RN
Clinical Assistant Professor
University of Michigan-Flint
Flint, Michigan
USA

Marilyn A. Ray, PhD, RN, CTN-A, FAAN
Professor Emeritus
Florida Atlantic University
Boca Raton, Florida
USA

Nancy R. Riggs, MSN, RN, ANP-BC, ACHPN
Adult Nurse Practitioner
Saint Joseph Mercy Health System- Palliative Care
Ann Arbor, Michigan
USA

Priscilla Limbo Sagar, EdD, RN, ACNS-BC, CTN-A
Professor, School of Nursing
Mount Saint Mary College
Newburgh, New York
USA

Cecily W. Strang, PhD, RN
Adjunct Faculty, King University, School of Nursing
Bristol, Tennessee
USA
Adjunct Faculty, Presbyterian University of East
Africa, Kenya
Community Health Worker
Maasailand, Kenya
East Africa

Helene Vossos, DNP, ARNP, ANP-BC, PMHNP-BC
Director of PMHNP-DNP Program and Assistant
Professor
Brooks College of Health
University of North Florida
Jacksonville, Florida
USA

Hiba B. Wehbe-Alamah, PhD, RN, FNP-BC, CTN-A
Professor
School of Nursing
University of Michigan-Flint
Flint, Michigan
USA

Mary T. Weiss, RN, MS, CTN-A
Associate Professor of Nursing
University of Alaska
School of Nursing - Bethel Outreach Site
Bethel, Alaska
USA

Foreword

Drs. Marilyn R. McFarland and Hiba B. Wehbe-Alamah are the foremost leaders, scholars, and experts in the world on Madeleine M. Leininger's *Theory of Culture Care Diversity and Universality* (also referred to as the *Culture Care Theory*), the Ethnonursing Research Method, and culturally congruent and competent nursing and health care. They are also pioneers in using metasynthesis to analyze ethnonursing studies guided by the Culture Care Theory to discover new and exciting benefits and values of the theory to advance transcultural nursing knowledge and skills. Their metasynthesis investigations also are instrumental in opening opportunities for interprofessional collaboration in research, education, and practice.

Prior to her passing in 2012, Dr. Leininger personally entrusted Drs. McFarland and Wehbe-Alamah with the honor and responsibility of writing future editions of her internationally acclaimed books. In 2015, Drs. McFarland and Wehbe-Alamah published a comprehensive, fully updated third edition of *Leininger's Culture Care Diversity and Universality: A worldwide Nursing Theory*. Prolific and facile writers, Drs. McFarland and Wehbe-Alamah worked diligently to complete the fourth edition of Dr. Leininger's popular *Transcultural Nursing: Concepts, Theories, Research, and Practices*. Dr. Leininger was a mentor colleague and friend to both the authors for many years, and their close relationship enables them to provide unique insights into the history, focus, and significance of transcultural nursing and examine key concepts, principles, guidelines, and policy statements relative to culturally congruent and competent health care. Drs. McFarland and Wehbe-Alamah provide the most comprehensive and authoritative compendium of Leininger's theory, research findings, cultural assessment, and other enablers or instruments that are available.

The fourth edition of *Transcultural Nursing* is a must-have text for the professional library of nurses and health care providers in other disciplines who strive to provide care to clients of diverse and similar cultures in meaningful, safe and beneficial ways—commonly referred to as *culturally congruent* or *culturally competent* care. Nursing and others in health-related fields will find a wellspring of information that will guide them in their quest for knowledge, understanding, and care of people from various cultures around the world. This is an authoritative, substantive, comprehensive text with both theoretical and practical information on transcultural nursing that will be useful for nurses and other health care providers in clinical practice, education, research, administration, and consultation.

I congratulate Dr. McFarland and Dr. Wehbe-Alamah on this outstanding contribution to transcultural nursing and health care.

Margaret M. Andrews, PhD, RN, CTN-A, FAAN
Interim Dean and Professor
School of Nursing
University of Michigan-Flint

Preface

The field of transcultural nursing has seen many major advances and breakthroughs since the publication of the third edition of this text in 2002. The purpose of the fourth edition of this book is to present readers with new transcultural nursing theoretical conceptualizations, discoveries, and applications as well as future directions for the discipline of transcultural nursing. The goal of this new edition is to promote the provision of culturally congruent transcultural health care for individuals, families, groups, communities, and organizations from diverse cultures locally, nationally, and globally. Since the first and second editions of this book were authored by Dr. Madeleine Leininger in 1978 and 1995, and the third edition co-authored with Dr. Marilyn McFarland in 2002, many transcultural nursing developments have inspired this fourth edition.

Six decades after Dr. Leininger pioneered the discipline of transcultural nursing, followed by later contributions from other transcultural nursing scholars, nursing and health care have been transformed. Much progress has been made in developing the body of transcultural nursing knowledge with concepts, principles, and research findings to guide nurses and other health care providers in caring for culturally diverse and similar people and populations around the world. Transcultural nursing theories supported by research findings are now being used to guide translational science practice innovation projects. These implementation projects introduce evidence-based care practices to nurses and others to prepare them to provide culturally congruent, sensitive, and meaningful care.

This fourth edition has three sections and 25 new chapters. In the first section, two chapters discuss the importance and historical evolution of transcultural nursing and the development of new transcultural nursing care concepts, principles, guidelines, and policies. In addition, major features and updates to the Theory of Culture Care Diversity and Universality, Ethnonursing Research Method, Sunrise Enabler, and other enablers are presented. The trailblazing influences of the Culture Care Theory on the development of other transcultural nursing theories and models are also discussed. Further, covered in this book is new content on the globalization of transcultural health care; cultural assessments and transcultural communications; generic and professional health care practices; transcultural food functions, beliefs, and practices; as well as the biocultural basis for transcultural nursing including genetic and genomic influences on care and health.

In the second section, special transcultural topics are presented including culturally congruent approaches for mental health care, the integration of culturally based care and caring into nursing practices, culturally congruent care for Haitians, and the relevance of Ayurvedic medicine in transcultural care practices. Also, an updated presentation of transcultural nursing and health care in Taiwan is shared; the role of the transcultural nurse in the global environment is explicated; and the application of the Culture Care Theory for transcultural conflict resolution for nurse administrators is described.

The third section focuses on research and practice. It presents the use of the Culture Care Theory in translational science through the process of engagement during cultural immersion experiences; culturally competent research practice about malaria care with the Maasai in Kenya is richly explicated; and it describes the lived experiences of urban-dwelling African-American women receiving transcultural care from nurse practitioners. Culture care research findings are also presented about the native Yupit people of southwest Alaska, the culture care needs of Appalachian mothers experiencing homelessness, Mexican-American women during the postpartum experience, and the culture care of Syrian Muslims in the midwestern United States.

This fourth edition expands previous transcultural nursing knowledge from prior editions to the present. The book reflects the work of experts and scholars in the discipline of transcultural nursing.

Their extensive experiences and actively sustained leadership render this book a substantive, authoritative, and credible contribution to transcultural nursing. The discipline of transcultural nursing remains a global imperative for study and practice for nurses and other health care providers.

Dr. Leininger passed the torch to us for the continued development of the Culture Care Theory and related contributions to the discipline of transcultural nursing. Through this book and other publications, we hope that we are successfully fulfilling her fervent wish *that the cultural needs of people in the world will be met by nurses prepared in transcultural nursing.*

Marilyn R. McFarland
Hiba B. Wehbe-Alamah

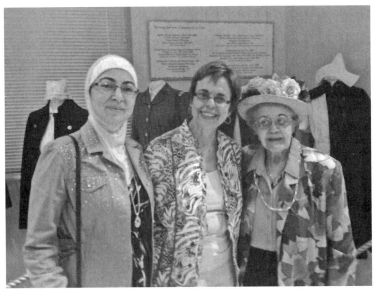

© 2010 Hiba B. Wehbe-Alamah

Picture of Drs. Hiba B. Wehbe-Alamah, Marilyn R. McFarland, and Madeleine M. Leininger taken in 2010 at the Leininger Library dedication, Florida Atlantic University, Boca Raton, Florida.

Dedication and Acknowledgment

This fourth edition is dedicated to Dr. Madeleine Leininger and the many nursing students, clinicians, faculty, scholars, researchers, administrators, and leaders who have been and remain actively committed to make transcultural nursing knowledge and practices a reality in human caring. These students and colleagues have blazed new pathways in the use of research-based transcultural nursing knowledge along with major concepts, principles, and practices to develop culturally congruent ways to provide meaningful and beneficial culture care. The book is also dedicated to our families, who have been understanding and caring as we have spent many days and nights on this major publication. We thank them for their patience and support.

Very special thanks go to our outstanding contributors. These transcultural nurse experts have shared their knowledge and practices to make this book truly a definitive, major, and substantive publication. The contributors' scholarship and expertise are clearly evident in their work, which has been drawn from their extensive in-depth experiences and use of theoretically based research knowledge to explicate the uses and practices of transcultural nursing. Their thoughtful work, genuine interest, and suggestions for the book have been much appreciated.

We are most grateful to Dr. Margaret Andrews for her willingness to write the foreword to this book. Her colleagueship, leadership, and friendship are deeply appreciated. We wish to acknowledge the McGraw-Hill staff for their unwavering dedication and support throughout the preparation and publication process. We also thank our colleague, Marilyn Eipperle, for her thoughtful and precise editing, incomparable organizational and communication skills, and her devotion to the integrity of the Culture Care Theory and the work of the late Dr. Madeleine Leininger. Marilyn, we could not have done this *second* book without you! Once again, we are truly grateful.

Finally, we thank the many cultural informants in Western and non-Western cultures. They have inspired the authors and editors to expand the discipline of transcultural nursing and the provision of culturally congruent quality care to diverse cultures worldwide.

Marilyn and Hiba

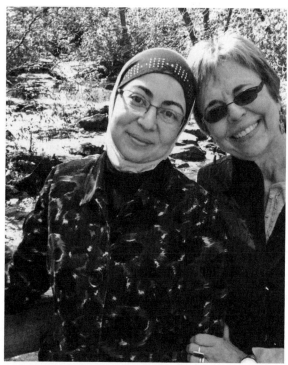

© 2010 Hiba B. Wehbe-Alamah

Picture of Drs. Hiba B. Wehbe-Alamah and Marilyn R. McFarland at Smoky Mountain National Park in Gatlinburg, Tennessee, following a Cultural Competence Training Workshop delivered at The University of Tennessee, Knoxville College of Nursing, Knoxville, Tennessee.

Transcultural Nursing: Essential Nursing Knowledge

CHAPTER 1

Transcultural Nursing: History, Focus, and Future Directions

Marilyn R. McFarland

> *Transcultural nursing has been defined as a formal area of study and practice focused on comparative human-care (caring) differences and similarities of the beliefs, values, and patterned lifeways of cultures to provide culturally congruent, meaningful, and beneficial health care to people (Leininger, 2002b, pp. 5-6).*

■ HISTORY OF TRANSCULTURAL NURSING

Madeleine M. Leininger, the founder of transcultural nursing, was the first professional nurse with graduate preparation in nursing to hold a PhD in cultural and social anthropology. While working at a child guidance home in the mid-1950s in Cincinnati, Leininger discovered that the staff lacked understanding of the cultural factors influencing the behavior of children. She observed differences in responses to care and psychiatric treatments among children from diverse cultural backgrounds, noting that traditional psychoanalytical therapy strategies did not seem to help them. Sometime thereafter, Leininger shared her observations and discussed the potential interrelationships between nursing and anthropology with Margaret Mead. Leininger asked Dr. Mead whether *she* saw any relationship between nursing and anthropology and "theoretical notions" to which Mead replied, "Well, that is something for you to discover" (Leininger, 1991).

During the 1950s and 1960s, Leininger (1970, 1978) identified some common areas of interest and scholarly work between the disciplines of nursing and anthropology, which inspired her in formulating transcultural nursing concepts, theory, principles, and practices. As doctoral student, Leininger studied the Gadsup people of the Eastern Highlands of New Guinea in the mid-1960s when she lived for two years with these indigenous people and undertook an ethnographic and ethnonursing study in their villages (Leininger, 1966, 1995, 1996). Not only was she able to observe the unique care views, beliefs, and practices of the culture, she also observed a number of striking differences between Western and non-Western cultures related to *care* and *health* practices. During her PhD dissertation study and first-hand experiences with the Gadsup people (1966), Leininger began to develop her *Theory of Culture Care Diversity and Universality* (*Culture Care Theory*) and the *Ethnonursing Research Method* (Leininger, 1978, 1991, 1995). Her research and theory have since guided nurses and nursing students in their study toward understanding the cultural differences and commonalities in how people care for themselves and their families during health and illness. Her enthusiasm and interest in developing the field of transcultural nursing with a care focus that sustained her in her mission for more than six decades.

In 1974, Leininger was appointed Dean and Professor of Nursing at the College of Nursing and Adjunct Professor of Anthropology at the University of Utah in Salt Lake City where she developed the first master's and doctoral programs in transcultural nursing (Leininger, 1978). These programs were the first in the world to offer substantive courses focused specifically on transcultural nursing. That same year, Leininger also founded the International Transcultural Nursing Society and remained an active leader in the organization throughout her lifetime.

Leininger's book, *Nursing and Anthropology: Two Worlds to Blend* (1970), laid the foundation for developing the field of transcultural nursing, the Culture Care Theory, and culturally-based health care. Her next book, *Transcultural Nursing: Concepts, Theories, and Practice* (1978), identified major concepts, theoretical ideas, and practices in transcultural nursing and was the first definitive publication on transcultural nursing. During the next 60 years, Leininger established, explicated, and used the Culture Care Theory to study many cultures within the United States and worldwide. She developed the Ethnonursing Research Method to fit and be used with the theory and to discover the insider or emic view of cultures (Leininger, 1991; Leininger & McFarland, 2002, 2006). The Ethnonursing Research Method was the first open inquiry research method designed for nurse researchers to study and discover culture care phenomena from the viewpoints of the person and their family as well as from the perspective of healthcare professionals (Leininger, 1978, 1985, 1990, 1991, 1995; Leininger & McFarland, 2002, 2006; McFarland & Wehbe-Alamah, 2015).

In the 1980s when Dr. Leininger joined the faculty at Wayne State University as a Professor of Nursing and Anthropology, she developed several courses and seminars in transcultural nursing, care, and qualitative research methods for baccalaureate, master's, doctoral, and postdoctoral nursing and non-nursing students. In addition to directing the transcultural course offerings at Wayne State University, she taught and mentored many students and nurses in qualitative research studies focused on transcultural nursing and continued to teach these methods at various universities in the United States and worldwide for 30 years. Leininger wrote or edited more than 30 books in her lifetime.

Dr. Leininger's last works on the Culture Care Theory were publications in peer-reviewed professional journals. She co-authored an interview piece for *Nursing Science Quarterly* (Clarke, McFarland, Andrews, & Leininger, 2009) in which she discussed the history and future of transcultural care, the nursing profession, and global health care. In 2011, she authored a reflective article about her ongoing research about father protective care in the *Online Journal of Cultural Competence in Nursing and Healthcare.* She conducted this retrospective comparative study of three Western and one non-Western culture (Old Order Amish Americans, Anglo Americans, Mexican Americans, and the Gadsup of the Eastern Highlands of New Guinea) in order to obtain in-depth knowledge about father protective care beliefs and practices with the goal of using that knowledge to provide culturally congruent care. She reported on culture care decision and action modes of similar and diverse care findings that were discussed with the informant fathers as potential ways they might integrate their cultural values and care practices to help their sons. Leininger then began work on a new culture care construct, *collaborative care*, which she co-presented with this author via a keynote video cast at the 37th Annual Conference of Transcultural Nursing Society in October 2011.

Dr. Madeleine Leininger died on August 10, 2012 in Omaha, Nebraska. She continued to work until shortly before her passing, collaborating with colleagues on contributions to several projects and other publications in progress as well as revisions to her website. Among these works was a chapter contribution, "Leininger's Father Protective Care" to the 2015 third edition of the theory book, *Leininger's Culture Care Diversity and Universality: A Worldwide Nursing Theory* by McFarland and Wehbe-Alamah. During her lifetime, Dr. Leininger influenced and inspired many nurses to continue to explore new transcultural directions, theories, educational approaches, and areas of scholarship.

■ TRANSCULTURAL NURSING, CROSS-CULTURAL NURSING, AND INTERNATIONAL NURSING

Leininger (2002b) distinguished between *transcultural nursing* and *cross-cultural nursing.* The former refers to nurses prepared in transcultural nursing who are committed to developing knowledge and integrating the values, beliefs, patterns, and worldview of cultural groups into nursing practices, whereas *cross-cultural nursing* refers to nurses who use medical anthropological concepts (Leininger, 1995; Leininger & McFarland, 2002, 2006; McFarland & Wehbe-Alamah, 2015). She also identified that *international nursing* and transcultural nursing are also different. *International nursing* occurs when nurses travel to or have nursing practice or service-learning experiences in other nations or countries; however, transcultural nursing involves multiple *cultures* and has comparative theoretical and practice-based foci (Leininger, 1995; Leininger & McFarland, 2002, 2006; McFarland & Wehbe-Alamah, 2015). Leininger described the transcultural nurse *generalist* (now known as certified transcultural nurse-basic or CTN-B), as a nurse prepared at the baccalaureate level who is able to apply transcultural nursing concepts, principles, and practices that are generated by transcultural nurse specialists (Leininger, 1991, 1995; Leininger & McFarland, 2002, 2006; McFarland & Wehbe-Alamah, 2015). The transcultural nurse *specialist* (now referred to as a certified transcultural nurse-advanced or CTN-A) is prepared in graduate programs and receives in-depth preparation and mentorship in transcultural nursing knowledge and practice. The CTN-A has competency skills acquired through post baccalaureate education and research-based knowledge about selected cultures in sufficient depth (values, beliefs, and lifeways) to provide high quality, safe, and effective transcultural nursing care (Leininger, 1991, 1995; Leininger & McFarland, 2002, 2006; McFarland & Wehbe-Alamah, 2015). The CTN-A therefore serves as an expert transcultural field practitioner, teacher, researcher, and consultant with respect to select cultures. This individual also values and uses nursing theory to develop and advance knowledge within the discipline of transcultural nursing, the field Leininger predicted must be the focus of all nursing education and practice (Leininger, 1991, 1995; Leininger & McFarland, 2002, 2006; McFarland & Wehbe-Alamah, 2015).

Transcultural nursing education has thus become an imperative for all nurses worldwide. Transcultural nurse certification by the Transcultural Nursing Society has provided a major step toward ensuring safe and culturally competent nursing practices (Leininger, 1991, 1995; Leininger & McFarland, 2002, 2006; McFarland & Wehbe-Alamah, 2015). Accordingly, more nurses are seeking transcultural certification so

as to be able to provide culturally congruent care for their clients. The *Journal of Transcultural Nursing, the Online Journal of Cultural Competence in Nursing and Healthcare,* and other transculturally focused professional journals have also provided published research and theoretical perspectives about numerous diverse cultures worldwide to guide nursing practices.

■ FURTHER DEVELOPMENT OF TRANSCULTURAL NURSING AS A DISCIPLINE

Present and future theories and studies in transcultural nursing will be essential to meet the needs of culturally diverse people. As the seminal theory in transcultural nursing, the Culture Care Theory will only continue to grow in importance worldwide. Universal and diverse care knowledge are both extremely important to establish a substantive body of transcultural nursing knowledge, and to support nursing as a transcultural profession and discipline. Leininger's theory has gained global interest and use because it is holistic, relevant, and futuristic and deals with specific *and* abstract care knowledge (Leininger, 1991, 1995; Leininger & McFarland, 2002, 2006; McFarland & Wehbe-Alamah, 2015).

Leininger believed that all professional nurses worldwide need to be prepared in transcultural nursing and demonstrate competencies in transcultural nursing (Leininger, 1988a, 1988b, 1995; Leininger & McFarland, 2002, 2006; McFarland & Wehbe-Alamah, 2015; Mixer, 2008). Transcultural nursing must become an integral part of education and practice for nurses to be relevant in the 21st century. Currently, the demand for prepared transcultural nurses far exceeds the numbers of nurses, faculty, and clinical specialists in the world. It is a transcultural imperative that every nurse have a basic knowledge about diverse cultures in the world and in-depth knowledge about two or three cultures at minimum (Leininger, 1995, 1996; Leininger & McFarland, 2002, 2006; McFarland & Wehbe-Alamah, 2015). Leininger believed that transcultural nursing research had already begun to lend some highly promising and different approaches to advanced nursing education and practice (Leininger, 1991, 1995; Leininger & McFarland, 2002, 2006; McFarland & Wehbe-Alamah, 2015). Health disciplines including medicine, pharmacy, and social work have transitioned toward integrating transcultural health knowledge and practices into their programs of study (Leininger, 1995). This trend has consequently created an increased demand for culturally competent faculty to teach transcultural health care.

■ CONTRIBUTIONS BY TRANSCULTURAL NURSING THEORISTS, RESEARCHERS, AND SCHOLARS

Leininger (2002b) stated that significantly greater numbers of transcultural nurse theorists, researchers, and scholars are also urgently needed to keep pace with and continue to develop new genres of transcultural knowledge as well as to further transform nursing education and practice.

> As transcultural nursing with its standards, policies, and certification continue [forward], all professional nurses will be expected to practice transcultural nursing worldwide by 2020…. As educational and service exchanges occur among all health disciplines, there will be very great demands for transcultural health education, research, and practice and the need to evaluate the outcomes and problems. (Leininger, 2002b, p. 30)

Since 2002, several transcultural nurse authors have published textbooks, which have been used worldwide to address Leininger's concerns about the need for further development of transcultural nursing knowledge, research, practice, and education. These contributions to the discipline of transcultural nursing represent a substantive body of work based on many years of transcultural study and research. Important contemporary transcultural models and guides include Sagar's *Transcultural Nursing Theory and Models: Application in Nursing Education, Practice and Administration* and her text *Transcultural Nursing Education Strategies;* Jeffreys' *Teaching Cultural Competence in Nursing and Health Care: Inquiry, Action, and Innovation*; Purnell's *Model of Cultural Competence*; Campinha-Bacote's *The Process of Cultural Competence in the Delivery of Healthcare Services*; Giger and Davidhizar's *Transcultural Assessment Model*; Basuray's *Culture & Health: Concept and Practice*; Ray's *Transcultural Caring Dynamics in Nursing and Health Care*; and the Andrews and Boyle *Nursing Assessment Guide for Individuals and Families.*

In 2012, Dr. Priscilla Sagar published her book, *Transcultural Nursing Theory and Models: Application in Nursing Education, Practice, and Administration* in which she presented a scholarly overview of Leininger's Culture Care Theory, Sunrise Enabler, and Ethnonursing Research Method as well as Leininger's culture care research. She also described Leininger's many other visionary publications and presentations focused on the evolving development of transcultural nursing and healthcare education, practice, and administration. In 2014, Sagar published *Transcultural Nursing Education Strategies,* wherein evidence-based and best practices in transcultural nursing education for students and professional staff were discussed in-depth. She acknowledged the valuable mentorship by Dr. Madeleine Leininger who was the inspiration for her work.

Dr. Marianne Jeffreys published the third edition of her book, *Teaching Cultural Competence in Nursing and Health Care: Inquiry, Action, and Innovation,* in 2016. This book emphasized a comprehensive approach toward cultural competence education for nurses and other healthcare professionals in educational programs of study as well as throughout their professional lives. Jeffreys used Leininger's three culture care modes of decisions and actions as guides for nurses in the provision of culturally congruent care. The modes are an essential part of professional practice for nurses and other health professionals. Jeffreys concurred with Leininger that the goal of culturally congruent care can only be achieved through the process of learning and teaching cultural competence (2016, p. 15).

Dr. Larry Purnell published the fourth edition of *Transcultural Healthcare: A Culturally Competent Approach* in 2014 and in that same year published a third edition of its companion, *Guide for Culturally Competent Healthcare.* These books provided an overview of the *Purnell Model of Cultural Competence* and its usefulness as an organizing framework for individual and family assessment, planning, and intervention in health promotion, maintenance, and restoration. In these two latest editions, Purnell has made a significant contribution to presenting insight to the beliefs and practices of diverse cultural or heritage groups with large populations in North America, such as African American, Appalachian, Cuban, Mexican, and Jewish persons. He also presented information about more recent immigrant groups to the United States such as people from Arab, Bosnian, Hmong, Somali, and Vietnamese cultures. In 2008, the American Association of Colleges of Nursing (AACN) chose Purnell's model along with Leininger's Culture Care Theory as well as several other transcultural models as the basis for the development of toolkits for cultural competence in baccalaureate, master's, and doctoral nursing education (AACN, 2008).

Dr. Josepha Campinha-Bacote published her text, *The Process of Cultural Competence in the Delivery of Healthcare Services: The Journey Continues* in 2007. In this volume, Campinha-Bacote discussed her first model, *Culturally Competent Model of Care* in conjunction with her later model, *The Process of Cultural Competence in the Delivery of Healthcare Services*. She had previously had acknowledged Leininger's early work in transcultural nursing (TCN; 1978), which was used to develop the first version of her own model (Camphina-Bacote, 2002). The key constructs of *cultural awareness, cultural skill, cultural knowledge, cultural encounters*, and *cultural desire* (ASKED) have been widely embraced throughout nursing practice and education. These concepts along with their associated assessment tools have been valuable contributions to transcultural nursing.

In 2017, Dr. Joyce Giger published the seventh edition of *Transcultural Nursing Assessment and Intervention* with presentation of the *Giger and Davidhizar Transcultural Assessment Model* (p. 6). Previous editions of this text were written with Dr. Ruth Davidhizar, her transcultural colleague and friend, who died in 2008. In the current edition, Dr. Giger has acknowledged Leininger as the impetus for nurses to develop cultural insight and deeper appreciation for human life and cultural values perspective (Leininger, 2007, as cited by Giger, 2017, p. 121). In the current book, Giger has made the significant transcultural nursing contribution of the six cultural phenomena in her model: *communication; space; social organization; time; environmental control;* and *biologic variation*. These phenomena are recommended for the assessment of multicultural populations (Giger, 2017). She discussed the application of these phenomena in the assessment of diverse cultural groups in the United States and throughout the world.

In 2012, Dr. Joanna Basuray (Maxwell) published *Culture and Health: Concept and Practice*. She described having organized her text using an integrated approach to the learning of theoretical and application components about cultural diversity based on Leininger's Culture Care Theory and Sunrise Enabler so as to provide clinicians and students with a solid grounding in the underlying concepts about culturally competent care (p. ix). In this work, Basuray provided significant insights into transcultural education and practice.

Dr. Marilyn Ray published the second edition of *Transcultural Caring Dynamics in Nursing and Health Care* in 2016. She acknowledged and thanked her teacher, mentor, colleague, and friend, Dr. Madeleine Leininger, who remains recognized as the mother of transcultural nursing and the inspiration for the development of nursing as a *human science*, and links this construct to *caring as the essence of nursing* (Ray, 2016). Ray's *Transcultural Caring Dynamics in Nursing and Health Care Theoretical Model* was developed as a *human rights theory* to empower people in their own lives and to help develop more resilient nations (2016, p. 21). Ray stated that a fundamental assumption for transcultural caring is that *caring itself is the human mode of being*, and cited Leininger's seminal work that deemed *caring as the most unifying, dominant, and central intellectual and practice focus in nursing* around the world (2016, p. 22).

In Andrews and Boyle's 2016 seventh edition of *Transcultural Concepts in Nursing Care*, the authors credit TCN founder Dr. Madeleine Leininger for using the concepts of *care* and *culture* to establish TCN as an evidence-based formal area of specialization within the discipline of nursing (p. 3). The authors give attention to Leininger's work and theory in their book but also introduce their *Transcultural Interprofessional Practice Model* (TIP) as a theory-based framework for delivering client-centered, high-quality nursing and health care that are culturally congruent, competent, and affordable for people from diverse cultures across the lifespan (p. 10). The TIP Model focuses on the importance of collaboration and communication among interdisciplinary professional colleagues within health care as well as folk and traditional healers from diverse cultural groups (p. 14).

■ FOUR EVOLUTIONARY PHASES OF TRANSCULTURAL NURSING

In the 2002 third edition of this book, Leininger described three evolutionary phases of transcultural nursing knowledge and uses (2002b, p. 28). In Phase I, the nurse gains cultural awareness and sensitivity of culture care differences and similarities. This is only the beginning phase toward becoming culturally competent. Sensitivity to another person, situation, or event is helpful but the nurse must gain evidence-based cultural knowledge to support culturally congruent nursing decisions and actions. In Phase II, the nurse gains in-depth knowledge about transcultural nursing concepts and principles to guide thinking and practices. A course in transcultural nursing and a mentor to discover culture care similarities and differences of clients is often essential in this phase. Transcultural holding knowledge of concepts, principles and theories are essential for cultural assessments of clients. The Culture Care Theory can serve as a guide to discover unknowns about individuals and groups of a particular culture. In Phase III, the nurse uses observations, experiences, and knowledge documented with clients to provide culturally congruent care. The nurse documents and evaluates the outcomes with patients when providing culturally-based care and uses theory-based knowledge along with transcultural nursing principles and evidence-based research findings to provide meaningful, safe, beneficial, and culturally congruent care. In this third phase, the nurse first identifies her/his own biases and then assesses their own cultural competence as well as areas that need to be strengthened. Leininger (2002b) stated that all three phases help to assess how one is becoming "… a knowledgeable, competent, and confident" transcultural nurse (p. 28).

This author now proposes that there is an evolving Phase IV (Refer to Figure 1.1) of transcultural nursing focused on evidence-based culturally congruent practice and translation science, which provides a basis for effective implementation care strategies to promote adoption of evidence-based transcultural practices in real-world clinical settings.

> … the nursing profession has provided major leadership for improving care through the application of research findings in practice. Nurses are now leading the way in translation science and EBP and, as a result, the scientific body of knowledge translation and the application of evidence in healthcare are growing. (Titler, 2014, p. 271)

In 2015, the American Nurses' Association (ANA) published the third edition of the *Nursing Scope and Standards of Practice*. This edition included a new standard (Standard 8) entitled *Culturally Congruent Practice*, stated as being "… the nursing care that is in agreement with the preferred values, beliefs, worldview, and practices of the healthcare consumer" (ANA, 2015, p. 31). In August 2015, the American Association of Colleges of Nursing (AACN) released a white paper that clarified the scholarship focus for the Doctor of Nursing Practice (DNP) degree, wherein practice-focused graduates are prepared to generate new knowledge through the innovation of practice change, translation of evidence, and implementation of quality improvement processes in specific practice settings, systems, organizations, or with specific population groups to improve health or healthcare outcomes. "An emerging body of knowledge in translation science provides an empirical base for guiding the selection of implementation strategies to promote the adoption of EBPs in real-world settings" (Titler, 2014, p. 270). New knowledge generated through practice innovations related to culturally congruent care for patients and the cultural competence of nurses in a clinical site, for example, could be of value in and transferred to other practice settings and/or to other organizations such as hospitals, nursing homes, and primary care clinics. The ANA (2015) has addressed culturally congruent practice for graduate-prepared nurses and advanced practice nurses as "… leading interprofessional teams to identify the cultural and language needs of the consumer" (p. 70). To discover and explore the foci of completed DNP scholarly projects, Murphy, Madgic, and Allison (2017) conducted an informal Internet search and categorized elements of identified projects by population, setting, and topic; in the area of *cultural and international focus*, ten projects were found (p. 237). African Americans were the predominant minority group identified as a population of interest, followed by Latinos, American Indian/ Alaskan natives, and Native American tribes from the Northwestern United States. International projects included studies conducted in Germany, Nigeria, Central Russia, Costa Rica, and Haiti (Murphy, Madgic, & Allison, 2017, p. 237).

There has been a renewed call to action regarding Leininger's three phases of evolutionary transcultural nursing knowledge that includes continued awareness of culture care similarities and differences; transcultural theory and research-based knowledge

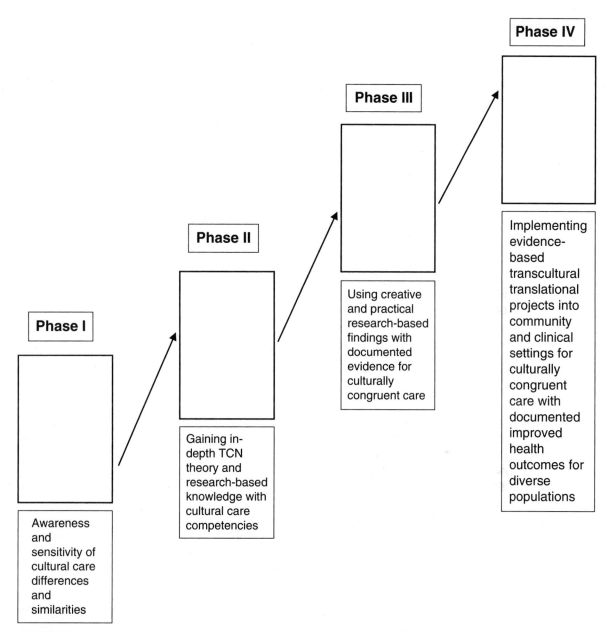

FIGURE 1.1 • Evolutionary Phases of Transcultural Nursing Knowledge. © M. R. McFarland (2017).
Adapted from M. M. Leininger and M. R. McFarland (Eds.), Transcultural nursing: Concepts, theories, research, practice (3rd ed., p. 28).
New York, NY: McGraw-Hill. Copyright M. M. Leininger (2002).

of culture care and cultural competence; implementation of culturally congruent care practices with health outcome measurements; as well as the proposed fourth phase of TCN evolution. This fourth phase focuses on the implementation of culturally congruent nursing practices by culturally competent nurses that transcends all clinical, educational, and research settings. Nurse researchers and nursing organizations have responded by designing translational transcultural projects for implementation in community and clinical settings (AACN, 2015, pp. 22-23) that can be beneficial for populations from diverse cultures to improve their health and quality of life (Marion et al., 2015).

■ SUMMARY

The discipline of transcultural nursing has continued to evolve for nearly seven decades. Leininger's predictive logo statement for transcultural nursing endures as the central goal and challenge for nursing, that "… the cultural care needs of people in the world will be met by nurses prepared in transcultural nursing" (2002b, p. 26). Since publication of the prior edition of this book, nurses worldwide have responded to Leininger's challenge. In their practice, education, research, administration, and scholarship nurses have continued to recognize, value, and develop the discipline of transcultural nursing and are seeking and integrating evidence-based culture care practices for individuals, families, groups, communities, organizations, and institutions around the globe. The chapters in this book are the contributions of knowledgable and dedicated authors who have been inspired by Leininger's work with the Culture Care Theory and who collectively have made significant contributions to the discipline and practice of transcultural nursing across all four of the evolutionary phases of transcultural nursing.

■ DEDICATION

This chapter is dedicated to my visionary friend and mentor, Dr. Madeleine M. Leininger, to whom I remain deeply indebted.

■ ACKNOWLEDGEMENTS

I wish to acknowledge with gratitude each of the transcultural authors cited in this chapter and our textbook contributing authors. Your valuable work is greatly appreciated.

■ DISCUSSION QUESTIONS

1. Discuss the contributions of transcultural nursing theorists/theories to the discipline and practice of nursing.
2. Discuss why transcultural nursing knowledge and practices are important in the provision of health care.
3. Describe at least three areas where transcultural theory/knowledge can be applied in nursing practice.

■ REFERENCES

American Association of Colleges of Nursing. (2008). *Cultural competency in nursing education* [Toolkits]. Retrieved from http://www.aacnnursing.org/Education-Resources/Tool-Kits/Cultural-Competency-in-Nursing-Education

American Association of Colleges of Nursing. (2015, August). *The doctor of nursing practice: Current issues and clarifying recommendations*. Report from the task force on the implementation of the DNP (pp. 22-23). Washington, DC: Author.

American Nurses' Association. (2015). *Nursing scope and standards of practice* (3rd ed., pp. 31, 70). Silver Spring, MD: Author.

Andrews, M. M., & Boyle, J. S. (2016). *Transcultural concepts in nursing care* (7th ed.). Philadelphia, PA: Wolters Kluwer.

Basuray (Maxwell), J. M. (2014). *Culture and health: Concept and practice* (2nd ed.). Ronkokoma, NY: Linus.

Campinha-Bacote, J. (2002). The process of cultural competence in the delivery of healthcare services: A culturally competent model of care. *Journal of Transcultural Nursing, 13*(3), 181-184.

Campinha-Bacote, J. (2007). *The process of cultural competence in the delivery of healthcare services: The journey continues*. Cincinnati, OH: Transcultural CARE Associates.

Clarke, P. N., McFarland, M. R., Andrews, M. M., & Leininger, M. M. (2009). Caring: Some reflections on the impact of the culture care theory by McFarland & Andrews and a conversation with Leininger. *Nursing Science Quarterly, 22*(3), 233-239.

Giger, J. N. (2016). *Transcultural nursing assessment and intervention* (7th ed.). St. Louis, MO: Mosby.

Jeffreys, M. R. (2016). *Teaching cultural competence in nursing and health care: Inquiry, action, and innovation* (3rd ed.). New York, NY: Springer.

Leininger, M. M. (1966). *Convergence and divergence of human behavior: An ethnopsychological comparative study of two Gadsup villages in the Eastern Highlands of New Guinea*. Doctoral dissertation. Seattle, WA: The University of Washington.

Leininger, M. M. (1970). *Nursing and anthropology: Two worlds to blend*. New York, NY: John Wiley & Sons.

Leininger, M. M. (Ed.). (1978). *Transcultural nursing: Concepts, theories, and practice*. New York, NY: John Wiley & Sons.

Leininger, M. M. (Ed.). (1981). *Caring: An essential human need*. Thorofare, NJ: Charles B. Slack.

Leininger, M. M. (Ed.). (1984). *Care: The essence of nursing and health*. Thorofare, NJ: Charles B. Slack.

Leininger, M. M. (1985). Transcultural care diversity and universality: A theory of nursing. *Nursing and Health Care, 6*(4), 202-212.

Leininger, M. M. (Ed.). (1988a). Care: The essence of nursing and health. Detroit, MI: Wayne State University Press.

Leininger, M. M. (Ed.). (1988b). *Caring: An essential human need.* Detroit, MI: Wayne State University Press.

Leininger, M. M. (1990). Ethnomethods: The philosophic and epistemic bases to explicate transcultural nursing knowledge. *Journal of Transcultural Nursing, 1*(2), 40-51.

Leininger, M. M. (Ed.). (1991). *Culture care diversity and universality: A theory of nursing.* New York, NY: National League for Nursing Press.

Leininger, M. M. (1995). *Transcultural nursing: Concepts, theories, and practice* (2nd ed.). Columbus, OH: McGraw-Hill College Custom Series.

Leininger, M. M. (1996). Culture care theory, research and practice. *Nursing Science Quarterly, 9*(2), 71-78.

Leininger, M. M. (2002a). Essential transcultural nursing concepts, principles, examples, and policy statements. In M. M. Leininger and M. R. McFarland (Eds.), *Transcultural nursing: Concepts, theories, research, & practice* (3rd ed., pp. 45-69). New York, NY: McGraw-Hill Medical Publishing Division.

Leininger, M. M. (2002b). Transcultural nursing and globalization of health care: Importance, focus, and historical aspects. In M. M. Leininger and M. R. McFarland (Eds.), *Transcultural nursing: Concepts, theories, research, & practice* (3rd ed., pp. 3-43). New York, NY: McGraw-Hill Medical Publishing Division.

Leininger, M. M. (2011). Leininger's reflection on the ongoing father protective care research. *The Online Journal of Cultural Competence in Nursing and Healthcare, 1*(2), 1-13.

Leininger, M. M. (2015). Leininger's father protective care. In M. R. McFarland and H. B. Wehbe-Alamah (Eds.), *Leininger's culture care diversity and universality: A worldwide nursing theory* (3rd ed., pp. 119-136). Burlington, MA: Jones and Bartlett Learning.

Leininger, M. M., & McFarland, M. R. (Eds.). (2002). *Transcultural nursing: Concepts, theories, research, & practice* (3rd ed.). New York, NY: McGraw-Hill Medical Publishing Division.

Leininger, M. M., & McFarland, M. R. (Eds.). (2006). *Culture care diversity and universality: A worldwide theory of nursing* (2nd ed.). Sudbury, MA: Jones & Bartlett.

Marion, L., Douglas, M., Lavin, M., Barr, N., Gazaway, S., Thomas, L., & Bickford, C. (2016). Implementing the new ANA Standard 8: Culturally congruent practice. *The Online Journal of Issues in Nursing, 22*(1). doi: 10.3912/ojin.vol22no01ppt20

McFarland, M. R. (with M. M. Leininger via videotape). (2011, October 20). *The culture care theory and a look to the future for transcultural nursing.* Keynote Address presented at the 37th Annual International Conference of the of Transcultural Nursing Society, Las Vegas, NV.

McFarland, M. R., & Webhe-Alamah, H. B. (Eds.). (2015). *Leininger's culture care diversity and universality: A worldwide theory of nursing* (3rd ed.). Burlington, MA: Jones and Bartlett Learning.

Mixer, S. J. (2008). Use of the culture care theory and ethnonursing method to discover how nursing faculty teach culture care. *Contemporary Nurse, 28*(2), 23-36.

Murphy, M. J., Madgic, K. S., & Allison, T. L. (2017). Measuring outcomes of doctor of nursing practice. In R. M. Kleinpell (Ed.), *Outcome assessment in advanced nursing practice* (4th ed.). New York, NY: Springer.

Purnell, L. D. (2014). *Transcultural healthcare: A culturally competent approach* (4th ed.). Philadelphia, PA: FA Davis.

Purnell, L. D. (2014). *Guide for culturally competent healthcare* (3rd ed.). Philadelphia, PA: FA Davis.

Ray, M. A. (2016). *Transcultural caring dynamics nursing and health care* (2nd ed.). Philadelphia, PA: FA Davis.

Sagar, P. L. (2012). *Transcultural nursing theory and models: Application in nursing education, practice, and administration.* New York, NY: Springer.

Sagar, P. L. (2014). *Transcultural nursing education strategies.* New York, NY: Springer.

Titler, M. G. (2014). Overview of evidence-based practice and translation science. *Nursing Clinics of North America, 49*(3), 269-274.

CHAPTER 2

Essential Transcultural Nursing Care Concepts, Principles, Guidelines, and Policy Statements for Culturally Congruent and Competent Health Care Practice, Education, and Research

Hiba B. Wehbe-Alamah

> *"The time is now to prepare health professionals to incorporate transcultural concepts into our educational and service programs. Ultimately, the goal is to serve people of different cultural lifestyles in an understanding and competent manner"* *(Leininger, 1994, p. 73).*

■ INTRODUCTION

Transcultural nursing is a growing and highly relevant area of study and practice that has great significance for nurses living and functioning in a multicultural world. It often leads to the discovery of entirely different ways of knowing and helping people of diverse cultures. With a transcultural focus, nurses caring for clients of different cultural backgrounds strive to learn about and integrate into their professional practice the knowledge about and an ability to accommodate to cultural differences and similarities as well as special needs and prohibitions. As nurses discover each client's particular cultural beliefs, practices, and values, they develop ways to provide sensitive, compassionate, and competent care that is beneficial and satisfying for that client. Gaining a deeper appreciation for cultures with their commonalties and differences is one of the primary goals of transcultural nursing. At the same time, the nurse will also discover many nursing insights about his or her own cultural background and how to use such knowledge

appropriately with clients in community, home, or health care settings. Transcultural nursing opens many new windows of cultural knowledge and competency previously unknown by nurses.

In this chapter, major and essential transcultural nursing concepts are defined and presented along with specific examples to help guide transcultural nursing practices. Transcultural nursing care principles, policies, standards of practice, and guidelines for integrating culturally congruent care into nursing clinical practice, management, education, and research are individually presented.

■ MAJOR THEORETICAL CONCEPTS AND DEFINITIONS IN TRANSCULTURAL NURSING

It is essential for nurses to understand the major concepts, constructs, theories, and principles of transcultural nursing. The term *construct* is used to indicate several concepts embedded in phenomena such as *care* or *caring* (Leininger, 2002). *Concept* refers to a single idea, thought, or object (Leininger, 2002). Transcultural nursing leaders have identified, studied, defined, and explicated a number of care concepts and constructs so that nurses can use these ideas in meaningful and appropriate ways. Such fundamental knowledge can assist nurses to communicate more effectively with others and thereby avoid conflicts or troublesome interactions. It is, therefore, essential that nurses and nursing students study these concepts before applying them to real-life situations (Leininger, 2002).

Transcultural Nursing

Although the general definition of transcultural nursing was presented in the theory chapter, its essential features require further examination. Leininger (1978a, 1994, 1995, 2002) defined transcultural nursing as a *substantive area of study and practice focused on comparative cultural care (caring) values, beliefs, and practices of individuals or groups of similar or different cultures…with its goal to provide culture-specific and universal nursing care practices for the health and wellbeing of people or to help them face disability, illness, or death in culturally meaningful ways.* This definition of transcultural nursing contains many important ideas, such as *the focus on discovering culture-care values, beliefs, and practices of specific cultures or subcultures to assist people with their daily health care needs.* This comparative viewpoint is emphasized so as to identify *both* differences and similarities between or among cultures. It is this comparative viewpoint that enables the nurse to identify specifics and commonalities of care for cultural clients or groups. The major goal of transcultural nursing is to provide nursing care that reasonably fits the client's culture-specific expectations and care needs to achieve beneficial health care outcomes as well as to identify both universal and diverse care practices. Thus defined, *culturally congruent care* is the desired and ultimate goal of transcultural nursing.

Human Care as Essence of Nursing and Transcultural Nursing

Beginning in the late 1940s, Leininger held that:

- *Care is an essential human need and the essence of nursing* on which the profession should be focusing (Leininger 1990a, 1991b, 2002; McFarland & Wehbe-Alamah, 2015);

- Nursing is a *caring profession and discipline* that directs nurses to discover and provide knowledgeable and skilled care to clients (Leininger, 2002); and
- *Nursing is a learned, humanistic, and scientific profession and discipline focused on human care phenomena and caring activities in order to assist, support, and facilitate or enable individuals or groups to maintain or regain their health or wellbeing in culturally meaningful and beneficial ways, or to help individuals face disabilities, illnesses, or death* (Leininger, 1978b, 1994, 2002).

These definitions reinforce the idea of *care as the essence and fundamental focus of nursing and transcultural nursing.*

In regarding nursing as a caring profession and discipline, it is important to remember that as a profession, nursing has a *societal mandate to serve people.* The professional nurse is challenged to serve others who need the assistance of a person prepared and qualified to respond to or who can anticipate their actual or covert care needs. Nurses are ultimately held responsible for and accountable to people in a particular society or culture to provide *care* that will help people regain and maintain their health and prevent illnesses. Nurses, however, function best when they know and understand diverse cultures in relation to their own experiences, human conditions, and cultural care values, beliefs, expressions, and practices.

All nurses need to be culturally prepared to provide effective and beneficial care to their clients. As a professional healthcare discipline, nursing has its own culturally defined modes of functioning and being that have been and remain subject to change over time. However, the culture of nursing dictates that nurses discover and use distinctive knowledge that explains and interprets nursing's unique focus and essence (Leininger, 1980). Most importantly, regarding nursing as a discipline implies that there is a *substantive body of knowledge* to guide its members' thinking, decisions, and actions. The discipline of nursing needs to focus more on care/caring to explain health and wellbeing among diverse or similar cultures. Leininger (1995, 2002) maintained that care, health, and wellbeing are central to what nursing is or should be. Transcultural nurses contribute new, unique, and significant knowledge to nursing from a comparative care focus including ways to use this knowledge to serve people of a specific culture or society worldwide. A number of publications, Leininger (1981, 1988a, 1988b, 1990b, 1991c, 2002); Gaut & Leininger, 1991; and McFarland & Wehbe-Alamah, 2015, discussed human care and caring as the central, distinct, and dominant focus to explain, interpret, and predict nursing as a discipline and profession and provided the following definitions:

- *Care* refers to an abstract or concrete phenomenon related to assisting, supporting, or enabling experiences or behaviors for others with evidence for anticipated needs to ameliorate or improve a human condition or lifeway (Leininger, 2002; McFarland & Wehbe-Alamah, 2015).
- *Caring* refers to actions, attitudes, practices, and activities directed toward assisting, supporting, or enabling another individual or group with evident or anticipated needs to ease, heal, or improve a human condition or lifeway or to face death or disability (Leininger, 2002; McFarland & Wehbe-Alamah, 2015).
- *Human care* refers to a specific *phenomenon* that is characterized to assist, support, or enable another human being or group to achieve one's desired goals or to obtain assistance with certain human needs (Leininger, 2002).
- *Human caring* refers to the *action aspect* or *activities* to provide service to other human beings. Differences in the meanings of care (noun) and caring (an action mode) are extremely important in understanding and practicing transcultural nursing caring as a professional art (Leininger, 2002).

These definitions of care and caring within a cultural context are the foundational constructs of transcultural nursing and characterize the nature and focus of the nursing discipline. They guide nurses in discovering care knowledge and ways to provide direct and holistic patient care. Care is an integral part of culture and nurses are challenged to understand both care and culture together to practice transcultural nursing.

Culture and Subculture

Culture is derived from the discipline of anthropology. Culture has been defined and used by anthropologists and other social scientists for more than 100 years. The term *culture*, however, was limitedly used and was neither valued nor explicated in nursing until the mid-1950s when Leininger played a leading role in raising awareness of culture as a crucial and major dimension of nursing. Gradually, culture began to be discussed and used in a variety of ways, disciplines, and contexts. Definitions are important in any discipline, and thus Leininger developed the following definitions for transcultural nursing:

- *Culture* refers to the learned, shared, and transmitted knowledge of values, beliefs, norms, and lifeways of a particular group that are generally transmitted intergenerationally and influence thinking, decisions, and actions in patterned ways (Leininger, 1978b, 1995, 2002; McFarland & Wehbe-Alamah, 2015).
- *Subculture* is closely related to culture, but refers to subgroups who deviate in certain ways from a dominant culture in values, beliefs, norms, moral codes, and ways of living with some distinctive features that characterize their unique lifeways (Leininger, 1978, 2002).

Both cultures and subcultures are developed by people over time with distinct values, beliefs, and lifeways. They are preserved and usually transmitted intergenerationally. Transcultural nurses are expected to study both cultures and subcultures as these groups have different care and health needs. Culture is a major construct for gaining understanding in transcultural nursing and it is also a key construct in anthropology, which has been studied since the 19th century. However, it is bringing culture and care *together* that provides new perspectives to understand and serve people of different lifeways (Leininger, 2002).

In transcultural nursing, culture and care are conceptualized as *bound together* to provide special insights valuable to nursing. *Culture care is a synthesized construct* that is the foundational basis for understanding and helping people of different cultures through culturally congruent nursing practices (Leininger, 2002). Anthropologically speaking, culture is the broadest and most holistic and comprehensive view of people; however, one can focus on specific ideas and practices to gain an understanding of people. Culturally based care was woefully missing in nursing until transcultural nursing came into focus and—slowly but surely—gained increased recognition for its value in nursing and other health care disciplines.

Features of Cultures

Important features of cultures need to be understood and are therefore explicated as follows:

First, cultures reflect shared and learned values, ideals, and meanings that guide human thoughts, decisions, and actions. Within shared cultural values and norms, individuals and groups tend to uphold the rules for living in a culture because doing so engenders security, order, and expected behavior. Cultural values usually transcend individual values and are influenced by groups and symbols. Cultural beliefs, values, and norms (or rules of behavior) are learned from others and are not considered to be genetically or biologically transmitted. Cultural values and practices have a powerful influence on others and embody ethical and moral standards that carry obligations and responsibilities.

Second, cultures have *manifest* (readily recognized) and *implicit* (covert and ideal) rules of behavior and expectations. Manifest cultural norms or rules of behavior are the obvious and readily known beliefs and expressions of a culture such as greeting another person by a handshake or a bow. Implicit and ideal values are usually covert rules that are difficult to see or understand. They have, however, important influences on decisions and actions such as nodding one's head as yes or no to accept or reject medications.

Third, human cultures have material items or symbols such as artifacts, objects, mode of dress, and actions that have special meaning in a culture. Cultures also have nonmaterial expressions, beliefs, and ideas such as the "evil eye" or having "good and bad spirits." Nonmaterial cultural symbols, such as certain hand gestures or words that are used when one wants to receive care, are important considerations for provision of culturally congruent care. Material symbols like crosses, rosaries, and special religious or cultural relics may be used for healing and protection or prevention from illnesses and harm. Human beings are unique for their symbolic thinking and reasoning and use of material objects for various reasons. Nurses should learn about material and nonmaterial symbols of caring, their meanings in different cultures, and how they influence healing, wellbeing, and illness.

Fourth, cultures have traditional ceremonial practices such as religious rituals, food feasts (Refer to Color Insert 2-A), and other activities that are transmitted intergenerationally and reaffirm family or group ties and caring ways. Cultural rituals are also found in nursing and medicine and serve certain purposes. For example, nurses have morning and evening chart report rituals to keep nurses informed and united on care goals. Physicians have the ritual of "grand rounds" in a hospital to share information about patients. Cultural groups such as the Taiwanese have healing rituals rooted in their ethnohistory (Refer to Color Insert 2-B). Such rituals usually have therapeutic value and need to be known and respected.

Fifth, members of cultures have local or emic (insider's) views and knowledge about their culture that are extremely important for nurses to discover and understand for meaningful care practices. Emic ideas and beliefs are often viewed as secrets and may not be willingly shared with cultural strangers or outsiders such as nurses or physicians unless the stranger is trusted. Transcultural nurses are expected to tease out emic data when trusting relationships have been established. It is *emic* (inside cultural) knowledge that nurses try to obtain from their clients. In contrast, *etic* (outsider's) knowledge, such as the nurse's professional ideas, may be very different from emic views and experiences. Both emic and etic knowledge are important to assess in order to guide nurses' thinking, decisions, and actions with clients (Leininger, 1995).

Sixth, all human cultures have some intercultural variations between and within cultures. *Cultural variation is an important concept to keep in mind when studying individuals and different cultures.* For example, both African-Americans and Italian-Americans show cultural variations in their emic daily lifeways regarding food choices, communication, dress, and response to illness and death (Leininger, 2002). Although slight and great variations within and between cultures exist, one can usually find some common patterns of expressions and lifeways within each culture. In transcultural nursing, *inter*cultural and *intra*cultural variations are important to observe in the responses of persons in one's care. The nurse remains alert to expressions of cultural variations while using commonalities of values, beliefs, and lifeway patterns to guide care. Individual and group variability is always taken into consideration to prevent stereotyping and to avoid treating individuals in a rigid and fixed way.

Cultural Diversity and Cultural Universals

Cultural diversity refers to the *variations and differences among and between cultural groups resulting from differences in lifeways, language, values, norms, expressions, and other cultural aspects* (Leininger, 2002). Cultural diversity was one of the first concepts emphasized in transcultural nursing, largely due to Leininger's observation in the 1950s that nurses seemed to ignore cultural differences and treated *all clients alike* as if belonging to the same culture (Leininger, 2002). By identifying cultural differences between and among cultures, nurses gradually learn to value such differences and to provide culture-specific care. However, Leininger (2002) wanted nurses to discover and respond appropriately to both the *diverse* and *universal* features of cultural beings. She held that both dimensions were major foci in her development of the Culture Care Theory as a means to arrive at culturally congruent care practices (Leininger, 1991c). By taking into account the cultural differences of individuals and groups, the transcultural nurse can prevent stereotyping, which results from viewing everyone as alike. Viewing and regarding clients in fixed cultural ways and ignoring cultural differences are detrimental to most clients. Recognizing and embracing cultural diversity helps nurses to value differences and provide culture-specific and culturally congruent care practices that are acceptable, meaningful, and beneficial to clients.

Cultural universals refer to *the commonalities among human beings or humanity* [in general] *that reflect the similarities or dominant features of humans. Universality* refers to *the nature of a being or an object that is held as common or universally found in the world as part of humanity* (Leininger, 2002). With universals, one seeks to discover and understand *commonalities* as opposed to *absolute* universals. The Theory of Culture Care Diversity and Universality is focused on discovering what is *universal* and *diverse* about human caring within cultural perspectives. The purpose of the theory is to discover similarities and differences about care and culture and to explain the relationship and reasons for such findings (Leininger, 1991c). Discovering commonalties and differences in lifeways, values, and norms among cultures is essential for nurses in an increasingly multicultural world, for it is both the commonalties and differences among cultures that keep nurses alert to humanistic care practices.

Cultural Values

Leininger (1995, 2002) maintained that it is essential to understand *cultural values* in transcultural nursing because values greatly influence human beliefs, actions, and lifeways. *Cultural values refer to the powerful internal and external directive forces that give meaning and order to the thinking, decisions, and actions of an individual or group* (Leininger, 1995, 2002; McFarland & Wehbe-Alamah, 2015). Discovering and understanding a culture's values are essential in transcultural nursing because they are major indicators of what cultures do, how they act, and what one can expect from them. Understanding culture-specific values becomes an important reflection or *holding knowledge* to consider when assisting a client and in developing culturally congruent nursing decisions and actions.

Unfortunately, cultural values are usually neither readily identified nor revealed to strangers until a trusting relationship is developed. Some cultures may not want to share their values out of fear of rejection because their values may be different from those of others, such as those held by nurses practicing in hospitals or clinics. However, while cultures have values that guide their lives in sickness and in health, some cultures are more open than others about sharing their values with outsiders. For example, most Americans value their independence, freedom of speech, and freedom of choice, and usually want to see these values respected. The Malawi people of Africa greatly value the presence of extended family and children and feel lost when they are not near them whether they are ill or well (Leininger, 2002). The Old Order Amish also value community living and praying together to maintain health (Wenger, 1991).

Cultural values are *powerful forces* that guide nurses in caring for people of diverse and similar cultures. Observing and actively listening to clients are critical for learning about cultural values in addition to having prior holding knowledge about cultures. Cultural values tend to be stable as they are learned thoroughly over time and provide security to members of that culture. Accordingly, the transcultural nurse must remain sensitive to cultural values and usually should not try to change them unless they cause harm to self or others.

Uniculturalism and Multiculturalism
Uniculturalism or *monoculturalism* refer to the belief that one's universe is largely constituted, centered upon, and functions from a *one-culture perspective*

and reflects excessive ethnocentrism. *Multicultural-ism* refers to a perspective of reality that there are *many different cultures and subcultures* in the world that need to be recognized, valued, and understood for their *differences and similarities* (Leininger, 2002). Multiculturalism helps people to appreciate the many cultures in a changing world. This viewpoint is essential in developing respect for the world's cultures.

Cultural Relativism

Cultural relativism refers to the position that cultures are *unique* and must be evaluated, judged, and helped according to their *own particular values and standards* (Haviland, 1993; Leininger, 2002). Cultural relativists often believe in firmly upholding a practice of a particular culture and consider all cultures as completely unique. Some relativists take the extreme position that one culture should not be judged by the values and lifeways of another culture. As a result, rigid cultural relativists encounter difficulties accepting commonalities and universal truths and often fight to protect what they perceive as unique cultural values (Leininger, 2002).

Cultural relativism may have both beneficial and less beneficial outcomes. Cultural relativism may be desired by some cultures for security and political reasons. On the other hand, strong relativism upholds that there are no universal norms, beliefs, or practices and that everything is relative to each situation, event, or happening. Such attitudes often lead to religious conflicts. Transcultural nurses remain open to discover what is both *particularistic* and *universal* as found in the philosophy of the Theory of Culture Care Diversity and Universality (also known as the Culture Care Theory or CCT). They monitor excessive cultural relativistic positions affecting health care and religious beliefs and deal with them in culturally sensitive ways by relying on their holding and professional knowledge. Most importantly, they can do so without relinquishing their own religious beliefs (Leininger, 2002).

Cultural Blindness

Cultural blindness is another term Leininger (2002) coined in the late 1950s to refer to *the inability of an individual to understand another culture mainly because of an inability to recognize or see one's own* *lifestyle, values, and modes of acting as those based largely on prejudices and ethnocentric and biased tendencies.* It may seem strange to think that some people are so "blind" that they fail to see and understand their own as well as other ways of living, believing, doing, or valuing. The nurse with cultural blindness needs mentorship to help him/her become sensitive and responsive to other ideas and ways that are different and beneficial.

Culture Shock

Culture shock is another key concept derived from anthropology and used in transcultural nursing. It refers to *an individual who is disoriented or unable to respond appropriately to another person or situation because these new lifeways are so strange and unfamiliar* (Leininger, 2002). Culture shock may leave one feeling helpless and confused. Nurses, clients, families, and researchers experience cultural shock in a variety of ways when they are unable to know what to say or how to act in a given cultural situation that is truly shocking to them. In the hospital setting, nurses may be shocked to relate to cultures that are different from their own (such as immigrants or refugees) or to situations that are drastically different. For example, a nurse may be surprised to find a Taiwanese client eating home-cooked chicken feet.

Leininger (1966) reported experiencing culture shock herself when conducting the first ethnonursing study in the non-Western culture of Papua, New Guinea. The lack of running water, electricity, and having to sleep in a hut with snakes and then later having to partake in a feast of cooked python caused her to feel momentarily disoriented and to question culturally appropriate responses. Culture shock may limit one's ability to function with strangers or in unfamiliar settings. When in a state of cultural shock, nurses often experience feelings of helplessness, depression, and not knowing what to do (Leininger, 2002). One can overcome and limit cultural shock by acquiring some holding knowledge about the people of a certain culture and their lifeways in advance of working with them.

Ethnocentrism

Ethnocentrism strongly influences one's thinking, decisions, and actions and is therefore an important concept in transcultural nursing. *Ethnocentrism* refers to

Leininger's Sunrise Enabler to Discover Culture Care
CULTURE CARE

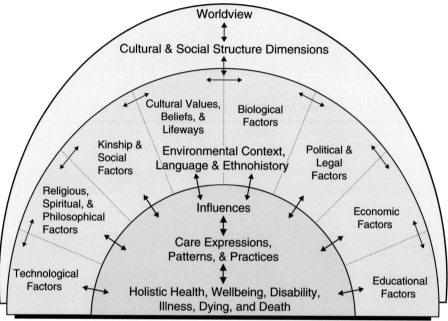

Worldview

Cultural & Social Structure Dimensions

Cultural Values, Beliefs, & Lifeways

Biological Factors

Kinship & Social Factors

Environmental Context, Language & Ethnohistory

Political & Legal Factors

Religious, Spiritual, & Philosophical Factors

Influences

Economic Factors

Care Expressions, Patterns, & Practices

Technological Factors

Educational Factors

Holistic Health, Wellbeing, Disability, Illness, Dying, and Death

Focus: Individuals, Families, Groups, Communities, or Institutions in Diverse Health Contexts of

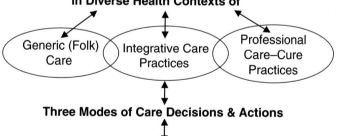

Generic (Folk) Care

Integrative Care Practices

Professional Care–Cure Practices

Three Modes of Care Decisions & Actions

**Culture Care Preservation and/or Maintenance
Culture Care Accommodation and/or Negotiation
Culture Care Repatterning and/or Restructuring**

Code: ←→ (Influencers)

© M. R. McFarland &
H. B. Wehbe-Alamah (2018)

Culturally Congruent Care for Holistic Health, Wellbeing, Disability, Illness, Dying, and Death

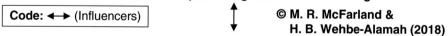

Leininger's Sunrise Enabler to Discover Culture Care. Used with permission. McFarland, M. R., & Wehbe-Alamah, H. B. (2018).

Color Insert 2-A

Color Insert 2-A

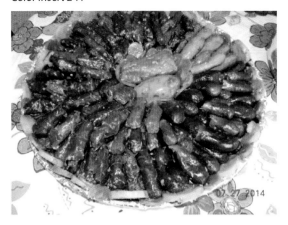

Lebanese homemade stuffed grape leaves, zucchini, and eggplant— favorite cultural foods. © H. B. Wehbe-Alamah (2018).

Color Insert 2-B

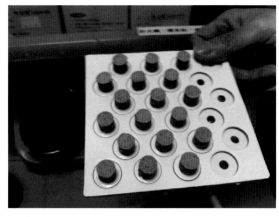

Moxibustion. Photograph taken at Chinese Medicine Clinic in Taipei, Taiwan, in 2011. © H. B. Wehbe-Alamah (2018).

Color Insert 3

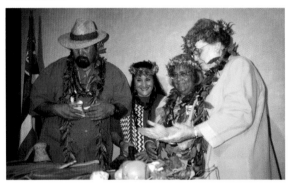

Polynesian traditional healers and carers sharing their knowledge at Transcultural Nursing Conference.

Color Insert 5

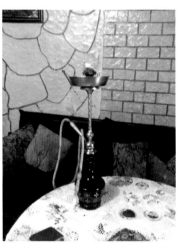

Argeeleh (also known as Water Pipe or Hookah). © H. B. Wehbe-Alamah (2018).

Color Insert 4

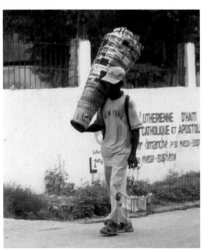 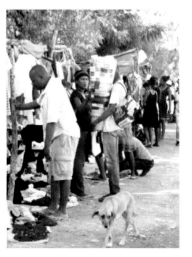

Examples of "Walking Pharmacies" with unregulated medications for sale: Note the "cones" of different blister packages. © Robert Kelch (2018).

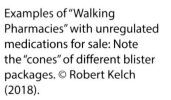

the belief that *one's own ways are the best, most superior, or preferred* ways to act, believe, or behave. Leininger (2002) maintained that ethnocentrism is a universal phenomenon in that most people tend to believe that their ways of living, believing, and acting are right, proper, and morally correct. However, excessive or strong ethnocentric attitudes can become a serious problem when dealing with others. When one holds too firmly to one's own beliefs, values, and standards, and is unwilling to accommodate or consider someone else's views, problems occur (Leininger, 2002).

Learning to value, appreciate, and understand *why* other cultures do and act differently within their particular viewpoints is essential in transcultural nursing. It is this knowledge and awareness of *other's views* that leads to finding creative ways to serve people and understand oneself. Beliefs that seem bizarre or strange may be common and important to one culture but differ greatly from other cultures. Strong ethnocentric views that are acted on can be destructive or harmful to other cultures and can limit professional growth and success. Modifying or changing one's own strong beliefs is often essential for an effective professional relationship with clients, staff, and organizational systems. An example of rigid ethnocentrism is a nurse who believes that there is only one way to make a hospital bed appropriately, which is to ensure that the bottom corners are folded in a way that keeps the client's feet tucked snugly in bed. When such a technique is used for a bed occupied by a tall Danish client who desires plenty of wiggle room for his feet, the client is rendered uncomfortable. Clients faced with ethnocentric tendencies will often challenge such views. This may lead to dissatisfaction, lack of trust, and cultural conflicts.

Excessive ethnocentrism is often a major concern for transcultural nurses because it can lead to cultural clashes, stresses, and negative outcomes. Some nurses may be so ethnocentric that they constantly misinterpret what is said or done by clients of a different cultural background. Rigid ethnocentric practices and attitudes by nurses generally lead to unfavorable client-care practices. Transcultural mentoring is essential to assess and prevent strong ethnocentrism. Sometimes problems continue because no one wants to deal with ethnocentric biases and practices. Leininger (2002) maintained that while all humans have some degree of ethnocentrism, it is the narrow, biased, and nonrespectful ones that cause difficulties.

Cultural Imposition

Cultural imposition refers to "the tendency of an individual or group to impose their beliefs, values, and patterns of behavior on another culture for varied reasons" (Leininger, 1991a, 2002). Cultural imposition remains a major serious and largely unrecognized problem in nursing as a result of cultural ignorance, blindness, ethnocentric tendencies, biases, racism, and other factors. In the health care system, cultural imposition occurs when health care providers (such as nurses and physicians) hold considerable power, influence, status, or authority over clients. A desire for expediency in performing a certain task or procedure may also result in cultural imposition. In addition, ethnocentric beliefs about what may be considered preferable compared to what is perceived as strange, bizarre, or nondesirable views often form the basis for practices steeped in cultural imposition.

Clients of some cultures—especially non-Western cultures—are vulnerable and often perceive that they have virtually no rights, power, or influence over individuals with authority or some degree of power. Cultural imposition often leaves these clients feeling helpless, angry, or frustrated. Transcultural nurses need to act as client advocates in sensitive and meaningful ways to prevent or address cultural imposition practices whenever they are encountered.

Cultural Pain

Cultural pain is a concept that Leininger (1997) developed while caring for people from diverse cultures who reported experiencing pain because nurses and physicians failed to recognize their cultural needs, discomforts, or prohibitions (taboos). Cultural pain refers to *suffering, discomfort, or* [the state of] *being greatly offended by an individual or group who shows a great lack of sensitivity toward another's cultural experience* (Leininger, 2002). Nurses are taught mainly about psychophysical pain, but seldom learn that cultural pain exists and may be extremely hurtful. Transcultural nurses are in a good position to identify cultural pain as they listen to and observe clients of different cultures. Cultural pain may be manifested through crying or other psychophysical expressions.

Nurses can induce cultural pain by verbalizing comments or engaging in actions that are offensive and hurtful to their culturally diverse clients. For example, demeaning comments about someone's faith, body size, physical features such as skin color, or *uncommon* cultural practices may lead to cultural pain. Ignoring requests for cultural accommodations and breeching cultural taboos may also cause cultural pain. Cultural pain stems from hurtful cultural offenses and goes beyond physical and psychological pain.

It is important also to be aware of the different ways cultures respond to or express physical and emotional pain. Some cultures are very sensitive and vocal in their response to physical pain and tend to quickly and loudly respond to even the slightest pin prick, injury, or bodily discomfort. Other cultures are very stoic in their response to physical pain and exhibit controlled stances. For example, some female Jewish and Italian clients in labor may express their pain more loudly than Russian, Lithuanian, German, or Slovenian clients. Pain expressions are often culturally learned; children are taught early on how to respond to or ignore physical injuries. Accepting pain may also be linked to religious beliefs such as observing a stoic and accepting attitude to gain spiritual graces known as *redemptive suffering* by Roman Catholics or as *atonement of sins* for Arab Muslims (Leininger, 2002; Wehbe-Alamah, 2015).

Transcultural nurses learn to be aware of how and why cultural expressions vary for physical and cultural pain with children and adults. Such holding knowledge helps nurses to respond appropriately to cultural pain differences in therapeutic and sensitive ways and to not assume everyone experiences physical, emotional, and cultural pain in the same manner or at the same level of intensity. It is especially important to go beyond psychophysical pain to include cultural pain when assessing clients' discomfort. The important principle to remember is that what constitutes pain for one culture or individual is largely culturally learned and patterned across the lifespan.

Cultural Bias

Cultural bias is closely related to ethnocentrism. It refers to *a firm position or stance that one's own values and beliefs must govern the situation or decisions* (Leininger, 2002). A culturally biased person usually fails to recognize their own biases and persists in making their biases known to others. Nurses with cultural bias are often rigid in their thinking and may get into problems working with diverse cultures (Leininger, 2002). Strong cultural biases usually lead to open resistance and negative relationships with others such as clients and staff.

Race, Ethnicity, and Culture

Culture is often defined according to ethnicity or race. This understanding is not only erroneous but very limiting. Culture is a much more holistic and comprehensive term that goes beyond ethnicity, which is based wholly or in part on selected racial features or national origins of people. It is important to understand how culture, ethnicity, and race differ and how they overlap.

Accordingly, *ethnicity* refers to *learned cultural and social identity* of particular groups related to specific ancestral features (such as language, customs, mode of dress, and religion); it is often but not always associated with inherited physical characteristics such as skin color or body shape (adapted from Leininger, 2002). The United States government (U. S. Office of Personnel Management, 2014, p. A137) recognizes the following ethnicities:

- Hispanic or Latino: A person of Cuban, Mexican, Puerto Rican, South or Central American, or other Spanish culture or origin, regardless of race.
- Not Hispanic or Latino: A person *not* of Cuban, Mexican, Puerto Rican, South or Central American, or other Spanish culture or origin.

Race refers to *social* classification of *inherited* biological physical, or genetic traits such as skin color, hair texture, and other physical features (adapted from Leininger, 2002). The United States government recognizes five race categories (U. S. Office of Personnel Management, 2014, pp. A137- A138):

- American Indian or Alaska Native: A person having origins in any of the original peoples of North and South America (including Central America), and who maintains tribal affiliation or community attachment (p. A-137).
- Asian: A person having origins in any of the original peoples of the Far East, Southeast Asia, or the Indian subcontinent including (in part), Cambodia, China, India, Japan, Korea, Malaysia, Pakistan, the Philippine Islands, Thailand, and Vietnam.
- Black or African-American: A person having origins in any of the black racial groups of Africa.
- Native Hawaiian or Pacific Islander: A person having origins in any of the original peoples of Hawaii, Guam, Samoa, or other Pacific Islands.
- White: A person having origins in any of the original peoples of Europe, the Middle East, or North Africa.

Racism and Related Concepts

The literature is abundant with numerous definitions for *racism*. The Merriam-Webster online dictionary (n.d.) defines racism as a *belief that race is the primary determinant of human traits and capacities and that racial differences produce an inherent superiority of a particular race.* Essed (1990, p. 11) defined racism as the *definitive attribution of inferiority to a particular racial/ethnic group and the use of this principle to propagate and justify the unequal treatment of this group.* Racism is defined by Bonilla-Silva (1997) as a *social system involving ethnoracial categories and some form of hierarchy that produces disparities in life chances between ethnoracial groups* (Berman & Paradies, 2008, p. 3). In recent times, there has been a push by some psychiatrists to recognize *racism* as a mental illness with a Diagnostics and Statistics Manual classification (Thomas, 2014). While the American Psychiatric Association has thus far refused to consider racism as a medical pathology, racism has already acquired several clinical names such as *prejudiced personality, intolerant personality disorder,* and *pathological bias* (Thomas, 2014).

Racism is derived from the concept of race, and race is generally defined as a biological factor of a discrete group whose members share distinctive genetic, biological, and other factors from a common or claimed ancestor (Leininger, 1991c). Leininger (2002) further held that focusing on outward or phenotype appearances such as skin color to define or describe race was not adequate because culture and genetic features needed to be included to understand race. For example, Native Americans are not red, yellow, or white and yet they are often referred to as *the red race.* Similarly, black skin has also various hues and thus the term *black* cannot be used to describe only Africans because many cultures have dark to lighter hues of color such as the Maori, Fijians, Southeast Indians, Native Australian Aborigines, Mayans, Aztecs, and others.

Kottak (1991) held that people often talk about *social races* rather than *genetic or biological races* in their public discourse (Leininger, 1991c). Social attitudes and perceived differences often precede prejudices, discrimination, and labels of racism. Racism often denotes subordination and the oppressive use of authority over others such as minorities, refugees, women, and religious groups. The term *people of color*

is still used in nursing practice and literature. Leininger (2002) believed that this term was misleading, ambiguous, imprecise, and that using it could lead to distorted or negative views.

Racism and racial profiling can lead to discrimination and/or vicious labelling of people with unsupported accusations especially between white and black peoples or religious groups worldwide (Leininger, 2002; American Civil Liberties Union [ALCU], n.d.). It can also lead to overt violence, cultural backlash, and prolonged alienation and legal suits. In nursing, racist discrimination practices do exist and therefore need to be proactively addressed to prevent harm to clients and to any people involved. Marked interpersonal tensions, isolation, violence, and other destructive behaviors can occur wherever racism is allowed to prevail. All nurses and health professionals need to address racism and discrimination problems and to discover their sources, reasons, and various factors that lead to or aggravate its occurrence.

Learning about cultural differences in values, beliefs, patterns, and lifeways and understanding *the why* of these differences is crucial. In addition, one needs to seek information about the roots of institutional racial beliefs, gender biases, disruptive behaviors, and prolonged animosities between different cultures. Transcultural nurses prepared through graduate/formal programs can be very helpful in dealing with these major concerns and problems worldwide.

Prejudice, Discrimination, and Stereotyping

Given that the terms *prejudice, discrimination,* and *stereotyping*—although closely related—are not often used correctly, the following definitions have been developed and used in transcultural nursing (Leininger, 2002):

- *Prejudice* refers to preconceived attitudes, ideas, beliefs, or opinions about an individual, group, or culture that limit a full and accurate understanding of the individual, culture, gender, event, or situation. Examples of prejudice include homophobia, Islamophobia, and anti-Semitism.
- *Discrimination* refers to overt or covert actions or ways that limit opportunities, choices, or life experiences of others based on feelings or on racial biases.
- *Stereotyping* refers to classifying or placing people into a narrow, fixed view with rigid, or inflexible,

boxlike characteristics. Stereotyping is often used as a "quick fix" to classify people without understanding individual and group cultural differences. When nurses stereotype clients, they usually fail to recognize any individual or group cultural variations and cultural beliefs.

Limited knowledge and understanding of cultures usually leads to stereotyping, discrimination, prejudices, racism, and biases. It is therefore important to acquire holding knowledge of diverse cultural beliefs, practices, expressions, and lifeways as well as to learn transcultural concepts, theories, models, communication, and assessment techniques to provide culturally sensitive care to clients of different cultural backgrounds and to avoid falling into the pitfalls of prejudice, bias, discrimination, and stereotyping. When allowed to become unleashed, stereotyping and prejudice can lead to racism, discrimination, and even violence or hate crimes (ACLU, n.d.).

Cultural Backlash

Cultural backlash refers to *negative feedback*, hostile responses, *or unfavorable outcomes* associated with ignoring or disrespecting cultural values, beliefs, practices, or taboos. V*isiting nurses who* fail to *provide care that fits with the needs, beliefs, and practices of* members of their *host culture* may experience cultural backlash. Typically this negative backlash is triggered by visiting nurses' decisions and actions that are enmeshed in ethnocentrism, bias, and cultural imposition practices or expressions. This phenomena makes one aware of the importance of providing care that *fits the culture* and is devoid of ethnocentrism and cultural imposition practices or expressions, thus avoiding a cultural backlash. Cultural backlash usually occurs with nurses who have not been prepared in transcultural nursing, or it may occur because of political reasons or conflicts that develop suddenly in the host country (Leininger, 2002).

Cultural Overidentification

Another related phenomenon that can occur in serving other countries or cultures is *cultural overidentification* which refers to *becoming too involved, overly sympathetic, or too compassionate with the people, situation, or a human condition of a certain culture* (Leininger, 2002). As a consequence, one is unable to be helpful to the culture or individual resulting in nontherapeutic or inappropriate actions. Sometimes this occurs when nurses have deeply sympathetic, biased, and emotional feelings about a culture or situation they experience such as working with poverty stricken, homeless, abused, oppressed, or battered individuals. The nurse's beliefs, attitudes, and actions become ineffective and can often be labelled by the host culture as *too compassionate* or *too emotionally involved* with members of the culture. The nurse needs to remain aware of overidentification tendencies when providing transcultural care.

Cultural Safety

The term *cultural safety* was first introduced by researchers from New Zealand as a means to highlight and address *the relationship and effect of power relations, racism, prejudice, social inequality, and discrimination in the health of minority groups* (Arieli, Mashiach, Hirschfeld, & Friedman, 2012). The term is widely used in New Zealand, Canada, and Europe. The Nursing Council of New Zealand (2011, p. 7) defined cultural safety as:

> The effective nursing practice of a person or family from another culture, and is determined by that person or family. Culture includes, but is not restricted to, age or generation; gender; sexual orientation; occupation and socioeconomic status; ethnic origin or migrant experience; religious or spiritual belief; and disability.
>
> The nurse delivering the nursing service will have undertaken a process of reflection on his or her own cultural identity and will recognise the impact that his or her personal culture has on his or her professional practice. *Unsafe cultural practice comprises any action which diminishes, demeans, or disempowers the cultural identity and wellbeing of an individual* [emphasis added].

Bioculturalism

Bioculturalism refers to *biological and physical expressions in different physical environments or cultural contexts related to care, health, illness, and disability* (Leininger, 2002). It also refers *to the acknowledgement that biological diversity is linked with cultural diversity in knowledge, language, and practice, and that sustaining both is necessary for ecological and cultural wellbeing* (Sullivan, 2011, p. 16). Humans are born and live within biophysical environments that influence their health and illness factors. Genetic, biocultural, and physical factors influence each other in different ecologies and cultural environments. Leininger's transcultural study conducted in 1960 on bioecological variability in two Gadsup villages was an early nursing and anthropological research study focused on health care (Leininger, 1966). Nurses work with clients in their biophysical and cultural settings and need to give attention to these factors and how they can influence caring practices and use of biocultural resources.

Culture-bound Illness or Syndrome

The concept of culture-bound illness or syndrome is another essential concept to understand in transcultural nursing. *Culture-bound* refers to *specific care, health, illness, and disease conditions that are particular, quite unique, and usually specific to a designated culture or geographical area* (Leininger, 2002). For example, in the Eastern Highlands of Papua New Guinea, *kuru* was discovered as a culture-bound illness in the early 1960s when Leininger was conducting her field study with the people of that area (Leininger, 1978). Kuru is a degenerative neurological disorder condition unique to the Eastern Highlands of New Guinea region—in which adult females died within approximately nine months of diagnosis—and was largely related to biocultural, viral, and other factors (Kottak, 1991). Kuru is believed to be related to the now extinct cultural practice of mortuary cannibalism or consumption of the dead. In Malaysia, one encounters the culture-bound syndrome *Amok* characterized by "periods of brooding with subsequent aggressive behaviour followed by amnesia or exhaustion" (Ehrmin, 2016, p. 288).

Anthropologists have studied these and other culture-bound conditions for many decades with findings revealing specific conditions confined to cultural, local, or regional areas. Culture-bound phenomena may be essentially new to nurses and many health professionals due to their lack of culture-specific knowledge. Transcultural nurses learn to be alert for occurrences of culture-bound expressions and conditions so as to identify related unique cultural care needs.

■ THE FIVE BASIC INTERACTIONAL CONCEPTS

Nurses working in transcultural contexts need to be clear about five basic concepts, namely: *Culture encounter; assimilation; acculturation; enculturation; and socialization.* Leininger (2002) held that these concepts came largely from anthropology and are essential to know and understand in transcultural nursing.

1. *Culture encounter or contact* refers to *a situation in which a person from one culture meets or briefly interacts with a person from another culture* (Leininger, 2002). A nurse having brief encounters with people from another culture seldom grasps and understands strangers and their cultural lifeways and does not become an "expert" or an authority on the culture. Nurses who rely on brief cultural encounters as a source of expertise without adequate accumulation of holding knowledge to publish, give lectures, or engage in different projects may find themselves on the receiving end of *cultural backlash* and embroiled in ethical issues should local cultures discover that their culture was not understood or presented accurately (Leininger, 2002).

2. *Acculturation* refers to *the process by which an individual or group from a culture* (Culture A) *learns how to take on many (but not all) values, behaviors, norms, and lifeways of another culture* (Culture B) (Leininger, 2002). An individual may retain and use some traditional values and practices from the old culture (Culture A), and take on new culture norms (from Culture B). When many values and lifeways of a different culture (Culture B) are evident, the individual (from Culture A) is usually regarded as acculturated (into Culture B). With acculturation, one generally becomes attracted to another culture for various reasons and almost unintentionally learns to take on the lifeways of the new culture in dress, talk, and daily living. Few cultures become fully acculturated to another lifeway. Instead, people are *selective* in *what they choose to change and retain.* It is important that transcultural nurses assess individuals or families to determine *if* they are living by traditional and/or new cultural values to achieve quality care outcomes.

3. *Socialization* refers to *the social process whereby an individual or group from a particular culture learns how to function within the larger society (or country); that is, to know how to interact appropriately with others and how to survive, work, and live in relative harmony within a society* (Leininger, 2002). For example, new immigrants learn about becoming a United States citizen and how to buy goods, interact, and communicate with Americans and others in the American society. This is commonly referred to as *taking on the new ways.* Socialization is different from acculturation because the goal of socialization is to learn how to adapt to and function in a large society with its dominant values, ethos, or national lifeways. It is not necessarily becoming acculturated to a particular local culture or another culture. *Socialization* entails becoming an accepted participant within the dominant and larger society (Leininger, 2002).

4. *Enculturation* refers to *the process by which one learns to take on or live by a particular culture with its specific values, beliefs, and practices* (Leininger, 2002). One can speak of a child becoming enculturated in learning how to become an Italian, Anglo-American, Amish, or whatever the parents or individual lives by or chooses. The child becomes enculturated when he or she shows acceptable behavior of the cultural values, beliefs, and actions. Nurses are also enculturated within the nursing profession by learning the norms (rules of behavior), values, and other expectations of the nursing culture. It is important that nursing students become enculturated into nursing values, norms, and lifeways to survive, function, and fully become professional nurses. Nurses become enculturated into the cultures of local hospitals, community agencies, and other health services in order to accept and maintain practice expectations. Some clients may become enculturated into a healthcare institution, especially if they stay in the institution over a long period of time such as with chronic illnesses or disabilities. However, not all children, clients, students, and nurses become enculturated into fully accepting the culturally desired or preferred values, norms, and practices. One needs to perform a self-assessment to determine whether one is or has become enculturated to another lifeway.

5. *Assimilation* refers to *the way (or process) by which an individual or group voluntarily chooses or is forcibly compelled to take on the traits of dominant culture to the extent where one's own ethnic cultural characteristics become indistinguishable from those of the dominant culture.* A new immigrant who willingly and eagerly fully embraces the cultural way of life, language, mode of dress, customs, and other cultural characteristics of the dominant or host culture in replacement of his or her own ethnic cultural characteristics demonstrates voluntary cultural assimilation. An example of forced assimilation is when a dominant culture forces indigenous minority cultures to assimilate into the mainstream (dominant) culture by coercing them into abandoning their ethnic cultural characteristics such as religious practices, mode of dress, and language in favor of those of dominant cultures. An example of this would be the forced assimilation of Native American tribal peoples (the children, in particular) in the United States during the latter half of the 19th century.

These five concepts are important for nurses and others to understand to assess, interpret, and work effectively with both diverse and similar cultures.

■ CULTURE CARE: A CENTRAL CONSTRUCT WITH RELATED CONCEPTS

Culture Care

A *construct* represents *many* embedded thoughts or ideas whereas a *concept* reflects *only one* (Leininger, 2002). In the early 1960s, Leininger (1991c) developed the construct of culture care as central to the Culture Care Theory. She defined *culture care* as *the cognitively learned and transmitted professional and indigenous folk values, beliefs, and patterned lifeways that are used to assist, facilitate, or enable another individual or group to maintain their wellbeing or health or to improve a human condition or lifeway* (Leininger, 2002, p. 57). This construct is central to transcultural nursing knowledge and practices.

Culture care is focused on discovering and learning about the meanings, patterns, and uses of care within cultures. Identifying patterns of care and their uses provides data that are beneficial to clients. Culture and care are tightly linked together and interdependent.

Both are needed to know and help people diverse cultures. From studies about culture care have come care subtypes such as *protective care.* For example, American Gypsies value and use *protective care* for their daily survival to remain well and prevent illness. For this culture, protective care refers to *being very watchful of strangers or outsiders who could harm or be noncaring* to Gypsies. It is the Gypsy males who are active in maintaining protective care. *Comfort care* is another major idea discovered in some cultures that is essential for healing and wellbeing. Many additional new discoveries have been made, such as *touching care, reassurance care,* and *filial care* as well as other culture-specific and holistic constructs (Leininger, 2002). These constructs have many embedded ideas that can guide nursing decisions and actions and serve as new ways to practice nursing (Leininger, 1991c & 2002).

Culture-Specific Care/Caring

The idea of *culture-specific care/caring* comes from culture care but refers to *very specific or particular ways* [by which] *to have care fit client's needs* (Leininger, 2002, p. 57). Leininger coined this term in the mid-1960s to help nurses focus on and provide care that fits the client's specific cultural needs and lifeways. To be culturally helpful to clients, care needs to be tailor-made and used in specific ways so that the client can experience its benefits in meaningful and therapeutic ways. Examples include *protective care* being used and maintained with the Gadsup Akuna of New Guinea or *touching care* with many Anglo-American children (Leininger & Wehbe-Alamah, 2015).

Generalized Culture Care

The construct of *generalized culture care* was also coined and developed by Leininger (1991c) at the same time as culture-specific care. It refers to *commonly shared professional nursing care techniques, principles, and practices that are beneficial to several clients as a general and essential human care need* (Leininger, 2002, p.57). Generalized culture care can be used in several cultures, such as the construct of *respectful care* discovered in several cultures. Generalized care tends to be valued by many cultures as a more common or even a universal care need. The nurse considers both *culture specific* and *generalized culture* care when practicing nursing (Leininger, 2002).

Culturally Congruent Care

The nursing goal is to provide *culturally congruent nursing care,* which is defined as *those assistive, supportive, facilitative, or enabling decisions and actions that include culture care values, beliefs, and lifeways to provide meaningful, beneficial, and satisfying care for the health and wellbeing of people, or for those facing disabilities, illness, or death* (Leininger, 1991c & 2002). Culturally congruent care remains the central focus and goal of the Theory of Culture Care Diversity and Universality and is the desired outcome of all transcultural nursing practices.

Cultural Care Conflict and Cultural Care Clashes

Cultural care conflict in nursing typically occurs when nurses work with mainly unknown cultures. *Culture care conflict* refers to *signs of distress, concern, and nonhelpful nursing care practices that fail to meet a client's cultural expectations, beliefs, values, and lifeways* (Leininger, 2002, p. 58). It is also closely related to *cultural care clashes* except that with cultural care clashes *obvious and known situations arise that are tense and cause overt problems.* Both client and nurse are usually fully aware of cultural care clashes, but may be less so with cultural care conflicts. In both situations, the client may be uncooperative, emotionally upset, and/or dissatisfied with the care offered (Leininger, 2002). Cultural clashes can be frequently observed in clinical and community settings between staff and clients from diverse cultures (Leininger, 1990c & 2002). For example, a Muslim female client from Afghanistan refused nursing care from a male nurse and became resistant and uncooperative. To this particular client, being cared for by a male stranger when a female alternative was present clashed with her cultural and religious beliefs. Some clients remain silent and use a "conspiracy of silence" to show their dislike for nursing or medical care when it clashes with their cultural values and beliefs. To prevent such potential cultural clashes, the nurse needs to know and understand the client's culture and the reasons for being nonadherent, tense, and resistant (Leininger, 2002).

Cultural Exports and Cultural Imports

Two closely related but different concepts to understand are cultural exports and cultural imports. *Cultural exports* refers to the *sending of ideas, techniques, material goods, or symbolic referents to another culture in order to improve lifeways or to advance practices* (adapted from Leininger, 2002). On the other hand, *cultural imports* refers to *taking in or receiving ideas, techniques, material goods, or other items that are perceived as useful or helpful to one's culture* (adapted from Leininger, 2002). Sometimes these exports and imports are useful, but sometimes they fail to fit the values, beliefs, or care practices of the recipient culture and become troublesome or dysfunctional to the people. Additional thought and knowledge are needed in nursing about cultural exports and imports in order to achieve beneficial or desired uses and to prevent unethical practices (Leininger, 2002).

Cultural Context

Cultural context refers to the *totality of shared meanings and life experiences—in particular social, cultural, and physical environments—that influence attitudes, thinking, and patterns of living* (Leininger, 2002, p. 60). Cultural context in nursing was first discussed by Leininger in a 1970 publication as an important concept for nurses to understand. Understanding the meanings and responses associated with cultural context is highly important. Cultural context that includes the cultural values, social structure, and environmental factors provides a holistic and totality view of the client within an environmental setting. It is the cultural context that gives meaning to understanding situations and clients and provides a powerful guide for nursing decisions and actions.

Generic and Professional Care/Caring

In developing the transcultural nursing field, two very important concepts identify different kinds of care: *generic care* (also referred to as indigenous, traditional, lay, or folk care) and *professional nursing care,* both of which were based largely on *emic* and *etic* care discoveries.

Generic care (caring) refers to *culturally learned and transmitted lay, indigenous traditional, and largely emic folk knowledge and skills used by cultures* (Leininger, 2002, p. 61). In contrast, *professional (nursing) care (caring)* refers to *formally and cognitively learned etic knowledge and practice skills that have been taught and used by faculty and clinicians to provide professional care* (Leininger, 2002, p. 61). Generic care has been and continues to be derived from the term *emic*

(meaning within the culture) and is typically transmitted inter-generationally. Professional care or etic care is derived largely from outside specific cultures from professional and institutional sources. Both have been identified as means to provide assistive, supportive, and facilitative care for the health and wellbeing of people or to help people face disability, illness, or death (Leininger, 1994, 1995, 2002).

During the past six decades, these two types of care have been studied by transcultural nurse researchers worldwide to discover new insights about the human care of diverse cultures. These terms were coined and developed by Leininger (2002) to discover whether and how differences and similarities exist among and between cultures from the *emic* viewpoint of cultures (insider's view) and the *etic* (outsider's view). Generic or indigenous emic care had not been studied in-depth or used in nursing until Leininger introduced the concepts in the 1960s. Professional nursing care ideas and skills were mainly used but not generic care knowledge and practices.

Leininger (2002) predicted that such differences in care could lead to different outcomes in the quality of care provided. With focus on comparative generic (folk) and professional care, a wealth of new knowledge has been forthcoming from research studies and practice experiences with major contrasts discovered about these two types of care. Table 2.1 presents some major differences between generic (emic) folk and professional (etic) data from cultural informants. These differences and many others presented in chapter eight of this text entitled "Integrating Generic and Professional Health Care Practices" are findings that merit urgent consideration by professional nurses to provide culturally congruent, safe, and responsible care. Both generic (emic) and professional (etic) care need to be explicitly taught, further researched, and brought into care practices for the therapeutic healing and satisfying care of clients of diverse and similar cultures.

Several important constructs and concepts have been presented as essential and relevant to transcultural nursing. In recent decades, a wealth of new and valuable culture care knowledge has been discovered from specific cultures such as *comfort care, nurturant care, continuity care,* and *respectful care* (Leininger, 2002). The reader is encouraged to study these care constructs in this text and other publications to appreciate the deep richness of *culture care.*

TABLE 2.1. Cultural Informants' Views of Comparative Generic and Professional Care/Cure.

Generic *(Emic)* Care/Cure	Professional *(Etic)* Care/Cure
• Humanistically oriented	• Scientifically oriented
• People based with practical and familiar referents	• Clients to be acted on with unfamiliar techniques and strangers
• Holistic and integrated approach with focus on social relationship, language, and lifeways	• Fragmented and nonintegrated services with focus on physical body and mind
• Focus is largely on caring	• Focus is largely on curing, diagnosis, and treatments
• Largely nontechnological using folk remedies and personal relationships	• Largely technological with many diagnostic tests and scientific treatments
• Focuses on prevention of illnesses, disability, & maintaining lifeways	• Focuses on treating diseases, disabilities, and pathologies
• Uses *high*-context communication modes	• Uses *low*-context communication modes
• Relies on traditional and familiar folk caring and healing	• Relies on biophysical and emotional factors to be assessed and treated

■ PRINCIPLES, POLICY STATEMENTS, STANDARDS, POSITION STATEMENTS, CODES, AND GUIDELINES

In this section, selected transcultural nursing principles, policy statements, standards, position statements, codes, and guidelines are presented in historical/chronological order of their inception so as to provide the reader with guides for developing culturally congruent and competent nursing decisions and actions in clinical practice, education, consultation, management, and research. Each entry is supplemented with an explication of its context and rationale for use.

Transcultural Nursing Care Principles

In 1990, Leininger shared what she termed as *essential transcultural nursing principles* that serve as *holding knowledge* to guide students, faculty, practitioners, administrators, and consultants in their thinking and deliberations toward providing beneficial nursing care practices or for having interactions with people of different cultures. Leininger (2002) envisioned the following transcultural nursing care principles as reflective guides that influence transcultural nurses' thinking, decisions, and actions as they provide culturally congruent care to individuals, families, groups, and institutions of diverse cultural backgrounds (p. 62):

1. Human caring with a transcultural care focus is essential for the health, healing, and wellbeing of individuals, families, groups, and institutions.

2. Every culture has specific beliefs, values, and patterns of caring and healing that need to be discovered, understood, and used in the care of people of diverse or similar cultures.

3. Transcultural nursing knowledge and competencies are imperative to provide meaningful, congruent, safe, and beneficial health care practices.

4. It is a human right that cultures have their cultural care values, beliefs, and practices respected and thoughtfully incorporated into nursing and health services.

5. Culturally based care and health beliefs and health practices vary in diverse and similar cultures and can change over time.

6. Comparative cultural care experiences, meanings, values, and patterns of culture care are fundamental sources of transcultural nursing knowledge to guide nursing decisions and actions.

7. Generic (emic, traditional, indigenous, folk, or lay) and professional (etic) care knowledge and practices often have different knowledge and experience bases that need to be assessed and understood before using the information in client care.

8. Holistic and comprehensive knowledge in transcultural nursing necessitates understanding *emic* and *etic* perspectives related to worldview; language; ethnohistory; kinship; religion or spirituality; technology; economic and political factors; and specific cultural values, beliefs, and practices bearing upon care, wellbeing, health, disability, illness, and death or dying.

9. Different modes of learning, living, and transmitting culture care and health across the lifespan are major foci of transcultural nursing education, research, and practice.
10. Transcultural nursing necessitates an understanding of one's self, one's culture, and one's ways of entering a different culture and helping others.
11. Transcultural nursing theory, research, and practice are interested in both universalities (commonalities) and diversities (differences) to generate new knowledge and to provide beneficial humanistic and scientific care practices.
12. Transcultural nursing decisions and actions are based largely on evidence-based research care and health knowledge derived from in-depth study of cultures and the use of this knowledge in professional caring.
13. Culture care lifespan patterns, values, and practices of cultures are valuable means to help sustain or maintain the health and wellbeing of people, or deal with other human conditions.
14. Transcultural nursing necessitates coparticipation of client and nurse for effective transcultural decisions, actions, practices, and outcomes.
15. Transcultural nursing uses culture care theories to generate new knowledge and then to disseminate, use, and evaluate outcomes in practice.
16. Observation, participation, and reflection are essential modalities to discover and respond to clients of diverse and similar cultures with their care needs and expectations.
17. Verbal and nonverbal language with their meanings and symbols are important to know, understand, and use in formulation of culturally congruent and therapeutic care outcomes.
18. Transcultural nurses respect human rights and are alert to unethical or illegal practices, health disparities, social injustices, cultural needs, and taboos or prohibitions.
19. Understanding the cultural context of the client is essential to assess and respond appropriately to clients and their holistic healthcare needs and concerns.
20. Culture care is needed for people who have experienced cultural pain, have been deeply hurt, insulted, or dehumanized because of cultural ignorance or non-caring attitudes and practices.

Policy Statements to Guide Transcultural Nursing Standards and Practices

Transcultural nurses know that while cultures are relatively stable, they are fluid and can change over an extended period of time. Therefore, it is important to have some general guidelines to initiate and maintain standards and policies for safe, meaningful, and effective care practices. *Policy statements* are *directive guides for decision and action making to maintain, protect, and ensure quality-based consumer services* (Leininger, 2002, p. 66). The Merriam-Webster online dictionary (n.d.) defines policy as *a definite course or method of action selected from among alternatives and in light of given conditions to guide and determine present and future decisions.* According to Leininger (1995, 2002), policy statements serve several important functions such as:

- Serving as an explicit guide with standards to provide and evaluate quality-based transcultural nursing by educators, practitioners, consultants, and researchers.
- Providing some commonly shared policy and standard statements to maintain culture care competencies and beneficial transcultural nursing practices.
- Serving to provide standards to guide transcultural nursing decisions, actions, and practices.
- Providing some explicit philosophical position of values, beliefs, and standards held by transcultural nursing experts.
- Providing a policy document for use by public officials such as legislators, the public, and others interested in knowing and understanding transcultural nursing in relation to consumer care services.

In 1998, members of the Board of Trustees of the Transcultural Nursing Society, which included Leininger as founder and permanent member, developed and published 20 policy statements to guide transcultural nursing standards and practices (Board of Trustees of the Transcultural Nursing Society, 1998) to generally support the common good or welfare of clients from diverse and similar cultures. Four years later, Leininger (2002) published 16 policy statements derived from the previously published standards in addition to knowledge learned from her extensive study and leadership work in transcultural nursing.

The revised 16 policy statements were offered as *directive guides* to help nurses reflect on and arrive at culturally congruent and appropriate decisions and actions in the best interest and safety of human beings. They also were intended to serve as a means to establish, improve, maintain, protect, and evaluate practices related to culturally congruent, meaningful, and beneficial care, decisions, and actions for people of diverse or similar cultures. Leininger (2002) maintained that these policies and standards supported the philosophical and epistemic premises of transcultural nursing along with established concepts, principles, ethical considerations, and research theory-based knowledge and practices. These 16 revised policy statements (Leininger, 2002, pp. 67-68) are:

1. Consumers of health care have a right to have their culture-care values, norms, and practices known, understood, and respected by nurses and other health care providers caring for people of diverse cultures.

2. Immigrants, refugees, oppressed individuals and groups, vulnerable groups, minorities or underrepresented cultural groups, the poor, and the homeless have a *right* to have their cultural and general health care needs understood and responded to in ways that are meaningful, helpful, and congruent with their beliefs, values, and practices, and to help improve their general health and wellbeing or to face disability, illness, or death.

3. Transcultural nursing needs to be grounded in *emic* (culture or people-centered) and *etic* (professional) humanistic and scientific research and theory-based knowledge to ensure culturally competent, congruent, safe, and responsible care to people of diverse or similar cultures.

4. Transcultural philosophical and epistemic findings hold that care, health, wellbeing, disability, illness, and dying are embedded in culture-care values, beliefs, and normative lifeways of cultures and subcultures which are essential to know and explicitly use to guide transcultural nursing decisions and actions for beneficial and therapeutic outcomes.

5. Transcultural care *diversities* (differences) and *universalities* (commonalties or similarities) exist within and among cultures and necessitate that nurses discover and assess their meanings and uses for culturally based care and to guide creative and culturally congruent decisions and actions with clients in different institutions or contexts.

6. Effective and beneficial policies for consumers of diverse or similar cultures necessitates that policy makers are aware of their prejudices, biases, racial stance, and ethnocentric tendencies in providing respectful and ethically sound policies and practices.

7. Transcultural nursing policies and standards require comprehensive knowledge of cultural consumers to prevent narrow and partial perspectives of culturally based people care.

8. Given that transcultural care is culturally constituted and rooted in the peoples' generic (emic or, local, folk, indigenous, or insiders') knowledge *and* appropriate professional (etic) knowledge, it is imperative that effective cultural policies reflect research-based data to attain culturally congruent care practices.

9. Ethical and moral transcultural knowledge, as well as human rights principles, must be integrated into or given full consideration for culturally based health care policies.

10. Transcultural health care policies need to be supported by theoretical and research-based knowledge to sustain sound policy decisions and actions, especially for consultation practices.

11. Transcultural health care policies and standards need to consider the community and institutional contexts in which [these] policies are [to be] used and evaluated over time.

12. The users of transcultural health and nursing care policies must consider [seeking the assistance of mentors] who are knowledgeable and skilled to [guide] the use [and application] with cultures.

13. National, regional, and local community hospitals, clinics, or other types of health care organizations should be grounded in transcultural or relevant anthropological insights to ensure sensitive, appropriate, effective, and culturally congruent healthcare practices.

14. Nursing faculty, administrators (academic and clinical), practitioners, researchers, and consultants who use and evaluate transcultural policies and standards should be prepared in transcultural nursing [in order to be able] to intelligently and wisely use them.

15. Transcultural nursing expert leadership and/or mentors are usually needed to guide government officials, practitioners, academic and clinical administrators, faculty, researchers, consultants, minorities, and others who are unprepared in transcultural nursing or transculturalism.
16. Financial support is essential to initiate, maintain, and evaluate policy and standard outcomes.

Standards for Culturally Competent and Congruent Care

An unpublished report entitled *Standards for Transcultural Nursing* was prepared by the Transcultural Nursing Society's Committee on Certification and Recertification (as cited by Leininger, 2002). Subsequently, Leininger (2002) published 12 *Standards for Culturally Competent and Congruent Care*, an adaptation of the *1998 Policy Statement to Guide Transcultural Nursing Standards and Practices* (Board of Trustees of the Transcultural Nursing Society, 1998). Leininger (2002a, pp. 132-133) viewed standards as *criteria* that guide policies. These 12 standards for culturally competent and congruent care are:

1. Consumers of diverse cultures have a right to have transcultural care standards used to protect and respect their generic (folk) values, beliefs, and practices and to have health personnel incorporate appropriate ways into professional practices.
2. Nurses assessing and providing care to diverse cultures or subcultures have a moral obligation to be prepared in transcultural nursing to provide knowledgeable, sensitive, and research-based care to the culturally different.
3. Cultural assessments and practices need to demonstrate the use of transcultural nursing concepts, principles, theories, and research findings and competencies to ensure safe, congruent, and competent practices.
4. Nurses need to show sensitivity and ways to use cultural and care knowledge with competence for clients of diverse cultures.
5. Nurses as caregivers have an ethical, moral, professional obligation and responsibility to study, understand, and use relevant research-based transcultural care for safe, beneficial, and satisfying client or family outcomes.
6. Providing culturally competent and congruent care should reflect the caregiver's ability to assess and use culture-specific data without bias, prejudice, discrimination, or related negative outcomes.
7. Nurses caring for clients of diverse cultures should seek to provide holistic care that is comprehensive and takes into account the client's worldview and includes ethnohistory; religion (or spirituality); moral/ethical values; specific cultural care beliefs and values; kinship ties (sociocultural); economic; and political (legal) factors with references to their environmental living or working context.
8. Nurses practicing transcultural nursing give evidence in their decisions and actions of being able to deal with intercultural prejudices, biases, racism, and other expressions that are destructive or nonbeneficial to clients of diverse cultures.
9. Nurses demonstrating cultural competence and congruent care maintain an open, learning, flexible attitude and desire to expand their knowledge of diverse cultures and caring lifeways.
10. Nurses with transcultural competencies show evidence of being able to use local, regional, and national resources for beneficial care outcomes.
11. Nurses with transcultural competencies demonstrate leadership skills to work with other nurses and interprofessional colleagues who need help to provide culturally safe and congruent client practices, thus preventing cultural imposition, cultural pain offenses, cultural conflicts, and many other negative and destructive outcomes.
12. Nurses with transcultural competencies are active to defend, uphold, and improve care to clients of diverse cultures and to share their research findings and competency experiences in public and professional arenas.

Transcultural Nursing Society Position Statement on Human Rights

In 2006, the Transcultural Nursing Society (TCNS) developed a position statement on human rights for people of all cultures worldwide (Miller, et al., 2008). The TCNS statement is as follows:

Regardless of race, ethnicity, national origin, religious and philosophical beliefs, gender, sexual orientation, cultural values, age, and other diversities, people have the following universal human rights:

- Access to quality care, including qualified health care professionals, organizations, and resources;
- Access to culturally and linguistically competent health care providers;
- Respectful care with recognition of the importance of personal dignity, privacy, and confidentiality;
- Informed participation in one's own health care;
- Involvement of family members and significant others in health care delivery and decision making, if desired by the care recipient;
- The ability to accept or refuse care and negotiate with health care providers to achieve culturally congruent care;
- Freedom from health care treatments that involve coercion, bribery, and illicit activities that place one's wellbeing at risk;
- Receipt of care in an environment in which physical, psychological, spiritual, and cultural safety is assured for the person, his or her family, and significant others; and
- Receipt of care without putting oneself or loved ones in jeopardy or harm's way. (Miller, et al., 2008, pp. 6-7)

Standards of Practice for Culturally Competent Nursing Care

Twelve standards of practice for culturally competent nursing care were developed in 2009 through a collaboration between members of the American Academy of Nursing Expert Panel on Global Nursing and Health and the Transcultural Nursing Society with participation by members of the American Academy of Nursing Expert Panel on Cultural Competence; they were again revised in 2011 (Douglas, et al., 2009, 2011). These standards (Refer to Table 2.2) were based on a framework of social justice and developed as a means to initiate discussion regarding a set of universally applicable standards of practice that could be used by nurses worldwide to guide culturally competent clinical practice, research, education, and administration.

Nursing Code of Ethics

The International Council of Nurses (ICN) Code of Ethics for Nurses (2012) outlined the standards of

ethical conduct for nurses and advocated for respect for human rights which included cultural rights, the right to dignity, and the right to be treated with respect. Additionally, the code specifically promoted that nursing care should be *respectful of and unrestricted by considerations of age, colour, creed, culture, disability or illness, gender, sexual orientation, nationality, politics, race or social status* (ICN, 2012, p. 1). Under the first element of the code, "Nurses and People," nurses were directed to promote an environment of care characterized by equity, social justice, and respect for human rights, customs, and spiritual beliefs of individuals, families, and communities.

The *Code of Ethics for Nurses with Interpretive Statements* (also known as *the Code*) by the American Nurses' Association (ANA, 2015) is a guide that establishes ethical standards for the nursing profession in the U. S. The Code contains nine provisions that address nursing ethical values, obligations, duties, and professional ideals. Provision 1 of the Code states: *The nurse practices with compassion and respect for the inherent dignity, worth, and unique attributes of every person* (ANA, 2015, p. 1). Accordingly, nurses must consider the needs and respect the values of all individuals in diverse settings, establish relationships of trust, and tailor services to each person's needs while setting aside any bias or prejudices (ANA, 2015). Nurses must additionally consider the culture, value systems, religious or spiritual beliefs, lifestyle, social support system, sexual orientation or gender expression, and primary language when planning individual, family, and population-centered care (ANA, 2015).

Provision 8 of the Code states: *The nurse collaborates with other health professionals and the public to protect human rights, promote health diplomacy, and reduce health disparities* (ANA, 2015, p. 31). Thus, health is a universal human right with economic, political, social, and cultural dimensions (ANA, 2015). As a result, nurses must engage in "… creative solutions and innovative approaches that are ethical, respectful of human rights, and equitable in reducing health disparities … Nurses must recognize that health care is provided to culturally diverse populations in [the U.S.] and across the globe. Nurses must collaborate to create a milieu that is sensitive to diverse cultural values and practices" (ANA, 2015, p. 32).

TABLE 2.2. **Standards of Practice for Culturally Competent Nursing Care.**

Standard	Description
Standard 1: Social justice	Professional nurses shall promote social justice for all. The applied principles of social justice guide nurses' decisions related to the patient, family, community, and other health care professionals. Nurses will develop leadership skills to advocate for socially just policies.
Standard 2: Critical reflection	Nurses shall engage in critical reflection of their own values, beliefs, and cultural heritage to have an awareness of how these qualities and issues can affect culturally congruent nursing care.
Standard 3: Knowledge of cultures	Nurses shall gain an understanding of the perspectives, traditions, values, practices, and family systems of culturally diverse individuals, families, communities, and populations they care for, as well as a knowledge of the complex variables that affect the achievement of health and well-being.
Standard 4: Culturally competent practice	Nurses shall use cross-cultural knowledge and culturally sensitive skills in implementing culturally congruent nursing care.
Standard 5: Cultural competence in health care systems and organizations	Health care organizations should provide the structure and resources necessary to evaluate and meet the cultural and language needs of their diverse clients.
Standard 6: Patient advocacy and empowerment	Nurses shall recognize the effect of health care policies, delivery systems, and resources on their patient populations and shall empower and advocate for their patients as indicated. Nurses shall advocate for the inclusion of their patient's cultural beliefs and practices in all dimensions of their health care.
Standard 7: Multicultural workforce	Nurses shall actively engage in the effort to ensure a multicultural workforce in health care settings. One measure to achieve a multicultural workforce is through strengthening of recruitment and retention effort in the hospital and academic setting.
Standard 8: Education and training in culturally competent care	Nurses shall be educationally prepared to promote and provide culturally congruent health care. Knowledge and skills necessary for assuring that nursing care is culturally congruent shall be included in global health care agendas that mandate formal education and clinical training, as well as required ongoing, continuing education for all practicing nurses.
Standard 9: Cross-cultural communication	Nurses shall use culturally competent verbal and nonverbal communication skills to identify client's values, beliefs, practices, perceptions, and unique health care needs.
Standard 10: Cross-cultural leadership	Nurses shall have the ability to influence individuals, groups, and systems to achieve outcomes of culturally competent care for diverse populations.
Standard 11: Policy development	Nurses shall have the knowledge and skills to work with public and private organizations, professional associations, and communities to establish policies and standards for comprehensive implementation and evaluation of culturally competent care.
Standard 12: Evidence-based practice and research	Nurses shall base their practice on interventions that have been systematically tested and shown to be the most effective for the culturally diverse populations that they serve. In areas where there is a lack of evidence of efficacy, nurse researchers shall investigate and test interventions that may be the most effective in reducing the disparities in health outcomes.

Reproduced, with permission from Douglas, M. K., Pierce, J. U., Rosenkoetter, M., Pacquiao, D., Callister, L. C., Hattar-Pollara, M., . . . Purnell, L. (2011). Standards of practice for culturally competent nursing care: 2011 update. *Journal of Transcultural Nursing, 22*(4), 317-333. doi: 10.1177/1043659611412965.

The National Culturally and Linguistically Appropriate Services (CLAS) Standards

The Office of Minority Health at the U.S. Department of Health and Human Services developed the first set of National CLAS Standards in 2000, which were later revised in 2013, in an effort to address health inequities and disparities by mandating that care and services be respectful of and responsive to the cultural and linguistic needs of individuals; respond to current and projected demographic changes in the United States; eliminate long-standing disparities and social injustice in the health status of people of diverse racial, ethnic and cultural backgrounds; and improve the quality of services and primary care outcomes. The enhanced National Standards for Culturally and Linguistically Appropriate Services in Health and Health Care (Refer to Table 2.3), known as the enhanced National CLAS Standards, were intended to advance health equity,

TABLE 2.3. The Enhanced National Standards for Culturally and Linguistically Appropriate Services.

Principal Standard:
  1. Provide effective, equitable, understandable, and respectful quality care and services that are responsive to diverse cultural health beliefs and practices, preferred languages, health literacy, and other communication needs.

Governance, Leadership, and Workforce:
  2. Advance and sustain organizational governance and leadership that promotes CLAS and health equity through policy, practices, and allocated resources.
  3. Recruit, promote, and support a culturally and linguistically diverse governance, leadership, and workforce that are responsive to the population in the service area.
  4. Educate and train governance, leadership, and workforce in culturally and linguistically appropriate policies and practices on an ongoing basis.

Communication and Language Assistance:
  5. Offer language assistance to individuals who have limited English proficiency and/or other communication needs, at no cost to them, to facilitate timely access to all health care and services.
  6. Inform all individuals of the availability of language assistance services clearly and in their preferred language, verbally and in writing.
  7. Ensure the competence of individuals providing language assistance, recognizing that the use of untrained individuals and/or minors as interpreters should be avoided.
  8. Provide easy-to-understand print and multimedia materials and signage in the languages commonly used by the populations in the service area.

Engagement, Continuous Improvement, and Accountability:
  9. Establish culturally and linguistically appropriate goals, policies, and management accountability, and infuse them throughout the organization's planning and operations.
 10. Conduct ongoing assessments of the organization's CLAS-related activities and integrate CLAS-related measures into measurement and continuous quality improvement activities.
 11. Collect and maintain accurate and reliable demographic data to monitor and evaluate the impact of CLAS on health equity and outcomes and to inform service delivery.
 12. Conduct regular assessments of community health assets and needs and use the results to plan and implement services that respond to the cultural and linguistic diversity of populations in the service area.
 13. Partner with the community to design, implement, and evaluate policies, practices, and services to ensure cultural and linguistic appropriateness.
 14. Create conflict and grievance resolution processes that are culturally and linguistically appropriate to identify, prevent, and resolve conflicts or complaints.
 15. Communicate the organization's progress in implementing and sustaining CLAS to all stakeholders, constituents, and the general public.

Source: Office of Minority Health. (2013). *National Standards for Culturally and Linguistically Appropriate Services in Health and Health Care: A Blueprint for Advancing and Sustaining CLAS Policy and Practice.* Retrieved from http://www.integration.samhsa.gov/Enhanced-CLASStandardsBlueprint.pdf.

improve quality, and help eliminate health care disparities by providing a blueprint for individuals and health and healthcare organizations to implement culturally and linguistically appropriate services (U.S. Department of Health and Human Services, Office of Minority Health, 2013, p. 9).

Guidelines for Implementing Culturally Competent Nursing Care.

A collaborative taskforce comprising members of the American Academy of Nursing (AAN) Expert panel on Global Nursing and Health and the Transcultural Nursing Society developed 10 guidelines for

TABLE 2.4. Guidelines for Implementing Culturally Competent Nursing Care.

Guideline	Description
1. Knowledge of Cultures	Nurses shall gain an understanding of the perspectives, traditions, values, practices, and family systems of culturally diverse individuals, families, communities, and populations they care for, as well as knowledge of the complex variables that affect the achievement of health and well being.
2. Education and Training in Culturally Competent Care	Nurses shall be educationally prepared to provide culturally congruent health care. Knowledge and skills necessary for assuring that nursing care is culturally congruent shall be included in global health care agendas that mandate formal education and clinical training, as well as required ongoing, continuing education for all practicing nurses.
3. Critical Reflection	Nurses shall engage in critical reflection of their own values, beliefs, and cultural heritage in order to have an awareness of how these qualities and issues can impact culturally congruent nursing care.
4. Cross-Cultural Communication	Nurses shall use culturally competent verbal and nonverbal communication skills to identify client's values, beliefs, practices, perceptions, and unique health care needs.
5. Culturally Competent Practice	Nurses shall utilize cross-cultural knowledge and culturally sensitive skills in implementing culturally congruent nursing care.
6. Cultural Competence in Health Care Systems and Organizations	Health care organizations should provide the structure and resources necessary to evaluate and meet the cultural and language needs of their diverse clients.
7. Patient Advocacy and Empowerment	Nurses shall recognize the effect of health care policies, delivery systems, and resources on their patient populations, and shall empower and advocate for their patients as indicated, Nurses shall advocate for the inclusion of their patient's cultural beliefs and practices in all dimensions of their health care.
8. Multicultural Workforce	Nurses shall actively engage in the effort to ensure a multicultural workforce in health care settings. One measure to achieve a multicultural workforce is through strengthening of recruitment and retention efforts in the hospitals, clinics, and academic settings.
9. Cross-Cultural Leadership	Nurses shall have the ability to influence individuals, groups, and systems to achieve outcomes of culturally competent care for diverse populations. Nurses shall have the knowledge and skills to work with public and private organizations, professional associations, and communities to establish policies and guidelines for comprehensive implementation and evaluation of culturally competent care.
10. Evidence-Based Practice and Research	Nurses shall base their practice on interventions that have been systematically tested and shown to be the most effective for the culturally diverse populations that they serve. In areas where there is a lack of evidence of efficacy, nurse researchers shall investigate and test interventions that may be the most effective in reducing the disparities in health outcomes.

Reproduced, with permission from Douglas, M. K., Rosenkoetter, M., Pacquiao, D. F., Callister, L. C., Hattar-Pollara, M., Lauderdale, J., . . . Purnell, L. (2014). Guidelines for implementing culturally competent nursing care. *Journal of Transcultural Nursing, 25*(2), 109-121. doi: 10.1177/1043659614520998.

implementing culturally competent nursing care in clinical practice, research, education, and administration (Douglas, et al., 2014). These guidelines (Refer to Table 2.4) were endorsed by the International Council of Nurses (ICN); the American Academy of Nursing (AAN) Expert Panel on Global Nursing and Health; the AAN Expert Panel on Cultural Competence; and the Transcultural Nursing Society (Douglas, et al., 2014). These guidelines were based on the principles of social justice and human rights and designed to be adapted into the sociocultural context and care settings in which they would be applied. Providing culturally competent care within a social justice framework, which involves integrating emic cultural beliefs into professional care and expanding healthcare access to vulnerable groups, serves to reduce health disparities and protect the dignity of the people.

■ SUMMARY

A number of very important and fundamental transcultural nursing concepts, definitions, and constructs have been presented in this chapter. Understanding the comparative nature of transcultural nursing and the essential value about why nurses need to know and understand the differences between generic (emic) and professional (etic) care were discussed. The fascinating and unique history of transcultural nursing with the many reasons the field needed to come into the discipline of nursing are crucial to understand. Specific transcultural nursing principles, standards, policy statements, and guidelines were also presented in chronological/historical order for nurses to use as guides toward attaining and maintaining culturally competent and responsible care practices worldwide. Understanding this content is essential for nurses and others so as to grasp the nature, scope, and important reasons why transcultural nursing was established and continues to be needed to facilitate the provision of culturally congruent care to diverse individuals, families, groups, communities, and institutions worldwide.

■ DISCUSSION QUESTIONS

1. Discuss examples from the media that have relevance to concepts and constructs presented in this chapter.

2. Discuss the relationships between the concepts of *stereotype*; *bias*; prejudice; *racism*; and *discrimination*.

3. Locate pictures that depict examples of some concepts presented in this chapter. Discuss how these pictures depict the chosen concepts and why.

4. In small groups, discuss how the standards or guidelines shared in this chapter could help nurses and others to improve clinical practice, education, research, consultation, and/or management.

5. Discuss the relationship between *culturally competent care* and *nursing ethics*.

■ REFERENCES

American Civil Liberties Union. (n.d.). *Racial profiling: Definition*. Retrieved from https://www.aclu.org/racial-profiling-definition

American Nurses' Association. (2015). *Code of ethics for nurses with interpretive statements*. Retrieved from http://nursingworld.org/MainMenuCategories/EthicsStandards/CodeofEthicsforNurses

Arieli, D., Mashiach, M., Hirschfeld, M., & Friedman, V. (2012). Cultural safety and nursing education in divided societies. *Nursing Education Perspectives*, 33(6), 364-368.

Berman, G., & Paradies, Y. (2008). Racism, disadvantage and multiculturalism: Towards effective anti-racist praxis. *Ethnic and Racial Studies* (pp. 1-19). doi: 10.1080/01419870802302272. Retrieved from http://bmw.curtin.edu.au/pubs/2009/Berman_etal_2008.pdf

Board of Trustees of the Transcultural Nursing Society. (1998). Policy statements to guide transcultural nursing standards and practices. *Journal of Transcultural Nursing*, 9(2), 75-77. doi: 10.1177/104365969800900214

Bonilla-Silva, E. (1997). Rethinking racism: Toward a structural interpretation. *American Sociological Review*, 62(3), 465-480.

Douglas, M. K., Pierce, J. U., Rosenkoetter, M., Callister, L. C., Hattar-Pollara, M., Lauderdale, J., . . . Pacquiao, D. (2009). Standards of practice for culturally competent nursing care: A request for comments. *Journal of Transcultural Nursing*, 20(3), 257-269.

Douglas, M. K., Pierce, J. U., Rosenkoetter, M., Pacquiao, D., Callister, L. C., Hattar-Pollara, M., . . . Purnell, L. (2011). Standards of practice for culturally competent nursing care: 2011 update. *Journal of Transcultural Nursing*, 22(4), 317-333. doi: 10.1177/1043659611412965

Douglas, M. K., Rosenkoetter, M., Pacquiao, D. F., Callister, L. C., Hattar-Pollara, M., Lauderdale, J., . . . Purnell, L. (2014). Guidelines for implementing culturally competent nursing care. *Journal of Transcultural Nursing*, 25(2), 109-121. doi: 10.1177/1043659614520998

Ehrmin, J. T., (2016). Transcultural Perspectives in Mental Health Nursing. In Andrews, M. & Boyle, J. (Eds.), *TransConcepts in Nursing Care*, (pp. 272-316). Philadelphia, PA: Wolters Kluwer.

Essed, P. (1990). *Everyday Racism: Reports from women of two cultures*. Alameda, CA: Hunter House.

Gaut, D., & Leininger, M. M. (1991). *Caring: The compassionate healer*. New York, NY: New York Press.

Haviland, W. (1993). *Cultural Anthropology* (7th ed.). Orlando, FL: Harcourt Brace Jovanovich College Publishers.

International Council of Nurses. (2012). *The ICN code of ethics for nurses*. Retrieved from http://www.integration.samhsa.gov/EnhancedCLASStandardsBlueprint.pdf

Kottak, P. (1991). *Anthropology: The exploration of human diversity*. New York, NY: McGraw-Hill Inc.

Leininger, M. M. (1966). *Convergence and divergence of human behavior: An ethnopsychological comparative study of two Gadsup villages in the Eastern Highlands of New Guinea* [Unpublished doctoral dissertation]. University of Washington, Seattle.

Leininger, M. M. (1970). *Nursing and anthropology: Two worlds to blend*. New York, NY: John Wiley & Sons.

Leininger, M. M. (1978a). Transcultural nursing: A New and Scientific Subfield of Study in Nursing. In M. M. Leininger (Ed.), *Transcultural nursing: Concepts, theories and practices* (pp. 8-12). New York, NY: John Wiley & Sons.

Leininger, M. M. (1978b). *Transcultural nursing: Concepts, theories, and practices*. New York, NY: John Wiley & Sons.

Leininger, M. M. (1980). Care: A central focus of nursing and health care services. *Nursing and Health Care*, 1(3), 135-143.

Leininger, M. M. (1981). *Caring: An essential human need*. Thorofare, NJ: Slack.

Leininger, M. M. (1988a). *Care discovery and uses in clinical and community nursing*. Detroit, MI: Wayne State Press.

Leininger, M. M. (1988b). *Care: The essence of nursing and health*. Detroit, MI: Wayne State University Press.

Leininger, M. M. (1990a). *Care: The essence of nursing and health*. Detroit, MI: Wayne State University Press.

Leininger, M. M. (1990b). *Ethical and moral dimensions of care*. Detroit, MI: Wayne State University Press.

Leininger, M. M. M. (1990c). The significance of cultural concepts in nursing. *Journal of Transcultural Nursing*, (2)1, 52-59.

Leininger, M. M. (1991a). Becoming aware of types of health practitioners and cultural impositions. *Journal of Transcultural Nursing*, 2(2), 32-39.

Leininger, M. M. (1991b). *Caring: An essential human need*. Detroit, MI: Wayne State University Press.

Leininger, M. M. (1991c). *Culture care diversity and universality: A theory of nursing*. New York, NY: National League for Nursing Press.

Leininger, M. M. (1994). *Transcultural nursing: Concepts, theories, and practices*. Columbus, OH: Greyden Press.

Leininger, M. M. (1995). *Transcultural nursing: Concepts, theories, research, and practice*. Blacklick, OH: McGraw-Hill College Custom Series.

Leininger, M. M. (1997). Understanding cultural pain for improved health care. *Journal of Transcultural Nursing*, 9(1), 32-35.

Leininger, M. M. (1998). Special research report: Dominant cultural care (emic) meanings and practice findings from Leininger's theory. *Journal of Transcultural Nursing*, 9(2), 45-49.

Leininger, M. M. (2002). Essential transcultural nursing care concepts, principles, examples, and policy statements. In M. M. Leininger and M. R. McFarland (Eds.), *Transcultural nursing: Concepts, theories, research, & practice* (3rd ed., pp. 45-70). New York, NY: McGraw-Hill.

Leininger, M. (2002a). Culture care assessments for congruent competency practices. In M. Leininger, and M. McFarland (Eds.), *Transcultural nursing concepts, theories, research, and practice* (pp.117-144). New York, NY: McGraw-Hill.

Leininger, M. M., & Wehbe-Alamah, H. B. (2015). Leininger's father protective care. In M. R. McFarland and H. B. Wehbe-Alamah (Eds.), *Culture care diversity and universality: A worldwide nursing theory* (3rd ed., pp. 119-136). Burlingame, MA: Jones and Bartlett Learning.

McFarland, M. R., & Wehbe-Alamah, H. B. (2015). Culture care diversity and universality theory. In McFarland, M. R. and Wehbe-Alamah, H. B. (Eds.), *Culture care diversity and universality theory and ethnonursing research method* (pp. 1-34). Burlingame, MA: Jones and Bartlett Learning.

Miller, J. E., Leininger, M., Leuning, C., Pacquiao, D., Andrews, M., Ludwig-Beymer, P., & Papadopoulos, I. (2008). Transcultural nursing society position statement on human rights. *Journal of Transcultural Nursing*, 19(1), 5-7. doi: 10.1177/1043659607309147

Nursing Council of New Zealand. (2011). *Guidelines for cultural safety: The treaty of Waitangi and Maori health in nursing education and practice*. Wellington, New Zealand: New Zealand Psychologists' Board. Retrieved from www.nursingcouncil.org.nz/.../Guidelines%20for%20 cultural%20safety

Policy. (n.d.). *Merriam-Webster.com*. Retrieved from http://www.merriam-webster.com/dictionary/policy

Racism. (n.d.). *Merriam-Webster.com*. Retrieved from http:// www.merriam-webster.com/dictionary/racism

Sullivan, S. (2011). On bioculturalism, shamanism, and unlearning the creed of growth. *Geography and You*, *11*(65), 15-19. Retrieved from https://siansullivan.files. wordpress.com/2011/04/3_sullivan.pdf

Thomas, J. M. (2014). Medicalizing racism. *Contexts*, *13*(4), 24-29. doi: 10.1177/1536504214558213

U.S. Department of Health and Human Services, Office of Minority Health. (2013). *National standards for culturally and linguistically appropriate services in health and health care: A blueprint for advancing and sustaining CLAS policy and practice*. Retrieved from http://www.integration. samhsa.gov/EnhancedCLASStandardsBlueprint.pdf

U.S. Office of Personnel Management. (2014). *The guide to data standards part A: Human resources*. Retrieved from http://www.opm.gov/policy-data-oversight/data-analysis-documentation/data-policy-guidance/reportingguidance/part-a-human-resources.pdf

Wehbe-Alamah, H. (2015). Folk care beliefs and practices of traditional Lebanese and Syrian Muslims in the Midwestern United States. In McFarland, M. R. and Wehbe-Alamah, H. B. (Eds.), *Culture care diversity and universality theory and ethnonursing research method* (3rd ed., pp. 137-182). Burlingame, MA: Jones and Bartlett Learning.

Wenger, A. F. (1991). The culture care theory and Old Order Amish. In M. M. Leininger (Ed.), *Culture care diversity and universality: A theory of nursing* (pp. 147-178). New York, NY: National League for Nursing Press.

The Theory of Culture Care Diversity and Universality

Marilyn R. McFarland

> "*The goal of the theory…is to provide culturally congruent care that would contribute to the health or wellbeing of people or to help them face disabilities, dying, or death*" *(Leininger, 2002d, p. 76).*
>
> "*The theory with its focus on care and culture [was] held by Leininger as the heart and soul of nursing and essential for developing new transcultural nursing knowledge and practices and to move nursing into a predicted multicultural and global world*" *(Leininger, 2006a, p. 7).*

■ ETHNOHISTORY OF THE THEORY

Leininger's first book, *Nursing and Anthropology: Two Worlds to Blend* (1970), laid the foundation for her creation of the Theory of Culture Care Diversity and Universality (known as the Culture Care Theory or CCT) and the subsequent integration of culturally-based care into the healthcare system as well as the evolutionary development of the field of transcultural nursing. Her next book, *Transcultural Nursing: Concepts, Theories, and Practice* (1978), identified major concepts, theoretical ideas, and practices in transcultural nursing and was the first definitive publication to describe transcultural nursing. During the next 60 years Leininger established, explicated, and used the Culture Care Theory to study many cultures across the United States and worldwide. She developed the Ethnonursing Research Method to fit and be used with the theory and to qualitatively discover insider or emic views about the care beliefs, views, and practices of diverse cultural groups (Leininger, 1991b, 2002d, 2006d; Wehbe-Alamah & McFarland, 2015b). The

Ethnonursing Research Method was the first qualitative research method designed for nurse researchers to study and discover culture care phenomena (Leininger, 1978, 1985, 1991b, 1995b, 2002d, 2006d; Wehbe-Alamah & McFarland, 2015b).

In 1981, Leininger was recruited by Wayne State University in Detroit and was appointed Professor of Nursing and Adjunct Professor of Anthropology and Director of Transcultural Nursing Offerings, where she remained until her semi-retirement in 1995. In 1989, Leininger launched the *Journal of Transcultural Nursing*, serving as its first editor until her retirement. While at Wayne State, she developed several courses and seminars in transcultural nursing, caring constructs, and qualitative research methods for baccalaureate, master's, doctoral, and postdoctoral nursing and non-nursing students. During her years at Wayne, she taught and mentored many students and nurses in transcultural nursing research guided by the Culture Care Theory using the Ethnonursing Research Method. She continued teaching and consulting about transcultural nursing and the Culture Care Theory at various universities across the United States and worldwide throughout her retirement.

Leininger wrote or edited more than 30 books during her lifetime; among the most significant were those that explicated her theory and the ethnonursing method more fully and focused on the discipline of transcultural nursing. They included *Nursing and Anthropology: Two Worlds to Blend* (1970); *Transcultural Nursing: Concepts, Theories, and Practice* (1978); *Culture Care Diversity and Universality: A Theory of Nursing* (1991a); *Transcultural Nursing: Concepts, Theories, Research, and Practice* (Leininger & McFarland, 2002); and *Culture Care Diversity and Universality: A Worldwide Theory of Nursing* (Leininger & McFarland, 2006). In 2012, Dr. Leininger charged Dr. Marilyn McFarland and Dr. Hiba Wehbe-Alamah to carry on her work with the Culture Care Theory, and the ethnonursing method, and in transcultural nursing. Dr. Leininger remained an active contributor to works bearing her name until her death in August 2012. In 2015, the third edition of *Leininger's Culture Care Diversity and Universality: A Worldwide Nursing Theory* by McFarland and Wehbe-Alamah included two chapters that Dr. Leininger had written before her death.

■ PURPOSE AND GOAL OF THE THEORY

The purpose of the Theory of Culture Care Diversity and Universality is to discover, document, know, and explain the interdependence of care and culture phenomena with differences and similarities between and among cultures (McFarland & Wehbe-Alamah, 2015b, pp. 5-6). Using the ethnonursing research method with the CCT, the researcher is challenged to discover the similarities and diversities about human care among cultures. The theory was predicted to help guide the nurse researcher to discover new meanings, patterns, expressions, and practices related to culture care that have influenced the health and wellbeing of individuals, families, and cultural groups. In the discovery process, both similarities (commonalities) and diversities (differences) can be identified as culture-specific modalities to provide as culturally congruent care related to the desired goal of health or wellbeing (Wehbe-Alamah & McFarland, 2015b, p. 39).

The goal of the theory is to provide culturally congruent care that contributes to the health and wellbeing of people or to help them face disabilities, dying, or death using the three modes of culture care decisions and actions. Ultimately, the goal is to establish a body of transcultural nursing knowledge for current best care practices for future generations of nurses in a global world. Such knowledge is essential for current and future professional nursing care practice as well as for use by other healthcare providers. This body of knowledge continues to change and transform nursing and health care with benefits to people from similar and diverse cultures (McFarland & Wehbe-Alamah, 2015b). The theory has guided nurses and other healthcare providers toward explicating care meanings so that culture care values, beliefs, and lifeways can serve as accurate and reliable bases for co-participatively making culture-specific care decisions and actions as well as to identify universal or common features about care (Leininger, 1994; McFarland & Wehbe-Alamah, 2015a). The theory states that nurses cannot separate worldviews, social structure factors, and cultural beliefs or practices (lay/folk/generic and professional) from health, wellness, illness, or care when working with cultures because these factors are closely linked and interrelated (Leininger, 1994; McFarland & Wehbe-Alamah, 2015a). Social structure factors such as religion, politics, culture, economics, and kinship are significant forces affecting care and influencing illness patterns and wellbeing (Leininger, 2006a, pp. 17-18). The theorist and others have long believed that discovering all forms of generic care beliefs, values, and expressions held by cultures and combining them with professional care practices to be of essential importance for the provision of culturally congruent care (Leininger, 1991a, 1995b; Leininger & McFarland, 2002, 2006; McFarland & Wehbe-Alamah, 2015a). Ethnonursing studies that have supported this premise include Gunn and Davis (2011); Lee (2012); Liang (2002); Mixer, McFarland, Andrews, and Strang (2013); Morris (2012); Moss (2014); Outwater, Tarimo, Miller, and Campbell (2012); Schumacher (2010); Strang and Mixer (2015); Wanchi, Armer, and Stewart (2015); and Wolf et al. (2014).

■ TENETS OF THE THEORY

Tenets are the positions held or the givens set forth by the theorist for use with a theory. In developing the Culture Care Theory, the following four major tenets were conceptualized and formulated by Leininger:

- Culture care expressions, meanings, patterns, and practices are diverse and yet there are shared commonalities and some universal attributes;

- Worldview, multiple social structure factors, ethnohistory, environmental context, language, and generic and professional care are critical influencers of culture care patterns to predict health, wellbeing, illness, healing, and ways people face disabilities and death;
- Generic emic [folk] and etic [professional] health factors in different environmental contexts greatly influence health and illness outcomes; and
- From an analysis of the above influencers, three major decision and action modes [culture care preservation and/or maintenance; culture care accommodation and/or negotiation; and culture care repatterning and/or restructuring] were predicted to provide ways to provide culturally congruent, safe, and meaningful health care to cultures. (McFarland & Wehbe-Alamah, 2015b)

In conceptualizing the theory, a major and central theoretical tenet was "…care diversities (differences) and universalities (commonalities) existed among and between cultures in the world" (Leininger, 2002d, p. 78). However, Leininger asserted that culture care meanings and uses first had to be *discovered* so as to establish a body of transcultural knowledge. Transcultural nurses conducting ethnonursing research guided by the CCT have discovered care diversities and universalities in both care themes and care patterns in their study findings. However, more *universal* than *diverse* care themes and patterns have been discovered and reported. Leininger commented that care diversities may be more covert and embedded in informant data/descriptors than are universalities (M. M. Leininger, personal communication, January-August, 2012). Studies with universal as well as diverse findings include McFarland and Zehnder's (2006) study about German-American elders; Mixer's (2011) study about nursing faculty teaching culture care; Embler, Mixer, and Gunther's work (2015) about end-of-life care with the Yup'ik people of Alaska; and Morris' (2015) book chapter about the subculture of urban African American adolescent gangs.

A second major theoretical tenet was that the "…worldview; social structure factors such as religion, economics, education, technology, politics, kinship (social), ethnohistory, environment, language; and generic care and professional care factors would greatly influence culture care meanings, expressions, and patterns in different cultures" (Leininger, 2002d, p. 78). Leininger (2002d) maintained that knowing the cultural and social structure factors [of a particular culture or group] was necessary in order to provide meaningful and satisfying care to people, and predicted they would be powerful influencers on culturally-based care (p. 78). She stated these factors also needed to be discovered directly from cultural informants to confirm them as being influencing factors related to health, wellbeing, illness, and death.

A third major theoretical tenet was "…both generic (emic or the insider's view) and professional (etic) health factors in diverse environmental contexts greatly influence health and illness outcomes" (McFarland & Wehbe-Alamah, 2015b, p. 7), and that these "…need to be taught, researched, and brought together into care practices for satisfying care for clients, which leads to their health and wellbeing" (Leininger, 2002d, 2006a). This tenet was added by Leininger in 2006a based on supporting data from published studies about resident care in a culturally-focused nursing home (McFarland & Zehnder, 2006) as well as other community settings (Leuning, Small, & van Dyk, 2002) and was later supported by additional studies (Strang & Mixer, 2015).

A fourth major theoretical tenet was the conceptualization of the three major culture care modes of decisions and actions [previously stated] to arrive at culturally congruent care for the general health and wellbeing of clients, or to help them face death or disabilities (Leininger & McFarland, 2002, 2006; McFarland & Wehbe-Alamah, 2015a). These decision and action modes were predicted to be *key* for the provision of culturally congruent, meaningful, and acceptable care and beneficial outcomes. When using the modes, individuals, families, groups, communities, or institutions are assessed and responded to in dynamic and participatory nurse-client relationships (Eipperle, 2015). These social structure factors need to be studied, assessed, and responded to in a dynamic and co-participatory nurse-client relationship. The researcher or clinician then draws upon findings from the social structure factors; generic care and professional practices; and other influences to develop individualized approaches in the plan of care using the three culture care modes with the care recipients/clients to provide culturally-based and culturally congruent care for the individual, family, or group (Eipperle, 2015; Leininger, 1991a; Leininger & McFarland, 2002, 2006; McFarland & Wehbe-Alamah, 2015a).

■ ASSUMPTIVE PREMISES OF THE THEORY

The major theoretical tenets of the theory led to the formulation of specific theoretical hunches or assumptions that a researcher could use with diverse cultural groups in different geographical locations. Major assumptions of The Theory of Culture Care Diversity and Universality presented here were derived from Leininger's definitive works on the theory and subsequent evolving changes that were discovered and/or confirmed by her and other researchers. For example, in her 2011 study, Mixer used five assumptive premises from the CCT to guide her research with faculty teaching transcultural nursing in the southeastern United States. Strang and Mixer (2015) stated five assumptions from the Culture Care Theory to guide a study of Malaria care among the Maasai of southern Kenya. These researchers reported that the assumptive premises derived from the CCT were supported by discoveries from both studies, which contributed the building of nursing theory (Mixer, 2011; Strang & Mixer, 2015). These findings also supported Leininger's statement (based on the 5th assumptive premise) that the universality of care reflects the common nature of human beings and humanity, whereas the diversity of care reflects the discovered variability and unique features of human beings. The assumptive premises of the CCT are:

- Care is the essence and central dominant, distinct, and unifying focus of nursing
- Humanistic and scientific care is essential for human growth, wellbeing, health, survival, and to face dying, death, and disabilities;
- Care (caring) is essential to curing or healing for there can be no curing without caring (this assumption was held to have profound relevance worldwide);
- Culture care is the synthesis of two major constructs [culture and care] that guide the researcher to discover, explain, and account for health, wellbeing, care expressions, and other human conditions;
- Culture care expressions, meanings, patterns, processes, and structural forms are diverse but some commonalities (universalities) exist among and between cultures;
- Culture care values, beliefs, and practices are influenced by and embedded in the worldview, social structure factors (e.g., [spirituality] religion,

philosophy of life, kinship, politics, economics, education, technology, biological factors [new revision/addition], and cultural values) and the ethnohistorical and environmental contexts;
- Every culture has generic [lay, folk, naturalistic; mainly emic] and usually some professional [etic] care to be discovered and used for culturally congruent care practices;
- Culturally congruent and therapeutic care occurs when culture care values, beliefs, expressions, and patterns are explicitly known and used appropriately, sensitively, and meaningfully with people of diverse or similar cultures;
- Leininger's three theoretical modes of care offer new, creative, and different therapeutic ways to help people of diverse cultures;
- The Ethnonursing Research Method and other qualitative research paradigmatic methods offer important means to discover largely embedded, covert, epistemic, and ontological culture care knowledge and practices; and,
- Transcultural nursing is a discipline with a body of knowledge and practices to attain and maintain the goal of culturally congruent care for health and wellbeing. (McFarland & Wehbe-Alamah, 2015b, pp. 8-9)

■ CENTRAL CONSTRUCTS OF THE CULTURE CARE THEORY

For several decades, transcultural nursing has been defined as *a discipline of study and practice focused on comparative culture care differences and similarities among and between cultures in order to assist human beings to attain and maintain meaningful and therapeutic healthcare practices that are culturally-based* (Leininger, 1991b, 2002d, 2006a; McFarland & Wehbe-Alamah, 2015b). Transcultural nursing researchers continue to identify and use comparative care discoveries, practices, and guidelines to help human beings in beneficial ways by delivering culturally congruent care to similar and increasingly diverse and vulnerable populations (Douglas et al., 2014).

Several central constructs used in the Culture Care Theory have been described and defined in numerous ethnonursing studies (Leininger, 1991a, 1995b; Leininger & McFarland, 2002, 2006; McFarland & Wehbe-Alamah, 2015b). These constructs were adapted in several ethnonursing research studies, which were subsequently published, including Farrell (2006); McFarland and Zehnder (2006); Mixer (2011); Schumacher (2010); Strang and Mixer (2015); and Wolf et al. (2014). The theory definitions are orientational and not operational as in quantitative studies. The orientational definitions were adapted from the theory definitions in order for the researchers to be open to discovering new dimensions of the theory constructs and to encourage discovery of new qualitative knowledge from cultural groups. This is a major difference between the Culture Care Theory and other nursing theories that have pre-determined definitions that usually reflect the researchers' interests or viewpoints.

Care

Care refers to both an abstract and/or a concrete phenomenon. Leininger defined *care* as those *assistive, supportive, and enabling experiences or ideas toward others* (Leininger, 1995a, 2002d, 2006a; McFarland & Wehbe-Alamah, 2015b). *Caring* refers to *actions, attitudes, and practices to assist or help others toward healing and wellbeing* (Leininger, 1995a, 2002d, 2006a; McFarland & Wehbe-Alamah, 2015b).

Care as a major construct of the theory includes both *folk care* and *professional care* and has been predicted and supported to influence and explain the health or wellbeing for similar and diverse cultures (Leininger, 1978). Based on the current research findings, care is a largely embedded and invisible phenomenon often taken for granted that is sometimes challenging for nurses to quickly identify or understand with in-depth meaning (Leininger, 1991b, 2002c, 2002d, 2006a; McFarland & Wehbe-Alamah, 2015b). However, over the past six decades many books, articles, and research studies have become accessible to nurses, enabling them to discover and know different care meanings from both similar and diverse cultures. Some relevant study exemplars include Farrell (2006); Gunn and Davis (2011); Leininger (2002c, 2006b); McFarland (2002a); Mixer (2011); Moss (2014); Strang and Mixer (2015); Wehbe-Alamah (2011, 2015); and Wolf et al. (2014).

Care has cultural and symbolic meanings such as *care as protection* (Leininger, 2002c, 2006b, 2015a); *care as respect* (Morris, 2012); and *care as presence* (Leininger as cited by McFarland, 2002b, p. 111 [Table 3.7]; Leininger, 2006c, p. 289). These care linkages are essential for the provision of culture-specific care and are often also gender linked.

Many research studies have discovered transcultural care meanings within and between cultures (Refer to Table 3.1). Most of these studies were conducted by doctorally-prepared transcultural nurse researchers who teased out covert and in-depth care meanings in scientific and authentic ways for clinical care practices. The updated Table 3.1 lists care constructs discovered and supported in numerous studies guided by the Culture Care Theory from 1960 to 2016. Among these newer constructs are *collaborative care* (McFarland & Leininger, 2011; M. M. Leininger, personal communication, October 20-22, 2011); *collective care* (McFarland & Zehnder, 2006); *father protective care* (Leininger, 2015a); *mentoring and co-mentoring* (Mixer, 2011); and *herbs as care, community as care,* and *praying to/for* (Strang & Mixer, 2015).

In addition, some researchers identified and confirmed culture care constructs in their studies that had been discovered in earlier ethnonursing research guided by the CCT. In her doctoral study about faculty teaching culture care, Mixer (2011) supported six care constructs previously discovered by Leininger and others; these were *respect*; *praying with*; *listening*; *collective care*; *reciprocal care*; and *surveillance care*. Strang and Mixer (2015) also reported confirmation for the formerly discovered care constructs of *respect for/about lifeways*; *acceptance*; *purging*; and *interest in and about*.

Culture

Culture is another major construct central to the Theory of *Culture* Care Diversity and Universality. Leininger (1991b, 2002d, 2006a) defined culture as the *learned, shared, and transmitted values, beliefs, norms, and lifeways of a particular culture that guide thinking, decisions, and actions in patterned ways*. From an anthropological perspective, culture is usually viewed as *the broadest and most comprehensive means to know, explain, and predict people's lifeways over time and in different geographic locations*. Moreover, culture is more than social interaction and symbols. Culture can be viewed as the blueprint for guiding human actions and decisions and includes material and nonmaterial features of any group or individual. It has been a major construct in anthropology for nearly a century. Culture is more than ethnicity or social relationships. Cultural phenomena distinguish human beings from nonhumans (Leininger as cited by McFarland & Wehbe-Alamah, 2015b, p. 10).

TABLE 3.1. Care/Caring Constructs.

1	Acceptance		51	Dependence
2	Accommodating		52	Direct help to others
3	Accountability		53	Discernment
4	Action (ing) for/about/with		54	Doing for/with
5	Adapting to		55	Eating right foods
6	Affection for		56	Enduring
7	Alleviation (pain/suffering)		57	Embodiment
8	Anticipation (ing)		58	Emotional support
9	Assist (ing) others		59	Empathy
10	Attention to/toward		60	Enabling
11	Attitude toward		61	Engrossment in/about
12	Being nonassertive		62	Establishing harmony
13	Being authentic (real)		63	Experiencing with
14	Being aware of others		64	Expressing feelings
15	Being clean		65	***Faith (in God)****
16	Being genuine		66	Faith (in others)
17	Being involved		67	Family involvement
18	Being kind/pleasant		68	Family support
19	***Being listened to**		69	**Father protective care****
20	Being orderly		70	Feeling for/about
21	Being present		71	Filial love
22	Being watchful		72	Generosity toward others
23	Bribing		73	Gentle (ness) & firmness
24	Care (caring)		74	Giving to others in need
25	*Caritas* (charity)		75	Giving comfort to
26	Cleanliness		76	Group assistance
27	Closeness to		77	Group awareness
28	Cognitively knowing		78	Growth promoting
29	Collaborative care**		79	Hands on
30	**Collective care****		80	Harmony with
31	Comfort (ing)		81	Healing
32	Commitment to/for		82	Health instruction
33	Communication (ing)		83	Health (wellbeing)
34	Community awareness		84	Honor (ing)
35	***Community as care**		85	Hope (fullness)
36	Compassion (ate)		86	Hospitality
37	Compliance with		87	Improving conditions
38	***Concern for**/about/with		88	Inclined toward
39	Congruence with		89	Indulgence from
40	Connectedness		90	Instruction (ing)
41	Consideration of		91	Integrity
42	Consultation (ing)		92	Interest in/about
43	Controlling		93	Intimacy/intimate
44	Communion with another		94	Involvement with/for
45	Cooperation		95	Kindness (being kind)
46	Coordination (ing)		96	Knowing of culture
47	Coping with/for		97	Knowing (another's reality)
48	Creative thinking/acts		98	Know cultural values/taboos
49	Culture care (ing)		99	**Language as protective care****
50	Cure (ing)		100	Limiting (set limits)
			101	Listening to/about

TABLE 3.1. Care/Caring Constructs.

102	***Love (kinship)**	145	Responding appropriately
103	Loving (love others)—Christian love	146	Responding to context
104	Maintaining harmony	147	Responsible for others
105	Maintaining privacy	148	Restoration (ing)
106	Maintaining reciprocity	149	Sacrificing
107	***Malaria**	150	Saving face
108	**Mentoring/co-mentoring****	151	Self-reliance (reliance)
109	Ministering to others—filial love	152	Self-responsibility
110	Need fulfillment	153	Sensitivity to others needs
111	Noncaring	154	Serving others (*caritas*)
112	Nurturance (nurture)	155	Sharing with others
113	Obedience to	156	Silence (use of)
114	Obligation to	157	Speaking the language
115	Orderliness	158	Spiritual healing
116	Other-care (ing)/non self-care	159	Spiritual relatedness
117	Patience	160	Stimulation (ing)
118	Performing rituals	161	Stress alleviation
119	Permitting expressions	162	Succorance
120	Personalized acts	163	Suffering with/for
121	Physical acts	164	Support (ing)
122	Praying with	165	Surveillance (watch for)
123	Presence (being with)	166	Symbols (ing)
124	Preserving (preservation)	167	Sympathy
125	Prevention (ing)	168	Taking care of environment
126	Promoting	169	Technical skills
127	Promoting independence	170	Techniques
128	***Praying to/for**	171	Tenderness
129	**Protective care**/protecting (other/self)**	172	Timing actions/decisions
130	Purging	173	Touch (ing)
131	Quietness	174	***Trust (Confidentiality)**
132	Reassurance	175	***Unconditional giving for the purpose of recovery from illness and wellbeing**
133	Receiving		
134	Reciprocity	176	Understanding
135	Reflecting goodness	177	Use of folk foods/practices
136	Reflecting with/about	178	Use of limit setting
137	Rehabilitate	179	Using nursing knowledge
138	Regard for	180	Valuing another's ways
139	Relatedness to	181	Watchfulness
140	Respect	182	Wellbeing (health)
141	Respect for/about lifeways	183	Wellbeing (family)
142	Respecting	184	Wholeness approach
143	Respecting privacy/wishes	185	**Worthiness****
144	Respecting sex differences		

* Indicates new constructs with current publication of table.
** Indicates new care constructs described in 2015 (Jones & Bartlett) publication of table.

Adapted and revised, with permission, from: McFarland, M. R., & Wehbe-Alamah, H. B. (2015). The theory of culture care diversity and universality. In M. R. McFarland and H. B. Wehbe-Alamah (Eds.), *Leininger's Culture Care Diversity and Universality: A Worldwide Nursing Theory* (3rd ed., pp. 11-13). Burlington, MA: Jones & Bartlett Learning. www.jblearning.com.

Culture Care

Transculturally-prepared nurses are advancing culture care knowledge in many ways by uniting culture and care together conceptually and for research purposes. This approach in nursing is encouraging. The powerfulness of the *culture care* dual construct to discover and understand illness, wellness, and other human health expressions remains an important focus in transcultural nursing. The theorist held that culture care phenomena conceived and linked together have great power to explain health and/or illness. Leininger (1978) conceptualized culture care as synthesized and closely linked phenomena with interrelated ideas. Both culture and care require rigorous and full study with attention to their embedded and constituted relationship to each other as human care phenomena (McFarland & Wehbe-Alamah, 2015b).

Emic and Etic

The constructs *emic* and *etic* care are also major parts of the Culture Care Theory. Leininger (1978, 1991b, 2002d, 2006a) wanted to identify differences and similarities among and between cultures and to differentiate the client's insider knowledge, in contrast with the researcher's outsider or professional knowledge. She also believed it was desirable to know what was universal [or common] and what was different [or diverse] among cultures with respect to care. The term *emic* refers to the local, indigenous, or insider's cultural knowledge and view of specific phenomena; *etic* refers to the outsiders' or stranger's—and often health professional's—views and the institutional knowledge about culture care phenomena (Leininger, 1991b, 2002d, 2006a; McFarland & Wehbe-Alamah, 2015b).

The terms *emic* and *etic* were derived from linguistics but were reconceptualized by Leininger (1978) within her theoretical perspectives to discover contrasting culture care phenomena. These two dual constructs, emic and etic, have been invaluable in explicating the differences and similarities among cultural informants' and professional nurses' knowledge and practices over the past several decades (Leininger, 1991b, 2002d, 2006a; Morris, 2012).

In transcultural nursing, emic and etic—when coupled with generic and professional care—are formally defined as:

- **Generic (emic) care** refers to the learned and transmitted lay, indigenous, traditional, or local folk (emic) knowledge and practices that are assistive, supportive, enabling, and facilitative acts for or toward others with evident or anticipated health needs in order to improve wellbeing or to help with dying or other human conditions (Leininger, 2002d, 2006a; McFarland & Wehbe-Alamah, 2015b).
- **Professional (etic) care** refers to formal and explicit cognitively learned professional care knowledge and practices obtained generally through educational institutions. These constructs are taught to nurses and other healthcare professionals so as to enable them to provide assistive, supportive, enabling, or facilitative acts for or to another individual or group in order to improve their health, prevent illnesses, or to help with dying or other human conditions (Leininger, 2002d, 2006a; McFarland & Wehbe-Alamah, 2015b).

The construct of *Integrative Care* is a recently added central construct of the CCT that emerged through further development and evolution of Leininger's earlier work (Leininger, 2002e; M. M. Leininger and H. B. Wehbe-Alamah, personal communications, October 20-22, 2011). This new central construct blends professional care and generic care and replaces *Nursing Care Practices* as the linking construct between *Generic* (folk) and *Professional Care-Cure Practices* in recognition of the integrative nature of culturally congruent care that transculturally-prepared nurses currently provide. This evolutionary change is now reflected in the revised 2016 Sunrise Enabler (Refer to Figure 3.1 and Color Insert 1).

In 2002e, Leininger discussed the construct of *integrative care* as the desired outcome of generic and professional care when appropriately and meaningfully used in therapeutic practices. She defined *integrative care* to refer to *safe, congruent, and creative ways of blending together holistic, generic, and professional care knowledge and practices so that the client experiences beneficial outcomes for wellbeing or to ameliorate a human condition or lifeway* (pp. 148-149).

Culturally Congruent Care

Culturally congruent care refers to *culturally-based care knowledge, acts, and decisions used in sensitive and knowledgeable ways to appropriately and meaningfully fit the cultural values, beliefs, and lifeways of clients for their health and wellbeing, or to prevent illness, disabilities, or death* (Leininger, 2006a). To provide culturally congruent care has been the major goal of the Culture Care Theory (Schumacher, 2010).

Leininger's Sunrise Enabler to Discover Culture Care
CULTURE CARE

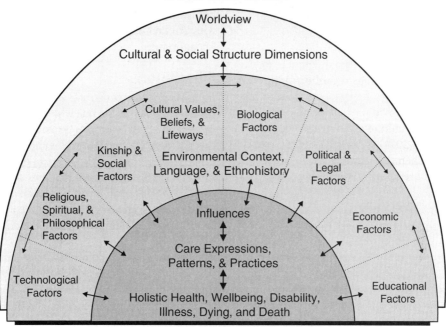

Focus: **Individuals, Families, Groups, Communities, or Institutions**
in Diverse Health Contexts of

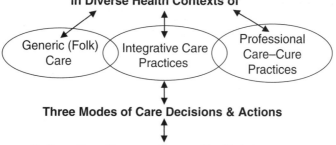

Three Modes of Care Decisions & Actions

Culture Care Preservation and/or Maintenance
Culture Care Accommodation and/or Negotiation
Culture Care Repatterning and/or Restructuring

Code: ←→ (Influencers)   © M. R. McFarland &
                                  H. B. Wehbe-Alamah (2018)

Culturally Congruent Care for Holistic Health, Wellbeing, Disability,
Illness, Dying, and Death

FIGURE 3.1 • Leininger's Sunrise Enabler to Discover Culture Care.
Used with permission. McFarland, M. R., & Wehbe-Alamah, H. B. (2018).

Strang and Mixer (2015) found that the Maasai voiced preferences for culturally congruent care that included education about professional malaria care to be combined with generic or traditional care that was safe and offered in a respectful manner. Lee (2012) alluded to *safe and respectful care* as culturally congruent care when she described the challenges mothers faced when providing care for their children within the context of family homelessness. She advocated for nurses to influence policies for safe and affordable housing for those persons who are homeless. Morris (2012) also discussed the concept of safety in the context of culturally congruent care among African American adolescent gang members within and for their community.

Culture Care Diversity

Culture care diversity refers to the differences or variabilities among human beings regarding culture care meanings, patterns, values, lifeways, symbols, or other features related to providing beneficial care to clients of a designated culture (Leininger, 2002d, 2006a, 2015a). Wolf et al. (2014) identified gender based differences in care when they studied the culture care of Somali immigrant refugees in Minnesota

Culture Care Universality

Culture care universality refers to the commonly shared or similar culture care phenomena features of individuals or groups with recurrent meanings, patterns, values, lifeways, or symbols that serve as a guide for caregivers to provide assistive, supportive, facilitative, or enabling people care for healthy outcomes (Leininger, 2006a, 2015b).

Another major theoretical tenet of the CCT states that *culture care expressions, meanings, and practices are **diverse yet also have shared commonalities** between and among cultures* (McFarland & Wehbe-Alamah, 2015b). Leininger further explained that many researchers have only reported on discovered care findings that are *common or universal* but have reported less often about those that are *diverse* (M. M. Leininger, personal communication, June 2012). However, Mixer (2011) described both universal and diverse care patterns within her overarching theme about faculty teaching culture care.

Health

Health refers to *a state of wellbeing that is culturally defined, valued, and practiced, and which reflects the ability of the individuals or groups to perform their daily role activities in culturally expressed, beneficial, and patterned lifeways* (Leininger, 1991b, 2015a). It is a *restorative state of wellbeing that is culturally constituted, defined, valued, and practiced by individuals or groups that enables them to function in their daily lives* (Leininger, 2002d, 2015a). These definitions of health have been confirmed by numerous ethnonursing researchers in their culture care studies including

Gunn & Davis (2011) who studied healing with botanicals among elderly African Americans in the Mississippi Delta region; Lee (2012) who studied family homelessness in urban Appalachia; and Moss (2014) who studied the care and health practices of rural Ecuadorians.

Ethnohistory

Ethnohistory is a construct of the theory that comes from anthropology but one which the Leininger (1978) reconceptualized within a nursing perspective. The theorist defined *ethnohistory* as the *past facts, events, instances, and experiences of human beings, groups, cultures, and institutions that occur over time in particular contexts that help explain past and current lifeways about culture care influencers of health and wellbeing or the death of people* (Leininger, 1991b, 2002d, 2006a, 2015a). Ethnohistory is another essential dimension to consider when providing culturally congruent care. Special past and current events and conditions within the historical context of cultures and their caring modalities are important caring practices to discover and know as transcultural nursing knowledge, especially when studied within the context of care and wellbeing. Wolf et al. (2014) explained how the ethnohistory of the cultural group of Minnesotan Somali refugees who had fled a 20-year civil war profoundly influenced their care access and treatment for mental illness. Moss (2014) also described how healthcare beliefs and practices of *mestizo* Ecuadorians living in rural and remote areas were influenced by their ethnohistory, which included a past intertwined with the indigenous people of Ecuador (the Inca) and Spaniards who ruled present day Ecuador from the 1500s to the 1800s.

Environmental Context

Environmental context refers to *the totality of an event, situation, or particular experience that gives meaning to people's expressions, interpretations, and social interactions within particular geophysical, ecological, spiritual, sociopolitical, and technologic factors in specific cultural settings* (Leininger, 1991b, 1995a, 2002d, 2006a; McFarland & Wehbe-Alamah, 2015b). Strang and Mixer (2015) in their article about the Maasai in Kenya shared the discovery about how the environmental context was both a *facilitator* and *barrier* influence to effective malaria care outcomes. These issues included the geographic environment and location; the expectation to first use traditional care; knowledge of care options; financial resources; and use of insecticide-treated sleeping nets to prevent transmission of malaria from bites of the Anopheles mosquito (Strang & Mixer, 2015).

Worldview

Worldview refers to the way people tend to look out upon their world or their universe to form a picture or value stance about life or the world around them (Leininger, 1978, 1991b, 2002d, 2006a). Worldview provides a broad perspective about one's orientation to life, people, or groups that influence care or caring responses and decisions. Worldview guides one's decisions and actions, especially related to health and wellbeing as well as care decisions and actions. Lee (2012) described how urban and rural Appalachian mothers who were homeless found a sense of faith and hope that allowed them to look toward the future. Wehbe-Alamah (2008, 2011) studied folk care beliefs of traditional Lebanese and Syrian Muslims in the Midwestern United States, discovering worldviews that were diversely and universally embedded in their Islamic religious as well as unique cultural beliefs and practices. The author later compared and further explicated these findings in a follow-up synthesis work (Wehbe-Alamah, 2015).

■ CULTURE CARE MODES OF DECISIONS AND ACTIONS

In the Culture Care Theory, Leininger (2002b) postulated three culture care decision and action modes for providing culturally congruent nursing care. The three modes were highly innovative and unique in nursing and health care. Leininger (1991b) held that nurses needed creative and different approaches to make care and culture needs meaningful and helpful to clients. These three theoretically predicted decision and action modes of the Culture Care Theory are defined as:

- *Culture care preservation and/or maintenance,* which refers to those assistive, supportive, facilitative, or enabling professional acts or decisions that help cultures to retain, preserve, or maintain beneficial care beliefs and values or to face illness, disability, dying, and or death;
- *Culture care accommodation and/or negotiation,* which refers to those assistive, accommodating, facilitative, or enabling creative provider

care actions or decisions that help cultures adapt [accommodate] to or negotiate with others for culturally congruent, safe, and effective care for their health, wellbeing, or to deal with illness, injury, disability, or dying; and

- *Culture care repatterning and/or restructuring,* which refers to those assistive, supportive, facilitative, or enabling professional actions and mutual decisions that would help people to reorder, change, modify, or restructure their lifeways and institutions for better (or beneficial) healthcare patterns, practices, or outcomes. (Eipperle, 2015; Leininger, 2006a)

The modes have substantively guided nurses to provide culturally congruent nursing care and thereby fostered the development of culturally competent nurses. Nurses practicing in large urban centers typically care for clients from many different cultures or subcultures. Leininger's Culture Care Theory provides practicing nurses with an evidence-based, versatile, useful, and helpful approach to guide them in their daily decisions and actions regardless of the number of clients under their care or the complexity of their care needs.

The three culture care modes of decisions and actions are essential for care/caring and need to be used with discoveries from ethnonursing research studies guided by the CCT. The Culture Care Theory has challenged nurses to discover specific and holistic care as known and used by cultures over time and in different contexts. Both *care* and *culture* are held to be central and critical for the discipline and practice of nursing. *Nursing interventions* is a term that is seldom used in the Culture Care Theory or in transcultural nursing. This term has often been used inappropriately and is viewed by several cultures as too controlling or all-knowing. When used by nurses, this term may lead to interferences through words or actions with the cultural lifeways, values, and practices of others. This is because the term [nursing interventions] is sometimes viewed as or represents *cultural imposition nursing practices* used when providing care to clients, which may be offensive or in conflict with their lifeways (Eipperle, 2015; Leininger, 2006a).

Leininger proposed that *culture care preservation and/or maintenance* should in most circumstances be considered first, as many times people are doing meaningful and acceptable care for their families and others that leads to beneficial health outcomes. Many nurses from Western cultures are focused on interventions so as to make changes, believing that care should be based solely on professional nursing knowledge. However, it is important to *first* consider what people are doing right in caring for themselves and their families. Many times people are providing exquisite care in their homes or in institutional, community, or primary settings (Eipperle, 2015; Gunn & Davis, 2011; Lee, 2012; McFarland & Zehnder, 2006; Outwater et al., 2014; Wanchai, Armer, & Stewart, 2015; Wehbe-Alamah, 2011).

These generic caring decisions and actions should be maintained and supported and sometimes combined with professional/integrative care by nurses, educators, and students to provide culturally congruent care for people (Leininger, 2002e). In international service-learning courses, preserving and/or maintaining care that is therapeutic is an essential lesson for nurses and nursing students (Knecht & Sabatine, 2015). They need to be guided by the care modes and in most circumstances consider *first* what caring actions should be maintained or preserved; then consider what should be accommodated or negotiated; and only as a final decision consider what should be changed—repatterned and/or restructured (Eipperle, 2015).

■ SUNRISE ENABLER AND THE CULTURAL AND SOCIAL STRUCTURE DIMENSIONS

The cultural and social structure dimensions refer to the dynamic, holistic, and interrelated patterns of structured features of a culture (or subculture) that include but are not limited to technology factors; religious and philosophical factors; biological factors [new revision/addition]; kinship and social factors; cultural values, beliefs, and lifeways; political and legal factors; economic factors; and educational factors as well as environmental context, language, and ethnohistory (Wehbe-Alamah & McFarland, 2015a, p. 75).

Cultural and social structure dimensions are other major features of the Culture Care Theory (Leininger, 1978). Social structure phenomena provide broad, comprehensive, and special factors influencing care expressions and meanings. Social structure factors of clients include religion (spirituality); kinship (social ties); politics; legal issues; education; economics;

technology; political factors; philosophy of life; and cultural beliefs and values with gender and class differences. The theorist predicted that these diverse factors must be understood as they directly or indirectly influence health and wellbeing (Leininger, 1978). In the past, social structure factors were not explicitly studied in nursing nor in reference to care until the advent of transcultural nursing (Leininger, 1978, 1991a). The use of Leininger's CCT has helped nurses to study these dimensions for a holistic or total view of clients. The study of these influencing factors has provided a wealth of invaluable insights about culturally-based care addressing health, wellness, or illness (McFarland & Wehbe-Alamah, 2015b, pp. 17-18).

The following discussion of the social structure dimensions presents substantive research findings, which can serve as resources for valuable technological, religious and spiritual, kinship and social, cultural political and legal, educational, economic, and technological factors discovered by transcultural nurse researchers who used the CCT to guide their ethnonursing studies.

Technological Factors

Leininger (2006b) studied the Gadsup Akuna of New Guinea in the 1960s and discovered that they had no Western technology for health care or daily lifeways. Their care was based on making cultural artifacts for family members and the rest of the community. Women demonstrated care by making infant and garden string bags and tending gardens to produce healthy foods for their families and the village community. Men made wooden vessels for cooking foods and decorative amulets for ceremonial functions. The Gadsup depended heavily on generic care rather than the professional care and technological interventions available 25 miles away at a small hospital.

In 1997, McFarland discovered that elderly African Americans and Anglo American elders residing in a long-term care facility preferred receiving health care at the small clinic located within the facility rather than being transferred to a large medical center with state-of-the-art technology located just a few blocks way. Most residents *cautiously* considered the discussed potential for better health outcomes from treatment obtained at the medical center, and often still elected to receive their care at the long-term care facility.

Kelch (2015) conducted a translational research project in Haiti, implementing a chronic disease management program based on the provision of culturally congruent care for health workers and ancillary staff with hypertension or Type 2 diabetes employed at a remote primary care clinic. He was able to bring the technology of HgbA1C testing to this remote tropical area despite not having the necessary climate-controlled storage or work spaces where blood sample testing took place (Kelch, Wehbe-Alamah, and McFarland, 2015). This challenge was addressed by storing blood samples in a portable cooler filled with reusable ice packs and a thermometer from the clinic to monitor temperatures. Thus, a climate-controlled environment was created for storing blood samples for testing. However, healthcare workers who were diagnosed with Type 2 diabetes were treated with oral medications only, given that insulin rapidly degraded in the excessive heat and most Haitians living in remote areas lacked the technologies of refrigeration or air conditioning.

Religious, Spiritual, and Philosophical Factors

Strang and Mixer (2015) discovered that spiritual factors among the Kenyan Maasai were important influencers on malaria care. The Maasai often prayed to God for healing before taking medicine offered by professional care providers. Gunn and Davis (2011) in their study about healing botanicals used by elderly African Americans in the Mississippi delta region reported that their caring practices in modern times were rooted in healing from God rather than depending on herbs, roots, and plants as was done in by-gone eras. Morris (2012) in her study of urban adolescent gang members discovered spiritual and religious beliefs were a means for them to ameliorate the harsh realities of the urban environment and to promote personal, group, and community wellbeing.

Kinship and Social Factors

Wolf et al. (2014) in their study of Minnesotan Somali immigrant refugees discovered that tribe and family involvement in care influenced their healthcare access and experiences. One informant described that female family members were never left alone in the hospital; she stated that Somalis would like nurses to understand that practice and allow extended family visits. Wehbe-Alamah (2006, 2015) discovered in her studies

with Lebanese and Syrian Muslims in the Midwestern United States that both groups relied on community members as extended caregivers and that husbands took on a more active role in the caregiving process due to the absence of immediate and extended family members.

Cultural Values, Beliefs, and Lifeways

Cultural values, beliefs, and lifeways as a factor has been studied extensively by transcultural nurse researchers using the CCT as a guide to discover how this factor influences and is influenced by the provision of culturally congruent care and health and wellbeing. This central placement of this factor in the enabler reflects its importance as a key influencer upon the other factors (rays of the sun) and culture care expressions, patterns, and practices, which in turn affect the provision of culturally congruent care, and thereby health and wellbeing. The discovery of cultural values, beliefs, and practices by diverse cultural groups were central to finding out how to provide culturally congruent care to rural Dominicans (Shumacher, 2010); African Americans in the Mississippi delta region (Gunn & Davis, 2011); urban African American gang members (Morris, 2012); homeless urban and rural Appalachian women and their children (Lee, 2012); bereaved Tanzanian relatives of homicide victims (Outwater et al., 2014); breast cancer survivors in northern Thailand (Wanchai et al., 2015); Somali refugee immigrants in Minnesota (Wolf et al., 2014); rural *mestizo* Ecuadorians (Moss, 2014); the Kimana Maasai of Kenya (Strang & Mixer, 2015); and rural healthcare workers in Haiti (Kelch et al., 2015).

Biological Factors

Biological factors are a developing construct—first referred to by Leininger (2002b, p. 53)—that emerged from studies guided by the CCT where physical conditions, illnesses, and syndromes were a major care focus of the cultural group under study. Among the more recent studies where biological factors were identified as key influencers on care were Strang and Mixer (2015) who studied malaria care with the Kenyan Maasai; Wolf et al. (2014) who studied immigrant Somalis in Minnesota and mental health; and Kelch et al. (2015) who studied hypertension and diabetes among multicultural healthcare workers in Haiti. *Biological factors* has been added as a central construct to the Sunrise

Enabler under *Cultural and Social Structure Dimensions* and above *Care Expressions, Patterns, and Practices* to emphasize the importance of assessing hereditary and genetic illnesses as well as culture-bound syndromes. This placement was done in recognition of the fact that biological factors influence and are influenced by cultural and social structure dimensions and the other factors depicted within the rays of the sun in the Sunrise Enabler, all of which thereby influence and are influenced by generic and professional care expressions, patterns, and practices (H. B. Wehbe-Alamah, personal communication, October 2015).

Political and Legal Factors

Political and legal factors exert influence through regulatory and legislative actions that affect access to and the professional provision of care at both the social structure and individual levels (Miller, 2002). Outwater et al. (2012) studied the care practices of bereaved relatives of homicide victims in Tanzania and found that care practices differed in rural areas compared to modern urban areas. If a person was murdered in a village without police, the assailant would be followed and the murder solved by the cooperative efforts of the local people as an expression of care. In her study of rural and urban families [women with children] who were homeless in Appalachia, Lee (2012) recommended that nurses move their advocacy efforts beyond the scope of providing direct care services to advocacy in the public policy arena seeking more substantive and lasting solutions to issues such as housing and employment reforms.

Economic Factors

Many transcultural nursing research studies guided by the CCT documented the importance of economic factors and their influences on the quality of generic and professional care provided to diverse cultural groups. Gunn and Davis (2011) addressed the economic woes of African Americans living in a rural county in the Mississippi delta region where the majority of households earn an income well below the poverty line, placing the population at greater risk for poor health outcomes. Kelch et al. (2015) discussed poor health outcomes for rural Haitians who chew on sugar cane stalks and eat cookies made with mud [dirt] and salt to alleviate their hunger. Morris (2012) discovered that senior African American adolescent gang members in a large Midwestern city in the United States encouraged younger children to become gang members as a means to earn a living.

Educational Factors

Educational factors have influenced care and caring through nursing education and encouraging young people to enter into healthcare professions (Leininger, 1995b). Educational levels also influence health literacy, which affects patients' ability to understand and navigate the healthcare system, and thereby has a direct bearing on health outcomes (Schumacher, 2010). Gunn and Davis (2011) discussed the uneducated workforce in the Mississippi delta as one reason for the high unemployment rate in the local community; industries were not willing to locate where there was not a population with skilled potential employees. Kelch et al. (2015) discussed educating local healthcare workers about nutrition and healthy local foods such as the indigenous fruits and vegetables available to Haitians. Such educated healthcare workers knowledgeable about the Haitian culture could provide nutritional information for patients in a culturally congruent and acceptable way. Mixer (2011) focused her research on how nursing faculty educated nursing students to become culturally competent to provide care to clients from diverse backgrounds.

■ SUMMARY/CONCLUSION

In reviewing studies for this chapter, it came to this author's attention that there were gaps in the extant knowledge base of the discipline that provide opportunities for future ethnonursing research using the Culture Care Theory. Such studies could address the culture care needs of immigrant and refugee populations; how technology is used in and/or affects the ways cultures seek or use health care; and the healthcare needs of people in developed and developing regions of the world experiencing local or globally occurring healthcare crises, disparities, or communicable disease epidemics.

The Theory of Culture Care Diversity and Universality has increasingly become used by transcultural nurses as a guide to study diverse cultures worldwide. Practicing nurses can use culturally-based research findings to provide culturally congruent care for clients from diverse and similar cultures. In addition, the theory can be used as a cultural guide to study current health issues related to problems in diverse communities in the world facing serious health challenges. Examples of this include animal-borne diseases that have been passed to humans and become epidemic such as the Ebola virus in West Africa and Zika virus in Puerto Rico and Florida in the United States (U. S. Department of Health and Human Services [USDHHS], 2015; Freiden, Schuchat, & Peterson, 2016).

In addition, forced displacement of persons has increased (34,000 people every day) to the extent that by the end of 2015, 65.3 million individuals were forcibly displaced worldwide (refugee or stateless persons), with more than half of these people coming from just three countries—the Syrian Arab Republic, Afghanistan, and Somalia (United Nations Refugee Agency [UNHRC], 2016). Among the displaced are nearly 21.3 million refugees (persons forced to flee their homes or homelands because of conflict or persecution), over half of whom are under the age of 18 (UNHRC, 2016). There are also 10 million stateless people being denied a nationality and access to basic human rights such as education, health care, employment, and freedom of movement (UNHRC, 2016). At the end of 2015, UNHRC reported that the world was poised to experience its highest recorded level of displaced persons known in history (UNHRC, 2015).

Many displaced people dwell in 'temporary' refugee camps where multiple urgent and often serious (life altering and/or life-threatening) healthcare needs are endured while they wait for durable solutions to their refugee status (UNHCR, 2014). Effective prevention, treatment, and eventual eradication of such easily transmittable communicable diseases and attending to the myriad health challenges faced by refugees will require transculturally-prepared nurses and other healthcare professionals to integratively address the influencing cultural and social factors at individual, community, institutional, and national levels (Leininger, 2002d).

One of the strategies used to control the spread of Ebola in West Africa has been to remove infected people from their communities where traditionally *family care* is provided for the sick (USDHHS, 2015). "…A CDC staffer discovered *30 unreported cases* [emphasis added] in one remote village in Sierra Leone; the health official in the village thought Ebola was witchcraft and intentionally kept their outbreak a secret" (USDHHS,

2015). It seems evident that shifting from treating the physiological or physical disease to integrating major social structure dimensions about cultures, caring, and health-and-illness values, beliefs, and practices would provide the broad cultural perspective essential to providing care/caring for and serving these individuals (Leininger 2002d). The study of culturally congruent and specific care beliefs and practices is *key* to prevent further illness, promote healing, maintain health, and be of help in the recovery from this and other epidemic illnesses (Leininger, 2002d, p. 73).

The sexual transmission of Zika, a mosquito-borne virus associated with human birth defects, has been reported in 60 countries or territories including Puerto Rico and the state of Florida in the United States (Freiden et al., 2016). Access to contraceptives and sensitive counseling for women who have had confirmed positive laboratory tests for the Zika virus is a pressing, imperative need. Further, active engagement with the people in the affected or at-risk communities is also urgently needed to promote understanding and gain support for interventions such as travel limitations, mosquito protections, and vector eradication programs (Freiden et al., 2016).

Using the three culture care modes of decisions and actions (*culture care preservation and/or maintenance*; *culture care accommodation and/or negotiation*; and *culture care repatterning and/or restructuring*) to engage people to participate in requisite strategies that will effect changes for healthy outcomes is vital for meaningful and lasting health and satisfying cultural lifeways. Co-participative and collaborative care decisions and actions are essential to effectively prevent, treat, and eradicate disease as well as to meet the evolving healthcare needs of cultures worldwide (Eipperle, 2015; Leininger, 2002a, 2015b).

■ DEDICATION

This chapter is dedicated to Madeleine M. Leininger, my teacher, mentor, colleague, and friend.

■ DISCUSSION QUESTIONS

1. Review the constructs of *culture, care and caring*, and *culture care*. Reflect upon and discuss what your beliefs and perceptions about them were before reading the chapter compared to what your

perceptions are now. How will this affect your interactions with patients?

2. Discuss how you can integrate (not add) culturally congruent care into your practices.

3. Discuss how the Theory of Culture Care Diversity and Universality is applicable to health care in the context of current national and global events.

4. Drawing from your own professional experiences, discuss how you might apply the three modes of culture care decisions and actions to past, present, or future client situations. How would the outcomes have been or be different?

5. Discuss how the Theory of Culture Care Diversity and Universality, the Sunrise Enabler, the three modes of culture care decisions and actions, and the Ethnonursing Research Method can be used by transcultural nurses and other healthcare providers to influence how governments and nongovernmental agencies could more effectively address prevention, intervention, and treatment for current and emerging global communicable disease crises and other healthcare issues worldwide.

■ REFERENCES

Douglas, M. K., Rosenkoetter, M., Pacquiao, D. F., Callister, L. C., Hattar-Pollara, M., Lauderdale, J., … Purnell, L. (2014). Guidelines for implementing culturally competent nursing care. *Journal of Transcultural Nursing*, 25(2), 109-121.

Eipperle, M. K. (2015). Application of the three modes of culture care decisions and actions in advanced practice primary care. In M. R. McFarland and H. B. Wehbe-Alamah (Eds.), *Leininger's culture care diversity and universality: A worldwide nursing theory* (3rd ed., pp. 317-344).

Embler, P., Mixer, S. J., & Gunther, M. (2015). End-of-life culture care practices among Yup'ik Eskimo. *Online Journal of Cultural Competence in Nursing and Healthcare*, 5(1), 36-49. doi:10.9730/ojccnh.org/v5n1a3

Farrell, L. S. (2006). Culture care of the Potawatomi Native Americans who experienced family violence. In M. M. Leininger and M. R. McFarland (Eds.), *Culture care diversity and universality: A worldwide theory of nursing* (2nd ed., pp. 207-238). Sudbury, MA: Jones & Bartlett.

Freiden, T. R., Schuchat, A., & Peterson, L. R. (2016, August 8). Zika virus 6 months later [Editorial]. *Journal of the American Medical Association* 316(14),1443-1444. doi:10.1001/jama.2016.11941

Gunn, J., & Davis, S. (2011). Beliefs, meanings, and practices of healing with botanicals recalled by elder African American women in the Mississippi Delta. *Online Journal of Cultural Care in Nursing and Healthcare*, 1(1), 37-49.

Kelch, R. H., Wehbe-Alamah, H. B., & McFarland, M. R. (2015). Implementation of hypertension and diabetes chronic disease management in an adult group in Les Bours, Haiti. *Online Journal of Cultural Competence in Nursing and Healthcare*, 5(1), 50-63. doi:10.9730/ojccnh.org/v5n1a4

Knecht, L., & Sabatine, C. (2015). Application of culture care theory to international service learning experiences in Kenya. In M. R. McFarland and H. B. Wehbe-Alamah (Eds.), *Leininger's culture care diversity and universality: A worldwide nursing theory* (3rd ed., pp. 475-501). Burlington, MA: Jones and Bartlett Learning.

Lee, R. C. (2012). Family homelessness viewed through the lens of health and human rights. *Advances in Nursing Science*, 35(2), e47-e59.

Leininger, M. M. (1970). *Nursing and anthropology: Two worlds to blend.* New York, NY: John Wiley & Sons.

Leininger, M. M. (Ed.). (1978). *Transcultural nursing: Concepts, theories, and practice.* New York, NY: John Wiley & Sons.

Leininger, M. M. (Ed.). (1985). Qualitative research methods in nursing. New York, NY: Grune & Stratton.

Leininger, M. M. (Ed.). (1991a). *Culture care diversity and universality: A theory of nursing.* New York, NY: National League for Nursing Press.

Leininger, M. M. (1991b). The Theory of Culture Care Diversity and Universality. In M. M. Leininger (Ed.), *Culture care diversity and universality: A theory of nursing* (pp. 5-68). New York, NY: National League for Nursing Press.

Leininger, M. M. (1994). Quality of life from a transcultural nursing perspective. *Nursing Science Quarterly*, 7(1), 22-28.

Leininger, M. M. (1995a). Overview of Leininger's Culture Care Theory. In M. M. Leininger (Ed.), *Transcultural nursing: Concepts, theories, and practice* (2nd ed., pp. 93-114). Columbus, OH: McGraw-Hill College Custom Series.

Leininger, M. M. (Ed.). (1995b). *Transcultural nursing: Concepts, theories, and practice* (2nd ed.). Columbus, OH: McGraw-Hill College Custom Series.

Leininger, M. M. (2002a). Culture care assesments for congruent competency practices. In M. M. Leininger and M. R. McFarland (Eds.), *Transcultural nursing: Concepts, theories, research, & practice* (3rd ed., pp. 117-143).

Leininger, M. M. (2002b). Essential transcultural nursing concepts, principles, examples, and policy statements. In M. M. Leininger and M. R. McFarland (Eds.), *Transcultural nursing: Concepts, theories, research, & practice* (3rd ed., pp. 45-69).

Leininger, M. M. (2002c). Life-cycle culturally based care and health patterns of the Gadsup of New Guinea: A non-Western culture. In M. M. Leininger and M. R. McFarland (Eds.), *Transcultural nursing: Concepts, theories, research, & practice* (3rd ed., pp. 217-237). New York, NY: McGraw-Hill Medical Publishing Division.

Leininger, M. M. (2002d). Part I. The theory of culture care and the ethnonursing research method. In M. M. Leininger and M. R. McFarland (Eds.), *Transcultural nursing: Concepts, theories, research, & practice* (3rd ed., pp. 71-98). New York, NY: McGraw-Hill Medical Publishing Division.

Leininger, M. M. (2002e). Part I. Toward integrative generic and professional health care. In M. M. Leininger and M. R. McFarland (Eds.), *Transcultural nursing: Concepts, theories, research, & practice* (3rd ed., pp. 145-154). New York, NY: McGraw-Hill Medical Publishing Division.

Leininger, M. M. (2006a). Culture Care Diversity and Universality Theory and evolution of the Ethnonursing Method. In M. M. Leininger and M. R. McFarland (Eds.), *Culture care diversity and universality: A worldwide theory of nursing* (2nd ed., pp. 1-41). Sudbury, MA: Jones & Bartlett.

Leininger, M. M. (2006b). Culture care of the Gadsup Akuna of the Eastern Highlands of New Guinea: The first transcultural nursing study [revised reprint]. In M. M. Leininger and M. R. McFarland (Eds.), *Culture care diversity and universality: A worldwide theory of nursing* (2nd ed., pp. 115-157). Sudbury, MA: Jones & Bartlett.

Leininger, M. M. (2006c). Selected culture care findings of diverse cultures using the Culture Care Theory and ethnomethods [Revised reprint]. In M. M. Leininger and M. R. McFarland (Eds.), *Culture care diversity and universality: A worldwide theory of nursing* (2nd ed., pp. 281-305). Sudbury, MA: Jones & Bartlett.

Leininger, M. M. (2006d). The Ethnonursing Research Method and enablers. In M. M. Leininger and M. R. McFarland (Eds.), *Culture care diversity and universality: A worldwide theory of nursing* (2nd ed., pp. 43-81). Sudbury, MA: Jones & Bartlett.

Leininger, M. M. (2011). Leininger's reflection on the ongoing father protective care research. *The Online Journal of Cultural Competence in Nursing and Healthcare, 1*(2), 1-13.

Leininger, M. M. (2015a). Leininger's father protective care. In M. R. McFarland and H. B. Wehbe-Alamah (Eds.), *Leininger's culture care diversity and universality: A worldwide nursing theory* [Revised by H. B. Wehbe-Alamah] (3rd ed., pp. 119-136). Burlington, MA: Jones and Bartlett Learning.

Leininger, M. M. (2015b). The benefits of the Culture Care Theory and a look to the future of transcultural nursing. In M. R. McFarland and H. B. Wehbe-Alamah (Eds.), *Leininger's culture care diversity and universality: A worldwide nursing theory* (3rd ed., pp. 101-118). Burlington, MA: Jones and Bartlett Learning.

Leininger, M. M., & McFarland, M. R. (Eds.). (2002). *Transcultural nursing: Concepts, theories, research, and practice* (3rd ed.). New York: McGraw Hill.

Leininger, M. M., & McFarland, M. R. (Eds.). (2006). *Culture care diversity and universality: A worldwide nursing theory* (2nd ed.). Sudbury, MA: Jones & Bartlett.

Liang, H-F. (2002). Understanding culture care practices of caregivers of children with cancer in Taiwan. *Journal of Pediatric Oncology Nursing, 19*(6), 205-217.

Leuning, C. J., Small, L. F., & van Dyk, A. (2002). Elder care in urban Nambian families: An ethnonursing study. In M. M. Leininger and M. R. McFarland (Eds.), *Transcultural nursing: Concepts, theories, research, & practice* (3rd ed., pp. 347-362). New York, NY: McGraw-Hill Medical Publishing Division.

McFarland, M. R. (1997). Use of cultural care theory with Anglo and African American elders in a long-term care setting. *Nursing Science Quarterly, 10*(4), 186-192.

McFarland, M. R. (2002a). Culture Care Theory and elderly Polish Americans. In M. M. Leininger and M. R. McFarland (Eds.), *Transcultural nursing: Concepts, theories, research, & practice* (3rd ed., 385-401). New York, NY: McGraw-Hill Medical Publishing Division.

McFarland, M. R. (2002b). Part II. Research findings from the Culture Care Theory. In M. M. Leininger and M. R. McFarland (Eds.), *Transcultural nursing: Concepts, theories, research, & practice* (3rd ed., pp. 99-116). New York, NY: McGraw-Hill Medical Publishing Division.

McFarland, M. R. (with M. M. Leininger via videotape). (2011, October 20). *The culture care theory and a look to the future for transcultural nursing.* Keynote Address presented at the 37th Annual International Conference of the Transcultural Nursing Society, Las Vegas, NV.

McFarland, M. R., & Wehbe-Alamah, H. B. (Eds.). (2015a). *Leininger's culture care diversity and universality: A worldwide nursing theory* (3rd ed.). Burlington, MA: Jones and Bartlett Learning.

McFarland, M. R., & Wehbe-Alamah, H. B. (2015b). The theory of culture care diversity and universality. In M. R. McFarland and H. B. Wehbe-Alamah (Eds.), *Leininger's culture care diversity and universality: A worldwide nursing theory* (3rd ed., pp. 1-34). Burlington, MA: Jones and Bartlett Learning.

McFarland, M. R., & Zehnder, N. (2006). Culture care of German American elders in a nursing home context. In M. M. Leininger and M. R. McFarland (Eds.), *Culture care diversity and universality: A worldwide nursing theory* (2nd ed., pp. 181-205). Sudbury, MA: Jones & Bartlett.

Mixer, S. J. (2011). Use of the Culture Care Theory to discover nursing faculty care expressions, patterns, and practices related to teaching culture care. *The Online Journal of Cultural Competence in Nursing and Healthcare, 1*(1), 3-14.

Mixer, S. J., McFarland, M. R., Andrews M. M., & Strang, C. W. (2013). Exploring faculty health and wellbeing: Creating a caring scholarly community. *Nurse Education Today, 33*(12), 1471-1476. Retrievable from http://dx.doi.org/10.1016/j.nedt.2013.05.019

Morris, E. J. (2012). Respect, protection, faith, and love: Major care constructs identified within the subculture of selected urban African American adolescent gang members. *Journal of Transcultural Nursing, 23*(3), 262-269.

Morris, E. J. (2015). An examination of subculture as a theoretical construct through an ethnonursing study of urban African American adolescent gang members. In M. R. McFarland and H. B. Wehbe-Alamah (Eds.), *Culture care diversity and universality: A worldwide nursing theory* (3rd ed., pp. 255-285). Burlington, MA: Jones and Bartlett Learning.

Moss, J. A. (2014). Discovering the healthcare beliefs and practices of rural mestizo Ecuadorians: An ethnonursing study. *Investigación y Educación en Enfermería, 32*(2), 326-336.

Outwater, A. H., Tarimo, E. A M., Miller, J. E., & Campbell, J. C. (2012). Meanings of care by bereaved relatives of homicide victims in Dar es Salaam, Tanzania: Implications for nursing. *Journal of Transcultural Nursing, 23*(4), 397-405.

Schumacher, G. (2010). Culture care meanings, beliefs, and practices in rural Dominican Republic. *Journal of Transcultural Nursing, 21*(2), 93-103.

Strang, C. W., & Mixer, S. J. (2015). Discovery of the meanings, expressions, and practices related to malaria care among the Maasai. *Journal of Transcultural Nursing, 27*(4), 333-341. Advance online publication. doi: 10.1177/1043659615573841

The United Nations Refugee Agency. (2014). *Global strategy implementation report.* New York, NY: Author. Retrieved from http://www.unhcr.org/en-us/public-health.html

The United Nations Refugee Agency. (2015). *2015 likely to break records for forced displacement—study* [Webpage]. New York, NY: Author. Retrieved from http://www.unhcr.org/en-us/news/latest/2015/12/5672c2576/2015-likely-break-records-forced-displacement-study.html

The United Nations Refugee Agency. (2016, June 20). *Global trends 2015: Figures at a glance.* New York, NY: Author. Retrieved from http://www.unhcr.org/en-us/figures-at-a-glance.html

U. S. Department of Health and Human Services, Centers for Disease Control and Prevention. (2015). *The road to zero: CDC's response to the West African Ebola epidemic (2014-2015).* Atlanta, GA: Author. Retrieved from http://www.cdc.gov/about/pdf/ebola/ebola-photobook-070915.pdf

Wanchai, A., Armer, J. M., & Stewart, B. R. (2015). Thai nurses' perspectives on the use of complementary and alternative medicine among Thai breast cancer survivors in northern Thailand. *International Journal of Nursing Practice, 21*(2), 118-124. doi:10.1111/ijn.12231

Wehbe-Alamah, H. B. (2006). Generic care of Lebanese Muslims in the Midwestern United States. In M. M. Leininger and M. R. McFarland (Eds.), *Culture care diversity and universality: A worldwide nursing theory* (2nd ed., pp. 307-325). Sudbury, MA: Jones & Bartlett.

Wehbe-Alamah, H. B. (2008). Bridging generic and professional care practices for Muslim patients through the use of Leininger's culture care modes. *Contemporary Nurse, 28*(2), 83-97.

Wehbe-Alamah, H. B. (2011). The use of Culture Care Theory with Syrian Muslims in the Midwestern United States. *Online Journal of Cultural Competence in Nursing and Healthcare, 1*(3), 1-12.

Wehbe-Alamah, H. B. (2015). Folk care beliefs and practices of traditional Lebanese and Syrian Muslims in the Midwestern United States. In M. R. McFarland and H. B. Wehbe-Alamah (Eds.), *Culture care diversity and universality: A worldwide nursing theory* (3rd ed., pp. 137-182). Burlington, MA: Jones and Bartlett Learning.

Wehbe-Alamah, H. B., & McFarland, M. R. (2015a). Leininger's enablers for use with the ethnonursing research method. In M. R. McFarland and H. B. Wehbe-Alamah (Eds.), *Culture care diversity and universality: A worldwide nursing theory* (3rd ed., pp. 73-100). Burlington, MA: Jones and Bartlett Learning.

Wehbe-Alamah, H. B., & McFarland, M. R. (2015b). The ethnonursing research method. In M. R. McFarland and H. B. Wehbe-Alamah (Eds.), *Culture care diversity and universality: A worldwide nursing theory* (3rd ed., pp. 35-71). Burlington, MA: Jones and Bartlett Learning.

Wolf, K. M., Zoucha, R., McFarland, M. R., Salman, K., Dagne, A., & Hashi, N. (2014). *Somali immigrant perceptions of mental health and illness: An ethnonursing study. Journal of Transcultural Nursing, 24*(4), 349-358. Advance online publication. doi: 10.1177/1043659614550487

CHAPTER 4

The Ethnonursing Research Method: Major Features and Enablers

Hiba B. Wehbe-Alamah

> *"Now and in the future, nurses prepared in transcultural studies will serve as leaders to guide nurses in the development of this new subfield [transcultural nursing discipline]"* (Leininger, 1994, p. 14).

■ INTRODUCTION

The Ethnonursing Research Method (ERM) was specifically developed by Dr. Madeleine Leininger, founder and leader of the academic field of transcultural nursing, to facilitate the discovery of data focused on the theory of Culture Care Diversity and Universality, also known as the Culture Care Theory (CCT). The term *ethnonursing* was coined and developed by the theorist in the mid-1960s (Leininger, 1985a, 1990, 1991b, 2002). Ethnonursing is defined as "*a qualitative nursing research method focused on naturalistic, open discovery and largely inductive (emic) modes and processes with diverse strategies, techniques, and enabling guides to document, describe, explain, and interpret people's worldview, meanings, symbols, life experiences, and other related aspects, as they bear on actual or potential nursing care phenomena*" (Wehbe-Alamah & McFarland, 2015b, p. 37).

The research method embodies an open inquiry approach designed to discover emic (insider) and etic (outsider) knowledge and practices related to holistic health (physical, mental, emotional, psychological, social, and spiritual) care, wellbeing, illness, disability, and death and dying as well as other actual or potential areas of interest to nurses and other health care professionals and researchers interested in discovering and providing culturally sensitive and congruent care to people of diverse cultural backgrounds. The method facilitates the discovery of care and health knowledge related to areas such as worldview; cultural and social structure dimensions; environmental context; language; ethnohistory; generic (folk) and professional care practices; integrative care (combination of generic and professional care); and other additional areas of the informant's cultural lifeways.

■ ETHNONURSING TERMINOLOGY

Researchers interested in conducting ethnonursing studies must familiarize themselves with the appropriate language of the method and its foundational theory. Readers are encouraged to review concepts and terminology related to the Culture Care Theory previously introduced in the first three chapters of this text. Additional language associated with Ethnonursing Research Method includes:

- **Informant** refers to the study participant or person being interviewed. In situations where the term *informant* is associated with negative interpretations that may adversely affect the course or outcome of the study, researchers may use the term *participant* instead.
- **Key informant** *is the* individual purposefully and thoughtfully selected by the gatekeeper or other study participants (members of the culture or subculture under study) and identified as *most* knowledgeable about the domain of inquiry of the research. Key informants are well-informed about the values, beliefs, norms, and general lifeways of the culture under study. They form the central foundation with whom the researcher, using direct observations and participant experiences, checks and rechecks collected data in relation to internal (emic) and external (etic) relevance, meanings, accuracy, and dependability (Wehbe-Alamah & McFarland, 2015a).
- **General informant** *refers to the* individual purposefully and thoughtfully selected by the gatekeeper or other study participants (members of the culture or subculture under study) and identified as *less* knowledgeable than the key informant about the domain of inquiry of the research. General informants offer relevant cultural insights and reflections that assist the researcher to identify diversities and universalities of findings or themes collected or abstracted from data obtained from key and general informants (Wehbe-Alamah & McFarland, 2015a).
- **Gatekeeper** refers to the person who facilitates or grants entry into the research site. It is often an individual who is highly respected or holds a leadership or authority status. For example, the gatekeeper may be a CEO, member of a management team, school principal, priest, or community leader.

■ HISTORICAL DEVELOPMENT AND RATIONALE

There are several major features and reasons why the Ethnonursing Research Method was developed for use with the Culture Care Theory. In the 1950s, Leininger noted that nurse theorists and researchers borrowed heavily from the statistical formulas, research tools, scales, and instruments of other disciplines to quantify or reduce nursing phenomena and findings which, in her opinion, limited the nurses' abilities to fully discover caring and other data related to nursing insights and practices (Wehbe-Alamah & McFarland, 2015a). She maintained that it was difficult to obtain findings of specific cultures and especially full, comprehensive, meaningful data using quantitative reductionistic and empirical research methods. She expressed concern that such quantitative approaches did not allow for the discovery of in-depth data about human care, health, ethnohistory, cultural values and lifeways, accurate culture-care interpretations, or meaningful nursing knowledge and phenomena (Leininger, 1991b, 2002).

As a result, Leininger embarked on what was considered at that time a bold and different step in nursing and a new breakthrough approach by developing the Ethnonursing Research Method within the qualitative paradigm to fit with her Culture Care Theory. After 20 years of studying nearly 25 different qualitative methods, she wrote and published the first qualitative nursing research book to guide nurses in using a different paradigm and a different method to discover nursing phenomena (Leininger, 1991a). Her philosophy and intent was for nurses to develop research methods that fit with or were meaningful to their theories to obtain credible and full data *and* to not rely totally on reductionistic modes of testing or data outcomes about nursing phenomena. To her, it was important to have nursing research methods that fit or were congruent with the discipline of *nursing* to discover complex, hidden, and covert nursing phenomena as they related to care and health in diverse cultures.

Leininger believed that qualitative and quantitative paradigms have different philosophies, purposes, goals, methods, and desired outcomes, and as a result, should not be viewed as the same or used in the same ways. She maintained that the two research paradigms and methods should not be mixed as doing so would violate the philosophy, purposes, and integrity of each paradigm and lead to questionable outcomes. She upheld that qualitative research methods and findings can stand alone to study and explain findings, and quantitative methods with statistical treatments are not necessary or appropriate to justify qualitative studies. According to Leininger, one does not have to add or mix many methods within the qualitative paradigm unless the researcher has good reasons and can justify using multiple methods. Most importantly, the researcher must know each qualitative method being used and analyze them fully within the stated research purposes. The ethnonursing qualitative research method was thoughtfully developed after studying the purposes and uses of both the *qualitative* and *quantitative* research paradigms (Leininger, 2002). Today, many nurse researchers use a mixed method approach when conducting nursing research.

The first ethnonursing research study, which is considered a classic today, took place in in the early 1960s in the Gadsup Akuna and Arona villages in Eastern Highlands of Papua New Guinea (Leininger, 2006; Wehbe-Alamah & McFarland, 2015b). Leininger, pursuing a doctorate in anthropology, developed the Ethnonursing Research Method and tested it during the course of her studies. Since its inception nearly six decades ago, the Ethnonursing Research Method continues to develop and evolve largely due to input from doctoral students working under Dr. Leininger's guidance and mentorship and who have since become transcultural research experts and mentors themselves. As a result, new enablers were created, original enablers were refined, terms and research processes were better defined, and the method gained increased awareness and usage across the field of transcultural nursing worldwide. More recently, researchers from diverse health care and social disciplines outside of nursing have expressed interest in learning about and/or using the Ethnonursing Research Method.

■ PURPOSES OF THE ETHNONURSING RESEARCH METHOD

The central purpose of the Ethnonursing Research Method is "*to establish a naturalistic and largely emic open inquiry discovery method to explicate and study nursing phenomena related to the Theory of Culture Care Diversity and Universality*" (Wehbe-Alamah & McFarland, 2015b, p. 39). Additional purposes of this research method include:

- To discover largely unknown or vaguely known complex nursing phenomena bearing on care, wellbeing, holistic health, disability, illness, death, and related cultural knowledge.

- To facilitate the researcher's ability to enter the people's emic (insider's) cultural world and learn from them first-hand about their beliefs, values, experiences, and lifeways about human care and health.
- To gain in-depth knowledge about the care meanings, expressions, beliefs, practices, symbols, metaphors, and daily night-and-day factors influencing health, wellbeing, disability, illness, and death as depicted in the Sunrise Enabler.
- To use standard and new enablers to tease out covert or embedded care and nursing knowledge related to the Culture Care Theory from emic and etic data findings.
- To use a rigorous, detailed, and systematic method of qualitative data analysis that would preserve naturalistic cultural and contextual data related to the theory.
- To use qualitative criteria (not quantitative) for accurate, meaningful, and credible analysis of findings.
- To identify the strengths and limitations of the Ethnonursing Research Method in advancing transcultural nursing science knowledge and outcomes (Leininger, 2002).

Leininger (2002) maintained that the ethnonursing purposes seemed urgently needed in nursing, especially to establish a body of transcultural nursing knowledge to guide culture care practices. The goal of ethnonursing research is to discover in-depth findings that can guide provision of culturally sensitive, congruent, safe, and beneficial care to people of diverse cultural backgrounds through the use of the three modes of culture care decisions and actions.

■ DOMAIN OF INQUIRY

The domain of inquiry (DOI) is a succinct tailor-made statement focused directly and specifically on culture care, health phenomenon, or any other area or domain under study. The DOI identifies the focus of investigation or discovery. For example, a DOI might be stated as: *Mexican Families and Care Meanings and Practices.* Another DOI would be: *Culture Care of Somali Refugees.* Excellent examples of domains of inquiry are found in several research studies by transcultural nurses in this text as well as other publications.

ENABLERS TO FACILITATE IN-DEPTH DISCOVERIES

To tap into the peoples' (or informants') world of knowing, the theorist developed several *enablers* (term coined by Leininger beginning in the 1960s) to tease out data bearing on culture care, health, disability, illness, death, and related nursing phenomena. *Enablers* are facilitators that assist with the examination of the major tenets of the theory and the domain of inquiry under study. They facilitate the discovery of informants' ideas and stories in natural and unstructured ways (Wehbe-Alamah & McFarland, 2015a, p. 74). Different enablers were developed to discover in-depth data of overt, covert, unknown, or ambiguous nursing phenomena. Leininger (2002) maintained that enablers sharply contrast with mechanistic devices such as *scales, measurement instruments*, and other impersonal *objective distancing tools* generally used in quantitative studies. She considered such tools as unnatural and frightening to cultural informants, especially to minorities, refugees, immigrants, homeless, poor, elderly, oppressed, and other vulnerable groups, as well as to cultures in general. The following are the most common enablers used in conjunction with the Ethnonursing Research Method (Wehbe-Alamah & McFarland, 2015a):

- The Sunrise Enabler to Discover Culture Care
- Leininger's Stranger-to-Trusted-Friend Enabler
- Leininger's Observation-Participation-Reflection Enabler
- Leininger's Semi-Structured Inquiry Guide Enabler to Assess Culture Care and Health
- Leininger's Acculturation Health Care Assessment Enabler for Cultural Patterns in Traditional and Nontraditional Lifeways
- Leininger's Phases of Ethnonursing Data Analysis Enabler for Qualitative Data
- The Leininger-Templin-Thompson (LTT) Ethnoscript Coding Enabler
- The Life History Health Care Enabler

The ethnonursing researcher often uses most (if not all) of the enablers listed above except for perhaps the Acculturation Enabler and the Life History Health care Enabler depending on the focus of the study. Enablers are used as a guide to gently tease out in-depth informant ideas and obvious facts related to a specific domain of inquiry under study. With enablers, informants are encouraged to talk out their ideas; tell stories; describe life experiences; and share pictures, tapes, and any materials they feel comfortable sharing related to the areas being discussed. The researcher remains alert to the informant's emic accounts and is an active and genuine listener. The researcher always *moves with the informant's line of thinking or flow of ideas.*

While the researcher unobtrusively uses each enabler as a guide to uncover specific knowledge areas related to the domain of inquiry, he/she does not give the Enabler to the informant to use. Throughout the use of the enablers, the ethnonursing researcher pays attention to his/her own etic responses, feelings, actions, and reactions reflecting on actual or possible influences of the researcher on the informant(s). Remaining in a nonintrusive role is desired, always sitting with the informant in a visiting style of relating to them and others. An explanation of enablers is provided to assist with appropriate and accurate use.

The Sunrise Enabler to Discover Culture Care

The Sunrise Enabler to Discover Culture Care, commonly referred to as the *Sunrise Enabler* (Color Insert 1), is a cognitive map of the Culture Care Theory and a visualization aid to see and to assess different holistic factors that tend to influence the care, health, wellbeing, disability, illness, death and dying of individuals, families, groups, communities, or institutions in their naturalistic settings. It is very useful for researchers seeking to tease out data related to multiple factors influencing care and health and for nurses and other health care providers conducting in-depth cultural assessments. The major areas for assessment embedded in the enabler are worldview; environmental context; language; ethnohistory; generic (emic) folk and professional (etic) beliefs and practices; and cultural and social structure dimensions (Leininger, 2002). The cultural and social structure dimensions include technological factors; spiritual, religious, and philosophical factors; kinship and social factors; cultural values, beliefs, and lifeways; political and legal factors; economic factors; and educational factors (Leininger, 2002). The environmental context includes but is not limited to physical and social features, food resources, cultural symbols, and home conditions (Leininger, 1970). The nurse assesses all of the above with a health care focus and draws on appropriate medical, nursing, liberal arts, and other knowledge relevant to professional care (Leininger, 2002). A new addition to the cultural and social structure dimensions is biological factors, which more explicitly addresses an area previously embedded in holistic health but often missed by clinicians or researchers.

In general, the Sunrise Enabler is an invaluable guide to discover new knowledge or to confirm knowledge about cultural informants/clients. There is no set or rigid approach where one begins in using the enabler. The discovery process may begin in the upper or lower part of the Sunrise Enabler according to the researcher's or clinician's focus, interests, knowledge, domain of inquiry, and competencies. Some users are more comfortable focusing first on professional and generic care; whereas those prepared in graduate transcultural nursing programs often focus initially on the worldview, social structure dimensions, and other areas in the upper part of the Sunrise Enabler, commonly referred to as *the Rays of the Sun*. Cultural informants/clients often have their own interests about what they want to talk about first and last, and the researcher/clinician tries to move with the informants'/clients' interests as much as possible to elicit in-depth data. Regardless of where one starts to use the Sunrise Enabler, one is expected to explore all dimensions or components with the particular domain being studied to obtain a holistic, comprehensive, and accurate data. For example, one may see an urgent need to assess the kinship and technology uses along with generic folk practices of concern to African mothers and their care needs during pregnancy. Accordingly, one would start with these areas of the enabler, but ultimately assess all factors in the enabler to get a comprehensive and accurate assessment (Leininger, 2002). The assessment is facilitated through the use of *The Semi-Structured Inquiry Guide Enabler to Assess Culture Care and Health*, explained later in this chapter.

As the researcher/clinician probes for care meanings, beliefs, values, expressions, and practices in relation to social structure, environment, and other factors with the informants, he/she remains alert to the different areas in the enabler and thinks about the commonalties among informants/clients—whether studying individuals, families, or groups. For example, studying the religious and care beliefs of Arab Muslims generally requires a focus on the religious beliefs and cultural value lifeways of the family or group to discover their culture care beliefs and practices. The researcher gently teases out religious data and remains cognizant of age, gender, and other factors influencing care. Physical, emotional, and other related knowledge that the informants share are important with regard to their specific meanings and expressions. Generally, a full picture of the life of each individual (or family) becomes apparent if the researcher/clinician remains genuinely interested and patient with informants while using the Sunrise Enabler (Leininger, 2002).

At all times the researcher/clinician is careful to withhold any judgments and his/her own professional nursing etic knowledge, but instead focuses on discovering emic knowledge from informants/clients. Teasing out embedded or concealed care practices with the informant's/client's emic meanings requires active listening, patience, and confirming with them whatever the researcher/clinician hears and sees. Listening to how care is linked to and explained using kinship, religion, economics, politics, cultural values and beliefs, and other general factors in the Sunrise Enabler are essential to in-depth cultural discovery. Informants and clients like to tell their story and are often pleased when the researcher or nurse caring for them remains interested in their world of telling and knowing. Obtaining informants'/clients' emic knowledge *first* is important before reflecting on etic professional knowledge.

When using the Sunrise Enabler to conduct an ethnonursing study or an in-depth cultural assessment, the researcher or clinician focuses on integrating generic care practices along with professional care-cure practices through the use of the three modes of culture care decisions and actions as may be appropriate for congruent, satisfying, safe, and beneficial to the people being studied or assessed. Because the theory has both abstract and practical features, professional nursing (and other disciplines') knowledge should be considered along with generic care data. It is, however, crucial to confirm discovered data with informants/clients related to the three culture care modes to identify and jointly develop congruent and meaningful nursing decisions and actions. The three modes of culture care decisions and actions that the nurse researcher or clinician examines and co-develops with informants are *culture care preservation and/or maintenance*; *culture care accommodation and/ or negotiation*; and *culture care repatterning and/or restructuring* (Leininger, 1991b, 2002).

Patient *problems* and *noncompliance* are terms often used in nursing, but seldom used in transcultural nursing because the underlying difficulties may not be client-derived but are more often associated with the nurse's lack of knowledge about important cultural issues. Such traditional linguistic nursing sayings are often troublesome to clients from different cultures and can lead to cultural resistance and nonadherent responses. When the researcher/clinician and the informant/client use a co-participant involvement approach and collaboratively determine appropriate care decisions and actions, this will often lead to acceptance and adherence to the proposed plan of care. The culture care modes, whether one or all, need to therefore reasonably fit with informants'/clients' cultural lifeways and may need to include some professional suggestions that may be beneficial to the informants/clients.

Carefully and sensitively teasing out care meanings, expressions, and practices from informants/clients with the Sunrise Enabler is generally informative and rewarding to the researcher/clinician and informants/clients. During the past six decades, the Sunrise Enabler—used in conjunction with the Culture Care Theory—has led to a wealth of largely unknown care and health knowledge to provide culturally congruent care to individuals, families, and groups and for health institutions, as is consistent with the goal of the theory. Care practice discoveries such as *protective care*, *supportive care*, *care as presence*, *care as respect*, and *care as family love* have been identified using the Culture care Theory and the Sunrise Enabler (Leininger, 1991b, 2002). The Sunrise Enabler and the Culture Care Theory can be used (with slight modifications) by other health care providers according to their particular discipline interests and therapeutic goals. Pharmacists, dental hygienists, physicians, social workers, health anthropologists, and others in the health care field have found that the Sunrise Enabler offers an excellent assessment guide to grasp the totality of the client's needs and lifeways (Leininger, 2002).

Leininger's Stranger-to-Trusted-Friend Enabler

Leininger's Stranger-to-Trusted Friend Enabler (Refer to Figure 4.1) is a sensitive guide that acts as an indicator to show how nurses move from a stranger to a trusted friend so as to get accurate, in-depth, and reliable data when conducting an in-depth cultural assessment or an ethnonursing research study. The goal of this enabler is to identify when the researcher becomes a *trusted friend* as he/she moves from the left side of the enabler (stranger or distrusted friend) to the right side of the enabler (trusted friend). Even if the researcher has previously functioned in the culture or is from the culture under study, use of this enabler will nonetheless be very helpful in identifying when the researcher has reached trusted friend status.

When a researcher enters a new or unfamiliar research environment, he/she is usually considered a *stranger* by informants participating in the research. As long as the researcher is not considered a trusted friend, informants may give false and/or distorted data and may not always be willing to share intimate and meaningful cultural knowledge and secrets. When signs of distrust exist, fear, doubt, and suspicion often prevail between researcher/clinician and informant/client, and the data becomes questionable and sparse and may often be inaccurate. Reaching the trusted friend stage is important as trust is essential for honest, credible, and in-depth data to be generated from informants.

Once one is a trusted friend, informants generally will more openly share their secrets and other insights than when one is a distrusted stranger. As a result, the credibility and accuracy of the discovered data increases as the researcher becomes trusted by the informants in the study. The *process* of moving from being a stranger to becoming a trusted friend takes time and sensitivity while showing a genuine interest in the informants and respecting their ideas, beliefs, responses, and cultural ideas. Looking anew at informants' ideas and responses, and not assuming that *one knows all about them and their culture*, remains extremely important in ethnonursing research.

This enabler is used early and throughout the research process to assess one's relationship with the informants to get the desired accurate data (Leininger, 1991b). It is also valuable for conducting culturalogical assessments. By focusing on studying the attributes in the right and left parts of the enabler, one can gauge and assess progress in moving from distrusted

The purpose of this enabler is to facilitate the researcher (or it can be used by a clinician) to move from mainly a distrusted stranger to a trusted friend to obtain authentic, credible, and dependable data (or establish favorable relationships as a clinician). The user assesses him or herself by reflecting on the indicators as he/she moves from stranger to friend.

Indicators of Stranger (Largely *etic* or outsider's views) Informant(s) or people are:	Date Noted	Indicators as a Trusted Friend (Largely *emic* or insider's views) Informant(s) or people are:	Date Noted
Active to protect self and others. They are "gate-keepers" and guard against outside intrusions. Suspicious and questioning.		Less active to protect self. More trusting of researchers (their "gatekeeping is down or less"). Less suspicious and less questioning of researcher.	
Actively watch and are attentive to what researcher does and says. Limited signs of trusting the researcher or stranger.		Less watching the researcher's words and actions. More signs of trusting and accepting a new friend.	
Skeptical about the researcher's motives and work. May question how findings will be used by the researcher or stranger.		Less questioning of the researcher's motives, work, and behavior. Signs of working with and helping the researcher as a friend.	
Reluctant to share cultural secrets and views as private knowledge. Protective of local life-ways, values and beliefs. Dislikes probing by the researcher or stranger.		Willing to share cultural secrets and private world information and experiences. Offers most local views, values, and interpretations spontaneously or without probes.	
Uncomfortable to become a friend or to confide in stranger. May come late, be absent, and with-draw at times from researcher.		Signs of being comfortable and enjoying friends and a sharing relationship. Gives presence, on time, and gives evidence of being a "genuine friend."	
Tends to offer inaccurate data. Modifies "truths" to protect self, family, community, and cultural lifeways. *Emic* values, beliefs, and practices are not shared spontaneously.		Wants research "truths" to be accurate regarding beliefs, people, values, and lifeways. Explains and interprets *emic* ideas so researcher has accurate data.	
*Developed and used since 1959.			

FIGURE 4.1 • Leininger's Stranger-to-Trusted-Friend Enabler.
Adapted from Leininger, M. M. (2002). The theory of culture care and the ethnonursing research method. In M. M. Leininger & M. R. McFarland (Eds.), *Transcultural nursing: Concepts, theories, research, and practice* (3rd ed., p. 91). New York: McGraw-Hill Companies, Inc.

to trusted researcher (or nurse clinician). This enabler is an essential requirement for conducting ethnon-ursing research. With this enabler, the researcher can learn much about him/herself and the different attitudes, behaviors, and expectations of the people under study as he/she moves from a stranger to a trusted friend. When using this enabler, it is essential to document what occurs as the researcher moves from being a stranger to becoming a friend. As the nurse studies and uses the Stranger-to-Trusted-Friend Enabler, self-awareness increases as interpersonal and intercultural factors are uncovered. Considerable personal and professional growth occurs with nurses and other health care professionals who use this enabler consistently and regularly.

Leininger first developed this enabler in the 1960s with her first transcultural nursing research study in the Eastern Highlands of New Guinea. It has since been used for six decades in transcultural nursing with many reliable and scientific truths and benefits. The enabler has proven to be enormously helpful to nurses working in any culture, but especially those working with non-Western and unknown cultures. The Stranger-to-Trusted friend Enabler helps to obtain a wealth of *emic* and *etic* cultural data, including cultural detailed information about the informants and their beliefs, values, and lifeways while learning about oneself as a researcher and stranger.

Leininger's Observation-Participation-Reflection Enabler

Leininger's Observation-Participation-Reflection Enabler (Refer to Figure 4.2), also known as the *OPR Enabler*, is regularly used as a most helpful and essential guide to enable the researcher to enter and remain with informants in the familiar or natural cultural context while one is observing and engaging in the study. With this enabler, the researcher moves gradually from an *observer and listener* role to a *participant and reflector* role with the informant(s) or with phenomena under study. The researcher moves in slowly and politely after seeking permission to be with the informant. The gradual entry helps the researcher to first observe what is occurring naturally in the environment and with the people before, during, and after contact. Gradual entry and ongoing observation leading to participation and reflection places the focus on the informant rather than the researcher. The enabler encourages the researcher to observe the whole or total situation/phenomena under study while remaining an active listener.

Identifying symbols, documenting facts and historical events, and reflecting on reactions and interactions are all essential to obtaining comprehensive ethnonursing data. The OPR Enabler allows the researcher to gradually move into center visibility while maintaining a more *passive* than *active doing* role. Once this has occurred, one begins to feel and experience the actual shared lifeways of the people and become part of the on-going situation and interaction. At all times the researcher encourages informants to explain and interpret what is being observed, done, or experienced. With this enabler, the researcher studies daily and nightly experiences or events. They are clarified with the informants on an ongoing basis while the researcher respects and values what is shared or explained.

It is a crucial principle of ethnonursing research that the researcher remains an active observer, listener, and reflector while focusing on the domain of inquiry. The researcher learns how to use long silence-listening periods with cultural informants and how to respect and document gender status, especially with the elders and children. Remaining patient and keeping focused on what is being said or not said is essential to get in-depth data that is meaningful, sequential, and authentic. The researcher documents specific and unusual events, cultural care offenses, taboos, and activities that are acceptable and nonacceptable. Past and present stories, incidents, and historical events about care giving and receiving are important sources of information. Throughout the use of this enabler, the researcher remains alert to the Culture Care Theory tenets and especially to cultural diversities (variabilities/differences) and universalities (commonalties/similarities).

The researcher also reflects on transcultural nursing concepts, principles, definitions, and holding knowledge

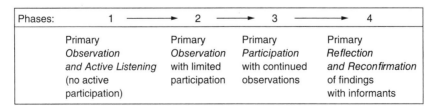

Phases:	1	2	3	4
	Primary *Observation and Active Listening* (no active participation)	Primary *Observation* with limited participation	Primary *Participation* with continued observations	Primary *Reflection and Reconfirmation* of findings with informants

FIGURE 4.2 • Leininger's Observation-Participation-Reflection Enabler.
Adapted from Leininger, M. M. (2002). The theory of culture care and the ethnonursing research method. In M. M. Leininger & M. R. McFarland (Eds.), *Transcultural nursing: Concepts, theories, research, and practice* (3rd ed., p. 90). New York: McGraw-Hill Companies, Inc.

about the culture to grasp what one observes and hears. Labeling, social profiling, or stereotyping are unacceptable in transcultural nursing and are, therefore, to be avoided. Transcultural nursing research mentors watch for these behavioral tendencies and discuss them with the researcher in an effort to prevent or address such propensities. This is often accomplished through the use of a researcher's daily journal or field log to record what has been observed, heard, and experienced with the enabler.

This enabler is also most valuable when conducting cultural assessments related to care and health practices. It should be noted that the *OPR Enabler* is quite different from the traditional participant-observation method used in anthropology in that the process is *reversed* and a reflection phase has been added. In addition, the OPR Enabler has explicit expectations to guide the researcher in each of its phases, which is different from the participant-observation method used in anthropology.

Leininger's Semi-Structured Inquiry Guide Enabler to Assess Culture Care and Health

This enabler (Refer to Figure 4.3), also referred to as *Leininger's Semi-Structured Inquiry Guide*, is used in ethnonursing research when conducting in-depth cultural assessments and interviews with key and general informants. It consists of a series of semi-structured, open ended inquiries, conceptualized around the Sunrise Enabler and the Culture Care Theory, with the aim of eliciting the cultural stories and emic perspectives of informants in relation to culture and care. This enabler can be adapted to fit the domain of inquiry for an ethnonursing study through the inclusion of culture-specific interview questions. The Semi-Structured Inquiry Guide assists the nurse to discover and understand the different dimensions related to cultural worldview, social structure, and all other domains of inquiry. *Holding knowledge* of these areas helps the nurse to reflect on what is seen and heard. With this enabler, factors such as ethnohistory and cultural and social structure dimensions are explored *with* the informant. This enabler offers some interview aids such as communication lead-ins and indirect suggestions to help nurses enter or follow along inside the informant's emic world by gently tapping into the

domains of inquiry. The nurse is encouraged to study this enabler in conjunction with the Sunrise Enabler as background preparation for a planned cultural assessment or interview.

When using this enabler, one must observe certain principles for conducting cultural assessments. Accordingly, the nurse remains open to the informant's ideas and leads. He/she makes nonobtrusive brief notations which are later processed in full using modern electronic data processing, qualitative data analysis software, and the Leininger-Templin-Thompson (LTT) Ethnoscript Coding Enabler. Throughout the interview process, the nurse seeks general cultural knowledge about different dimensions depicted in the Sunrise Enabler such as folk and professional care practices. He/she remains a very active listener and observer of both the informant and the context where the assessment occurs. The nurse constantly reflects on the different dimensions of the Sunrise Enabler and on how they help to discover aspects of care, health, wellbeing, disability, illness, or death. This process requires the nurse to focus on what he/she sees, hears, and discovers while permitting very little interference to the flow of the informant's ideas.

While doing so, the nurse must remain alert to and document any cultural-specific terms and meanings used by the informant(s). Nonverbal communication and use of space and language patterns (tone, style, and body gestures) need to also be identified. Keeping an open mind and a learning attitude are crucial to discover the informant's ideas and to avoid imposing one's own views and interpretations which may be ethnocentric. It is equally important to note subtle differences and commonalities about the informant's ideas and views in relation to others in the culture for a later comparative view. With each cultural assessment interview, the nurse increases and perfects his/her assessment skills and grasp of highly individualistic and comparative beliefs, practices, and needs.

Leininger's Acculturation Health Care Assessment Enabler for Cultural Patterns in Traditional and Nontraditional Lifeways

Leininger's Acculturation Health Care Assessment Enabler for Cultural Patterns in Traditional and

Instructions: The purpose of this enabler is to enter the world of the client and discover information to provide holistic, culture-specific care. Use broad and open inquiry modes rather than direct confrontational questions. Move with the client (or informant) to make the inquiry natural and familiar. These inquiry areas are examples for the inquiry and not exhaustive. Identify at the outset if assessing an individual, family, group, institution, or community. (This inquiry guide focuses on the individual). Identify yourself and the purpose of the inquiry to the client, e.g., to learn from the client about his/her lifeway to provide nursing care that will be helpful or meaningful.

Domains of Inquiry: Suggested Inquiry Modes

1. Worldview	I would like to know how you see the world around you. Could you share with me your views of how you see things are for you?
2. Ethnohistory	In nursing, we can benefit from learning about the client's cultural heritage, e.g., Korean, Philippine, etc. Could you tell me something about your cultural background? Where were you born and where have you been living in the recent past? Tell me about your parents and their origins. Have you and your parents lived in different geographic or environmental places? If so, tell me about your relocations and any special life events or experiences you recall that could be helpful to understand you and your needs. What languages do you speak? How would you like to be referred to by friends or strangers?
3. Kinship and Social Factors	I would like to hear about your family and/or close social friends and what they mean to you. How have your kin (relatives) or social friends influenced your life and especially your caring or healthy lifeways? Who are the caring or noncaring persons in your life? How has your family (or group) helped you to stay well or become ill? Do you view your family as a caring family? If not, what would make them more caring? Are there key family responsibilities to care for you or others when ill or well? Explain. In what ways would you like family members (or social friends) to care for you? How would you like nurses to care for you?
4. Cultural Values, Beliefs, and Lifeways	In providing nursing care, your cultural values, beliefs, and lifeways are important for nurses to understand. Could you share with me what values and beliefs you would like nurses to know to help you regain or maintain your health? What specific beliefs or practices do you find most important for others to know to care for you? Give me some examples of "good caring" ways based on your care values and beliefs.
5. Religious/Spiritual/Philosophical Factors	When people become ill or anticipate problems, they often pray or use their religion or spiritual beliefs. In nursing, we like to learn about how your religion has helped you in the past and can help you today. How do you think your beliefs and practices have helped you to care for yourself or others in keeping well or to regain health? How does religion help you heal or to face crisis, disabilities or even death? In what ways can religious healers and nurses care for you, your family or friends? What spiritual factors do we need to incorporate into your care?
6. Technological Factors	In your daily life, are you greatly dependent upon "high-tech" modern appliances or equipment? What about in the hospital to examine or care for you? (Explain.) In what ways do you think technological factors help or hinder keeping you well? Do you consider yourself dependent upon modern technologies to remain healthy or get access to care? Give some examples.
7. Economic Factors	One often hears "money means health or survival." What do you think of that statement? In what ways do you believe money influences your health and access to care or to obtain professional services? Do you find money is necessary to keep you well? If not, explain. How do you see the cost of hospital care versus home care cost practices? Optional: Who are the wage earners in your family? Do they earn enough to keep you well or help you if sick?

FIGURE 4.3 • Leininger's Semi-Structured Inquiry Guide Enabler to Assess Culture Care and Health.
Adapted and revised from Leininger, M. M. (2002). Culture care assessments for congruent competency practices. In M. M. Leininger & M. R. McFarland (Eds.), *Transcultural nursing: Concepts, theories, research, and practice* (3rd ed., pp. 137-139). New York: McGraw-Hill Companies, Inc.

8. Political and Legal Factors	Our world seems full of ideas about politics and political actions that can influence your health. What are some of your views about politics and how you and others maintain your wellbeing? In your community or home, what political or legal problems tend to influence your wellbeing or handicap your lifeways in being cared for by yourself or others? Explain.
9. Educational Factors	I would like to hear in what ways you believe education contributes to your staying well or becoming ill. What educational information, values or practices do you believe are important for nurses or others to care for you? Give examples. How has your education influenced you to stay well or become ill? How far did you go with formal education? Do you value education and health instruction? Explain.
10. Language and Communication Factors	Communicating with and understanding clients is important to meet care needs. How would you like to communicate your needs to nurses? What language(s) do you speak or understand? What is the primary language used in your family or cultural group? What barriers in language or communication influence receiving care or help from others. What verbal or nonverbal problems have you seen or experienced that influences caring patterns between you and the nursing staff? In what ways would you like people to communicate with you and why? Have you experienced any prejudice or racial problems through communication that nurses need to understand? What else would you like to tell me that would lead to good or effective communication practices with you?
11. Professional Care Beliefs and Practices	What professional nursing care practices or attitudes do you believe have been or would be most helpful to your wellbeing within the health care setting or at home? What types of professional care systems do you seek when ill? What professional care practices make sense to you or are most helpful? What professional care practices have contributed to your wellness? In what ways do health care professionals from different disciplines collaborate and communicate to provide your care? Have these been effective or helpful to you? If so, how? In what ways have your past or current experiences in the health care system influenced your recovery or health?
12. Generic (folk or lay) Care Beliefs and Practices	What home remedies, care practices, or treatments do you value or expect from a cultural viewpoint? I would like to learn about home healers or special healers in your community and how they help you. What does health, illness, or wellness mean to you and your family or culture? What folk practices make sense to you or are most helpful? Could you give some examples of healing or caring practices that come from your cultural group? What folk practices and food preferences have contributed to your wellness? What foods are taboo or prohibited in your life or in your culture? What other ideas should I know about what makes you well through good caring practices?
13. Biological Factors	What culture-bound syndromes are common in your culture? What illnesses/health issues are dominant in your culture? What genetic, physiological, chemical, or neurological conditions or phenomena are prevalent in your culture?
14. General and Specific Nursing Care Factors	In what ways would you like to be cared for in the hospital or home by nurses? What is the meaning of care to you or your culture? What do you see as the link between good nursing care and regaining or maintaining your health? Tell me about some of the barriers or facilitators to good nursing care. What values, beliefs or practices influence the ways you want nursing care? What stresses in the hospital or home need to be considered in your recovery or in staying well? What else would you like to tell me about ways to care for you? What community resources have helped you get well and stay well? Give some examples of nonhelpful care nursing practices. What environmental or home community factors should nurses be especially aware of to give care to you and your family? What cultural illnesses tend to occur in your culture? How do you manage pain and stress? Clarify. What else would you like to tell me so that you can receive what you believe is good nursing care? Give specific and general examples.

FIGURE 4.3 • *(Continued)*

Nontraditional Lifeways (Refer to Figure 4.4), often abridged as *The Acculturation Enabler,* is used when an examination of the extent of acculturation of the informants is desired or needed. This enabler assesses whether informants are *more traditionally or non-traditionally oriented in their values, beliefs, and general lifeways.* It is most frequently used when conducting culturalogical assessments and is also used during ethnonursing research studies. Acculturation is a critical factor in assessments to determine whether a client takes on or adopts the lifeways of another culture. This dimension of assessment is important so as to obtain the dominant patterns of caring and health practices, whether one is dealing with a traditional or new lifeway.

This enabler was developed and tested in several cultures since the early 1960s. It is one of the oldest and most continuous guides for assessing whether individuals are more traditionally or nontraditionally oriented to their cultures in diverse areas. This information influences how nurses and other health care providers plan care decisions and actions. Leininger's Acculturation Enabler was developed to obtain data with the Ethnonursing Research Method and the Culture Care Theory and has been used by several disciplines and health care providers to get credible, reliable, and meaningful assessment data about informants (Leininger, 1991b, 2002).

The strength of this enabler is that it allows for *holistic* assessments, especially when it is used with the Culture Care Theory and the Sunrise Enabler. It offers a systematic assessment of the person (or family) of a particular culture with respect to worldview, social structure factors, language use, environmental context, appearance, generic and professional care practices, and other areas. It is divided into two parts (Refer to Figure 4.4). In Part I, the nurse makes direct notations and uses this information in Part II to make a qualitative summary profile of the client regarding whether the person (or family) is more traditionally or nontraditionally oriented in cultural values, beliefs, and lifeways. The data are then used to develop guidelines or plans for nursing decisions and actions in collaboration with the client (or family) using the three modes of culture care decisions and actions, namely: *culture care maintenance and/or preservation; culture care accommodation and/or negotiation;* and *culture care repatterning and/or restructuring.*

It is crucial to document and describe the place where the assessment occurred such as the home, hospital, or another setting because the context can greatly influence the client's responses and their meanings. The nurse should jot down general observations about the home, setting, person, and environment as well as the narrative information shared by the client. The Acculturation Enabler is not intended to be used by the informant, but rather by the nurse who is responsible for the assessment and who uses the Culture Care Theory with the Sunrise Enabler. This enabler is also used as a research guide to analyze information in order to substantiate or refute theories related to the extent of acculturation by documenting past and present lifeways. It provides more qualitative data indicators than quantitative data, but has been used with both paradigms. This enabler provides a holistic picture or profile of cultural informants as related to care, health, and special needs of clients of diverse cultures.

Leininger's Phases of Ethnonursing Data Analysis Enabler for Qualitative Data

To facilitate systematic data analysis in ethnonursing and other qualitative research methods, Leininger developed *Leininger's Phases of Ethnonursing Data Analysis Enabler for Qualitative Data* (Refer to Figure 4.5) and confirmed its use with more than 100 studies over the past six decades (Leininger, 1991b, 1995). The four phases provide a systematic data analysis when thoughtfully, accurately, and rigorously used. This enabler is often used in conjunction with the *Leininger-Templin-Thompson (LTT) Ethnoscript Coding Enabler* to process the large amount of grounded raw qualitative data gathered from in-depth interviews (Leininger, Templin, & Thompson, 1990) with key and general informants, researcher observations, and other data collected throughout the research process. Data analysis is an ongoing process that begins with the initiation of the study. All gathered data is transcribed, processed through a computer using a qualitative research software, coded, and classified for ongoing analysis and abstraction at each phase of analysis that ultimately results in findings of universal and diverse themes (Wehbe-Alamah & McFarland, 2015b).

During the *first phase,* the researcher collects, describes, documents, and begins to analyze raw data related to the purposes of the study, the domain of inquiry (DOI) or questions under study. Collected

Name of Assessor: _____ Date: _____

Informants or Code No.: _____ Sex: _____ Age: _____

Place or Context of Assessment: _____

Directions: This enabler provides a general qualitative profile or assessment of traditional or nontraditional orientation of informants of their patterned lifeways. Health care influencers are assessed with respect to worldview, language, cultural values, kinship, religion, politics, technology, education, environment, and related areas. This profile is primarily focused on *emic* (local) information to assess and guide health personnel in working with individuals and groups. The *etic* (or more universal view) also may be evident. In Part I, the user observes, records, and rates behavior on the scale below from 1 to 5 with respect to traditional or nontraditionally oriented lifeways. Numbers are plotted on the summary Part II to obtain a qualitative profile to guide decisions and actions. The user's brief notations on each criterion should be used to support ratings and reliable profile. This enabler was not designed for quantitative measurements, but rather as a qualitative enabler to explicate data from informants.

....

Part I: Rating of Criteria to Assess Traditional and Nontraditional Patterned Cultural Lifeways or Orientations

Rating indicators:	Mainly Traditional 1	Moderate 2	Average 3	Moderate 4	Mainly Nontraditional 5	Rater Value No.

Cultural Dimensions to Assess Traditional or Nontraditional Orientations

1. Language, Communication, and Gestures (Native or Non-native). Notations: _____
    _____
    _____
    _____

2. General Environmental Living Context (Symbols, material, and nonmaterial signs). Specify: _____
    _____
    _____

3. Wearing Apparel and Physical Appearance. Notations: _____
    _____
    _____

4. Technology Being Used in Living Environment. Notations: _____
    _____
    _____

5. Worldview (How person looks out upon the world). Notations: _____
    _____
    _____

6. Family Lifeways (Values, beliefs, and norms). Notations: _____
    _____

FIGURE 4.4 • Leininger's Acculturation Health Care Assessment Enabler for Cultural Patterns in Traditional and Nontraditional Lifeways.

Rating indicators:	Mainly Traditional 1	Moderate 2	Average 3	Moderate 4	Mainly Nontraditional 5	Rater Value No.

7. General Social Interactions and Kinship Ties. Notations: _____
_____
_____

8. Patterned Daily Activities. Notations: _____
_____
_____

9. Religious (or Spiritual) Beliefs and Values. Notations: _____
_____
_____

10. Economic Factors (Rough cost of living estimates and income). Notations: _____
_____
_____

11. Educational Values or Belief Factors. Notations: _____
_____
_____

12. Political or Legal Influencers. Notations: _____
_____
_____

13. Food Uses and Nutritional Values, Beliefs, and Taboos. Specify: _____
_____
_____

14. *Folk* (Generic or Indigenous) *Health Care* (-*Cure*) Values, Beliefs
& Practices. Specify: _____
_____
_____

15. *Professional Health Care* (-*Cure*) Values, Beliefs, and Practices. Specify: _____
_____
_____

16. Care Concepts or Patterns that guide actions, (i.e., concern for, support, presence, etc.):
_____
_____
_____

17. Caring Patterns or Expressions: _____
_____
_____

18. Views of Ways to: a) Prevent illnesses: _____
b) Preserve or maintain wellness or health: _____
c) Care for self or others: _____
_____
_____

19. Other Indicators to support more traditional or nontraditional lifeways: _____
_____
_____
_____

FIGURE 4.4 • *(Continued)*

Part II: Acculturation Profile from Assessment Factors

Directions: Plot an X with the value numbers rated on this profile to discover the orientation or acculturation gradient of the informant. The clustering of numbers will give information of traditional or nontraditional patterns with respect to the criteria assessed.

Criteria	1 Mainly Traditional	2 Moderate	3 Average	4 Moderate	5 Mainly Nontraditional
1. Language and Communication Modes					
2. Physical Environment					
3. Physical Apparel and Appearance					
4. Technology					
5. World View					
6. Family Lifeways					
7. Social Interaction and Kinship					
8. Daily Lifeways					
9. Religious Orientation					
10. Economic Factors					
11. Educational Factors					
12. Political and Legal Factors					
13. Food Uses					
14. Folk (Generic) Care-Cure					
15. Professional Care-Cure Expressions					
16. Caring Patterns					
17. Curing Patterns					
18. Prevention/ Maintenance Factors					
19. Other Indicators					

Note: The assessor may total numbers to get a summary orientation profile. Use of these ratings with written notations provide a wholistic qualitative profile. Detailed notations are important to substantiate the ratings. This guide has been developed, refined, and used since early 1960s by Dr. Madeleine Leininger and other anthropologists and transcultural nurses. It has been useful to obtain informants' orientation to traditional or non traditional lifeways. It provides qualitative indicators to meet credibility, confirmability, meaning-in-context, and recurrent patterning criteria for qualitative studies.

FIGURE 4.4 • *(Continued)*

data includes interviews from key and general informants, identification of contextual meanings and symbols, and data related to the DOI or phenomenon under study mainly from an emic focus. Attention is given to etic ideas which are also recorded including researcher observations, field journals, accounts of participatory experiences, and preliminary data interpretations. All data are processed electronically into a computer in preparation for the second phase of ethnonursing data analysis.

During the *second phase*, all processed data are coded, categorized, and classified as they relate to the domain of inquiry, and sometimes, the research questions. Emic and etic descriptors are studied within ontexts and for similarities and differences. Recurrent components are studied for their cultural meanings. When large amounts of data are present, the coding process is simplified through the use of the *Leininger-Templin-Thompson (LTT) Ethnoscript Coding Enabler*, discussed later in this chapter. Data categorization and classification are

---

First Phase

Collecting, Describing, and Documenting Raw Data into a Computer

The researcher collects, describes, documents, and begins to analyze raw data related to the purposes, domain of inquiry, or questions under study. This phase includes recording data with emic foci such as interviews with key and general informants; identifying contextual meanings; and identifying symbols, as well as data with etic foci such as documenting observations and field journals; recording participatory experiences; and making preliminary interpretations. All data are processed directly into a computer.

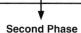

Second Phase

Identification and Categorization of Descriptors and Components

Data are coded and classified as related to the domain or inquiry and sometimes the questions under study. Emic and etic descriptors are studied within context and for similarities and differences. Recurrent components are studied for their meanings.

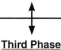

Third Phase

Pattern and Contextual Analysis

Data are scrutinized to discover saturation of ideas and recurrent patterns of similar or different meanings, expressions, structural forms, interpretations, or explanations of data related to the domain of inquiry. Data are also examined to show patterning with respect to meanings-in-context and along with further credibility and confirmability of findings.

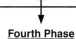

Fourth Phase

Major Themes, Research Findings, Theoretical Formulations, and Recommendations

This is the highest phase of data analysis, synthesis, and interpretation. It requires synthesis of thinking, configuration analysis, interpretation of findings, and creative formulation based on data from the previous phases. The researcher's task is to abstract and confirm major themes, research findings, recommendations, and sometimes make new theoretical formulations.

FIGURE 4.5 • Leininger's Phases of Ethnonursing Data Analysis Enabler for Qualitative Data.
Adapted and revised from Leininger, M. M. (2002). The theory of culture care and the ethnonursing research method. In M. M. Leininger & M. R. McFarland (Eds.), *Transcultural nursing: Concepts, theories, research, and practice* (3rd ed., p. 95). New York: McGraw-Hill Companies, Inc.

then facilitated through the use of a qualitative research software such as NVivo or ATLAS.ti.

The third and fourth phases of data analysis require that the researcher identify recurrent patterns (*third phase*) and themes (*fourth phase*). In the third phase, data are scrutinized to discover saturation of ideas and recurrent patterns of similar or different meanings, expressions, structural forms, interpretations, or explanations of data related to the domain of inquiry. Data are also examined to show patterning with respect to meanings-in-context along with further determining the credibility and confirmability of the findings. In the fourth phase, the researcher not only thoughtfully analyzes the patterns into abstracted themes but arrives at synthesized formulations of the findings derived from data gathered in the previous three phases.

The fourth phase requires the researcher to engage in the highest level of abstraction, *critical thinking* and *creative reflections*, to synthesize the findings into dominant care themes related to the domain of inquiry and theory tenets in order to arrive at succinct, accurate, and usually powerful explanatory themes from the mass of rich data processed. The researcher rechecks and does audits trails of all analysis themes ensure they are substantiated with grounded evidence and credibility from the raw data of the informants. The term *substantiation of findings* is used for reporting ethnonursing and other qualitative results rather than verification or generalization as the latter are used with quantitative research studies. These themes are clearly stated as the major dominant ones that guide nurses in providing culturally congruent and relevant care for cultures—the ultimate goal of the theory—to lead to optimal health and wellbeing and assist during disability, illness, or dying.

Transcultural nursing research mentors who are experienced with the ethnonursing method can be of great help to facilitate the researcher's thinking during the abstraction of the major themes in order to obtain high or powerful levels of formulations for meaningful analysis of themes. The ethnonursing researcher who has collected the data from informants becomes the key person to analyze the findings for credibility and accuracy. The unique feature of the Ethnonursing Research Method is that the findings are firmly grounded with the cultural informants, and in having both emic and etic findings. The researcher may share

his/her own responses, special views, and immersion experiences with the culture and informants. The researcher's narratives and ongoing extensive experiences over time are always of interest to readers so as to grasp the nature of the interactive transcultural research process. The comparative perspectives of diversities and similarities with emic and etic findings among informants are important to document. Special experiences of the researcher, informants, and community participants are important in revealing *humanistic* findings (Leininger, 2000).

During the final review of the Phases of Ethnonursing Data Analysis for Qualitative Data, the researcher rechecks the final themes to ensure that they are supported by the data discovered in all phases of the analysis. Such a rigorous and systematic analysis shows the study reader how the data were substantiated and how the themes and the conclusions were reached.

The Leininger-Templin-Thompson (LTT) Ethnoscript Coding Enabler

In 1985, the Leininger-Templin-Thompson (LTT) Ethnoscript Qualitative Software was developed to facilitate the collection, processing, and analysis of large amounts of data discovered in ethnonursing research studies as conceptualized within Leininger's Theory of Culture care Diversity and Universality (Leininger, 1987; Leininger, Templin, & Thompson, 1991). The software was refined and tested by several doctoral nursing students under Dr. Leininger's mentorship.

At that time, the software was a welcomed innovation that allowed for the analysis of large amounts of detailed qualitative data using (new) computer technology. It integrated a coding process structured around important tenets and elements of the Culture Care Theory (CCT) and the Sunrise Enabler such as worldview; cultural and social structure dimensions; language; ethnohistorical and environmental contexts; and generic (folk) and professional health care practices (Leininger, 1991b). While the LTT Ethnoscript Qualitative Software is no longer used, the coding system originally developed for it has been adapted and converted into *the Leininger-Templin-Thompson Ethnoscript Coding Enabler* (Refer to Figure 4.6) to assist ethnonursing researchers in coding and categorizing large amounts of study data within the framework of the CCT.

Code Numbers, Categories, and Domains of Information: (Includes processing of observations, interviews, interpretations, material, and nonmaterial data)

<u>**Code Numbers**</u>   <u>**Categories and Domains of Information**</u>

Category I: General Cultural and Holistic Domains of Inquiry

1	Worldview
2	Cultural–social lifeways and activities (typical day/night)
3	Ethnohistorical (includes chrono-data, acculturation, cultural contacts, etc.)
4	Environmental contexts (i.e., physical, ecological, cultural, social)
5	Linguistic terms and meanings
6	Cultural foods related to care, health, illness, and environment
7	Material and nonmaterial culture (includes symbols and meanings)
8	Ethnodemographics (numerical facts, dates, population size, and other numerical data)
9	*

Category II: Domain of Cultural and Social Structural Data

(Includes normative values, patterns, functions, and conflicts)

10	Cultural values, benefits, norms
11	Economic factors
12	Educational factors
13	Kinship (family ties, social network, social relationships, etc.)
14	Political and legal factors
15	Religious, philosophical, and ethical values and beliefs
16	Technological factors
17	Interpersonal relationships (individual groups or institutions)
18	*
19	*

Category III: Care, Cure, Health (Wellbeing), and Illness of Folk and Professional Lifeways and Systems

20	Folk (includes popular health and illness benefits, values, and practices)
21	Professional health
22	Human care/caring and nursing (general beliefs, values, and practices)
23	Folk care/caring (emic or indigenous beliefs, values, and lifeways)
24	Professional care/caring (etic beliefs, values, lifeways)
25	Professional nursing care/caring (etic and emic) lifeways (congruence and conflict areas)
26	Noncare/caring beliefs, values, and practices
27	Human cure/curing beliefs, values, and practices

FIGURE 4.6 • The Leininger-Templin-Thompson (LTT) Ethnoscript Coding Enabler.

Reproduced, with permission, from Wehbe-Alamah, H.B., & McFarland, M.R. (2015). Leininger's enablers for use with the ethnonursing research method. In M.R. McFarland, & H.B. Wehbe-Alamah (Eds.), *Culture care diversity and universality: A worldwide nursing theory* (3rd ed., pp. 92-94). Burlington, MA: Jones & Bartlett Learning, www.jblearning.com. Adapted from Leininger, M. M., Templin, T., Thompson, F. (1991). *The Leininger-Templin- Thompson Ethnoscript Qualitative Program User's Handbook* (pp. 16-19), Wayne State University (MI), the Madeleine M. Leininger Collection on Human Caring and Transcultural Nursing (ARC-008, Folder 6-29). Retrieved from the Archives of Caring in Nursing, Christine E. Lynn College of Nursing, Florida Atlantic University, Boca Raton, FL.

Code Numbers	Categories and Domains of Information
28	Folk and generic cure/curing (etic beliefs, values, and practices)
29	Professional cure/curing (etic and emic perspectives)
30	Alternative or emerging care/cure systems
31	*
32	*
33	*
34	*

Category IV: Health Care, Social Structure Institutions/Systems

(Includes administrative norms, beliefs, and practices with meanings-in-context)

35	Cultural–social norms, beliefs, values, and context
36	Political–legal factors
37	Economic factors
38	Technological factors
39	Environmental factors
40	Educational factors (formal and informal)
41	Social organization or structural factors
42	Decisions and action patterns
43	Inter- and multidisciplinary norms, values, and collaborative practices
44	Nursing specialties and features
45	Non-nursing specialties and features
46	Ethical/moral care-cure factors
47	*
48	*
49	*

Category V: Life Cycle with Inter- and Intragenerational Patterns

(Includes ceremonies, beliefs, and rituals)

50	Life cycle male and female enculturation and socialization processes
51	Infancy and early childhood years
52	Adolescence (or transitions) to adulthood
53	Middlescence years
54	Advanced years
55	Cultural life-cycle values, beliefs and practices
56	Cultural life-cycle intra and intergenerational conflict areas
57	Special life-cycle subcultures and groups
58	Life passages (includes birth, marriage, death)
59	*
60	*

FIGURE 4.6 • *(Continued)*

Code Numbers	Categories and Domains of Information
Category VI: Methodological, Reflections, Issues, and Research Features	
61	Specific methods or techniques used
62	Key informants
63	General informants
64	Enabling tools or instruments used
65	Problem areas, concerns or conflicts
66	Strengths, favorable and unanticipated outcomes of researcher or informants, subjective data and questions
67	Unusual incidents, interpretations, questions, etc.
68	Factors facilitating or hindering the study (time, staff, money, etc.)
69	Emic data methodological issues
70	Etic data methodological issues
71	Dialogue by interviewer
72	Dialogue by someone other than informant or interviewer
73	Additional contextual data (includes nonverbal symbols, total view, environmental features, etc.)
74	Informed consent factors
75-100	*

*Denotes areas where researcher adds own additional codes and descriptions

FIGURE 4.6 • *(Continued)*

1. Introduce yourself and explain that you would like to obtain the person's life and health history. Indicate how such a history could be helpful to health personnel and of interest to him or her. Answer questions or clarify concerns of the individual. Obtain written permission from the individual for the autobiographical or biographical health history study (clarify the differences in these methods).
2. If the individual wishes to write his or her own life history (an autobiography), encourage him to write in his own style, but ask him to include his views and experiences about health, care, and illness patterns in order to help him and others benefit from such knowledge. Clarify how you plan to use the research findings.
3. If you are writing the individual's health and care history biographical account, proceed as follows:
    A. Plan to record the information before initiating the interview. Use unobtrusive materials so that you do not distract the informant in telling his history. If you are using a tape recorder, choose one hour tapes to prevent disruption in the flow of the life history with the informant. Written permission must be obtained from the informant prior to any recording (follow the requirements of the committee for human subjects research). If you use ethnographic field notes, you may wish to use the guidelines already described by the author in this book, or use Spradley's suggestions for record keeping (Spradley, 1979, 1980). It is important to note that some informants are not comfortable with having their life history taped and their request must be respected. If an informant consents to taping, offer him or her a copy of the tape without cost. (Usually the informant does want a copy.) If taping is not agreed to, use a stenographer's pad and record words and an outline of what you are observing and talking about. Immediately after the history taking, write in detail what you observed, heard, and talked about. Do not wait hours or days, as recall is difficult and accuracy decreases.
    B. Use primarily the ethnographic open-ended type of interview method described in this book or in Spradley's book (1979) to encourage and promote an open flow of information. The researcher's introductory comment might be, "I would like to learn about you and how you have known and experienced health, caring, illness, or disabilities." "As

FIGURE 4.7 • The Life History Health Care Enabler.
Adapted, with permission, from MacNeil, J. (1994). Culture care: Meanings, patterns and expressions for Baganda women as AIDS caregivers within Leininger's theory (pp. 144-146). (Doctoral dissertation, Wayne State University). Available from ProQuest Dissertations & Theses database. (UMI No. 9519922).

a nurse, I am interested in your past and present lifeways so I can learn what has made you healthy or less healthy, and who you believe have been caring persons in your life." "Feel free to offer special stories or events as you recall ideas important to you." (Clarify as needed how this information may be helpful to nurses to improve nursing care.)

C.   Suggest some life history domains or topic areas on which to focus, using with leadin statements with a sequence, such as the following:

(1)   "Let us talk about where you were born and what you remember about your early days of growing up, keeping well, or experiencing illness."

(2)   "Can you recall special events, experiences, and health practices during childhood and adolescent years that were especially important to you in keeping well, or that limited your wellness or healthiness?"

(3)   "Let us talk about your special health care experiences that were particularly clear and pleasant (or unpleasant) to you regarding these periods in your life" (encourage use of folk stories, humorous tales, and descriptions of special events):
   a.   Early childhood days
   b.   Adolescent years
   c.   Midlife years
   d.   Older years

(4)   "Give some examples of healthy caring activities or ways of living by your family, cultural group, or significant people who helped you."

(5)   "As you think about your life experiences to date, what do you recall about these experiences and what did you value most or least about":
   a.   Going to school (primary, secondary, and college days) and your health status.
   b.   Employment experiences and how you viewed or experienced them as healthy or less healthy.
   c.   Marriage or remaining single throughout life (stresses or nonstresses).
   d.   Sudden (or gradual) death of loved persons and how such experiences influenced your thinking and health status.
   e.   Accident or illness events to you, your family, or friends and the care expressions.

(6)   "I would like to hear about your general philosophy of keeping well and how you believe your religion, political, and cultural values have helped (or hindered) your life goals and health. Can you tell me what beliefs or values have especially guided you to remaining well or become ill?" (Give examples.)

(7)   "Can you recall special folk or professional health and caring experiences that were most important to you during your life regarding the following topics?"
   a.   Staying well (or becoming ill).
   b.   Becoming disabled (and maintaining/getting well).
   c.   Experiencing or dealing with healthy patterns of living.
   d.   Recovering from a traumatic experiences as perceived by you.

(8)   "Can you recall who you believe were good caretakers in the past (and today) and what made them such good caretakers? What noncaring persons influenced your lifestyle or made life difficult or unhealthy for you? What caregivers were important in your life and what made them so? Can you tell me about nurses as caretakers?"

(9)   "Throughout your life, what factors seemed to keep you going, living, or establishing healthy patterns of living for yourself and others?"

(10)   "What have been some of the greatest rewards or joys in your life? The least rewarding and why? How are these joys related to health or illness?"

(11)   "Feel free to tell me other aspects of your life so I can understand it as fully as possible. You can tell me stories, jokes, healing practices, and any special events you believe I should know about to understand you."

D.   *Writing and Checking the History.* Covering the above life history points (and others the researchers wishes to include) will take several sessions–usually three to four. Upon completion of the history, you should carefully review and check the history, and then clarify vague points immediately while fresh in the mind of informant. Use the informants own words and account as much as possible. Thank the informant and make plans to confirm and share the written (biographical) account. If the account is autobiographical, return and go over the written account to be sure it is understandable and readable, suitable for reproduction as a written document. Express appreciation for the informant's time and information. Present a copy of the tape(s) to the informant. Be sure to provide sufficient time after you have written the account to clarify, confirm, re-examine, or explicate ideas from the informant.

FIGURE 4.7 • *(Continued)*

E.   *Analysis of Data.* Analyzing the data is a creative art and skill in that the researcher must consciously preserve the informant's statements, but still identify salient themes and synthesize life events in context. It is also an art and skill to both write a health and care life history and keep it accurate and interesting. The verbatim and sequenced account is preserved. Generally thematic, semantic, contextual, and general textual analyses of the data are done with life histories as part of the researcher's separate but special analysis. (See other chapters in this book on these methodological approaches.) Try to identify and analyze patterns of health, care, and illness (if present) so that a synthesis of ideas can be readily identified and used by research consumers. The researcher may wish to present the raw biographical data to the informant and retain theoretical and complex data for the researcher, still sharing dominant findings with the informant at the end of the study.

FIGURE 4.7 • *(Continued)*

The Life History Health Care Enabler

The Life History Health Care Enabler (Refer to Figure 4.7) is a guide that facilitates the discovery of longitudinal data about *the lived experiences of informants across their lifespan* while focusing on care, caring, and related nursing aspects (Wehbe-Alamah & McFarland, 2015a). This enabler was designed to discover a thorough and detailed description from informants about their healthy or less healthy caring lifeways and the care beliefs and practices that influence their wellbeing.

Use of this enabler has resulted in unearthing rich and comprehensive data with respect to human caring, expressions, meanings, and health values (Leininger, 1985b). When conducting ethnonursing research, the Life History Health Care Enabler assists in the discovery of longitudinal narratives about informants' experiences in generic (folk) and professional (etic) health care at the home and/or institutional settings. It also helps to tease out historical insights about health care values and practices across the lifespan.

Other Enablers Developed by Leininger

Over the years, Leininger also developed other enablers that were either used with specific studies or later on eventually became enfolded into some of the enablers previously described. Some examples of such enablers include: Audio-Visual Guide; Cultural Care Values and Meanings; Generic and Professional Care Enabler Guide; Cross-Cultural Interview Guide to Study Ethnonursing, Caring, and Related Aspects; Culturalogical [Cultural] Care Assessment Guide; and Ethnonursing Field Research Data Form (Leininger, 1985a, 1988; Wehbe-Alamah & McFarland, 2015a).

■ CRITERIA TO EVALUATE QUALITATIVE RESEARCH STUDIES

Realizing in the 1960s and 1970s that too few nurses were educated in qualitative methods and many were using quantitative criteria (such as validity, reliability, and other statistical criteria) to evaluate findings from qualitative investigations to have their research findings accepted by other colleagues, Leininger engaged in an intensive and extensive literature study and identified specific qualitative criteria for qualitative studies (Leininger, 1997a). Consequently, she developed six major criteria to evaluate qualitative paradigmatic investigations (including ethnonursing) that have been defined and used for the past six decades. These criteria, which have been supported by educational researchers such as Lincoln and Guba (1985), are as follows (Leininger, 1997b, 1991b):

• *Credibility* refers to the "truth," accuracy, and believability of findings that have been mutually established between the researcher and the informants as accurate, believable, and credible about the experiences and knowledge of phenomena (Wehbe-Alamah & McFarland, 2015b, pp. 56-57). Truths are sought as direct sources of emic evidence or information from the people within their environmental contexts and are held firmly as believable to them. The researcher's observations and documentation of meanings-in-contexts, specific situations, and events as well as the direct experiences with the people over time, *and* the people's interpretations or explanations, serve to substantiate the emic truths, beliefs, and values.
• *Confirmability* refers to repeated direct and documented objective and subjective data confirmed

with the informants, primarily through observed and primary informant source data, and recurrent explanations or interpretive data from informants about certain phenomena (Wehbe-Alamah & McFarland, 2015b, p. 57). Confirmability indicates that the researcher has confirmed with informants over time what he/she has heard, seen, or experienced with respect to the phenomena under study in familiar and natural living contexts.

- *Meaning-In-Context* refers to findings that are understandable to informants studied within their natural and familiar environmental contexts (Wehbe-Alamah & McFarland, 2015b, p. 57). The significance of interpretations and understanding of symbols, actions, events, communication, and other human activities within specific or cultural contexts is the fundamental aspect of this criterion.
- *Recurrent Patterning* refers to repeated instances, patterns of expressions, sequences of events, experiences, or lifeways that tend to recur over a period of time in designated ways and contexts (Wehbe-Alamah & McFarland, 2015b, p. 57). The documented evidence of repeated experiences, expressions, events, and acts over time reflect consistency in lifeways or patterned behaviors support this criterion.
- *Saturation* refers to the exhaustive search from informants of data relevant to the domain of inquiry in which no new findings are forthcoming from informants (Wehbe-Alamah & McFarland, 2015b, p. 57). This criterion is reached when informants no longer offer new findings and all gathered information is redundant or duplicated.
- *Transferability* refers to whether particular findings from a qualitative study can be transferred to another similar context or situation and still preserve the particularized meanings, interpretations, and inferences of the completed study (Wehbe-Alamah & McFarland, 2015b, p. 58).

Leininger's criteria for evaluation of qualitative research studies should be studied before beginning a qualitative investigation such as an ethnonursing study. They are specifically, thoughtfully, and discerningly used with qualitative data to arrive at accurate interpretations and credible findings. These criteria are documented during the study and rechecked in the final analysis as the researcher uses *The Phases of*

Quantitative Data Analysis Enabler (Leininger, 2002). The criteria are identified and documented while collecting data. The reader is encouraged to read other studies to understand the uses of the qualitative criteria to ensure accuracy from the beginning to the end of the research. The qualitative researcher needs to remain cognizant that the goal of qualitative studies is *not to produce generalizations* but rather to document, understand, and substantiate the meanings, attributes, patterns, symbols, metaphors, and other data features related to the domain of inquiry under study while drawing heavily on informant data. The researcher will find using these qualitative criteria most rewarding as they confirm and reaffirm their findings with the informants throughout the study and again during the final analysis and interpretation of findings.

■ GUIDE TO USING THE ETHNONURSING RESEARCH METHOD

In studying any theory, it is important to understand and use an appropriate research method to collect and analyze data. While the Culture Care Theory may be used with any qualitative research method, the Ethnonursing Research Method was developed specifically for use with the Culture Care Theory. Ethnonursing research embodies a very systematic and rigorous investigative process to ensure a sound study. For newcomers to the Culture Care Theory and ethnonursing research, it is wise to begin with studying individuals and then gradually master researching families, groups, communities, and institutions, which are more complex. The researcher needs to remain focused on the theory tenets and the domain of inquiry under study (the latter varies with each researcher). In this section, an overview of the ethnonursing research process is presented, but the reader is encouraged to study further the method by reading completed research studies. A review of the literature conducted in April 2017 using the search terms *Ethnonursing*, *Culture Care*, and *Leininger* resulted in the identification of 361 master's and doctoral studies, which are listed in chronological order in the Appendix at the end of this book.

The sequential steps for the Ethnonursing Research Method are explained below to guide the researcher in formulating and planning their own ethnonursing studies (adapted from Leininger, 2002; Wehbe-Alamah & McFarland, 2015b):

1. **Identify focus and general intent of study.**
   a. Identification of *domain of inquiry* (DOI): The first step in using the Ethnonursing Research Method is to clearly and succinctly state the DOI being studied by the researcher. *The DOI is the major focus of the research.* All key words stated in the DOI are thoughtfully selected as the researcher studies them comprehensively and in-depth with key and general informants. For example, some stated domains of inquiry might be: *Culture care meanings, expressions, and patterns of elderly Old Order Amish*; *Generic care practices of Chinese mothers living in a rural community*; or *Afro-British teenagers and their cultural needs in an urban context.* The researcher has the full responsibility to discover all aspects of the DOI under study. Superficial knowledge is inadequate and would fail to provide for a sound ethnonursing research investigation.
   b. Formulation of research questions: A few research questions are usually stated after the DOI to ensure that every idea in the domain is completely explicated and fully studied. An example of a DOI is presented next followed by its research questions. The DOI statement is: *Culture care meanings, expressions, and patterns of caring with Japanese families.* The related research questions are:

      - What is the meaning of care (caring) to Japanese families?
      - What are generic care practices used by Japanese families?
      - In what ways can nurses use the three modes of culture care decisions and actions to provide culturally congruent care to Japanese families?

   c. Stating the purpose(s) and goal(s) of the study: The researcher clearly states the purpose(s) and goal(s) of the study and identifies the potential relevance or significance of this study to advance transcultural nursing or related nursing knowledge and practice areas. In general, the purpose of an ethnonursing research study is discovery of aspects pertaining to the DOI while the goal is related to application of findings to the relevant setting [clinical practice, academic, or others]. Periodically, the researcher may need to clarify with informants the purposes or intent of the study to avoid misunderstandings.
   d. Consultation with ethnonursing research expert or mentor: The researcher consults with and discusses the research process, scope of the study, and DOI with a transcultural nursing research mentor or expert to ensure clear domains, theoretical ideas, and research plans. It is highly encouraged that the researcher—especially when new to the method—confer with an experienced transcultural nursing mentor to provide insights and to help the researcher hold personal biases or prejudices in check. To reduce transcultural nurse biases and prejudices, considerable time is spent in transcultural nursing courses learning to deal with such realistic concerns under the guidance of experienced transcultural nurse mentors.

2. **Identify the potential significance of the study to nursing practice, research, and education.** The researcher addresses the benefits and influences of the proposed study toward advancing the body of nursing knowledge in the areas of academia, practice, and research.

3. **Fully review the literature related to the domain of inquiry under study and other studies close to the DOI.** The researcher engages in a review of the literature (ROL) to gather holding knowledge that will assist with the conceptualization of a research plan and the development of interview questions. He/she identifies how these studies are similar to or different from his/her DOI. The ROL may include qualitative as well as quantitative studies related to the DOI. Holding knowledge derived from the ROL can also be integrated later in the discussion of study results.

4. **Conceptualize a research plan for the study.**
   a. Theoretical conceptualizations: The researcher conceptualizes orientational (not operational) definitions, theoretical interests, and assumptive premises derived from the CCT to study the DOI.
   b. Research site, barriers and facilitators, informed consent, and human subject considerations:

The researcher decides on appropriate research site and obtains permissions (from gatekeeper, institutions, organizations, or communities) needed to secure entry into the research site. The researcher seeks and obtains consent from institutions or community agencies necessary to protect informants' and institutional rights. Anonymity of informants is assured through the use of code names or code numbers in lieu of real names and to prevent the identification of the informants and institutions. Consent and other important forms are kept confidential and in locked files. The researcher addresses potential barriers and facilitators for conducting the research, as well as the informed consent procedures, and the informant's/participant's right to withdraw from the study at any point in time. Interestingly, very few withdrawals have occurred with ethnonursing studies as informants have usually liked the method and been eager to share their (emic) cultural stories and views, as well as past experiences with professional care practices. When use of a tape recorder and/or camera is desired to record interviews or take pictures and/or videos, obtaining permission from the informants is necessary to protect their rights. Members of some cultures may consider their spoken word better than a written document, and therefore refuse to sign the written forms, such as the Old Order Amish (Leininger, 2002).

c. Selection of enablers: The researcher decides on the appropriate selection of Leininger's enablers to use in the study. He/she may decide to develop additional study-specific enablers to guide his/her research. Some enablers, such as *The Observation-Participation-Reflection Enabler* and *The Stranger to-Trusted-Friend Enabler* are integral parts of the Ethnonursing Research Method and should therefore be used in all ethnonursing studies.

d. Informants' selection criteria and interview considerations: The researcher develops criteria for the selection of informants and thoughtfully and purposefully selects *key* and *general* informants after identifying potential participants for the study. *Key informants* are usually studied *in-depth*, while *general informants* are

studied for their reflections and for representations in the wider community or context. Generally, extensive and multiple sessions are held with key informants to elicit discoveries related to the DOI. In contrast, the researcher engages in fewer and shorter sessions with the general informants who provide *general ideas* about the DOI.

e. Criteria for maxi and mini studies: For a *maxi* ethnonursing study, usually 12 to 15 *key informants* are selected and approximately 20 to 25 *general informants* are needed. For a *mini* study (often done as a pilot study before conducting a maxi study) about six to eight key and 10 to 12 general informants are needed. The mini (or smaller) study helps the researcher to gain considerable skills and confidence for conducting a large or maxi study. Often, baccalaureate and master nursing students perform mini studies, whereas doctoral students are expected to conduct maxi investigations. Based on nearly six decades of research conducted by transcultural nurse research experts as well as many nursing students, the numbers of informants for both maxi and mini studies have been found to be reliable for reaching saturation *and* for meeting the six qualitative evaluation criteria for ethnonursing research findings.

f. Research timeline: How long one spends doing an ethnonursing study depends on the domain of inquiry and whether the research is a maxi or mini study. The researcher must communicate with the informants from the very beginning of the study the plan for exiting the research site upon conclusion of study.

g. Communication, field data, and ongoing reflection and data analysis: During the study, the researcher tries to maintain a nonobtrusive or nondominating position while observing, talking to, or participating with the people. Exhibiting a genuine interest and becoming immersed in the culture are important. Learning with "new ears and eyes" about the people and their culture care brings many knowledge rewards. It is the responsibility of the primary researcher to regularly and systematically document all observations and work throughout the study. The researcher frequently assesses his/her own attitude, verbal and nonverbal communication modes, gender focus/lens, and any other factors that may influence informants' responses. The researcher's personal and professional etic views should always be documented and studied for biases, racism, and for differences, similarities, conflicts, and other factors related to interpretation of what is seen or heard. The researcher maintains a field journal log or may process observations and reflections immediately after each session using a computer, audio-recorder, or paper note pad to document an accurate account and to prevent memory lapses. Nonverbal and verbal observations and participatory experiences along with the researcher's reflections are also documented. It is important for the researcher to record one's etic feelings, views, and responses which are usually entered into a separate log by date.

Historical documents, pictures, and other documents from informants are an important part of the ethnonursing collected data to be studied. Descriptions of the environmental context and any special language statements need to be dated and recorded.

Analysis of all collected data is ongoing from the beginning to the end of research process. During the study it is especially important for key informants to confirm, refute, or reconfirm findings with the researcher so that an accurate and truthful account is forthcoming. Key informants are usually interviewed and studied *first* and the general informants *near the end* of the study to confirm cultural representation of the findings. Frequent confirmation of findings with informants is crucial for credibility and confirmability of findings. Consultation with an expert in the research method will guide and facilitate this process. Use of *The Phases of Ethnonursing Data Analysis Enabler for Qualitative Data* and *The Leininger-Templin-Thompson (LTT) Ethnoscript Coding Enabler*, as well as an appropriate and reliable software for the qualitative data analysis, may assist the researcher with the coding and analysis of all raw data.

h. Criteria for evaluation of ethnonursing research findings: The previously defined six criteria to evaluate ethnonursing research findings are used by the researcher to guide, support, and substantiate the domain of inquiry throughout the ethnonursing study. The researcher provides evidence on the use and effect of the six criteria on the study findings. The six criteria (*credibility; confirmability; recurrent patterning; meaning in-context; saturation;* and *transferability*) should be used *daily* to document different contexts and findings while collecting and analyzing data rather than waiting until the end of the study. The *transferability* criterion is considered at the end of the study and requires very thoughtful consideration by the researcher to determine if the results are transferable to a *similar* context.

5. **Final analysis and writing of research findings.** Soon after completion of the study, the researcher conducts a final data analysis and then proceeds with finalizing or writing the research findings. The final report should state whether the theory (assumptive premises) and the domain of inquiry have been substantiated or refuted with substantive evidence.

6. **Dissemination of findings.** A summary of the major findings is shared first with interested informants. This is essential in ethnonursing research as informants are usually interested about the findings and should be aware of them before they are publicly presented or published. It also provides time for the researcher to personally thank the informants for their contributions to professional nursing knowledge and practices. The informant summary can be a brief report presented near the research site. The researcher then proceeds to publically disseminate the detailed research findings in the form of manuscripts and/or local, national, or international presentations. He/she discusses in published works how the study findings can guide use of the three modes of culture care decisions and actions to provide culturally congruent nursing care in practical ways (Leininger, 1993; McFarland, 1997). Both culturally diverse and universal findings

are reported with the theory and ethnonursing study findings. Strengths and limitations of the study are shared.

7. **Development of plans for future studies.** The researcher reflects on the study's findings and identifies plans and recommendations for future research.

8. **Becoming a mentor.** When the researcher becomes confident in his/her understanding and application of the CCT and Ethnonursing Research Method, he/she becomes a mentor to other novice researchers. In this role, the researcher serves as a guide and consultant in the design and implementation of other ethnonursing research studies.

■ SUMMARY

This chapter has presented an overview of the Ethnonursing Research Method and the theory enablers. The general features of the method were discussed to show the close and important relationship of the theory and the method for meaningful and congruent care outcomes. Many nurses are now using the Ethnonursing Research Method worldwide to discover crucial and long overdue cultural knowledge to help nurses function in our transcultural world. Leininger predicted that "… the Theory of Culture Care with the Ethnonursing Research Method has been probably the most significant breakthrough in nursing and will have even greater impact in this 21st century to improve culture care practices" (Leininger, 2002, p. 97).

■ DISCUSSION QUESTIONS

1. Discuss the rationale for using Leininger's Stranger-to-Trusted Friend Enabler in ethnonursing research.

2. Formulate a domain of inquiry and related research questions for a proposed ethnonursing research study.

3. Select a diverse culture; then develop a culture-specific adaptation of Leininger's Semi-Structured Inquiry Guide Enabler to Assess Culture Care and Health.

■ REFERENCES

Leininger, M. M. (1970). *Nursing and anthropology: Two worlds to blend.* New York, NY: John Wiley & Sons.

Leininger, M. M. (1985a). Ethnography and ethnonursing: Models and modes of qualitative data analysis. In M. M. Leininger (Ed.), *Qualitative research methods in nursing* (pp. 33-72). Orlando, FL: Grune & Stratton.

Leininger, M. M. (1985b). Life health care history: Purposes, methods, and techniques. In M. M. Leininger (Ed.), *Qualitative research methods in nursing* (pp. 119-132). Orlando, FL: Grune & Stratton.

Leininger, M. M. (1987). Importance and uses of ethnomethods: Ethnography and ethnonursing research. In M. Cahoon (Ed.), *Recent advances in nursing* (pp. 17, 23-25). London, U. K.: Churchhill Livingstone.

Leininger, M. M. (1988). *Caring: An essential human need.* Detroit, MI: Wayne State University Press.

Leininger, M. M. (1990). Ethnomethods: The philosophic and epistemic basis to explicate transcultural nursing knowledge. *Journal of Transcultural Nursing, 2*(1), 254-257.

Leininger, M. M. (1991a). *Culture care diversity and universality: Theory of nursing.* New York, NY: National League for Nursing.

Leininger, M. M. (1991b). Ethnonursing: A research method with enablers to study the theory of culture care. In M. M. Leininger (Ed.), *Culture care diversity and universality: Theory of nursing* (pp. 73-116). New York, NY: National League for Nursing.

Leininger, M. M. (1993). Culture care theory: The relevant theory to guide functioning in a multicultural world. In M. Parker (Ed.), *Patterns of nursing theories in practice* (pp. 103-122). New York, NY: National League for Nursing Press.

Leininger, M. M. (1994). *Transcultural nursing: Concepts, theories, and practices.* Columbus, OH: Greyden Press.

Leininger, M. M. (1995). *Transcultural nursing: Concepts, theories, research and practice* (2nd ed.). Blacklick, OH: McGraw-Hill College Custom Series.

Leininger, M. M. (1997a). Ethnonursing research method: Essential to discover and advance Asian nursing knowledge. *Japanese Journal of Nursing Research, 30*(2), 20-32.

Leininger, M. M. (1997b). Overview and reflection on the theory of culture care and the ethnonursing research method. *Journal of Transcultural Nursing, 118*(2), 32-53.

Leininger, M. M. (2000). Transcultural nursing to discovery of self and the world of others. *Journal of Transcultural Nursing, 11*(4), 312-313.

Leininger, M. M. (2002). Part 1: The theory of culture care and the ethnonursing research method. In M. M. Leininger & M. R. McFarland (Eds.), *Transcultural nursing: Concepts, theories, research, & practice* (3rd ed., pp. 71-98). New York, NY: McGraw-Hill.

Leininger, M., Templin, T., & Thompson, F. (1990). *The Leininger-Templin-Thompson Ethnoscript Qualitative Software program user's handbook* (pp. 16-19). Walter P. Reuther Library, Madeleine M. Leininger Collection on Human Caring and Transcultural Nursing (ARC-008, Folder 6-29). Archives of Caring in Nursing, Christine E. Lynn College of Nursing, Florida Atlantic University, Boca Raton, FL.

Lincoln, Y. S., & Guba, E. G. (1985). *Naturalistic inquiry.* Newbury Park, CA: Sage.

McFarland, M. R. (1997). Use of culture care theory with Anglo and African American elders in a long-term care setting. *Nursing Care Quarterly, 10*(4), 186-192.

Wehbe-Alamah, H. B., & McFarland, M. R. (2015a). Leininger's enablers for use with the ethnonursing research method. In M. R. McFarland & H. B. Wehbe-Alamah (Eds.), *Leininger's culture care diversity and universality: A worldwide nursing theory* (3rd ed., pp. 73-100). Burlington, MA: Jones and Bartlett Learning.

Wehbe-Alamah, H. B., & McFarland, M. R. (2015b). The ethnonursing research method. In M. R. McFarland & H. B. Wehbe-Alamah (Eds.), *Leininger's culture care diversity and universality: A worldwide nursing theory* (3rd ed., pp. 35-71). Burlington, MA: Jones and Bartlett Learning.

CHAPTER 5

Culture Care Theory: A Trailblazing Theory

Priscilla Limbo Sagar

> *"[A] cultural evolution has transformed nursing and health care so that clients of diverse cultures can benefit from transcultural nursing in many places in the world. This whole movement has been a significant development created by a small cadre of committed leaders....[with] considerable progress made over the past [six] decades in developing a body of transcultural nursing knowledge with concepts, principles, and research findings to guide nurses in working with the culturally different"* (Leininger, 2002c, p. xvii).

■ INTRODUCTION

As a nurse caring for children with mental-health problems, Madeleine Leininger realized in the 1950s that culturally congruent care was a missing component in health care (Leininger, 1995b; McFarland & Wehbe-Alamah, 2015). This realization directed her pioneer efforts in establishing the field of transcultural nursing (TCN) that created a huge body of knowledge for culturally congruent care (Sagar, 2014). Thus Dr. Leininger founded transcultural nursing (TCN), was its leader for six decades, and often has been referred to as its "mother" (Ryan, 2011). Leininger's Theory of Culture Care Diversity and Universality (also known as the Culture Care Theory or CCT), one of the earliest nursing theories, centers on human caring and focuses on similarities and differences among cultures (2002a, 2002b, 2006). The CCT is a visionary nursing theory, not borrowed, but an outcome of original thinking and careful refining for six decades (McFarland & Wehbe-Alamah, 2015).

Leininger's (1970) ground-breaking book, *Anthropology and Nursing: Two Worlds to Blend,* laid the foundation for transcultural nursing. With the end-goal of studying nursing phenomena in-depth, Leininger developed the ethnonursing method along with the CCT in the 1960s. At that time, the founder of TCN was concerned about nursing's heavy use of research tools and instruments from other disciplines and thereby concomitantly overlooking nursing insights and meanings (Leininger, 2002b, 2006).

The ethnonursing method—along with other qualitative methods such as grounded theory, ethnography, and phenomenology—is best suited to investigate lived experiences, cultural values, beliefs, and attitudes of diverse people. These and some quantitative methods may be employed in examining the vast research gaps toward addressing healthcare disparities in care access and health outcomes among minority populations such as African Americans, Native Americans, Hispanic Americans (Sullivan Commission, 2004), and Asian Americans (Agency for Health Research and Quality [AHRQ], 2011).

In this chapter, the author identifies and explains the influences of Leininger's Theory of Culture Care Diversity and Universality upon some subsequent transcultural scholars and theorists such as Andrews and Boyle; Campinha-Bacote; Giger and Davidhizar; Jeffreys; Pacquiao; Purnell; Ray; and Spector. Choi's Theory of Cultural Marginality, although not directly influenced by the CCT, is also included because it is a theory consistent with the premises of the CCT.

■ CULTURE CARE THEORY

The CCT is figuratively depicted by the Sunrise Enabler (**Color Insert 1**) used symbolically to help generate new knowledge in nursing. In the Sunrise depiction, seven sunrays shine upon factors that influence individuals, families, and groups for health and illness. These social structure factors are *technological; religious and philosophical; kinship and social; cultural values, beliefs, and lifeways; political and legal; economic;* and *educational* (Leininger, 1995a, 2002a, 2002b, 2006). There are 11 theoretical assumptions from the major tenets of CCT; the essence of two of those assumptions center on *caring as the essence of nursing* and *diversities and commonalities existing between cultures* (Leininger, 1995a, 2002b, 2006). In the Sunrise Enabler, nursing care is situated strategically beween generic folk care and professional care. This is most advantageous for achieving greater nursing influence and effectiveness in the assessment, planning, implementation, and evaluation of culturally congruent care (Sagar, 2012, 2014, 2015).

The CCT is applicable for care in nursing as well as by other health disciplines (Leininger, 1995a, 2002a, 2006; McFarland & Wehbe-Alamah, 2015). Social structure and kinship factors are special in planning holistic care. Some cultures are more individually oriented whereas others are family/group oriented (Leininger, 2006). It is imperative that healthcare professionals consider family dynamics in providing care to individuals, groups, and communities. Religion and spirituality vastly influence health and wellbeing (Andrews, 2012). Socio-economic factors have direct influence upon being able to access health care and the quality of that [received] healthcare (Leininger, 2006; McFarland & Wehbe-Alamah, 2015; Pacquiao, 2012).

Education serves as the gateway toward improving ones economic status and access to healthcare. Environmental factors can have long-lasting effects upon health and illness (McFarland & Wehbe-Alamah, 2015). Leininger (2006) emphasized that these factors were not explored when planning holistic care until the creation of TCN. More importantly, she stressed that these factors needed to be studied from cultural informants or *emic* (insider) perspectives that influence health, wellness, death and dying (Leininger, 2002b). According to Leininger (2002b, 2006), these perspectives consisted of *generic or traditional/folk care* which needs to be differentiated form *professional care*. Generic or folk care are those naturalistic care acts that people learn informally while whereas professional nursing care is acquired from formal knowledge and structured study (Leininger, 2006; McFarland & Wehbe-Alamah, 2015).

■ LEININGER'S THREE MODES OF CULTURE CARE DECISIONS AND ACTIONS

Leininger (2006) developed the three culture care modes of decisions and actions for the provision of culturally congruent care; they are *culture care preservation and/or maintenance; culture care accommodation and/or negotiation; and culture care repatterning and/or restructuring* (p. 8). These three culture care modes provide a guide for nurses in providing culturally congruent nursing care thus enhancing their development as culturally competent practitioners (McFarland & Wehbe-Alamah, 2015). More importantly, Leininger (2006) called upon nurses to be creative and to use wide-ranging approaches to ensure that care is "… meaningful and helpful to clients" (p. 8). Having been developed based on qualitative research findings, these three culture care modes are crucial for the provision of culturally congruent care and caring and must be used with clinical assessment information or research data discovered using the CCT (Leininger, 2006; Leininger & McFarland, 2006; McFarland & Wehbe-Alamah, 2015).

Culture care preservation and/or maintenance are professional approaches in assisting, supporting, or facilitating clients to preserve and retain care beliefs and values to maintain health and wellness, to cope with illness, or to face handicaps or death (Leininger, 2006). Preserving lifeways such as the generic care practices that maintain and promote health is essential when caring for all patients, groups, communities, and organizations. It has been widely documented that individuals use generic care alongside Western medicine for their health and wellness (Leininger, 2006).

Culture care accommodation and/or negotiation helps in blending generic practices and professional care in a way that is acceptable to people (Leininger, 2002b, 2006). Accommodation of practices for health and wellbeing can be integrated into the care of clients (Leininger, 2002b, 2006). In addition, this mode helps healthcare providers and organizations to fulfill the mandates, guidelines, and accreditation requirements of the U. S. federal government regarding the provision of culturally and linguistically appropriate health care.

Culture care repatterning and/or restructuring entail the use of professional care to assist and facilitate professional approaches and mutual decision-making when helping clients change or alter lifeways for better outcomes (Leininger, 1995, 2006). For example, the use of a "one stop shopping" approach in health care that provides transportation, social services, occupational training, among other services may enable disadvantaged families to access necessary care and services for all family members with less time off work for the parents. With the improved access to care and resources for clients and families thus facilitated, the interprofessional team may be more successful in addressing changes in client behavior for improved health outcomes.

■ THEORIES, MODELS, AND GUIDES INFLUENCED AND INSPIRED BY THE CCT

Funded by the California Endowment, the American Association of Colleges of Nursing (AACN, 2008) developed the *Cultural Competency in Baccalaureate Nursing Education: End-of-Program Competencies for Baccalaureate Nursing Program Graduates and Faculty Toolkit for Integrating These Competencies into Undergraduate Curriculum* guideline. This document—vital in promoting cultural competence among baccalaureate nursing graduates—uses Leininger's *Culture Care Theory* along with four nursing models, namely Campiha-Bacote's *The Process of Cultural Competence*

in the Delivery of Healthcare Services Model; Giger and Davidhizar's *Transcultural Assessment Model*; Purnell's *Model of Cultural Competence*; and Spector's *Health Traditions Model* (AACN, 2008). In 2009, the AACN published the *Toolkit for Cultural Competence in Master's and Doctoral Nursing Education*. Revised in 2011, this document utilized the CCT and the models cited, along with Jeffreys *Cultural Confidence Model,* as part of the baccalaureate toolkit (AACN, 2011).

Whether explicitly acknowledged or not, there are many areas of similarity among the focal points of these theories, models, or guides, such as communication; beliefs and values; environmental context; and biocultural variations.

Andrews and Boyle: Transcultural Nursing Assessment Guide for Individuals, Families, and Communities

Arising from a collaboration between faculty and students at the University of Utah and focused on clarifying the application of TCN in clinical practice, Andrews and Boyle initially published their *Transcultural Concepts in Nursing Care* textbook in 1989 and have consistently used a transcultural nursing framework and a developmental approach across the lifespan in each subsequent edition of their textbook. Many nursing schools that do not follow a specific TCN model use the Andrews and Boyle textbook to guide their transcultural curricular content (Boyle, 2007).

Andrews and Boyle (2012) developed the *Transcultural Nursing Assessment Guide for Individuals and Families (TCNGIF)* with aspects of Leininger's social structure factors integrated into its 12 major categories of cultural knowledge. The guide consists of *biocultural variations and cultural aspects of the incidence of disease; communication; cultural affiliations; cultural sanctions and restrictions; developmental considerations; economics; educational background; health-related beliefs and practices; kinship and social networks; nutrition; religion and spirituality; and values orientation* (Boyle & Andrews, 2012a, pp. 451–455). It is an effective tool for performing a thorough cultural and physical assessment, which is imperative for the provision of culturally congruent care (Sagar, 2012, 2014).

Centered on community and group assessment, Andrews and Boyle (2012) also created the

Andrews/Boyle Transcultural Nursing Assessment Guide for Groups and Communities (TCNAGGC). This guide has eight major categories: *Family and kinship systems; social and life networks; political or government systems; language and traditions; worldviews, value orientations, and cultural norms; religious beliefs and practices; health beliefs and practices;* and *healthcare systems* (Boyle & Andrews, 2012b, pp. 456-458). A thorough and structured cultural assessment of the community and other groups is necessary for effective partnerships and collaboration toward better health outcomes.

The cultural competence of an organization is dependent upon the knowledge and skills of each individual healthcare provider; this, too, calls for a lifetime journey and commitment to learning and self-growth (Ludwig-Beymer, 2012). Acknowledging the need to work toward becoming a culturally competent organization, Boyle, Andrews, and Ludwig-Beymer (2012) devised the *Andrews/Boyle Transcultural Nursing Assessment Guide for Health Care Organizations and Facilities.* The nine areas in this guide are *environmental context; language and ethnohistory; technology; religious/ philosophical; social factors; cultural values; political/ legal; economic;* and *education* (Boyle et al., 2012, pp. 459-461). This guide may be very applicable to use as healthcare organizations plan initiatives as part of program development, accreditation, or magnet designation. Content areas from within each of the three guides may be used to develop individualized assessment tools or the guides can be used in their original form.

Campinha-Bacote: The Process of Cultural Competence in the Delivery of Healthcare

Campinha-Bacote (2007) created the original version of her model, *A Culturally Competent Model of Care,* in 1991 by blending elements from the works of Leininger from 1978; Pedersen from 1988; Kleinman from 1978; and Law from 1993. The model was represented by the four interelated constructs of *cultural awareness, cultural knowledge, cultural skill,* and *cultural encounters* (Campinha-Bacote, 2007, 2011, p. 42). In 1998, *cultural desire* was added (Campinha-Bacote, 2014) and Campinha-Bacote renamed her model *The Process of Cultural Competence in the Delivery of Healthcare Services* (PCCDHS). The new model image depicted five overlapping Venn circles—aptly mirroring the interdependent relationships among those constructs (Campinha-Bacote, 2011,

2014). By 2005, she had also integrated ideas from the works of Chapman (2005) into the model (as cited by Campinha-Bacote, 2007).

In 2007, Campinha-Bacote developed two self-assessment tools to assess cultural competence: *The Inventory for Assessing the Process of Cultural Competence Among Healthcare Professionals-Revised* (IAPCC-R) and its version for student nurses, the *IAPCC-Student Version (IAPCC-SV).* Both tools have been widely used in nursing education, practice, administration, and research to measure [perceived] practitioner and student cultural competence (Sagar, 2014). Based on this work, Campinha-Bacote also developed *A Biblically Based Model of Cultural Competence in the Delivery of Healthcare Services* (BBMCCDHS, 2007) drawing again upon the 2006 works of Leininger and McFarland as well as her own (Campinha-Bacote, 2007) and that of others (Chapman, 2005; Cross et al., 1989; Kleinman, 1980; Law, 1993; Pederson, 1988; Wilkerson, 2002; Wood, 1998 as cited by Campinha-Bacote, 2014). When using the BBMCCDHS, Campinha-Bacote (2015) emphasized the crucial need for healthcare professionals to see the image of God ("Imago Dei") in their clients and to integrate love, caring, humility, and compassion as well as other virtues (para 1) such as justice and patience. In both Camphina-Bacote models, healthcare professionals must regard themselves as *becoming* culturally competent rather than *being* culturally competent (2011, 2014, 2015).

The *Culturally Competent Model of Care* has been highly regarded worldwide. The 1999 version of the model formed part of the basis for the Consortium of Institutes of Higher Education in Health and Rehabilitation in Europe (COHEHRE) cultural competence terminology framework along with Leininger (1991, as cited by Sairanen et al., 2013). In addition, the 2003 Inventory for Assessing The Process of Cultural Competence Among Healthcare Professionals–Revised (IAPCC-R) was translated and used for student assessment by a Swedish nursing program (Olt, Jirwe, Gustavsson, & Emami, 2010).

Jeffreys: Cultural Competence and Confidence Model

Jeffreys' (2010, 2016) *Cultural Competence and Confidence* (CCC) model is an evidence-based, highly applicable theoretical framework used globally by educators, researchers, and learners in various health professions. This theoretical model is used to "… interrelate concepts that explain, describe, influence, and/or predict the phenomenon of learning (developing) cultural competence and integrate the construct of *transcultural self-efficacy* (TSE or confidence) as a major influencing factor" (Jeffreys, 2010, p. 46). By definition, TSE is the "… perceived confidence for performing or learning" (p. 46) transcultural skills when working with diverse clients. In the CCC Model, Jeffreys (2010, 2016) underscored that cultural competence is a multidimensional learning process in transcultural nursing with three dimensions (*cognitive, practical,* and *affective*). It is chiefly influenced by TSE and directed toward *culturally congruent care.* Formal education and other learning experiences could positively affect the three dimensions of TSE as well as the development of individual cultural competence essential for the provision of culturally congruent care (Jeffreys, 2010, 2016).

Jeffreys (2010, 2016) explained that the *cognitive learning* dimension encompasses knowledge and comprehension about cultural factors that influence professional care for culturally diverse clients throughout their life span. Jeffreys also noted similarities between the *practical learning dimension* and the *psychomotor domain* of learning. In the context of TCN, this dimension refers to both verbal and nonverbal communication skills used when performing a cultural assessment. The *affective learning dimension* essential for professional value and attitude development involves "… attitudes, values, and beliefs" (Jeffreys, 2010, p. 52). *Optimal cultural competence* (going beyond minimum competence) involves an ongoing seven-step process of *self-assessment; active promotion; systematic inquiry; decisive action; measurement;* and *evaluation* (Jeffreys, 2016). Optimal cultural competence has been added to the core of the updated 2016 model to emphasize its significance.

Jeffreys (2010, 2016) developed her *Transcultural Self-Efficacy Tool (TSET)* in 1994. "The TSET is an 83-item questionnaire based on the CCC designed to measure and evaluate learners' confidence (transcultural self-efficacy) for performing general transcultural nursing skills among diverse client populations" (Jeffreys Toolkit, 2010, 2016). The TSET Multidisciplinary Health Provider (TSET-MHP) version is available for multidisciplinary health professionals. The

TSET had undergone multiple reliability and validity testings and has been administered to nurses, nursing students, physicians, and other healthcare clinicians and professionals (Jeffreys, 2010, 2016). *The Cultural Competence Clinical Evaluation Tool* (CCCET) was adapted from the TSET to gather data about the provision of cultural specific care, cultural assessments, and cultural sensitivity within clinical or educational settings (Jeffreys Toolkit, 2010, 2016); several CCCET versions are available. In addition, Jeffreys developed the *Clinical Setting Assessment Tool-Diversity and Disparity (CSAT-DD)* for data collection of diverse client populations (Part I) and clinical problems centered (Part II) on the focus areas of Healthy People 2020 (Jeffreys, 2010, 2016).

The CCC is highly applicable in nursing education, practice, administration, and research as well as in allied health disciplines. More than 50 quantitative and qualitative studies have utilized the TSET and/or CCC model and have validated the underlying assumptions of the model (Amerson, 2010; Sarafis, Michael, Chara, & Maria, 2014; Shattell et al., 2013). An example of an educationally-focused program application of the CCC is the use of the TSET by the Department of Nursing at the University of Michigan-Flint as a pre/post assessment of students' perceived cultural competence conducted to evaluate undergraduate and graduate outcomes for the nursing program.

Giger and Davidhizar: Transcultural Assessment Model

There was a dearth of cultural assessment tools in 1988 when Giger and Davidhizar (2004, 2008) pioneered their *Transcultural Assessment Model (TAM)* in response to challenges made by the transcultural nursing profession that students needed to provide culturally congruent and competent care to culturally diverse clients. The TAM (as cited by Giger, 2013; Giger & Davidhizar, 2004, 2008) was based on the groundbreaking work of Leininger (1978) as well as those of Spector (1996), and Orque, Bloch, and Monroy (1983).

The TAM embraces six cultural phenomena: *Biocultural variations; environmental control; time; social orientation; space;* and *communication* (Giger, 2013; Giger & Davidhizar, 2004, 2008). The TAM offers a means to perform a functional and thorough assessment in planning *culturally congruent care* for clients

(AACN, 2008; Giger, 2013). These cultural phenomena appear within each diverse culture, interact with each other, intersect with one another, and differ in their functionality and application (Giger, 2013; Giger & Davidhizar, 2008).

Over the past 20 years, the TAM has served as a guide for healthcare practitioners not just in nursing education, practice, administration, and research but also in allied fields such as medical imaging, dentistry, and hospital administration to guide the provision of culturally congruent care (Giger, 2013). In recognition of this, the American Academy of Nursing (AAN) honored it with their Edge Runner Award (Giger, 2013) and the National League for Nursing (NLN, 2009) utilized the TAM in its *Diversity Toolkit.* In 2008, the Royal College of Nursing in London, England, began using the TAM as one of their primary conceptual frameworks as the basis for caring in a global, diverse society (Giger, 2013). The U. S. Department of Health and Human Services (USDHHS) Office of Minority Health (OMH) used the TAM as one of the key frameworks when developing the federal guideline for culturally competent care (Giger, 2013).

Spector: Heritage Assessment Model

Spector's (2002, 2004a, 2009, 2013) textbook was initially published in 1977 to fulfill a promise to her students and has since undergone eight editions. In developing the *Health Traditions Model (HTM)* in 1993, Spector (2004a, 2004b, 2009) integrated Giger and Davidhizar's six cultural phenomena. The HTM first appeared in Potter and Perry's 1993 *Fundamentals in Nursing* textbook (Giger, 2013; Giger & Davidhizar, 2008). Spector (2004a) described her model as one that reflected the *personal health traditions of a unique cultural being.* Spector (2013) used the term *Cultural Care* to describe the concept of culturally and linguistically competent professional health care. To assess the depth of self-identification with one's own personal heritage, Spector (2004a) also developed a *Heritage Assessment Tool.* This tool is especially helpful to assess traditional beliefs and practices about health and illness among individuals and groups which are key for locating community services for support (Spector, 2013).

Spector (2013) regarded health as "… the balance of the person, both within one's beings—physical, mental, and spiritual—and in the outside world"

(p. 91). The *personal methods of maintaining health, protecting health,* and *restoring health* for each of the *physical, mental,* and *spiritual* facets of health thereby constitute the nine interrelated facets of health (Spector, 2013, p. 93). For example, to restore health an individual may use massage (physical), exorcism (mental), and meditation (spiritual). Such holistic approaches have gained greater acceptance in modern health care. Complementary and alternative methods such as acupuncture, yoga, and meditation are not only used along with Western medicine but their quantifiable benefits in promoting wellness and in the treatment and rehabilitation phases of some illnesses have been revealed through scientific medical research (Andrews, 2012; Basuray, 2013).

Pacquaio: Model for Culturally Competent Ethical Decisions

The Model for Culturally Competent Ethical Decision Making (Pacquaio, 2012) underscores universal principles of ethics and focuses on advocating for social justice and for protecting human rights. Social, safety, and health risks among certain cultural groups compromise their capacity for self-advocacy and for accessing a better quality of life (Pacquaio, 2012). The critical motivation, according to Pacquaio (2012), is compassion—compassion ignites the energy whereby advocates take on the challenges of complex risks and precious resources. Compassion compels one into action, to give voice to the voiceless such as people who are oppressed, disadvantaged, and/or marginalized.

Pacquaio (2012) outlined three action strategies for transforming an individual's compassion: *Collaboration, partnership,* and *advocacy* (p. 415). Collaborative partnerships with families, groups, and communities develop mutual understanding and foster empathy. These repeated, continuing encounters promote genuine concern and empathy in the professional. Advocacy for social justice and human rights require such partnerships and collaborations; they promote community empowerment. Furthermore, Pacquaio recommended strengthening the curricula of community health nursing to "… sensitize students to public health issues and social inequities affecting population health" (p. 415). Pacquaio's model is applicable with structured didactic and clinical experiences for nursing and allied health students during cultural encounters, collaborations, and partnerships with diverse and vulnerable populations. Pacquaio suggested seeking out both local and international experiences especially those involving homeless shelters, local churches, and advocacy groups.

Compassionate actions must be culturally congruent and competent to prevent disenfranchising others; the goal is to balance the rights of the disadvantaged with the rights of nondisadvantaged people (Pacquaio, 2012, p. 414). As Pacquio had previously stated:

> Culturally competent and ethical care begins with an appreciation of the significant role of culture in health and caring. Cultural appreciation prompts practitioners to examine their own values and biases and engage in fully understanding the clients' context of meanings. Respecting and accommodating their unique life context allow for switching frames of understanding in order to work with cultural differences and design care that minimizes disadvantages associated with being different. (Pacquaio, 2008, pp. 420-421)

As a direct influence from Leininger's Culture Care Theory (2002a, 2002b, 2006), Pacquaio integrated the three modes of culture care decisions and actions into her model: Culture care preservation and/or maintenance; culture care accommodation and/or negotiation; and culture care repatterning and/or restructuring. Pacquaio (2012) emphasized *maintaining core values and practices* (preservation); *working with them toward an effective health care* (accommodation); and *assisting them to change their way of life for healthier, safer existence* (repatterning; pp. 414-415) as strategies to follow when working with individuals and groups.

Purnell: Model of Cultural Competence

Purnell (2002, 2013) developed the *Purnell Model for Cultural Competence (PMCC)* in 1991. Initially intended as a framework for clinical assessment, the primary purpose of the PMCC is to serve as a tool for healthcare providers in interrelating "… characteristics of culture to promote congruence and … delivery of consciously sensitive and competent health care" (Purnell, 2013, p. 15). The major assumptions of the model include *healthcare professionals require similar information regarding diversity*; *cultures share core similarities*; and *differences are present within, among, and between cultures* (p. 15). The PMCC is configured with 12 wedge-shaped cultural domains surrounded

by four rims that signify *global society* (outside rim); *community* (second rim); *family* (third rim); and the *individual* (fourth [innermost] rim (Purnell, 2002, 2007, 2008, 2013a). The solid black center of the PMCC circle signifies what is *unknown* about cultures. The jagged line at the bottom of the model depicts the nonlinearity aspects of cultural consciousness (Purnell, 2013). The model can be used in its entirety, or any of the domains can be selectively applied individually or in various combinations.

Lipson and Desantis (2007) cited the PMCC as one of the most extensively utilized models in nursing curricula; its 12 cultural domains can be threaded into theoretical nursing courses as well as clinical course components (Sagar, 2012). This model is not only widely used in nursing education, practice, administration, and research but also in other health-related fields and international projects. Notably, the PMCC was the organizing framework of the Commission on Internationalization and Cultural Competence for the European Union project for the Bologna-Sorbonne-Salamanca World Health Organization declarations (Purnell, 2007).

Ray: Transcultural Caring Dynamics in Nursing and Health Care

Ray's (2010, 2016) *Transcultural Caring Dynamics in Nursing and Health Care (TCDNHC)* model was directly influenced by the work of Leininger (1978). As with the CCT, *caring* is a central nursing construct in this model. Ray's (2010, 2016) holistic model portrays culture as dynamic and complex; integrates understanding of the nursing meta-paradigms (Fawcett, 1984) and the four ways of knowing (Carper, 1978); and focuses on TCN caring, ethics, cultural context, and spirituality as the basis for "… awareness, understanding, and choice" (p. 20). The TCDNHC model was developed to answer questions arising when caring for clients from different cultures from a perspective of mutuality and co-participation (Ray, 2010) in areas that include *the meaning of caring*; *effects of culture on health, illness, healing, and caring*; *meaning of patient choices in terms of TCN*; and *perceptions of vulnerable individuals' negotiation for their health and wellbeing* (Ray, 2010, pp. 19-20). In 2016, Ray added the concept of *theory* to address the assumptions of transcultural caring in complex nursing, health care, and global contexts in a manner that corresponds to the model.

Ray's model is therefore applicable to healthcare professionals and patients in a mutual relationship of decision making about "… caring, health, illness, death, healing, and wellbeing" (2010, p. 21). The model has three main aspects: *explanation, illustration,* and *application* (Ray, 2010). The *explanatory aspect* of the model leads the healthcare professional to not only obtain knowledge toward understanding both the personal and relational natures of culture and multiculturalism, but also to reflect on how these elements affect the process of making choices (Ray, 2010). In the *illustrative aspect*, cultural materials contain information about the nature of caring, TCN ethics, context, and spirituality. The *applicability aspect* can be used as a guide toward achieving optimal health and care outcomes as health partnerships "…. co-create choices and the best possible future in the nurse-patient relationship in given transcultural situations" (p. 21). The model has been applied within a theory-guided research approach using quantitative and qualitative analysis to study Muslim Americans and Arab women (Martin, 2015).

Choi: Theory of Cultural Marginality

Choi (2008), as did Leininger, began the development of her theory while working with mentally and emotionally disturbed children. Also an immigrant, Choi (2013), conceived the *Theory of Cultural Marginality* (TCM) while working with immigrant adolescents in the United States when she noticed their unique situations resulting from the immigration process which in turn had affected their mental health (Choi, 2008, 2013). In a community-based study, Korean American adolescents showed considerably lower levels of self-esteem, coping skills, and higher levels of depression and somatic symptoms than their American counterparts (Choi, Stafford, Meininger, Roberts, & Smith, 2002). In an ensuing school-based research study, Asian American and Hispanic American adolescents also revealed higher levels of social stress, somatic symptoms, and depression compared to European American adolescents (Choi, Meininger, & Roberts, 2006).

The TCM has three major concepts: *Marginal living; across culture conflict recognition;* and *easing cultural tension* (Choi, 2008, 2013). *Marginal living* causes passivity and feelings of being in between two cultures—living and shaping new relationships in the midst of the old culture—and concurrently being in conflict and in promise (Choi, 2008, 2013). The *sensation of passivity* and the *push-pull tension* (or conflict) between two cultures are identifying attributes of marginal living (Choi, 2008, 2013). Park (1928, as cited by Choi, 2013) referred to marginal living as a condition of being doomed to live in two worlds in which the individual does not quite belong to either culture. *Cross-cultural conflict recognition* is the early understanding of differences between two contradicting sets of cultural values, customs, behaviors, and norms (Choi, 2008, 2013). Conflict surfaces when individuals face divergent value systems—each with its own associated expectations—and are required to make difficult choices (Choi, 2013). To resolve cross-cultural conflict, the individual copes by using positive adjustment responses.

Choi (2013, citing Weisberger, 1992) also modified the four responses from his research about marginality among German Jews: *Assimilation; reconstructed return; poise;* and *integration. Assimilation* entails absorption into the dominant culture by adopting its new language, customs, and lifeways (Choi, 2008, 2013). In *reconstructed return*, an individual opts to return to the original culture due either to conflicts with the new culture or as an aftermath of longing for the old culture (Choi, 2008, 2013). Overidentification with the original or new culture are common expressions in reconstructed return (Choi, 2008, 2013). The characteristic patterned response of *poise* is tentativeness, due to the potential return of the previous cycle of emotional conflicts and struggle (Choi, 2008, 2013). The response of *integration* denotes adjustment; the individual forms a new, third culture by blending the old and new cultures (Choi, 2008, 2013).

Choi's (2008, 2013) goal in developing the *TCM* was to foster understanding of the distinct experiences of immigrant persons who are living between two cultures. Choi called this complicated living the "straddling of cultures" (2008, p. 243). Choi (2008, 2013) was hopeful that TCM would offer healthcare professionals guideposts for the provision of culturally congruent care for immigrants. The image of an individual—whether an immigrant, a person of mixed race and/or heritage, or someone deciding to adopt a new culture—standing astride two cultures vividly portrays the difficulty, alienation, marginalization, and agony of the process. In 2013, Choi developed a 13-item *Cultural Marginality Scale (CMS)* tool to investigate the marginal living experiences of immigrant children in

South Korea. The CMS was adapted from the *Societal, Attitudinal, Familial, and Environmental Acculturative Stress Scale for Children* (SAFE-C; Chavez et al., 1997 as cited in Choi, 2013).

■ SUMMARY

In the future, many more theories will spring forth, be tested, and become validated. Leininger's Theory of Culture Care Diversity and Universality has had a lasting effect not only in the provision of culturally congruent care for diverse individuals, groups, and communities but also by influencing new theories, models, and guides. The Sunrise Enabler will continue to be used to guide health care as was envisioned by its founder (McFarland & Wehbe-Alamah, 2015).

As the healthcare system worldwide grapples with the challenges of providing culturally-based, culture-specific, and culturally congruent care, healthcare professionals will continue to use the CCT as well as other transcultural theories, models, and guides that have been influenced and inspired by Leininger's work. Use of these care models, theories, and guides is predicted to lead to better health and wellbeing outcomes for individuals, groups, communities, and organizations. And, as individuals and communities strive for cultural competence, applications of the CCT and other transcultural theories, models, and guides will be more deeply and broadly explored. So the journey begins—for each individual, group, community, and organization.

■ DEDICATION

This chapter is wholeheartedly dedicated to Dr. Madeleine Leininger. She has inspired, inspires, and will continue to inspire my future work. Her influence as the mother and founder of TCN has profoundly and firmly established this field of nursing. Mentoring in TCN will continue in the way she mentored so many; those she mentored are in turn mentoring others. The CCT has influenced many other theories, models, and guides in the areas of caring; health history and physical assessment; and culturally congruent care. The continuing diversity in the U. S. and the focus on globalization will further necessitate culturally-based

care. This thrust to cultural competence is additionally accelerated by government mandates, guidelines, and accreditation requirements. What Dr. Leininger envisioned many years ago—and worked ardently toward for six decades—is coming to full fruition.

■ DISCUSSION QUESTIONS

1. Discuss why Leininger's Cultural Care Theory (CCT) has been referred to as a "trailblazing theory." Explain at least two other theories or models that were inspired by the CCT. What specific aspects of these theories and models were influenced by the CCT?
2. How has the ethnonursing method generated and contributed to the body of knowledge in TCN? Give five examples of research studies conducted with the use of the ethnonursing method. Discuss areas where there are still gaps in knowledge that future studies could focus on.
3. As government mandates, guidelines, as well as accreditation requirements, center on cultural and linguistic competence, what further developments do you envision in TCN?
4. Discuss the Leininger influences upon the theories/models described in the chapter. Give three examples.

■ REFERENCES

Agency for Healthcare Research and Quality. (2011). AHRQ funded research on health care for Asian Americans/Pacific Islander. Retrieved from http://www.ahrq.gov/research/findings/factsheets/minority/aapifact/aapifact.pdf

American Association of Colleges of Nursing. (2008). *Cultural competency in baccalaureate nursing education*. Washington, DC: Author.

American Association of Colleges of Nursing. (2011). *Toolkit for cultural competence in master's and doctoral nursing education*. Washington, DC: Author.

American Nurses' Association. (2014). Public ranks nurses as most honest, ethical profession for 13th straight year: High ranking in Gallup poll coincides with ANA's Year of Ethics. Retrieved from http://nursingworld.org/FunctionalMenuCategories/MediaResources/PressReleases/2014-PR/Nurses-Most-Honest-Ethical-Profession-for-13-Years.html

Amerson, R. (2010). The impact of service-learning on cultural competence. *Nursing Education Perspectives, 31*(1), 18-22.

Andrews, M. M. (2012). The influence of cultural and health belief systems on health care practices. In M. M Andrews & J. S. Boyle). *Transcultural concepts in nursing care* (6th ed., pp. 73-88). Philadelphia, PA: Wolters Kluwer|Lippincott Williams & Wilkins.

Andrews, M. M., & Boyle, J. S. (2008). *Transcultural concepts in nursing care* (5th ed.). Philadelphia, PA: Wolters Kluwer|Lippincott Williams & Wilkins.

Andrews, M. M., & Boyle, J. S. (2012). *Transcultural concepts in nursing care* (6th ed.). Philadelphia, PA: Wolters Kluwer/Lippincott Williams & Wilkins.

Basuray, J. M. (2013). Health beliefs across cultures: Understanding transcultural nursing. In J. M. Basuray (Ed.), *Culture and health: Concept and practice* (Rev. Ed., pp. 57-84). Ronkonkoma, NY: Linus.

Boyle, J. S. (2007). Commentary on "Current approaches to integrating elements of cultural competence in nursing education." *Journal of Transcultural Nursing, 18*(1), 21S-22S.

Boyle, J. S., & Andrews, M. M. (2012a). Andrews/Boyle transcultural nursing assessment guide for individuals and families. In M. M. Andrews & J. S. Boyle (Eds.), *Transcultural concepts in nursing care* (6th ed., pp. 451-455). Philadelphia, PA: Wolters Kluwer|Lippincott Williams & Wilkins.

Boyle, J. S., & Andrews, M. M. (2012b). Andrews/Boyle transcultural nursing assessment guide for groups and communities. In M. M. Andrews & J. S. Boyle (Eds.), *Transcultural concepts in nursing care* (6th ed., pp. 456-458). Philadelphia, PA: Wolters Kluwer|Lippincott Williams & Wilkins.

Boyle, J. S., Andrews, M. M., & Ludwig-Beymer, P. (2012). Andrews/Boyle transcultural nursing assessment guide for health care organizations and facilities. In M. M. Andrews & J. S. Boyle (Eds.), *Transcultural concepts in nursing care* (6th ed., pp. 459-461). Philadelphia, PA: Wolters Kluwer|Lippincott Williams & Wilkins.

Campinha-Bacote, J. (2007). *The process of cultural competence in the delivery of healthcare services: The journey continues.* Cincinnati, OH: Transcultural C.A.R.E. Resources.

Campinha-Bacote, J. (2011). Coming to know cultural competence: An evolutionary process. *International Journal for Human Caring, 15*(3), 42-48.

Campinha-Bacote, J. (2014). The Process of Cultural Competence in the Delivery of Healthcare Services. Retrieved from http://www.transculturalcare.net/

Campinha-Bacote, J. (2015). A Biblically Based Model of Cultural Competence. Retrieved from http://transculturalcare.net/a-biblically-based-model-of-cultural-competence/

Carper, B. A. (1978). Fundamental patterns of knowing in nursing. *Advances in Nursing Science, 1*(1), 13-23.

Choi, H. (2008). Theory of cultural marginality. In M. J. Smith & P. R. Liehr (Eds.), *Middle range theory for nursing* (2nd ed., pp. 243-259). New York, NY: Springer.

Choi, H. (2013). Theory of cultural marginality. In M. J. Smith & P. R. Liehr (Eds.), *Middle range theory for nursing* (3rd ed., pp. 289-307). New York, NY: Springer.

Choi, H., Meininger, J. C., & Roberts, R. E. (2006). Ethnic differences in adolescents' mental distress, social stress, and resources. *Adolescence, 41*(162), 263-283.

Choi, H., Stafford, L., Meininger, J. C., & Roberts, R. E. & Smith, D. P. (2002). Psychometric properties of the DSM Scale for Depression (DSD) with Korean American youths. Issues in Mental Health Nursing, *28*(8), 735-756.

Fawcett, J. (1984). The metaparadigms of nursing: Present status and future refinements. *Journal of Nursing Scholarship, 16*(3), 84-87.

Gallup. (2014). Americans rate nurses highest on honesty, ethical standards. Retrieved from http://www.gallup.com/poll/180260/americans-rate-nurses-highest-honesty-ethical-standards.aspx

Giger, J. N. (2013). *Transcultural nursing: Assessment and interventions* (6th ed.). St. Louis, MO: Mosby Elsevier Health Science.

Giger, J. N., & Davidhizar, R. E. (2004). *Transcultural nursing: Assessment and intervention* (4th ed.). St. Louis, MO: Mosby Elsevier.

Giger, J. N., & Davidhizar, R. E. (2008). *Transcultural nursing: Assessment and intervention* (5th ed.). St. Louis, MO: Mosby Elsevier.

Jeffreys, M. R. (2010). A model to guide cultural competence education. In M. R. Jeffreys (Ed.), *Teaching cultural competence in nursing and health care* (2nd ed., pp. 45-59). New York, NY: Springer.

Jeffreys, M. R. (2016). *Teaching cultural competence in nursing and health care* (3rd ed.). New York, NY: Springer.

Leininger, M. M. (1970). *Anthropology and nursing: Two worlds to blend.* New York, NY: John Wiley & Sons.

Leininger, M. M. (1978). *Transcultural nursing: Concepts, theories, and practices.* New York, NY: John Wiley & Sons.

Leininger, M. M. (1995a). Overview of Leininger's culture care theory. In M. M. Leininger (Ed.), *Transcultural nursing: Concepts, theories, research, and practice* (2nd ed., pp. 93-114). New York, NY: McGraw-Hill.

Leininger, M. M. (1995b). Transcultural mental health nursing. In M. M. Leininger (Ed.), *Transcultural nursing: Concepts, theories, research, and practice* (2nd ed., pp. 279-293). New York, NY: McGraw-Hill.

Leininger, M. M. (2002a). Culture care theory: A major contribution to advance transcultural nursing knowledge and practices. *Journal of Transcultural Nursing, 13*(3), 189-192.

Leininger, M. M. (2002b). Part I. The Theory of Culture Care and the Ethnonursing Method. In M. M. Leininger & M. R. McFarland (Eds.), *Transcultural nursing: Concepts, theories, research, and practice* (2nd ed., pp. 71-98). New York, NY: McGraw-Hill.

Leininger, M. M. (2002c). Preface. In M. M. Leininger & M. R. McFarland (Eds.), *Transcultural nursing: Concepts, theories, research, and practice* (2nd ed., p. xvii). New York, NY: McGraw-Hill.

Leininger, M. M. (2006). Culture Care Diversity and Universality and evolution of the ethnonursing method. In M. M. Leininger & M. R. McFarland (Eds.), *Culture care diversity and universality: A worldwide nursing theory* (3rd ed., pp. 1-41). Sudbury, MA: Jones & Bartlett.

Leininger. M. M., & McFarland, M. R. (2006), *Transcultural nursing: Concepts, theories, research, and practice* (2nd ed.). New York, NY: McGraw-Hill.

Lipson, J. G., & Desantis, L. A. (2007). Current approaches to integrating elements of cultural competence in nursing education. *Journal of Transcultural Nursing, 18*(1), 10S-20S.

Ludwig-Beymer, P. (2012). Creating culturally competent organzations. In M. M. Andrews and J. S. Boyle (Eds), *Transcultural concepts in nursing care.* (6th ed., pp. 211-242). Philadelphia, PA: Wolters Kluwer/Lippincott Williams & Wilkins.

McFarland, M. R., & Wehbe-Alamah, H. B. (2015). The theory of culture care diversity and universality. In M. R. McFarland & H. B. Wehbe-Alamah (Eds.), *Leininger's culture care diversity and universality: A worldwide nursing theory* (3rd ed., pp. 1-34). Burlington, MA: Jones & Bartlett.

Martin, M. B. (2015). Gender equality and the empowerment of women in Arab countries: A transcultural caring perspective. *International Journal for Human Caring, 19*(1), 13-18.

National League for Nursing. (2009). *Diversity toolkit.* Retrieved from http://www.nln.org/facultyprograms/Diversity_Toolkit/diversity_toolkit.pdf

Orque, M. S., Bloch, B., & Monrroy, L. S. A. (1983). *Ethnic nursing care: A multicultural approach.* Maryland Heights, MO: Mosby.

Olt, H., Jirwe, M., Gustavsson, P., & Emami, A. (2010). Psychometric evaluation of the Swedish adaptation of the Inventory for Assessing the Process of Cultural Competence among Healthcare Professionals-Revised (IAPCC-R). *Journal of Transcultural Nursing, 21*(1), 55-64.

Pacquaio, D. F. (2008). Cultural competence in ethical decision making. In M. M. Andrews & J. S. Boyle (Eds.), *Transcultural concepts in nursing care* (5th ed., pp. 408-423). Philadelphia, PA: Wolters Kluwer|Lippincott Williams & Wilkins.

Pacquaio, D. F. (2012). Cultural competence in ethical decision making. In M. M. Andrews & J. S. Boyle (Eds.), *Transcultural concepts in nursing care* (6th ed., pp. 403-420). Philadelphia, PA: Wolters Kluwer|Lippincott Williams & Wilkins.

Purnell, L. D. (2002). The Purnell model for cultural competence. *Journal of Transcultural Nursing, 13*(3), 193-196.

Purnell, L. D. (2007). Commentary on "Current approaches to integrating elements of cultural competence in nursing education." *Journal of Transcultural Nursing, 18*(1), 23S-24S.

Purnell, L. D. (2008). The Purnell model for cultural competence. In L. D. Purnell & B. J. Paulanka (Eds.), *Transcultural health care: A culturally competent approach* (3rd ed., pp. 15-44). Philadelphia, PA: FA Davis.

Purnell, L. D. (2013). The Purnell model for cultural competence. In L. D. Purnell (Ed.), *Transcultural health care: A culturally competent approach* (4th ed., pp. 15-44). Philadelphia, PA: FA Davis.

Ray, M. A. (2010). *Transcultural caring dynamics in nursing and health care.* Philadelphia, PA: FA Davis.

Ray, M. A. (2016). *Transcultural caring dynamics in nursing and health care* (2nd ed.). Philadelphia, PA: FA Davis.

Ryan, M. (2011). A celebration of a life of commitment to transcultural nursing: Opening of the Madeleine M. Leininger Collection on Human Caring and Transcultural Nursing. *Journal of Transcultural Nursing, 22*(1), 97.

Sagar, P. L. (2012). *Transcultural nursing theory and models: Application in nursing education, practice, and administration.* New York, NY: Springer.

Sagar, P. L. (2014). *Transcultural nursing education strategies.* New York, NY: Springer.

Sagar, P. L. (2015). Nurses leading the fight against Ebola virus disease. *Journal of Transcultural Nursing, 26*(3), 322-326. doi: 10.1177/1043659615574326

Sairanen, R., Richardson, E., Kelly, H., Bergknut, E., Koskinen, L., Lundberg, P., …De Vliegerm, L. (2013). Putting culture in the curriculum: A European project. *Nurse Education in Practice, 13*(2013), 118-124.

Sarafis, P., Michael, I., Chara, T., & Maria, M., (2014). Reliability and validity of the transcultural self-efficacy tool questionnaire [Greek version]. *Journal of Nursing Measurement, 22*(2), e41-e51.

Shattell, M. M., Nemitz, E. A., Crosson, N., Zackeru, A. R., Starr, S., Hu, J., & Gonzales, C. (2013). Culturally competent practice in a pre-licensure baccalaureate nursing program in the United States: A mixed-methods study. *Nursing Education Perspectives, 34*(6), 383-389.

Spector, R. E. (1996). *Cultural diversity in health and illness* (3rd ed.). Norwalk, CT: Appleton & Lange.

Spector, R. E. (2002). Cultural diversity in health and illness. *Journal of Transcultural Nursing, 13*(3), 197-199.

Spector, R. E. (2004a). *Cultural diversity in health and illness* (6th ed.). Upper Saddle River, NJ: Pearson Education.

Spector, R. E. (2004b). *Cultural care guide to heritage assessment and health traditions* (3rd ed.). Upper Saddle River, NJ: Pearson Prentice Hall.

Spector, R. E. (2009). *Cultural diversity in health and illness* (7th ed.). Upper Saddle River, NJ: Pearson Education.

Spector, R. E. (2013). *Cultural diversity in health and illness* (8th ed.). Boston, MA: Pearson Education.

The Sullivan Commission. (2004). Missing persons: Minorities in the health professions: A report of the Sullivan Commission on diversity in the healthcare workforce. Retrieved from https://depts.washington.edu/ccph/pdf_files/Sullivan_Report_ ES.pdf

Wehbe-Alamah, H. B., & McFarland, M. R. (2015). The ethnonursing research method. In M. R. McFarland & H. B. Wehbe-Alamah (Eds.), *Leininger's Culture care diversity and universality: A worldwide nursing theory* (3rd ed., pp. 35-71). Burlington, MA: Jones & Bartlett.

6

The Globalization of Transcultural Nursing: Contributions to the Achievement of the Millennium Development and Sustainable Development Goals

Margaret M. Andrews

> *"...the nurse is challenged to use worldview, social structure, language expressions, environment, and folk practices.... to provide culture specific and culturally congruent care" (Leininger, 2006b, p. 152).*

■ HISTORICAL CONTEXT

In the mid-1960s, Dr. Madeleine Leininger lived with and studied the Gadsup people of the Eastern Highlands of New Guinea for the purpose of substantiating her Theory of Culture Care Diversity and Universality (also known as the Culture Care Theory or CCT) where she began to create the ethnonursing research method while studying childrearing, ethnocare, and ethnohealth in a non-Western culture (Leininger, 2006b). This study was the first transcultural, transnational, ethnonursing qualitative research study in nursing. From the inception of transcultural nursing, Leininger envisioned nursing as transcultural and global in nature (Leininger, 2006a). Since that time, transcultural nursing concepts, theories, research, and practices have increasingly spread worldwide. As predicted by Leininger (1978) when she established transcultural nursing as a formal area of study and practice, the discipline of transcultural nursing has transformed nursing from its previous unicultural, biomedical, and mind-body emphasis to a transcultural, comparative, multicultural, caring and curing focus on the prevention of illness and disabilities for and maintenance of the health and wellbeing of people globally (Leininger, 2015; Leininger & McFarland, 2002, 2006; McFarland & Wehbe-Alamah, 2015).

According to Leininger (2015), health care is a global human phenomenon and a cultural right and expectation. Humans live, exist, and function in a global world and are increasingly interdependent on one another for basic survival as well as for the health and wellbeing of individuals, groups, communities, and nations. Leininger posited that the ways humans stay well, become ill, and/or survive in a global world are only partially known, noting the endless cultural possibilities and numerous care modalities given that so many different cultures exist globally (2015). The world consists of many diverse cultural groups in different geographic locations with different languages, and changing political, economic, social, and religious environments within different cultural contexts and climates. Leininger encouraged nurses and other healthcare providers to think within a very broad worldview, advising them to examine *globalization* in a geographic scope with great diversity and complexity of cultures. She discovered in the course of her life-long global research that there were universal care values and diverse values such as respect, kindness, and attention that could be conceptualized as an integral component of globalization (Leininger & McFarland, 2006). Leininger stated that globalization means attention to local, regional, and international culture care values and practices in large or small cultural areas (2015). In addition, there were many culture care diversities that needed to be studied from a transnational comparative health outcome perspective. Furthermore, Leininger encouraged transcultural nursing researchers to consult and unite with scholars in other disciplines, such as anthropology and the social and geographic sciences, to define and refine care areas for globalization with particular focus on those areas that remain unknown or unexplored. As nurses expand their work globally, they will need research-based data about culture care phenomena with knowledge of climate changes as well as healthcare environments for children and the elderly to make meaningful global transformations (Leininger, 2015, p. 103).

Leininger identified the importance of nurses focusing on the culture care needs associated with increased migrations of immigrants and refugees settling in or leaving diverse places in the world. She indicated that knowledge of these migrations with respect to health care is critical to discover how "culturally congruent care can decrease or increase culture conflicts, stresses, killings, and criminal acts" (Leininger, 2015, p. 109). Leininger foreshadowed that population changes would have a major effect on health, illness, wellbeing, and accidents among cultures globally (2015). She also encouraged nurses to investigate immigration and healthcare practices that may lead to illnesses, increased culture care conflicts, and unfavorable illness outcomes including disability and death (Leininger, 2015). Leininger also predicted that globalization would require increased interdisciplinary cooperation among healthcare providers (2015).

Nurses with formal academic preparation in transcultural nursing substantively influenced the spread of transcultural nursing to Africa; Asia; Australia and the Pacific Rim; Europe; the Middle East; and throughout North, Central, and South America (Andrews, 2006). In the third edition of *Culture Care Diversity and Universality: A Worldwide Theory of Nursing*, several contributing authors described their use of the Culture Care Theory and ethnonursing research method in global contexts including Australia (Omeri, 2015; Raymond & Omeri, 2015); Greece (Larsen, 2015); Italy (Zoucha & Turk, 2015); and Kenya (Knecht & Sabatine, 2015) as well as immigrants (Raymond & Omeri, 2015; Wehbe-Alamah, 2015) and subcultures (Morris, 2015). In other texts, nurses focused on the application of the Culture Care Theory and transcultural nursing for the care of individuals, groups, and communities such as the Sudan (Baird, 2011) and Iraq (Goodman, Edge, Agazio, & Prue-Owens, 2015) in addition to specific diseases such as Ebola (Gray, 2015) or HIV/AIDS (Gardner, 2013; Grimsrud, Kaplan, Bekker, & Myer, 2014; Hensen et al., 2012). All of these authors illustrated ways in which both the theory and the method were globally applicable in clinical practice, education, and service.

■ THE MILLENNIUM DEVELOPMENT GOALS

Established in 1945, the United Nations (U. N.) is an international organization comprised of 193 member states (United Nations, n. d.-a). The mission and work of the United Nations are guided by the purposes and principles contained in its founding charter which includes taking action on the issues confronting humanity in the 21st century such as peace and security, climate change, sustainable development, human rights, disarmament, terrorism, humanitarian, international health, health emergencies, gender equality, governance, and food production (United Nations, n.d.-b). The U. N. also provides a forum for its members to express their views in the General Assembly, the Security Council, the Economic and Social Council, and other internal bodies and committees (See Figure 6.1). By enabling dialogue between its members and by hosting these negotiations, the organization has become a mechanism for governments to find areas of agreement and solve problems together (adapted from http://www.un.org/en/sections/about-un/overview/index.html). The overall management of

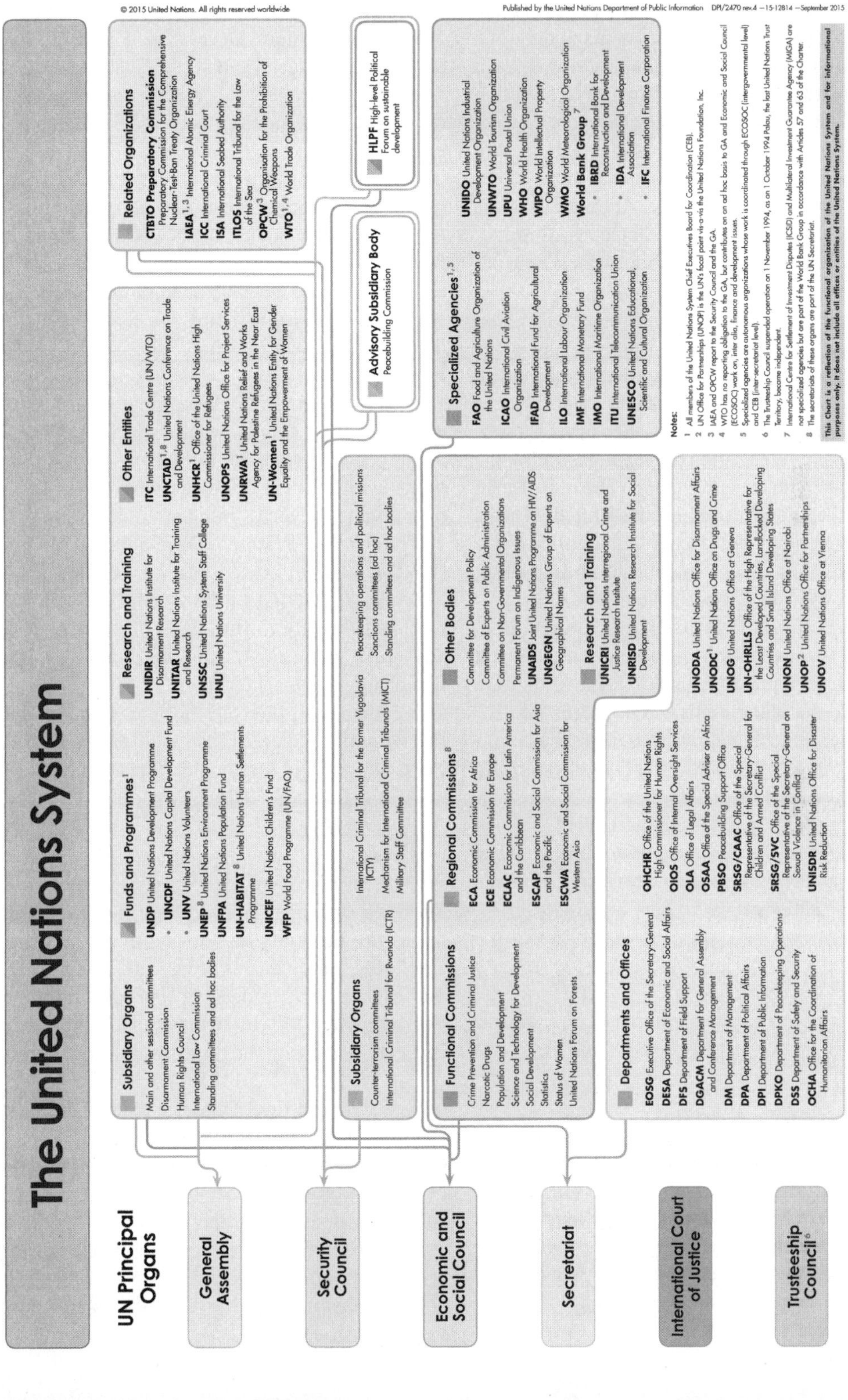

The United Nations System

UN Principal Organs
- General Assembly
- Security Council
- Economic and Social Council
- Secretariat
- International Court of Justice
- Trusteeship Council[6]

General Assembly

Subsidiary Organs
- Main and other sessional committees
- Disarmament Commission
- Human Rights Council
- International Law Commission
- Standing committees and ad hoc bodies

Funds and Programmes[1]
- UNDP United Nations Development Programme
  - UNCDF United Nations Capital Development Fund
  - UNV United Nations Volunteers
- UNEP[8] United Nations Environment Programme
- UNFPA United Nations Population Fund
- UN-HABITAT[8] United Nations Human Settlements Programme
- UNICEF United Nations Children's Fund
- WFP World Food Programme (UN/FAO)

Research and Training
- UNIDIR United Nations Institute for Disarmament Research
- UNITAR United Nations Institute for Training and Research
- UNSSC United Nations System Staff College
- UNU United Nations University

Other Entities
- ITC International Trade Centre (UN/WTO)
- UNCTAD[1,8] United Nations Conference on Trade and Development
- UNHCR[1] Office of the United Nations High Commissioner for Refugees
- UNOPS United Nations Office for Project Services
- UNRWA[1] United Nations Relief and Works Agency for Palestine Refugees in the Near East
- UN-Women[1] United Nations Entity for Gender Equality and the Empowerment of Women

Related Organizations
- CTBTO Preparatory Commission Preparatory Commission for the Comprehensive Nuclear-Test-Ban Treaty Organization
- IAEA[1,3] International Atomic Energy Agency
- ICC International Criminal Court
- ISA International Seabed Authority
- ITLOS International Tribunal for the Law of the Sea
- OPCW[3] Organisation for the Prohibition of Chemical Weapons
- WTO[1,4] World Trade Organization

HLPF High-level Political Forum on sustainable development

Security Council

Subsidiary Organs
- Counter-terrorism committees
- International Criminal Tribunal for Rwanda (ICTR)
- International Criminal Tribunal for the former Yugoslavia (ICTY)
- Mechanism for International Criminal Tribunals (MICT)
- Military Staff Committee
- Peacekeeping operations and political missions
- Sanctions committees (ad hoc)
- Standing committees and ad hoc bodies

Advisory Subsidiary Body
- Peacebuilding Commission

Economic and Social Council

Functional Commissions[8]
- Crime Prevention and Criminal Justice
- Narcotic Drugs
- Population and Development
- Science and Technology for Development
- Social Development
- Statistics
- Status of Women
- United Nations Forum on Forests

Regional Commissions[8]
- ECA Economic Commission for Africa
- ECE Economic Commission for Europe
- ECLAC Economic Commission for Latin America and the Caribbean
- ESCAP Economic and Social Commission for Asia and the Pacific
- ESCWA Economic and Social Commission for Western Asia

Other Bodies
- Committee for Development Policy
- Committee of Experts on Public Administration
- Committee on Non-Governmental Organizations
- Permanent Forum on Indigenous Issues
- UNAIDS Joint United Nations Programme on HIV/AIDS
- UNGEGN United Nations Group of Experts on Geographical Names

Research and Training
- UNICRI United Nations Interregional Crime and Justice Research Institute
- UNRISD United Nations Research Institute for Social Development

Specialized Agencies[1,5]
- FAO Food and Agriculture Organization of the United Nations
- ICAO International Civil Aviation Organization
- IFAD International Fund for Agricultural Development
- ILO International Labour Organization
- IMF International Monetary Fund
- IMO International Maritime Organization
- ITU International Telecommunication Union
- UNESCO United Nations Educational, Scientific and Cultural Organization
- UNIDO United Nations Industrial Development Organization
- UNWTO World Tourism Organization
- UPU Universal Postal Union
- WHO World Health Organization
- WIPO World Intellectual Property Organization
- WMO World Meteorological Organization
- World Bank Group[7]
  - IBRD International Bank for Reconstruction and Development
  - IDA International Development Association
  - IFC International Finance Corporation

Secretariat

Departments and Offices
- EOSG Executive Office of the Secretary-General
- DESA Department of Economic and Social Affairs
- DFS Department of Field Support
- DGACM Department for General Assembly and Conference Management
- DM Department of Management
- DPA Department of Political Affairs
- DPI Department of Public Information
- DPKO Department of Peacekeeping Operations
- DSS Department of Safety and Security
- OCHA Office for the Coordination of Humanitarian Affairs
- OHCHR Office of the United Nations High Commissioner for Human Rights
- OIOS Office of Internal Oversight Services
- OLA Office of Legal Affairs
- OSAA Office of the Special Adviser on Africa
- PBSO Peacebuilding Support Office
- SRSG/CAAC Office of the Special Representative of the Secretary-General for Children and Armed Conflict
- SRSG/SVC Office of the Special Representative of the Secretary-General on Sexual Violence in Conflict
- UNISDR United Nations Office for Disaster Risk Reduction
- UNODA United Nations Office for Disarmament Affairs
- UNODC[1] United Nations Office on Drugs and Crime
- UNOG United Nations Office at Geneva
- UN-OHRLLS Office of the High Representative for the Least Developed Countries, Landlocked Developing Countries and Small Island Developing States
- UNON United Nations Office at Nairobi
- UNOP[2] United Nations Office for Partnerships
- UNOV United Nations Office at Vienna

Notes:
1. All members of the United Nations System Chief Executives Board for Coordination (CEB).
2. UN Office for Partnerships (UNOP) is the UN's focal point vis-a-vis the United Nations Foundation, Inc.
3. IAEA and OPCW report to the Security Council and the GA.
4. WTO has no reporting obligation to the GA, but contributes on an ad hoc basis to GA and Economic and Social Council (ECOSOC) work on, inter alia, finance and development issues.
5. Specialized agencies are autonomous organizations whose work is coordinated through ECOSOC (intergovernmental level) and CEB (inter-secretariat level).
6. The Trusteeship Council suspended operation on 1 November 1994, as on 1 October 1994 Palau, the last United Nations Trust Territory, became independent.
7. International Centre for Settlement of Investment Disputes (ICSID) and Multilateral Investment Guarantee Agency (MIGA) are not specialized agencies but are part of the World Bank Group in accordance with Articles 57 and 63 of the Charter.
8. The secretariats of these organs are part of the UN Secretariat.

This Chart is a reflection of the functional organization of the United Nations System and for informational purposes only. It does not include all offices or entities of the United Nations System.

FIGURE 6.1 • Structure of the United Nations.
Source: From the United Nations Department of Public Information. © United Nations (2015). All rights reserved worldwide. Reprinted with the permission of the United Nations.

the U. N. is conducted by the Office of the Secretariat. "The Secretariat is one of the main organs of the U. N. and is organized along departmental lines, with each department or office having a distinct area of action and responsibility. Offices and departments coordinate with each other to ensure cohesion as they carry out the day-to-day work of the Organization in offices and duty stations around the world. At the head of the United Nations Secretariat is the Secretary-General" (http://www.un.org/en/sections/about-un/secretariat/index.html).

The World Health Organization (WHO) is a specialized agency of the United Nations concerned with the international public that was established in 1948. The WHO world headquarters are located in Geneva, Switzerland. For a comprehensive overview of its programs, projects and partnerships, follow the link http://www.who.int/entity/en/ (WHO, n. d.). In this chapter, the author examines the United Nations Millennium Development Goals (2000-2015) with special emphasis on Goal 4 (reduce child mortality); Goal 5 (improve maternal health); and Goal 6 (combat tuberculosis, HIV/AIDS, malaria, and other infectious diseases) as well as on the recently announced Sustainable Development Goals (2015-2030) that are the sequelae to the Millennium Development Goals.

In 2000, leaders of countries around the world met at the United Nations to establish a systematic approach to the reduction of extreme poverty. The plan for reducing poverty, laid out in the United Nations Millennium Declaration, was organized under eight goals known as the Millennium Development Goals (MDGs). The MDGs are:

1. Eradicate extreme poverty and hunger
2. Achieve universal primary education
3. Promote gender equality and empower women
4. Reduce child mortality
5. Improve maternal health
6. Combat HIV/AIDS, malaria, and other diseases
7. Ensure environmental stability
8. Develop partnership for development (U. N., 2015b)

The President of the Transcultural Nursing Society states that "… Transcultural nursing is a unique specialty that is not defined by a physical or geographic environment, specific technical skills, or a particular patient or learner population. Intrinsically, transcultural nurses are distinctively positioned to influence care within the global community. As such, the United Nations Millennium Development Goals, Post 2015 Development Agenda, and the Sustainable Development Goals can serve as a platform for the practice of transcultural nursing worldwide" (Marrone, 2016, p. 199).

Nurses with expertise in transcultural nursing practice, education, research, administration, and consultation—as well as those working with culturally competent interprofessional health care teams—contributed their transcultural nursing knowledge and experience toward assisting the United Nations and its global partners to achieve the MDGs (Amieva & Furguson, 2012).

Each Millennium Development Goal had a series of time-bound targets with a 2015 deadline. These eight goals were used by countries and development institutions around the world to guide efforts to mitigate poverty, hunger, and disease (U. N., 2015a; United Nations Development Programme [UNDP], 2015; United Nations Children's Emergency Fund [UNICEF], 2013, 2014). Goals 4, 5, and 6 related directly to the scope of practice of nurses and nurse practitioners and are therefore the foci of this chapter. The achievement of the other five goals also emphasized the roles of nurses and nurse practitioners, particularly those with expertise in transcultural nursing (Amievia & Furguson, 2012; Baird, 2011; Carmichael, 2011; Eipperle, 2015; Leuning, 2011; Marrone, 2011; WHO, 2013, 2015a).

Goal 4: Reduce Child Mortality

The focus of Target 4A under Goal 4 was to reduce the under-five mortality rate by two thirds between 1990 and 2015. Although this target was not on track to be met by 2015, the under-five mortality rate nonetheless declined by 47% by 2015 with 19% of participating countries achieving the target in their country (U. N., 2015c; Wang et al., 2014; WHO, 2015b). In 2015, 5.9 million children under age five died globally (WHO, 2015b). Inequality between high- and low-income countries remains large with low-income countries having 13 times the mortality rate for this age group compared to high-income countries (WHO, 2015a, 2015b). The WHO African Region had the highest under-five mortality rate with 81 per 1,000 live births, about seven times higher than the WHO European Region with 11 per 1,000 live births (U. N., 2015c;

WHO, 2015a, 2015b). However, the region also saw enormous gains in meeting this target goal. Most under-five deaths occur during the first 28 days of life; improving survival during this crucial period remains an enormous challenge in most low-income countries and requires a different set of technical skills and interventions (U. N., 2015b, 2015c; UNDP, 2013; UNICEF, 2014; Wang et al., 2014; WHO, 2015a, 2015b). Undernutrition causes an estimated 45% of deaths worldwide for children under the age of five but many countries were on target to meet 2015 target goals to reduce the number of underweight children (UNICEF, 2013, 2014; Wang et al., 2014; WHO, 2015b).

Measles is a highly contagious, viral disease that has largely been eradicated in the United States, Canada, and Europe through the immunization of children. In many low-income nations, measles remains one of the leading causes of death among young children, primarily due to complications such as pneumonia and encephalitis. In 2014, there were 13 measles-related deaths hourly worldwide (WHO, 2015c). In 2012, 84% of children had been vaccinated for measles and 66% of WHO member states had measles immunization rates of over 90%, a 22% increase of member states achieving this rate since 2000 (UNICEF, 2013; WHO, 2014). Globally, deaths from measles had also declined by 78% since 2000 (U. N. Secretariat, 2015; WHO, 2014, 2015c).

There is an ever-increasing need for transnational nurses with transcultural nursing and healthcare skills to respond to global needs with their expertise in addressing the MDGs related to maternal and child care (Prescott & Nichter, 2014; Wilson et al., 2013). Research has shown that the improvement in under-five mortality during the period from 2000-2015 can be attributed to childhood growth and development assistance, improvements to infrastructure, and the effects of efforts toward achieving the MDGs. Specific endeavors that contributed to success in this area were the reduction of mother-to-child transmission of HIV (Grimsrud et al., 2014; Hensen et al., 2012; Kohi et al., 2014; Ledikwe et al., 2014); increased male (infant) circumcision for HIV prevention in eastern and southern Africa (U. N., 2015c); and government policy changes, increased development assistance for health, and health system strengthening (Leffers & Mitchell, 2011; U. N., 2015c). Another important factor toward increased child survival is maternal education, which carries greater significance than income level (U. N., 2015a, 2015b, 2015c). Persistently high fertility rates in some countries made expansion of contraception/maternal education programs a priority for child survival goals, resulting in an increased worldwide contraceptive prevalence among women aged 15-49 from 55% in 1990 to 64% in 2015 (U. N., 2015c). Using Leininger's Culture Care Theory, Cortez and Zagal (2011) studied the global cultural implications of family planning and quality of life for women and their families to discover effective cultural care practices to improve the health and wellbeing of women during the childbearing and childrearing periods of their lives. The study involved training local traditional birth attendants to decrease complications of pregnancy before, during, and after delivery and other culturally congruent interventions. Moving forward, achieving MDG 4 required continued investments in maternal education, income growth, and the development and application of new health technologies (U. N. Secretariat, 2015; Wang et al., 2014; WHO, 2012, 2015a, 2015b).

In addition to their usual clinical roles in community health centers and hospitals, local nurses also played a large role in child survival programs, including the management of childhood illness; improvement of immunization techniques; and promoting healthy practices such as breastfeeding; early postnatal visitation by nurses, midwives, and indigenous and/or traditional women's health providers; managing and monitoring local child survival activities; capacity building; and supervising community health workers (Taylor, Hwenda, Larsen, & Daulaire, 2011). Providing maternal and child health and child survival homecare services that included prenatal outreach and educating cultural groups about reproductive health and family planning were also initiatives in which nurses actively participated (Cortez & Zagonel, 2011; UNICEF, 2013; U. S. Agency for International Development [USAID], 2012; WHO, 2012, 2014, 2015c).

Goal 5: Improve Maternal Health

Goal 5 had two main two targets. Target 5A was to "Reduce by three quarters, between 1990 and 2015, the maternal mortality ratio" and Target 5B to "Achieve, by 2015, universal access to reproductive health" (U. N., 2015a). Although the number of women dying due to complications during pregnancy and childbirth decreased by 50% worldwide since 1990, this target was not on track to reach global achievement by 2015 (U. N., 2015a). More than 71% of births were assisted by skilled health personnel globally in 2014, an increase from 59% in 1990 when the MDGs were initiated (U. N., 2015c; WHO, 2015b). Preventable deaths almost universally occurred in low- and middle-income countries where the critical obstacles to success in this area were lack of access to quality care before, during, and after childbirth (U. N., 2015a, 2015c). There continue to be large unmet needs for contraception especially in the WHO Africa region (WHO, 2014, 2015a, 2015b). Only 56% of pregnant women received the minimum recommended number of prenatal visits and in some low-income countries only 46% of births were attended by a skilled birth attendant (Dorwie & Pacquiao, 2014; Miller, Rashida, Tasneem, & Haque, 2012; Pereira, Mbaruku, Nzabuhakwa, Bergström, & McCord, 2011; Prata et al., 2011; Souza et al., 2013). High rates of adolescent pregnancy also contributed to the increased rates of maternal mortality (Alves, Wihlelm, de Souza, Ressel, 2013; UNICEF, 2014; WHO, 2014, 2015a, 2015b).

In a study of traditional birth attendants (TBAs) in Sierra Leone, Dorwie and Pacquiao (2014) found that TBAs were valued by mothers, health professionals, and the community because they provided accessible and affordable care to mothers who otherwise may not have had access to any health services. TBAs needed to receive training, supervision, and access to resources so as to provide effective care for expectant mothers. Systemic problems in the healthcare system created significant barriers independent of TBA practices that contributed to the continued high maternal and infant mortality rates (Dorwie & Pacquiao, 2014). This study and data from international health care organizations (WHO, 2014; U. N., 2015c) provide implications for broad public policy development toward improving maternal and child health in Sierra Leone and other less developed countries worldwide. Availability of essential obstetric services alone does not guarantee positive outcomes as these are highly dependent on the quality of the interventions provided. Obstacles to meeting Targets 5A and 5B included delayed or inappropriate implementation of interventions; failure to prevent and treat infections; and failure to promptly recognize the severity of maternal conditions (U. N., 2015a, 2015b, 2015c; WHO, 2015b). Future reductions in maternal mortality will depend upon the expansion of comprehensive emergency care and overall improvements in maternal health care (Souza et al., 2013; Wilson et al., 2013; WHO, 2015b).

Nurse-midwives played an important role in reducing maternal mortality by providing evidence-based, culturally competent, accessible, and affordable prenatal and delivery care. Nurses promoted health by encouraging the use of skilled birth attendants; repatterning and/or restructuring harmful cultural practices through client education; recognizing early warning signs during pregnancy and childbirth; and teaching family planning methods (Joshi, Sharma, & van Teijlingen, 2014; Lori & Boyle, 2011). Nurses collaborated with professional midwives and community health workers to encourage pregnant women to obtain appropriate prenatal care. As patient advocates, nurses ensured that maternity care was made available and accessible to as many diverse cultural groups as possible (Amieva & Ferguson, 2012; Tasçi-Duran, 2013).

Goal 6: Combat HIV/AIDS and Other Communicable Diseases

The three targets for Goal 6 were to halt HIV/AIDS and begin reversal of its spread by 2015; achieve universal access to treatment for HIV/AIDS for all those who need it by 2010; and halt and begin to reverse the incidence of malaria and other major diseases by 2015 (U. N., 2015).

HIV/AIDS

New HIV infections worldwide fell by approximately 40% between 2000 and 2013, from 3.5 million cases to 2.1 million, and people with HIV are living longer (U. N., 2015c).

MEDICATIONS Globally, fewer people die of HIV/AIDS each year, primarily as a result of access to the antiretroviral therapy (ART) medications and the concomitant and necessary patient educational programs (Matambo et al., 2014; U. N., 2015c; WHO, 2015b). ART refers to all medications used to treat HIV. These drugs do not kill the virus or cure the disease, but they are often able to reduce the viral load in patients' blood (Asfaw et al., 2014).

When taken in formulated combinations, these medications inhibit or disrupt the growth or replication of the virus. When the viral load is thus reduced, the health of infected person improves although the infection remains. Traditional cultural healers can be effective conduits to connecting HIV-positive patients with ART in African nations such as Uganda where the disease has become endemic. The importance of their active participation in HIV/AIDS prevention programs cannot be overstated (Horwitz et al., 2013).

The 2010 WHO strategy for the prevention of mother-to-child HIV transmission (PMTCT) set forth a comprehensive approach with four main components: Primary prevention of HIV infection; prevention of unintended pregnancies among women living with HIV; prevention of HIV transmission of a woman with HIV to her infant; and provision of appropriate treatment, care, and support to mothers living with HIV and their families (Kohi et al., 2014; van der Straten, Van Damme, Haberer, & Bangsberg, 2012; WHO, 2010). The WHO strategy provided guidelines for countries regarding the provision of ART to pregnant women and their infants to prevent vertical transmission of HIV during pregnancy, delivery, and breastfeeding (Walensky et al., 2012; WHO, 2012, 2014).

Critical to the prevention and treatment of HIV is the timely identification of HIV-positive individuals and counseling of all patients regarding their HIV status (U. N., 2015c). Although Kenya has approximately 1.4 million adults with HIV/AIDS and a national prevalence rate of approximately 7.4%, the majority of Kenyans are unaware of their HIV status (WHO, 2015a). This lack of awareness increases the likelihood of infecting others and spreading the disease. Gardner (2013) conducted a phenomenological study to explore HIV-positive women's experiences and perceptions about Voluntary Counseling and Testing (VCT) programs. In-depth interviews were conducted with 29 women residing in rural parts of Kenya. The following six themes emerged from the data: *Living in fear*; *making the decision to be tested*; *the journey toward acceptance*; *changing behavior*; *planning for the future*; and *encouraging others to be tested*. VCT programs are essential in attaining MDG goals related to the prevention and management of AIDS. The nurse-researcher who conducted the investigation explored the women's experiences, perceptions, and issues concerning AIDS, and their acceptance and use of VCT. The results of this study may be useful in providing more culturally congruent VCT programs in the future, thereby increasing the likelihood that Kenyan

women will participate and subsequently become aware of their HIV status (Gardner, 2013).

In another study, researchers discovered that by making HIV testing and counseling by trained health-care providers part of routine health care, the stigmas surrounding HIV/AIDS were reduced, more HIV-positive individuals were provided with appropriate care and treatment, and prevention messages for persons testing positive were reinforced (Roura, Watson-Jones, Kahawita, Ferguson, & Ross, 2013). When these and other related care services are provided in connection with prenatal care, their benefits include increased prevention of mother-to-child HIV transmission (Hensen et al., 2011; Kohi et al., 2014).

MALE CIRCUMCISION Since 2007, the WHO and its global health partner organizations and ministries have promoted voluntary medical male circumcision (VMMC) as a means for reducing heterosexual HIV transmission by approximately 60% (WHO, 2012, 2014). VMMC programs contributed to the development of innovative circumcision methods (such as the use of surgical devices that do not require injected local anesthesia or sutures) and also provided opportunities to present and/or reinforce HIV prevention education (Reed et al., 2012). Male circumcision is often highly bound to culture; overcoming cultural barriers to accepting this method of HIV prevention continued to pose significant challenges for public health professionals worldwide (Ledikwe et al., 2014; Reed et al., 2012). The target goal of performing 20 million male circumcisions by 2015 was estimated to have the potential to prevent 3.4 million new HIV infections and thereby also averting $16.5 billion in HIV treatment costs by 2025 (Reed et al., 2011).

PRE-EXPOSURE PROPHYLAXIS Among the foci of HIV prevention that continues to evolve is pre-exposure prophylaxis (PrEP) using the drug tenofovir (Walensky et al., 2012). One study estimated that PrEP could decrease mean lifetime risk of HIV infection among South African women from 40% to 27% but its cost effectiveness remained questionable (Walensky et al., 2012). Research about the factors affecting the efficacy and acceptability of PrEP have shown widely variable results that were likely influenced by regimen adherence and cultural acceptability of the various PrEP product components (van der Straten et al., 2012). Nurses and nurse practitioners played a significant role in HIV/AIDS prevention, care, and treatment during this era of increased task-shifting away from physicians toward nonphysician healthcare providers. In addition to traditional roles in health promotion and education, nurses took responsibility for initiating and managing ART and provided VMMC services (Fairall et al., 2012). Nurse-managed and nurse-initiated ART resulted in outcomes similar to those from physician-managed ART programs but at lower costs, increased accessibility, and potential reductions in loss to follow-up (Gardner, 2013; Grimsrud et al., 2014; Kredo, Adeniyi, Bateganya, & Pienaar, 2014). Research in Ethiopia found that ART service delivery provided by nurses and health officers was rated more highly by patients than that provided by physicians (Asfaw et al., 2014). A systematic review and meta-analysis of responsibilities task-shifted from medical doctors to nonphysician providers (including nurses) found that reported rates of adverse events were similar to those of physicians and specialists (Ford, Chu, & Mills, 2011).

Tuberculosis, Malaria, and Other Selected Diseases

New cases of tuberculosis (TB) have been declining for more than ten years with disease mortality falling 45% since 1990 (WHO, 2015b). However, the emergence of multidrug resistant TB poses a growing threat to undermining this achievement (WHO, 2015a). The global *incidence* of malaria has fallen by 25%, and by 31% in the WHO Africa region; in addition, the worldwide *mortality* from malaria decreased by 42% (WHO, 2015a). The incidence rates and mortalities related to untreated tropical diseases also declined. For example, leprosy has been eliminated from 119 of the 122 countries where it was previously endemic (WHO 2014, 2015a). However, rates of dengue fever continue to increase, thwarting efforts toward its eradication (WHO, 2014, 2015a).

Ebola virus disease (EVD), formerly known as Ebola haemorrhagic fever, is a severe, often fatal illness in humans. The first EVD outbreaks occurred in remote villages in Central Africa near tropical rainforests, but the most recent outbreak in West Africa has involved major urban as well as rural areas with occasional cases reaching the United States and Europe (WHO, 2016). The EVD virus is transmitted to people from wild animals and spreads in the human population through human-to-human transmission. The average EVD case fatality rate is around 50%, with case fatality rates ranging from 25% to 90% in past outbreaks.

Effective outbreak control relies on applying multiple interventions by nurses and others on the health care team including case management; surveillance and contact tracing; accurate laboratory services; and safe burial practices that prevent post mortem spread (World Health Organization, 2016). The contributions of transcultural nursing in providing culturally congruent and culturally competent care recently gained visibility when EVD reached the United States and sickened two nurses (Gray, 2015).

The United Nations Development Programme (UNDP) has been one of the leading organizations working to reach the MDG targets (UNDP, 2015). With its presence in more than 170 countries and territories, the UNDP-funded projects helped to fulfill goals and monitor progress toward achieving these outcomes (UNDP, 2015). The 15-year interval spanning the MDG implementation period recorded the fastest reduction in poverty in human history (U. N., 2015c). As a result of the MDG efforts, half a billion *fewer* people live *below* the internationally determined poverty line of $1.25 a day; child death rates decreased by more than 30%, saving approximately three million children's lives annually; and deaths from malaria were reduced by 25% compared to 2000 (U. N. Secretariat, 2015). This unprecedented progress in reducing poverty was driven by the combination of economic growth, improved public policies, and global commitment to the MDGs which were multi-faceted and problematic challenges for the entire world to address. Nevertheless, there remains significant ongoing global poverty.

■ PRIMARY CARE NURSE PRACTITIONERS' CONTRIBUTIONS TO ACHIEVEMENT OF THE MDGs

Nurses and other health-care leaders from countries with diverse levels of development have stated their collective goals toward improving primary healthcare services worldwide. These goals include: Increase the volume of primary care services offered; improve access and affordability to quality health care; and enhance the cultural competency knowledge and skills of primary care nurse practitioners for the provision of culturally congruent nursing and healthcare services (Eipperle, 2015).

The Transcultural Nursing Society (TCNS) Scholars group (http://www.tcns.org/Scholars.html) was established to promote the advancement of transcultural nursing knowledge, research, education, and practice in health care worldwide. The activities and contributions of TCNS Scholars in the promotion of culturally congruent and competent care through education, research practice, and administration in the global community are significant. For example, consistent with the purpose of the TCNS Scholars and the goal of the University of Brooklyn Hospital (UBH) Department of Nursing Services to expand its scope of influence and expertise for the delivery of nursing care globally, the UHB hosted 20 advanced practice nursing students and faculty from the Netherlands. The purpose of the USA-Dutch exchange was to discuss the delivery of culturally congruent and culturally competent care of vulnerable populations by advanced practice nurses (Marrone, 2011).

Common problems faced by both high-income and low-income countries include the growing epidemic of chronic disease; reappearance of previously controlled or eradicated infectious diseases; inadequate healthcare access; health outcome disparities; high-costs associated with end-of-life care; and lack of preventive care for infants and children (U. N., 2015c). These problems have led to the use of costly technological methods that may not be beneficial or acceptable, particularly in low-income countries that might lack critical infrastructure to consistently operate selected types of technology, such as access to electricity or other reliable energy sources; satellite connectivity; and support services necessary for the use of many contemporary technologies. One strategy for addressing these challenges is the increased use of nurse practitioners to provide primary care services. Decades of extensive research has documented that health outcomes are improved when nurse practitioners and other advanced practice nurses provide holistic, culturally congruent, and family-centered care, which is well-suited to meet the challenging healthcare needs of patients and families in the context of globalization (Courtney & Wolgamott, 2015; Eipperle, 2015; Fairall et al., 2012; Grimsrud et al., 2014; WHO, 2013). Barriers that prevent nurse practitioners (NPs) from practicing to the fullest extent of their education and experience in primary care (or other) settings include lack of standardized curricula and program outcomes for schools of nursing across national borders; lack of standardized scope of practice and regulatory body credentialing requirements within and between countries; varying levels of knowledge and expertise held by nurse practitioners across cultures, borders, and healthcare systems; transnational or global standardized titling; and uniform regulating processes for nurse practitioners. Some countries such as Australia, Canada, and the United States (where the majority of nurse practitioners work in primary care) have title standardization and protection, formal advanced graduate education programs, and regulating bodies that maintain licensure standards.

Task-shifting away from physicians toward primary care nurse practitioners was shown to be effective in numerous parts of the world including South Africa (Fairall et al., 2012). In 2014, the Global Advanced Practice Nursing Symposium called for role standardization that included adopting the 2002 International Council of Nurses definition for the advanced practice nurse (APN) role; enhancing education curricula through cultural respect; eliminating policies that prevent APNs from practicing to the fullest extent of their education and training; establishing funding mechanisms that support APN-based practice models; and disseminating research about APN care quality and patient outcomes across the globe. Not only will these efforts help to standardize the APN role but they will also help to create clarity within the profession while supporting healthcare reform and policy changes, which together promote all nurses' roles toward achieving the Millennium Development Goals.

■ SUSTAINABLE DEVELOPMENT GOALS

The people and countries of the world are more connected now than when the MDGs were established in 2000. The 2030 Agenda for Sustainable Development, unanimously adopted in September 2015 by leaders of all 193 United Nation member states, consists of 17 ambitious Sustainable Development Goals (SDGs) and 169 targets (U. N., 2015a). Leaders from United Nations member countries built on the many successes of the past 15 years, creating a common vision for the future

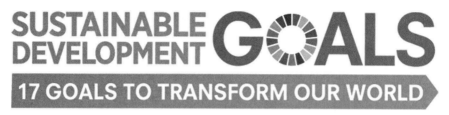

FIGURE 6.2 • United Nations. Sustainable Development Goals: 17 Goals to Transform Our World.
Retrieved from http://www.un.org/sustainabledevelopment/sustainable-development-goals/. Used with permission of the United Nations.

of the planet (UNDP, 2015) with a new set of goals based on respect for universal human rights to address current global issues. These aim to end poverty, hunger, inequality, and climate change by 2030 (U. N., 2015c). Recognizing the connection between people and planet, they also established goals that address how we will manage the land, the oceans, and waterways of our globe. The United Nations Secretary General referred to the SDGs as a plan of action for people, planet and prosperity (http://www.un.org/sustainabledevelopment/sustainable-development-goals/).

The SDGs are (Refer to Figure 6.2):

- No poverty
- Zero hunger
- Good health and wellbeing
- Quality education
- Gender equality
- Clean water and sanitation
- Affordable and clean energy
- Decent work and economic growth
- Industry, innovation, and infrastructure
- Reduced inequalities
- Sustainable cities and communities
- Responsible consumption and production
- Climate action
- Life below water
- Life on land
- Peace, justice, and strong institutions
- Partnerships for goal achievement

■ SUMMARY

Transcultural nurses with expertise in transcultural nursing and health care and culturally competent interprofessional teams have contributed significantly to the achievement of the Millennium Development Goals between the years 2000 to 2015. Although some goals were achieved in advance of the target date, progress toward many of the goals remains only partially completed in many areas of the world. As a result, the United Nations renewed its commitment to targeting women's and children's health, poverty, hunger, disease, and gender equality through the development of the Post-2015 Agenda and Sustainable Development Goals. Nurses with transcultural nursing expertise will play a pivotal role in bringing the Sustainable Development Goals to fruition by the year 2030 (WHO, 2013). The new development agenda applies to all countries; promotes peaceful and inclusive societies; creates better jobs; and tackles the environmental challenges of our time—particularly climate change. The Sustainable Development Goals must finish the work that remains from the Millennium Development Goals, address important new goals for the future of the planet, and leave no one behind (UNDP, 2015).

■ DISCUSSION QUESTIONS

1. Discuss how the Theory of Culture Care Diversity and Universality has been integrated into nursing theories or models for worldwide/global applications in health care by nurses and other professionals.
2. Discuss the influence of transcultural nursing and transnationalism upon the global incidence and prevalence of childhood morbidity and mortality during the 15-year period of the Sustainable Millennial Goal period.
3. Discuss the influence of transcultural nursing and transnationalism upon perinatal maternal health worldwide during the 15-year period of the Sustainable Millennial Goal period.

4. Discuss the influence of transcultural nursing and transnationalism upon the global incidence and prevalence of HIV/AIDs and other infectious diseases during the 15-year period of the Sustainable Millennial Goal period.
5. Discuss how reading this chapter may influence your *personal* viewpoints and perceptions about global events.
6. Discuss how reading this chapter may influence your *professional* viewpoints and perceptions about global health.
7. Discuss how reading this chapter may influence your *professional* viewpoints and perceptions about health volunteerism locally or globally (include mission work; service-learning; emergency response team; and/or educational preceptorships in your discussions).

■ REFERENCES

Alves, C. N., Wilhelm, L. A., de Souza, D. F., & Ressel, L. B. (2013). Nursing care provided to pregnant women from the cultural perspective: Introductory note. *Journal of Nursing UFPE/Revista De Enfermagem UFPE, 7*(7S), 5047-5050. doi: 10.5205/reuol.4700-39563-1-ED.0707esp201332

Andrews, M. M. (2006). The globalization of transcultural nursing theory and research. In M. M. Leininger & M. R. McFarland (Eds.), *Culture care diversity and universality: A worldwide nursing theory* (2nd ed., pp. 91-110). Sudbury, MA: Jones & Bartlett.

Amieva, S., & Ferguson, S. (2012). Moving forward: Nurses are key to achieving the United Nations Development Program's Millennium Development Goals. *International Nursing Review, 59*(1), 55-58. doi: 10.1111/j.1466-7657.2011.00944.x

Asfaw, E., Dominis, S., Palen, J. G. H., Wong, W., Bekele, A., Kebede, A., & Johns, B. (2014). Patient satisfaction with task shifting of antiretroviral services in Ethiopia: Implications for universal health coverage. *Health Policy and Planning, 29*(Suppl 2), ii50-ii58. doi: 10.1093/heapol/czu072

Baird, M. B. (2011). Lessons learned from translators and interpreters from the Dinka tribe of southern Sudan. *Journal of Transcultural Nursing, 22*(2), 116-121. doi: 10.1177/1043659610395764

Carmichael, T. B. (2011). Letter to the editor: Cultural competence: A necessity for the 21st century. *Journal of Transcultural Nursing, 22*(1), 5-6. doi: 10.1177/1043659610387155

Cortez, E. F., & Zagonel, I. S. (2011). Cultural implications in family planning and quality of life of the woman and family, and Leininger's theory. *Cogitare Enfermagem, 16*(2), 296-302.

Courtney, R., & Wolgamott, S. (2015). Using Leininger's theory as the building block for cultural competence and cultural assessment for a collaborative team in a primary care setting. In M. R. McFarland & H. B. Wehbe-Alamah (Eds.), *Leininger's culture care diversity and universality: A worldwide nursing theory* (3rd ed., pp. 345-368). Burlington, MA: Jones and Bartlett Learning.

Dorwie, F. M., & Pacquiao, D. F. (2014). Practices of traditional birth attendants in Sierra Leone and perceptions by mothers and health professionals familiar with their care. *Journal of Transcultural Nursing, 25*(1), 33-41. doi: 10.1177/1043659613503874

Eipperle, M. K. (2015). Application of the three modes of culture care decisions and actions in advanced practice primary care. In M. R. McFarland & H. B. Wehbe-Alamah (Eds.), *Leininger's culture care diversity and universality: A worldwide nursing theory* (3rd ed., pp. 317-344). Burlington, MA: Jones and Bartlett Learning.

Fairall, L., Bachmann, M. O., Lombard, C., Timmerman, V., Uebel, K., Zwarenstein, M., & Bateman, E. (2012). Task shifting of antiretroviral treatment from doctors to primary-care nurses in South Africa (STRETCH): A pragmatic, parallel, cluster-randomised trial. *Lancet, 380*(9845), 889-898. doi: 10.1016/S0140-6736(12)60730-2

Ford, N., Chu, K., & Mills, E. J. (2012). Safety of task shifting for male medical circumcision in Africa: A systematic review and meta-analysis. *AIDS, 26*(5), 559-566. doi: 10.1097/QAD.0b013e32834f3264

Gardner, J. (2013). The experiences of HIV-positive women living in an African village: Perceptions of voluntary counseling and testing programs. *Journal of Transcultural Nursing, 24*(1), 25-32. doi: 10.1177/1043659612462404

Goodman, P., Edge, B., Agazio, J., & Prue-Owens, K. (2015). Cultural awareness: Nursing care of Iraqi patients. *Journal of Transcultural Nursing, 26*(4), 395-401. doi: 10.1177/1043659614524794

Gray, J. (2015). Thoughts on transcultural nursing and Ebola. *Journal of Transcultural Nursing, 26*(1), 6-7. doi: 10.1177/1043659614561680

Grimsrud, A., Kaplan, R., Bekker, L., & Myer, L. (2014). Outcomes of a nurse-managed service for stable HIV-positive patients in a large South African public sector antiretroviral therapy programme. *Tropical Medicine & International Health, 19*(9), 1029-1039. doi: 10.1111/tmi.12346

Hensen, B., Baggaley, R., Wong, V. J., Grabbe, K. L., Shaffer, N., Lo, Y. J., & Hargreaves, J. (2012). Universal voluntary HIV testing in antenatal care settings: A review of the contribution of provider-initiated testing & counselling. *Tropical Medicine & International Health, 17*(1), 59-70. doi: 10.1111/j.1365-3156.2011.02893.x

Historicair, C. C. (n. d.). Structure of the United Nations [Figure]. Retrieved from https://commons.wikimedia.org/W/index.php?curid=4392031

Horwitz, R. H., Tsai, A. C., Maling, S., Bajunirwe, F., Haberer, J. E., Emenyonu, N., & Bangsberg, D. R. (2013). No association found between traditional healer use and delayed antiretroviral initiation in rural Uganda. *AIDS and Behavior*, *17*(1), 260-265. doi: 10.1007/s10461-011-0132-7

Joshi, R., Sharma, S., & van Teijlingen, E. (2014). Improving neonatal health in Nepal. *Health Science Journal*, *7*(3), 247-257.

Knecht, L., & Sabatine, C. (2015). Application of Culture Care Theory to international service learning experiences in Kenya. In M. R. McFarland & H. B. Wehbe-Alamah (Eds.), *Leininger's culture care diversity and universality: A worldwide nursing theory* (3rd ed., pp. 475-501). Burlington, MA: Jones and Bartlett Learning.

Kohi, T. W., Mselle, L. T., Mashauri, P. M., Mpandana, C., Vermond, N., & Mfalla, L. (2014). Using a collaborative approach to address task shifting during the HIV epidemic: The Tanzania experience. *African Journal of Midwifery and Women's Health*, *8*(2), 17-19.

Kredo, T., Adeniyi, F. B., Bateganya, M., & Pienaar, E. D. (2014). Task shifting from doctors to non-doctors for initiation and maintenance of antiretroviral therapy. *The Cochrane Database of Systematic Reviews*, *7*, CD0073.

Larsen, M. (2015). The Greek connection: Discovering the cultural and social structure dimensions of the Greek culture using Leininger's theory of culture care: A model for a baccalaureate study-abroad experience. In M. R. McFarland & H. B. Wehbe-Alamah (Eds.), *Leininger's culture care diversity and universality: A worldwide nursing theory* (3rd ed., pp. 503-520). Burlington, MA: Jones and Bartlett Learning.

Ledikwe, J. H., Nyanga, R. O., Hagon, J., Grignon, J. S., Mpofu, M., & Semo, B. (2014, October 8). Scaling-up voluntary medical male circumcision - what have we learned? *HIV/AIDS-Research and Palliative Care*, *6*, 139-146.

Leffers, J., & Mitchell, E. (2011). Conceptual model for partnership and sustainability in global health. *Public Health Nursing*, *28*(1), 91-102. doi: 10.1111/j.1525-1446.2010.00892.x

Leininger, M. M. (1978). The culture concept and its relevance to nursing. In M. M. Leininger (Ed.), *Transcultural nursing: Concepts, theories, and practices* (pp. 109-120). New York, NY: Wiley Medical.

Leininger, M. M. (2006a). Culture care diversity and universality theory and evolution of the ethnonursing research method. In M. M. Leininger & M. R. McFarland (Eds.), *Culture care diversity and universality: A worldwide nursing theory* (2nd ed., pp. 1-41). Sudbury, MA: Jones and Bartlett.

Leininger, M. M. (2006b). Culture care of the Gadsup Akuna of the Eastern Highlands of New Guinea: First transcultural nursing study [Revised reprint]. In M. M. Leininger & M. R. McFarland (Eds.), *Culture care diversity and universality: A worldwide nursing theory* (2nd ed., pp. 115-157). Sudbury, MA: Jones and Bartlett.

Leininger, M. M. (2015). Benefits of the culture care theory and a look to the future of transcultural nursing. In M. R. McFarland & H. B. Wehbe-Alamah (Eds.), *Leininger's culture care diversity and universality: A worldwide nursing theory* (3rd ed., pp. 101-118). Burlington, MA: Jones and Bartlett Learning.

Leininger, M. M., & McFarland, M. R. (Eds.). (2002). *Transcultural nursing: Concepts, theories, research, and practice* (3rd ed.). New York, NY: McGraw-Hill.

Leininger, M. M., & McFarland, M. R. (Eds.). (2006). *Culture care diversity and universality: A worldwide nursing theory* (2nd ed.). Sudbury, MA: Jones and Bartlett.

Leuning, C. J. (2011). Transcultural nursing scholars' corner: Advancing our practice, changing our world. *Journal of Transcultural Nursing*, *22*(4), 417-417. doi: 10.1177/1043659611414202

Lori, J. R., & Boyle, J. S. (2011). Cultural childbirth practices, beliefs, and traditions in post conflict Liberia. *Healthcare for Women International*, *32*(6), 454-473. doi: 10.1080/07399332.2011.555831

Marrone, S. R. (2011). Transcultural nursing scholars' corner: Promoting culturally competent care globally from within a service setting. *Journal of Transcultural Nursing*, *22*(3), 307. doi: 10.1177/1043659611404433

Marrone, S. R. (2016). President's message: Transcultural nursing in the global community. *Journal of Transcultural Nursing*, *27*(2), 199.

Matambo, S., Machakaire, E., Motswere-Chirwa, C., Legwaila, K., Letsholathebe, V., Dintwa, E., & Glenshaw, M. (2014). Quality assurance of prevention of mother-to-child transmission of HIV in Botswana. *African Journal of Midwifery and Women's Health*, *8*(3), 130-133.

McFarland, M. R., & Wehbe-Alamah, H. B. (2015). *Leininger's culture care diversity and universality: A worldwide nursing theory* (3rd ed.). Burlington, MA: Jones and Bartlett Learning.

Miller, P. C., Rashida, G., Tasneem, Z., & Haque, M. (2012). The effect of traditional birth attendant training on maternal and neonatal care. *International Journal of Gynaecology and Obstetrics: The Official Organ of the International Federation of Gynaecology and Obstetrics*, *117*(2), 148-152.

Njeuhmeli, E., Forsythe, S., Reed, J., Opuni, M., Bollinger, L., Heard, N., & Hankins, C. (2011). Voluntary medical male circumcision: Modeling the impact and cost of expanding male circumcision for HIV prevention in eastern and southern Africa. *PLoS Medicine*, *8*(11), 1-10 (e1001128). doi: 10.1371/journal.pmed.1001132

Omeri, A. S. (2015). Culture care diversity and universality: A pathway to culturally congruent practices in transcultural nursing education, research, and practice in Australia. In M. R. McFarland & H. B. Wehbe-Alamah (Eds.), *Leininger's culture care diversity and universality: A worldwide nursing theory* (3rd ed., pp. 443-474). Burlington, MA: Jones and Bartlett Learning.

Pereira, C., Mbaruku, G., Nzabuhakwa, C., Bergström, S., & McCord, C. (2011). Emergency obstetric surgery by non-physician clinicians in Tanzania. *International Journal of Gynecology and Obstetrics, 114*(2), 180-183. doi: 10.1016/j.ijgo.2011.05.004

Prata, N., Passano, P., Rowen, T., Bell, S., Walsh, J., & Potts, M. (2011). Where there are (few) skilled birth attendants. *The Journal of Health, Population, and Nutrition, 29*(2), 81-91. doi: 10.3329/jhpn.v29i2.7812

Prescott, M., & Nichter, M. (2014). Transnational nurse migration: Future directions for medical anthropological research. *Social Science & Medicine (1982), 107*, 113-123. doi: 10.1016/j.socscimed.2014.02.026

Reed, J. B., Njeuhmeli, E., Thomas, A. G., Bacon, M. C., Bailey, R., Cherutich, P., & Bock, N. (2012, August 15). Voluntary medical male circumcision: An HIV prevention priority for PEPFAR. *JAIDS: Journal of Acquired Immune Deficiency Syndromes, 60*(3S), S88-S95. doi: 10.1097/QAI.0b013e31825cac4e

Roura, M., Watson-Jones, D., Kahawita, T. M., Ferguson, L., & Ross, D. A. (2013). Provider-initiated testing and counselling programmes in sub-Saharan Africa: A systematic review of their operational implementation. *AIDS (London, England), 27*(4), 617.

Souza, J. P., Gülmezoglu, A. M., Vogel, J., Carroli, G., Lumbiganon, P., Qureshi, Z., … Say, L. (2013, May 18-24). Moving beyond essential interventions for reduction of maternal mortality (the WHO multicountry survey on maternal and newborn health): A cross-sectional study. *Lancet, 381*(9879), 1747-1755. doi: 10.1016/S0140-6736(13)60686-8

Tasçi-Duran, E., & Sevil, U. (2013). A comparison of the prenatal health behaviors of women from four cultural groups in Turkey: An ethnonursing study. *Nursing Science Quarterly, 26*(3), 257-266. doi: 10.1177/0894318413489180

Taylor, A. L., Hwenda, L., Larsen, B., & Daulaire, N. (2011). Stemming the brain drain—a WHO global code of practice on international recruitment of health personnel. *The New England Journal of Medicine, 365*(25), 2348-2351. doi: 10.1056/NEJMp1108658

Transcultural Nursing Society. (n. d.). Transcultural Nursing Society Scholars. Retrieved from http://www.tcns.org/Scholars.html

United Nations. (n. d.-a). *United Nations overview.* Retrieved from http://www.un.org/en/sections/about-un/overview/index.html

United Nations. (n. d.-b). *United Nations secretariat.* Retrieved from http://www.un.org/en/sections/about-un/secretariat/index.html

United Nations. (2015a). *Transforming our world: The 2030 agenda for sustainable development.* New York, NY: Author. Retrieved from https://sustainabledevelopment

United Nations. (2015b). *We can end poverty: Millennium development goals and beyond 2015.* Retrieved from http://www.un.org/millenniumgoals/

United Nations. (2015c). *The millennium development goals report 2015 summary.* Retrieved from http://www.un.org/millenniumgoals/2015_MDG_Report/pdf/MDG%202015%20rev%20%28July%201%29.pdf

United Nations Children's Emergency Fund. (2013). *Young child survival and development.* [Thematic Report] Retrieved from http://www.unicef.org/Young_Child_Survival_and_Development_2011.pdf

United Nations Children's Emergency Fund. (2014). *Delivery care: Skilled attendant at birth - percentage in 2014.* Retrieved from http://data.unicef.org

United Nations Development Programme. (2015). *A new sustainable development agenda.* Retrieved from http://www.undp.org/content/undp/en/home/mdgoverview.html

United Nations Secretariat, Department of Economic and Social Affairs, Inter-Agency and Expert Group on MDG Indicators. (2015). *Millennium development goals report: 2015.* New York, NY: Author. Retrieved from http://millenniumindicators.un.org/unsd/mdg/Resources/Static/Products/Progress2015/English2015.pdf

United Nations Sustainable Development Goals. (2015). Retrieved from http://www.un.org/sustainabledevelopment/ sustainable-development-goals/

U. S. Agency for International Development. (2012). *USAID's child survival and health grants program: Select information from five projects.* Washington, D. C.: Author. Retrieved from https://www.usaid.gov/mdg

van der Straten, A., Van Damme, L., Haberer, J. E., & Bangsberg, D. R. (2012). Unraveling the divergent results of pre-exposure prophylaxis trials for HIV prevention. *AIDS, 26*(7), F13-F19. doi: 10.1097/QAD.0b013e3283522272

Walensky, R. P., Park, J., Wood, R., Freedberg, K. A., Scott, C. A., Bekker, L., & Paltiel, A. D. (2012). The cost-effectiveness of pre-exposure prophylaxis for HIV infection in South African women. *Clinical Infectious Diseases: An Official Publication of the Infectious Diseases Society of America, 54*(10), 1504-1513. doi: 10.1093/cid/cis225

Wang, H., Liddell, C. A., Coates, M. M., Mooney, M. D., Levitz, C. E., Schumacher, A. E., … Idrisov, B. T. (2014). Global, regional, and national levels of neonatal, infant, and under-5 mortality during 1990-2013: A systematic analysis for the global burden of disease study 2013. *Lancet, 384*(9947), 957-979. doi: 10.1016/S0140-6736(14)60497-9

Wilson, A., Gallos, I. D., Plana, N., Lissauer, D., Khan, K. S., Zamora, J., & Coomarasamy, A. (2011, December 1). Effectiveness of strategies incorporating training and support of traditional birth attendants on perinatal and maternal mortality: Meta-analysis. *British Medical Journal, 343*(d7102), 1-10. doi: 10.1136/bmj.d7102

World Health Organization. (n. d.). *About the World Health Organization*. Retrieved from http://www.who.int/about/what-we-do/en/

World Health Organization. (2012). *Voluntary medical male circumcision for HIV prevention*. Retrieved from http://www.who.int/hiv/topics/malecircumcision/fact_sheet/en/

World Health Organization. (2013). *A universal truth: No health without a workforce*. Geneva, SZ: Author. Retrieved from http://www.who.int/workforcealliance/knowledge/resources/GHWA_AUniversalTruthReport.pdf

World Health Organization. (2014). *World health statistics 2014* (Annual No. 2014 IIS 4640-S2). Retrieved from http://www.who.int/gho/publications/world_health_ statistics/en/

World Health Organization. (2015a). *Global Health Observatory (GHO) data*. Retrieved from http://www.who.int/gho/en/

World Health Organization. (2015b). *Global Heath Observatory data: Under-five mortality*. Retrieved from http www.who.int/gho/child_health/mortality_under_five_mortality

World Health Organization. (2015c). *Measles fact sheet*. Retrieved from http://www.who.int/mediacentre/fact-sheets/ fs286/en/

World Health Organization. (2016). *Ebola virus disease*. Retrieved from http://www.who.int/mediacentre/fact-sheets/ fs103/en/

Zoucha, R., & Turk, M. (2015). Using the Culture Care Theory as a guide to develop and implement a transcultural global course for doctor of nursing practice students for study in Italy. In M. R. McFarland & H. B. Wehbe-Alamah (Eds.), *Leininger's culture care diversity and universality: A worldwide nursing theory* (3rd ed., pp. 521-535). Burlington, MA: Jones and Bartlett Learning.

CHAPTER 7

Cultural Assessments and Transcultural Communication for Culturally Congruent Care

Hiba B. Wehbe-Alamah

> *"The roots of cultural influence are deep and widespread. They require careful study and assessment to determine the regularities and irregularities of a particular culture as a sound basis for health care practices" (Leininger, 1994b, p. 85).*

■ INTRODUCTION

One of the greatest challenges for nurses is to discover how culturally based care factors can make a difference in providing meaningful, appropriate, and satisfying health care to the people we serve. To achieve this goal, nurses need both knowledge and skills to conduct effective cultural assessments. This means learning from the people about their cultural care values, beliefs, lifeways, contexts, and practices to understand their world, needs, taboos, and the most optimal ways to provide professional care practices. Conducting accurate and comprehensive cultural assessments can greatly expand the nurse's understanding of people and empower them to discover ways to practice culturally competent, congruent, sensitive, meaningful, and responsible care. When clients receive nursing care that is individually tailored to their cultural beliefs, needs, prohibitions, and lifeways—often through a partnership between the nurse and client—they are more satisfied with the type of care received, more committed to adhering to the care plan, and more trusting of the nurse-client relationship.

The purpose of this chapter is to identify and discuss culturally based healthcare assessments and transcultural communication techniques with the goal of providing culture-specific, meaningful care to people of different cultures including individuals, families, special groups, communities, institutions, and subcultures. To achieve this goal, the nurse enters the client's world to discover cultural knowledge that is often embedded within individual and family values and lifeways. The Sunrise Enabler (see Color Insert 1) enables the nurse to ascertain and assess what is valued, known, and practiced as well as what care preferences are desired but not always attained. Both emic (client) and etic (outside) factors are discovered and used in culturally based assessments.

Environmental context factors and the use of the principles presented in Chapter Two are extremely important for conducting any cultural assessment with individuals, families, groups, and institutions. Theoretical perspectives such as The Theory of Culture Care Diversity and Universality (also known as the Culture Care Theory or CCT) are kept in mind while using the Sunrise Enabler or other cultural enablers along with use of specific holding knowledge about the culture(s).

■ CULTURAL ASSESSMENTS FOR CULTURALLY CONGRUENT CARE

Definition, Purposes, Goal, and Historical Overview of Cultural Assessments

Definition

Cultural assessments refer to the *"systematic identification and documentation of culture care beliefs, meanings, values, symbols, and practices of individuals or groups within a holistic perspective which includes the world-view, life experiences, environmental context, ethnohistory, language, and diverse social structure influences"* (Leininger, 1978). Culturally based care assessments are directed toward obtaining a holistic or comprehensive picture of informants within the particular factors that are meaningful and important to them. Cultural assessments go beyond traditional nursing assessments that focus on partial views as psychomotor, physiological, or mental conditions to that of holistic, cultural, environmental, ethnohistorical, and social structure factors while still considering medical and nursing phenomena. Although the traditional nursing areas are given full attention, the nurse goes beyond them to tap into holistic or totality dimensions of living and functioning. Nurses are educated in transcultural nursing to use liberal arts and other broad areas of knowledge to obtain a realistic and accurate picture of people and their health needs or concerns.

Purposes

Over the span of six decades Leininger (2002a) identified several purposes of cultural assessments. They are as follows:

- To discover the client's culture care and health patterns and meanings in relation to the client's worldview, lifeways, cultural values, beliefs, practices, context, and social structure factors.
- To obtain holistic culture care information as a sound basis for nursing care decisions and actions.
- To discover specific culture care patterns, meanings, and values that can be used to make differential nursing decisions that fit the client's values and lifeways and to discover what professional knowledge can be helpful to the client.

- To identify potential areas of cultural conflicts, clashes, and neglected areas resulting from emic and etic value differences between clients and professional health personnel.
- To identify general and specific dominant themes and patterns that need to be known in context for culturally congruent care practices.
- To identify comparative cultural care information among clients of different or similar cultures, which can be shared and used in clinical, teaching, and research practices.
- To identify both similarities and differences among clients in providing quality care.
- To use theoretical ideas and research approaches to interpret and explain practices for congruent care and new areas of transcultural nursing knowledge.

Leininger (2002a) maintained that serving as a cultural broker is not the major purpose of a cultural assessment. The concept of *cultural broker* is derived from anthropology and refers to how one serves as a "mediator" or "broker" between two or more persons with different interests. In nursing, one would mediate between the client's cultural beliefs and values and the nurse's professional goals. While this concept has merit, the cultural assessment goes beyond this to a higher domain. Moreover, the nurse cannot be an effective cultural broker or mediator unless he/she is very knowledgeable about the client's culture and the diverse factors influencing the client's needs and lifeways. Health personnel with superficial, biased, or inaccurate views of a client's culture cannot function as effective cultural brokers because limited knowledge often leads to miscommunications, misinterpretations, and misunderstandings. For example, a Mexican nurse tried to serve as a cultural broker for an Arab Muslim patient. She failed because she was unaware of the client's cultural background, values, and practices. She also had many biases and misconceptions about Arab Muslims.

To be an effective cultural broker requires the nurse know general historical factors as well as political, religious, kinship, and other social structure factors as depicted in the Sunrise Enabler. The cultural broker who is prepared in transcultural nursing uses appropriate skills and holding knowledge to assess and be helpful to clients. Becoming a cultural broker necessitates that one understands the culture and that the client desires a mediator. The nurse can serve as a care provider in different ways as guided by the Culture Care Theory. As a culturally sensitive cultural broker, the nurse develops mutually agreed upon decisions and actions with the client to avoid ethical problems and cultural imposition practices.

Goal

The central goal of the cultural care assessment is to provide respectful, meaningful, and competent care to people of diverse cultures by obtaining a full and accurate account of beliefs, lifeways, needs, and taboos or prohibitions so that appropriate nursing care decisions and actions can be made collaboratively with the care recipient for their beneficial health outcomes. The major focus of the assessment is to identify culture care beliefs, values, patterns, expressions, practices, meanings, and lifeways related to the client's needs for obtaining or maintaining health and wellbeing or to face disability, acute or chronic illness, or death.

Historical Overview

Leininger's work in culturally based care and health assessments began in the early 1960s as she reflected upon anthropological, cultural, and caring ideas from within nursing (Leininger, 1978). The Sunrise Enabler, the Semi-Structured Inquiry Guide Enabler to Assess Culture Care and Health, the Short Assessment Guide, the Acculturation Assessment Enabler for Cultural Patterns in Traditional and Nontraditional Lifeways, and the Life History Healthcare Enabler were all developed to assist practicing nurses, nurse researchers, and nurse educators in assessing various cultural aspects necessary for the provision of holistic and culturally congruent care for people from diverse cultural backgrounds.

It was not, however, until *many* nurses were prepared in both transcultural nursing and in anthropology that these assessments were valued, understood, and used (Leininger, 1970). Cultural assessments continue to be increasingly viewed as essential in nursing practice to provide accurate, meaningful, and congruent care to members of diverse cultures. Psychomedical aspects traditionally emphasized in nursing assessments or histories are increasingly supplemented with cultural care dimensions. Nurses prepared in transcultural nursing who use the Culture Care Theory with the Sunrise Enabler are especially skilled in performing in-depth cultural assessments. These nurses know the great importance of a holistic

assessment and are able to explicate the many benefits to clients, other nurses, and consumers (Leininger, 1995).

Although Leininger played an instrumental role in raising awareness and establishing transcultural nursing as a professional discipline and field, she also helped pave the way for other transcultural nurses to develop their own models and assessment instruments or tools. As a result several models, views, and strategies for cultural assessments exist. Many of these have been inspired by or have integrated some components of Leininger's early work in transcultural nursing, her Culture Care Theory, and/or the Sunrise Enabler.

Examples of other cultural assessments include but are not limited to Andrews & Boyle's (2016) Transcultural Nursing Assessment Guide for Individuals and Families, Groups and Communities, and their companion guide for Health Care Organizations and Facilities; Campinha-Bacote's (2015) Inventory to Assess the Process of Cultural Competence Among Healthcare Professionals-Revised (IAPCC-R), the Inventory for Assessing a Biblically Based Worldview of Cultural Competence Among Healthcare Professionals (IABWCC), and the Inventory for Assessing the Process of Cultural Competence Among Healthcare Professionals in Mentoring (IAPCC-M); Giger and Davidhizer's (2004) Transcultural Assessment Model; Jeffreys' (2016) Transcultural Self-Efficacy Tool (TSET), the Cultural Competence Clinical Evaluation Tool (CCCET), and the Clinical Setting Assessment Tool-Diversity and Disparity (CSAT-DD); Purnell's (2014) Model for Cultural Competence; Schim's (2003) Cultural Competence Assessment Instrument (CCA); and Spector's (2016) Heritage Assessment Tool. The purposes, target audiences, and scopes of application or uses for these instruments vary. Therefore, potential users need to evaluate each to determine an appropriate fit for the intended purpose and audience.

Leininger's Enablers for Cultural Assessments

As discussed in the chapter covering the ethnonursing research method and enablers, Leininger developed numerous enablers to facilitate in-depth culture care discoveries. Some of these enablers have not been limited solely for use during ethnonursing research. Instead, they have and continue to be used for comprehensive cultural assessments in clinical practice. As a result, they have been enormously helpful to nurses and other health practitioners in assessing clients' cultural care needs, taboos or prohibitions, values, beliefs, behaviors, lifeways, patterns, and expressions. Readers are invited to revisit Chapter Four for a review of the following enablers: The Sunrise Enabler (Refer to Color Insert 1); Leininger's Semi-Structured Inquiry Guide Enabler to Assess Culture Care and Health (Refer to Figure 4.3); Leininger's Stranger-to-Trusted-Friend Enabler (Refer to Figure 4.1); Leininger's Acculturation Healthcare Assessment Enabler for Cultural Patterns in Traditional and Nontraditional Lifeways, (Refer to Figure 4.4); and the Life History Health Care Enabler (Refer to Figure 4.7).

Caring Rituals Important to Assess

In performing cultural assessments, there are special areas bearing on caring patterns and healing that provide valuable information. Nearly all cultures have caring rituals that are sequenced activities people use to maintain wellness, prevent illness, ease dying, or regain health. *Generic (folk) caring rituals* are learned and used in the home, but they may be in demand in hospitals or clinics because they are held to be therapeutic and essential by the clients. Generic caring rituals generally serve specific functions when used *thoughtfully* whether in the home or hospital. Nurses need to discover these particular rituals for their healing or other benefits with different cultures. Helpful caring rituals need to be preserved and/or maintained and when indicated and mutually agreed upon, they can also be accommodated and/or negotiated. Folk caring rituals should be assessed by the nurse to determine any potential for harm which can then be addressed using culture care restructuring and/or repatterning.

Cultures have care rituals for one's skin, hair, and body and for gaining or losing weight. For example, Africans have very special rituals for their hair and skin care. Such rituals have cultural functions such as reassurance, security, protection, and feeling good (Leininger, 2002a). Rituals provide a sense of wellbeing through activities that are important to be regularly performed each day or night. Healthcare professionals can learn these cultural rituals and develop ways to creatively use them in transcultural practices with the client or family. Most rituals have ascribed healing attributes with benefits that can be learned if one studies them with clients while using professional insights.

Some types of caring rituals that nurses ought to know or be ready to learn are described in the following passages.

Eating Rituals

All human beings have regular times and patterns of eating that are generally ritualized and expected to be respected. For example, British people tend to use their forks with prongs facing down whereas Americans use forks with prongs facing upward. Chinese individuals use chop sticks and other cultures (India, Africa, and the Middle East) may use their fingers in lieu of eating utensils (Leininger, 2002a). Halal dietary law (Muslims) and Kashrut dietary law (Jewish) prohibit the consumption of pork products. Pork consumption is also not acceptable for Seventh-day Adventists and Ethiopian Orthodox believers. Alcohol consumption is forbidden in Islam, Jainism, and Sikhism.

Certain foods are ritually prepared and only eaten on special occasions. Polish and Germans enjoy a special sausage cooked in special ritualized ways for festive occasions. The environmental setting and gender or class rules related to who may eat together are important in numerous cultures. In some non-Western cultures, women only eat after the men have eaten, and/or eat separately from them (Leininger, 2002a). These rituals should be respected and facilitated in the hospital as they can make a big difference in maintaining the person's health. The nurse needs to know about culturally important food rituals, culturally taboo foods, class or gender preferences, and ritually prepared cold and hot foods to assist clients in times of wellness or illness.

Daily and Nightly Ritual Care Activities

It is important and equally fascinating to observe the client's patterns of daytime/morning and bed or night time care rituals. Assessing daily personal exercises are helpful to know and may shed light on a person's health status or ways health may be improved. For example, traditional as well as many modern day Japanese maintain their early morning Tai Chi exercises for health and spiritual wellbeing. Americans may engage in early morning, noon, and evening running, walking, and other physical rituals to keep them well, to prevent cardiovascular or heart disease, and to keep them in good physical condition. Some people engage in nightly skin care rituals. Others favor daily morning showers and hair care. Such ritual activities need to be respected, assessed, and understood for their meaning and contribution to cultural health and wellbeing. Nurses can often accommodate these expected ritual activities in the daily care plan and facilitate them if beneficial.

Sleep and Rest Ritual Patterns

Cultures have patterns of sleep and rest that have usually been established early in life and maintained throughout the lifespan for personal health maintenance. Children and older adults especially tend to adhere to specific rituals of resting and sleeping. Children's bedtime stories and nightlights are a common norm among many Americans. In Japan and among Australian Aborigines, co-sleeping with other family members is an acceptable cultural practice for children (Lilley, 2010). Sleep and rest cultural patterns are especially important in the busy and pressured life-world of tasks and activities. Such rituals are usually important to providing culturally congruent care for client health maintenance and/or preservation.

Religious Rituals

Some cultures have prayer rituals such as the five obligatory daily prayers for Muslims. In the hospital setting, nurses may need to assist Muslims in their quest for fulfilling their religious rituals by providing them with a private space for prayer, positioning their beds in the *qiblah* direction (prayer direction pointing towards Makkah [Mecca] in Saudi Arabia (in the United States, the qiblah direction is North East) and assisting them with wudu' (ablution/washing) that precedes prayer (Wehbe-Alamah, 2008, 2015).

Roman Catholics, Protestants, Jewish, and other faith groups have prayer rituals for the sick and dying, which need to be respected and supported when priests, ministers, or other designated religious and/or family members carry out sacramental or spiritual rites with clients of diverse faiths. Male circumcision is a religious ritual for people who ascribe to Judaism, Islam, Coptic Christianity, and the Ethiopian Orthodox Church (Rukhman, Ladizinski, & Lee, 2014). Many cultures also have specific religious rituals associated with dying and burial. Assessing religious rituals and their effects on the clients' health is important and facilitates the delivery of culturally congruent care.

Lifespan Rituals

Transcultural nurses and anthropologists have been studying lifespan rituals in diverse cultures for many years to discover their commonalties and differences related to healing and health. *Lifespan rituals are especially crucial because they demonstrate patterns of caring for health and illness as well as generic folk lifeways.* Lifespan rituals can help nurses know and value care from birth to old age when identified and respected. Hence, lifespan rituals should be assessed and studied in cultures from birth and at special times such as marriage, death, illness, or injury for their therapeutic or nontherapeutic outcomes (Leininger, 2002a).

Some lifespan cultural rituals are stressful but most fit within the culture and are held by them as essential and beneficial. One of the oldest theories about rituals comes from Arnold van Gennep (1960) in his classic study, *The Rites of Passage*, originally published in 1909. The author hypothesized that there were major phases of human rites of passage identified as *a phase of separation*; *a phase of transition*; and *a phase of incorporation*. Persons experience these phases across the lifespan when changing positions or statuses such as being separated from their past role and taking on a new role. One moves into the second phase as a transitional phase but with uncertain role expectations. In the last phase, people learn to take on and integrate into a new role or position with the culture that gives them recognition or status such as being married or becoming a nurse, an elder, or a prisoner. Rites of passage and rituals are extremely important to study in every culture; they are often unique and yet can be found to have some commonalities when assessed with the Culture Care Theory and with van Gennep's (1960) cultural perspectives (Leininger, 2002a).

Nurse and Hospital Rituals

Nurses have many rituals that are often not recognized nor assessed and yet they exist in hospitals and other settings wherever nurses function or live (Leininger, 1994a). There are nursing rituals for administering medications, giving baths, assessing clients, and caring for those who are acute or chronically ill. Some rituals appear more beneficial to nurses than they do to clients. Clients assess nursing *task rituals* and what makes nurses *good* caregivers. Nursing rituals such as morning report and rounds with physicians tend to regulate the time when clients can expect to receive nursing care. New immigrants may not know these rituals and thus perceive their care as being less. Some clients may become upset if nursing rituals related to food, medicine, and basic care needs are not explained or offered (Leininger, 2002a).

Periodically, nurses need to assess their own rituals for their caring benefits and values to clients of diverse cultures. Rituals can have favorable or less favorable caring and therapeutic features for clients. For several decades transcultural nurses have studied some nursing rituals and how congruent they are with client needs. Some nursing rituals may have limited benefits to clients, but may be more helpful to nurses for the efficiency of tasks or other ritualized routines. Wolf (1990) and Leininger's (1988a, 1994a) studies of hospital rituals resulted in systematic discoveries that awakened nurses to their own rituals and resultant effects.

In addition, folk and professional rituals need to be assessed and compared to identify and prevent professional practices that may inadvertently cause folk illnesses. For example, many Mexicans believe that the *evil eye (mal de ojo)* may be triggered by nurses praising or envying a child (Leininger, 2002a). Therefore, a culturally competent nurse will refrain from enthusiastically admiring a hospitalized child or a newborn baby to avoid causing mal de ojo. In addition, nursing administration rituals in clinical and academic settings need to be assessed for their beneficial and non-beneficial features for students and consumers from different cultures. Assessment of these rituals can often provide some entirely new insights about nursing practices and outcomes. For example, a Native American Sioux viewed hospital admission rituals as punishing, demeaning, and non-caring when the nurses failed to obtain the client's story about what had happened on the reservation (Leininger, 2002a).

Cultural factors related to rituals have meaning for clients in different care contexts including the hospital setting. For example, in some cultures hospitalized individuals who are separated from their extended family may feel abandoned. In several cultures, the ritual of hospital admission often communicates to pediatric and older adult clients that the hospital is a place where they will die or be abandoned, and as a result, they are very reluctant to go to the hospital except as a last resort (Leininger, 2002a). In many cultures, when

a hospitalized client dies, the family may immediately begin engaging in mourning or dying rituals while still at the hospital. Since the early 1970s, transcultural nurses have been instrumental in establishing "mourning rooms" in hospitals for dying clients where family members can engage in their appropriate grieving rituals. This is especially important for Oceanians, Southeast Asians, and Native Americans (Leininger, 2002a). Mourning rooms have been most therapeutic and have become part of the modern hospital care context— another contribution from transcultural nursing.

There are additional cultural rituals related to folk healing and caring that need to be learned from clients and studied for their uses in professional caring. Integrated generic and professional rituals are an important part of transcultural nursing care. Knowing and respecting generic emic healing rituals are increasingly being reestablished by many cultures, and nurses are expected to know these rituals and help clients use them. If rituals are non-beneficial to a client, they need to be assessed and discussed with the client, family, and healthcare providers.

In general, cultural caring rituals of clients and nurses are powerful forces to know, understand, assess, and respectfully use. More and more nurses will be expected to integrate generic rituals into client care for congruent and beneficial care. Comparative studies about the caring rituals of different cultures have greatly expanded transcultural nurses' knowledge for several decades (Leininger, 2002a). They have provided valuable and specific care data for nurses who are attentive to diversities and universalities using culture care findings (Leininger, 1991b, 1998b), such as Chrisman's (1990) assessment and analysis of operating room rituals which provided new insights and practice implications for surgical nursing care. Transcultural care findings need to be used with the three modes of culture care decisions and actions, namely, *culture care maintenance and/or preservation; culture care accommodation and/or negotiation;* and *culture care repatterning and/or restructuring* so as to provide culturally competent and congruent care to clients in specific and therapeutic ways (Leininger, 1977, 1991a, 1991c, 1999b, 2002a).

Nurses are encouraged to study culture care rituals for their positive or less positive outcomes by using available scientific and humanistic transcultural nursing research findings. One must also remember that rituals can and do change over time, but usually slowly and partially because of their function for ensuring cultural security and consistency. Nursing faculty members and clinical textbooks often fail to recognize cultural differences in diverse caring rituals. If rituals are not known and used by nurses in their practices, client wellbeing, satisfaction, trust, and adherence to care regimens will be affected (Leininger, 2002a).

Principles for Comprehensive Cultural Assessments

The following principles for cultural assessments (Refer to Table 7.1) have been developed to guide nurses in preparing to engage in comprehensive, holistic, and therapeutic cultural assessments and to collect credible and meaningful data with clients.

- *Know thyself: Know own cultural values, beliefs, lifeways, biases, stereotypes, ethnocentric tendencies, and prejudices.*

The idea of knowing about a very different or strange culture was first introduced by Margaret Mead in the 1950s who held that one learned and remembered more about a "new" or different culture than a familiar one. Assessing sharp cultural differences and discovering why cultures are different or similar leads to breakthroughs in knowledge and practices. Similarities within and between cultures are important, but require astute observations that are often subtle or not clearly overt.

Prior to engaging in a cultural assessment of another, the nurse assesses his/her own cultural values, beliefs, lifeways, biases, prejudices, stereotypes, and ethnocentric views in relation to people or cultures different from one's self. Developing an awareness of one's own cultural heritage emphasizes the importance of significant cultural values and lifeways held by others and helps the nurse to make meaningful comparisons about commonalities or diversities among or between cultures.

Misconceptions, biases, prejudgments, and narrow views can greatly limit the accurate assessments of others. Engaging in a cultural self-assessment helps nurses to identify personal factors that may interfere with their effective assessments and understanding of clients. Some nurses may have lifelong strongly held or negative predetermined views or prejudices about a culture or group. Preconceived ideas may influence and distort what they see, hear, and interpret from clients (Leininger, 1995).

Biases are often related to cultural ignorance and blindness and limit reliable and accurate client assessment. When performing cultural assessments, nurses

TABLE 7.1. Principles for Comprehensive Cultural Assessments.

1	Know Thyself: Know own cultural values, beliefs, lifeways, biases, stereotypes, ethnocentric tendencies, and prejudices
2	Holding Knowledge: Acquire and reflect on learned evidence-based transcultural knowledge about the client's culture
3	Theoretical Framework: Study a holistic theoretical framework such as the Culture Care Theory and Sunrise Enabler to guide the cultural assessment of others
4	Clarification of cultural assessment purpose, goal, and process: Clarify and explain at the outset to the individual, family, or group the purpose, goal, and process of the cultural assessment, including times, location, and number of visits
5	Presence: Show a genuine and sincere interest while engaging in active listening and learning
6	Transcultural communication: Give attention to differences related to gender, age, class, interpersonal space, language, and other verbal and nonverbal communication modes
7	Environmental Context: Be observant of environmental context and its influence on health, wellbeing, disability, illness, and death or dying
8	Emic and etic perspectives: Discover and reflect on the clients' emic and the nurse's etic beliefs, values, lifeways, and culture care
9	Active and ongoing client-nurse collaboration: Actively involve the client in evaluation of assessment findings and development of a collaborative plan of care

need to remain vigilant about stereotyping. *Stereotyping* involves classifying people in rigid, fixed, or "*cookbook*" ways with prejudged views about them and their lifeways (Leininger, 2002a). Nurses need to avoid stereotyping and profiling people as these actions limit acceptance of individual variations and are often inaccurate, negative, and demeaning. There are many different role-playing exercises and games used in transcultural nursing to prevent stereotyping and prejudgments about cultures (Wehbe-Alamah & McFarland, 2015).

Practicing cultural care assessments in the classroom before working with clients is important for changing attitudes and developing new skills and insights. In clinical settings, transcultural nurse specialists can help staff nurses and interdisciplinary colleagues to identify and deal with stereotyping, long-standing prejudices, cultural discrimination, and injustice practices. Each nurse needs to frequently assess his/her own attitudes and viewpoints by him/herself and/or with a mentor to ensure objectivity during client assessments.

Students in transcultural nursing are required to know and deal with their own cultural biases under a mentor's supervision. Assessing a strange culture can make one keenly aware of one's own cultural differences and lifeway tendencies. Assessing a culture that is markedly different from one's own forces one to think anew, whereas a culture that is similar tends to make the nurse assume *they know all about the culture.* Major differences between cultures can lead nurses to experience culture shock or to avoid learning about the people.

A client's belief that nurses from his/her own culture are best suited to perform a cultural assessment with him/herself may not be always beneficial because such nurses may have their own cultural blindness or strong ethnocentric tendencies or may hold acculturated viewpoints for a culture that is entirely different from that of the client (Leininger, 2002a). When nurses have become acculturated to another culture, they may be unable to see and know their own traditional or heritage culture. If a person dislikes his/her own culture, s/he may not want to be identified with that culture and remain blind to it or deny it (Leininger, 2002a). Cultural blindness and cultural ignorance are two serious factors limiting effective nursing assessments and culture care practices. Cultural blindness is generally related to strong ethnocentrism, cultural ignorance, and a lack of transcultural knowledge about a culture.

It is crucial that nurses and other healthcare providers assess their own cultural values, lifeways, biases, stereotypes, ethnocentric tendencies, prejudices, and other factors that limit accurate cultural assessments. *Know Thyself* is a critical and essential principle in transcultural nursing that allows each nurse to examine his/her own competency and deficit areas and is an *essential* prerequisite to learning about other cultures' values, beliefs, and lifeways and for providing culturally competent care.

- *Holding Knowledge: Acquire and reflect on learned evidence-based transcultural knowledge about the client's culture.*

Acquiring some holding knowledge about a client's culture in advance of performing a cultural assessment helps the nurse to *identify key cultural linguistic terms, values, lifeways, generic care practices, and folk illnesses; formulate culture-specific assessment questions;* and *reflect upon or clarify findings directly with the client.* Statements such as "Tell me about *susto*" (a folk cultural fright illness common among Latin Americans) or "I would like to learn more about your experience with the evil eye" are gateways for in-depth assessment and allow for gaining a better understanding and for having a meaningful subsequent reflection about what has been said and shared (Leininger, 2002a). Reflections without cultural holding knowledge often lead to errors or misunderstandings. Using evidence-based holding knowledge and reflecting on what has been shared (such as the evil eye and susto) gives meaning and credibility to the findings.

- *Theoretical framework: Study a holistic theoretical framework such as the Culture Care Theory and Sunrise Enabler to guide the cultural assessment of others.*

The nurse uses a theory or theoretical perspective such as the holistic Culture Care Theory with use of the Sunrise and other enablers to guide the cultural assessment. A visual image of the Sunrise Enabler can serve as a road map and helps the nurse to ascertain that all relevant knowledge areas have been considered for conducting a holistic cultural assessment. The nurse stays alert to whatever the client wishes to share and explores these ideas while keeping focus on culture, care values, religion, kinship relationships, and other factors as depicted in the Sunrise Enabler (Leininger, 1984, 2002a).

Leininger (2002a) was adamant that one must be *"patient, persistent, and open to learn"* from others to discover rich and meaningful data about care, health, wellbeing, disability, illness, death or dying, and other areas with the Sunrise Enabler, the Culture Care Theory, and the Stanger-to-Trusted-Friend Enabler. According to Leininger (1991a, 1991c, 2002a), rich scientific data are often embedded in social structure factors such as family relationships, religion, politics, and economics. Such data requires time to tease out gently and sensitively and can be used with the three culture care modes of the CCT to arrive at culturally congruent and therapeutic health outcomes or to help with facing disabilities, illness, or death.

- *Clarification of cultural assessment purpose, goal, and process: Clarify and explain at the outset to the individual, family, or group the purpose, goal, and process of the cultural assessment, including times, location, and number of visits.*

Cultural assessments are quite different from physical assessments. Cultural assessments typically require an explication of rationale, more time with clients, patience, a broad holding knowledge base, and a reasonably quiet place with minimal disruptions to allow for ample time to talk about the different relevant areas in the Sunrise Enabler. Because a cultural care assessment may be a new experience for some clients, the nurse will often need to repeatedly clarify with the client as well as others in the care setting about the role cultural assessments play in providing culturally competent care.

The nurse shares with clients about his/her interest in learning about their cultural values, beliefs, and lifeways in order to provide them with high quality, holistic care. It is recommended that nurses begin the cultural assessment with comments such as: "I would like to learn about some of your ideas, experiences, and beliefs and about how you would like to be cared for while here" or "I would like to learn about your cultural heritage or family roots to better understand you and your care needs."

Clients generally like having cultural assessments as they value sharing ideas and stories about their culture, family folk care, and practices. The goal is for the nurse to integrate cultural findings into the development of professional care plans, to earn client trust

and cooperation, and to increase client satisfaction. It is important to keep in mind that the nurse is not expected to fully cover all the domains and details depicted in the Sunrise Enabler, but rather capture dominant themes and patterns from current and subsequent sessions with the client.

Cultural assessments in hospital settings often will need to fit into the client's busy hospital schedule. As a result, the nurse may need to arrange for several sessions. The initial session will typically last about 20 minutes. Assessing communication, the existence of any potential language barriers, and the possible need for qualified translators are typically completed before or during the first session. Subsequent visits are usually longer, especially if conducted at the client's home. Allowing sufficient time between sessions for the client to think about ideas related to cultural beliefs, care, or health values is important.

During the early sessions, some clients may test the nurse to determine if he/she can be trusted or is truly genuinely interested in the client's culture. Distrust indicators are usually reflected in client tension, caution, and sharing sparse and/or inaccurate information. Leininger (2002a) observed that during in-depth cultural assessments, negative experiences or stories are usually told at the end of the sessions along with valuable and "sacred cultural secrets" such as the use of generic local healers or cultural spiritualists. She deducted that the reason for this is so the client can evaluate whether the nurse can be a "genuinely trusted friend" who would respect their cultural secrets. The nurse needs to use the Stranger-to-Trusted-Friend Enabler (Refer to Figure 4.1) to assess how to become a trusted friend with the client, group, or family by using the indicators in the enabler.

- *Presence: Show a genuine and sincere interest while engaging in active listening and learning.*

Showing genuine interest and respect are most important throughout the entire assessment (Leininger, 1984, 2002a). The real secret for an effective cultural care assessment is to remain an *"active listener, learner, and reflector"* (Leininger, 2002a) about what the client has shared and deemed to be important. Throughout the assessment, the nurse maintains a flexible and open attitude while exhibiting a willingness *to listen and move with the client's* ideas and interpretations. After each session the nurse always thanks the client or family in a sincere way and provides an opening to bring forth new or reinforced ideas at a later time. The nurse keeps in mind that there are no rigidly prescribed steps or techniques for conducting a cultural assessment given that, by its nature, it is a sensitive process of dynamic discovery for grasping the client's world about cultural meanings of care, health, disability, illness, and lifeways.

- *Transcultural communication: Give attention to differences related to gender, age, class, interpersonal space, language, and other verbal and nonverbal communication modes.*

The nurse gives attention to gender, age, or class roles and to language, interpersonal space, and other verbal and nonverbal communication modes such as silence, eye contact, and need for professional translators. During the assessment, the nurse also remains alert for any intergenerational differences and similarities so as to discover potential changes in cultural values and practices influencing care practices over time. Intergenerational male and female role-taking differences are noted, especially in relation to human caring and health, along with social structure and historical factors influencing these changes (Leininger, 1984, 2002a). Intergenerational assessments take more time but can be very valuable for tracing culture care, health, and illness patterns. The informants are encouraged to be active sharers of comparative generational perspectives. Additional information about transcultural communication is provided in a later section of this chapter.

- *Environmental context: Be observant of environmental context and its influence on health, wellbeing, disability, illness, and death or dying.*

When the cultural assessment is performed in the client's home, the nurse has a wonderful opportunity to see the client's naturalistic environment and material culture items firsthand, meet with family members or guests, and observe kinship interactions (Leininger, 2002a). Seeing and documenting the client's cultural context, talking with family members about how they care for one another, and learning about their generic (emic) care practices provide some holistic understandings of the client's cultural lifeways and additional means for the nurse to grasp in-depth and accurate cultural meanings of care, health, and life experiences.

The Culture Care Theory helps the nurse to explain and obtain a holistic or total client picture in their natural and familiar home or work environments. The nurse uses nursing, medical, and humanistic knowledge sources to understand the client in his or her environment. Traditional medical and nursing views oriented to medical diseases, symptoms, medications, and treatment modes often fail to include environmental, cultural, and other factors depicted in the Sunrise Enabler and therefore result in a limited as opposed to holistic or comprehensive understanding (Leininger, 2002a).

Leininger (2002a) perceived cultural assessments conducted in the clinic or hospital usually require more time due to frequent interruptions by other health personnel for medical or other procedures. She similarly held that cultural minorities are often more cautious about talking openly in hospitals and clinics about their cultural secrets (such as folk practices) out of fear that recording such information in their medical charts may result in stereotypes and negative care repercussions.

- *Emic and etic perspectives: Discover and reflect on the client's emic and the nurse's etic beliefs, values, lifeways, and culture care.*

As the client shares information from an emic perspective, the nurse evaluates her etic views and reflects on the meanings of these findings with the client. The nurse uses a holistic perspective as depicted in the Sunrise Enabler for a total and accurate picture of client/family needs and expectations. The discovery of and subsequent reflection about the client's emic and the nurse's etic culture care beliefs, values, lifeways creates a climate that is trusting, safe, and beneficial for the client.

Some clients are more eager than others to share their cultural beliefs, lifeways, and experiences such as Italians, Jews, Eastern Europeans, and Anglo-Americans (Leininger, 2002a). The way the client wants to be cared for is important and should be taken into consideration by the nurse. Western clients are usually conditioned to report medical symptoms, diseases, and professional or over the counter treatments to healthcare providers. However, they may experience difficulty reporting or sharing their cultural lifeways, history, values, and beliefs. In contrast, non-Western clients view their family lifeways and folk caring practices as equally important to share (Leininger, 1995, 2002a).

Storytelling has long been valuable to non-Western and minority cultures, and has increasingly become considered as an ideal approach by Western healthcare practitioners. The nurse encourages the client to narrate his or her story, experiences, and ideas. Helping clients to become active sharers of their emic perspectives as well as co-participants in the etic assessment and development of plans of care is a transcultural art and skill.

- *Active and ongoing client-nurse collaboration: Actively involve the client in evaluation of assessment findings and development of a collaborative plan of care.*

Use of the assessment findings in sensitive, knowing, creative, and meaningful ways with clients input often results in beneficial and satisfying outcomes. Encouraging clients to reflect on their cultural beliefs, values, and lifeways frequently stimulates them to reexamine their values and to work collaboratively with nurses as they actively partner in the development of their professional plans of care.

When the client is an active co-participant in the cultural assessment, the nurse can obtain credible and accurate data and provide culturally specific and congruent care through the use of the three modes of culture care decisions and actions. Identifying and then validating with the client specific and general cultural care values, beliefs, and needs related to generic (emic) and professional (etic) data results in a more desired client-nurse collaboration, improved client satisfaction, and increased mutual trust.

Many clients want culturally congruent care that is not offensive or in conflict with their cultural values and practices. Cultural assessments help to avoid cultural misunderstandings, clashes, or conflicts. Many cultures, minorities, immigrants, and subcultures are increasingly aware of their rights and demanding to have *their* cultural practices respected. Transcultural nursing holds that all human beings are entitled to receive culturally sensitive and congruent care, an outcome that is facilitated by conducting cultural assessments and integrating findings collaboratively with the client into professional care decisions and actions.

The preceding principles as outlined and shown in Table 7.1 serve as a guide for nurses conducting in-depth cultural assessments. It is strongly recommended that nurses first engage in a self-assessment (Know Thyself) and acquire holding knowledge about the client's culture before conducting a cultural assessment. Cultural assessments must be congruent with the client's lifeways to be useable, beneficial, and acceptable to client's emic knowing world.

Generic (emic) and professional (etic) knowledge should be integrated or blended together to provide *culturally congruent care* as previously discussed and again in Chapter Eight. Effective cultural assessments provide the means to enter into the client's world while they experience a sense of control and power over their ideas in regard to what is caring and beneficial to them within their cultural orientation and lifeways. Transcultural nurses have led the way to show how and why cultural assessments are beneficial to clients as well as rewarding to care providers. Nurses who are unable to complete an in depth cultural assessment due to lack of time or other barrier are advised to ask their clients, when appropriate, a simple question: "What do I need to know about you to provide you with the best possible care?" A question of this nature may open the line for instant and future communication of important emic beliefs and practices that can be used by the nurse as he/she engages in culturally congruent integrative care.

Important Summary Points for Cultural Assessments

In this chapter several principles, standards, definitions, models, enablers, and guides have been presented to help nurses conduct culturally competent assessments to achieve high quality care outcomes. The following summary points are important to keep in mind:

- The Culture Care Theory with the Sunrise Enabler serve as the best and most reliable guides to obtain holistic views about an individual, family, or group and for institutional assessments of cultures (Leininger, 2002a). Their worldviews, cultural and social structure dimensions, ethnohistories, language uses, and environmental contexts are all essential areas for obtaining holistic, comprehensive, and culture-specific information. Some areas will be of more interest than others with specific cultures and to the assessor. For example, Mexicans,

Africans, Italians, and Arabs generally emphasize the importance of extended family care. In contrast, Anglo-Americans tend to emphasize individuality and their own specific needs and concerns about costs, technologies, and legal and political factors of health care. The nurse actively listens to and observes clients to enter their world and learn from them. Rather than narrow mind-body pathophysiological or emotional-symptom or disease foci, a broad and open view is maintained.

- Throughout the assessment the nurse remains an active listener, learner, and reflector rather than a teacher or "know it all" healthcare provider. The nurse refrains from using professional jargon or medical terms as this tends to suppress cultural data and inhibits informants from sharing their ideas. If the informant enquires about professional knowledge, the nurse responds but is careful not to practice cultural imposition or rigid ethnocentrism.

- The nurse is mindful to keep the assessment focused on the client's world of knowing (*the emic focus*) rather than on the nurse's views or professional (*the etic focus*) ideas about care, health, and lifeways. If the nurse is prone or eager to share ideas or sell products to the client, this can lead to cultural conflicts and clashes and thwart the client's participation and sharing of ideas.

- The nurse continually encourages the client or family to share their cultural care practices including health values, beliefs, and lifeways and how they use them in daily life. Clients usually like to share their values and lifeways through stories, special life experiences, photographs, letters, or tangible cultural symbols (such as religious medals, icons, talismans, or other symbolic items) or by talking about a "blue stone or bead" (to ward off the evil eye in some Middle Eastern cultures) or the "medicine bag" (for some Native Americans) that promote or hinder healing and wellbeing in their culture. Clients like to share both the tangible items and nontangible ideas that have the most meaning for them in their lives. Focusing on the meanings of clients' ideas for themselves during the assessment is extremely important. Some family members have diaries and videotapes to share their special life experiences with the nurse, especially during a home assessment. In the hospital, video and home artifacts have been seen less frequently; however,

with the availability of affordable portable electronic devices (e.g., "smart" telephones and tablets, picture frames, notepads, and DVD players) such sharing is encountered more often.

- Throughout the assessment, the nurse asks very few direct questions but instead uses indirect probing that focuses on areas of inquiry. Open-ended framing is used such as "Tell me about ____" or "I would like to have you to talk about yourself and your family" or "I need to learn more about the ways you care for children and elders." Encouraging the client to talk about their experiences is a good strategy. Also, it is important to clarify terms used as "comfort care." Eliciting ideas to help the nurses give "good care" from an emic perspective is nearly always welcome. The nurse tries to use the client's words and frame of reference rather than those of the nurse. This preserves the client's world of knowing and understanding and is a major approach toward developing culturally competent nursing skills.

- The nurse explores not only present-life experiences and values but also past historical events and future views related to the general assessment. These are discovered in relation to culture, care/caring, health, wellbeing, environmental context, and social structure domain factors influencing health or illness patterns.

- The nurse identifies and appreciates that most clients are capable of explaining and interpreting their own experiences related to care, health, illness, and maintaining wellness in their culture. Narratives, poems, cultural taboos, songs, pictures, and symbols have cultural meanings that the clients often may use to explain their ideas. The nurse should acknowledge that she or he is not the expert interpreter and analyzer, but that the client is the knower. The nurse's etic (outsider) views usually differ from the client's emic interpretations, so it is the responsibility of the nurse to withhold offering his or her ideas and interpretations. Knowledge of the language and being able to speak certain phrases or questions is critical for obtaining accurate assessments and interpretations. At the end of each assessment period (and there may be several), the nurse rechecks findings or data for accurate client interpretations and explanations.

- Tapping into the client's cultural secrets is done gently and sensitively. These are generally not shared unless the client believes that the nurse can be trusted, is genuinely interested in the client and the culture, and can protect cultural secrets and viewpoints from being misinterpreted or used inappropriately. Some clients fear that their cultural ideas and experiences might be demeaned or devalued by outsiders. *Respect as caring* is mindfully practiced when performing assessments. Spiritual, political, and legal ideas are usually guarded by clients and only shared when trust is evident.

- The client may want to wear traditional dress, adornments, or symbols for the assessment or bring items to tell "their story." The nurse respects and encourages these practices. Seeing the client in familiar dress and using certain tangible cultural items is valuable for helping the nurse to learn about the culture and their health, caring, and healing modes that then can serve as good talking cues.

- Making the client or family feel comfortable and able to enjoy sharing their ideas with the nurse is an important principle during assessments, and so therefore, is the selection of settings that will help the client share ideas, including confidential and special cultural secrets.

- Throughout the assessment process, the nurse seeks to assess whether the information he/she hears, sees, or observes is accurate or credible with the client's lifeways. The family and other representatives of the culture may also confirm such knowledge with the nurse. Individual and group variations always exist, and one must not generalize findings to other cultures.

- The nurse remains appreciative of the client's willingness to share ideas by gratefully thanking them after each session. Giving money or gifts for assessments is generally not practiced unless the assessment was part of a research study. However, the purpose and benefits (actual or potential) related to conducting the assessment do need to be discussed with participants both at the outset and at the end of each session.

In general, a cultural care assessment is a very creative and dynamic discovery and learning process that brings forth valuable knowledge. It is often filled with informational surprises about cultures that are generally limitedly known to most nurses and healthcare providers. The Culture Care Theory with the Sunrise Enabler and other enablers can make the journey an exciting and meaningful process with benefits for the client and rewarding experiences for the nurse or other healthcare professionals. Rich and valuable evidence-based cultural data have been discovered over the past six decades using the cultural care assessment process with the Culture Care Theory and its enablers.

■ TRANSCULTURAL COMMUNICATION FOR CULTURALLY CONGRUENT CARE

Transcultural Communication Modes

Transcultural communication is extremely important when conducting an assessment or providing care for immigrants, refugees, and many indigenous people who may be residing in a given country whether permanently or for short or long periods of time. Understanding clients' verbal and nonverbal communication patterns is imperative in an increasingly multicultural world.

According to the 2013 U. S. Census Bureau American Community Survey, 21% of the U. S. population (accounting for 61.8 million or one in five U. S. residents) speaks a language other than English at home (Camarota & Zeigler, 2014). Hispanics or Latinos account for 16.6% of the population and Asians represent 4.9% of U. S. residents (U. S. Department of Commerce, Census Bureau, 2015). In 2013, the largest *growth* in foreign languages spoken at home in the U. S. was Spanish, followed by Chinese, then Arabic, then Urdu [Pakistan]. The *most common* foreign languages spoken at home were Spanish, followed by Chinese, then Tagalog [Philippines], Vietnamese, French, Korean, and Arabic (Camarota & Zeigler, 2014).

While nurses work more directly and continually with clients in comparison to other healthcare professionals, there are no known statistics about the number or percentage of bilingual nurses in the U. S. However, "… the nation's health professions [including nurses] have not kept pace with changing [U.S.] demographics" (American Association of Colleges of Nursing [AACN], 2015, p. 2). According to the April 2000 report from the National Advisory Council on Nurse Education and Practice, a culturally diverse nursing workforce is critical to reduce the health disparities affecting minority populations and to meet the healthcare needs of the nation (AACN, 2015).

Understanding clients' verbal and nonverbal communication is imperative in an increasingly multicultural world. Leininger (2002a) held that nurses should speak at least two languages; language learning should begin in grade school and continue throughout the lifespan; nursing curricula should require language skills so nurses can provide better care for clients of diverse cultures in clinical practice, education, research, and consultation; and professional translators who are trained in transcultural care and cross-cultural communications should be used when nurses and other healthcare providers are unable to communicate verbally with clients in either their own or the client's native (or preferred) language.

Body language expression is a form of nonverbal communication and is usually culturally patterned. Nurses and other healthcare professionals need to learn about the meanings for transcultural nonverbal communication, especially when unable to speak the client's language. Anthropologists and linguistic scientists such as Birdwhistell (1970) and Hall (1974) studied different patterns of nonverbal communication and body/gesture language in many cultures over time and provided valuable information that nurses can account for as they perform cultural assessments. Nurses need to rely on literature and evidence-based data from scientists who have thoroughly studied and documented such findings and their meanings. Miscommunication of verbal and nonverbal expressions can lead to serious problems and destructive or harmful outcomes in client and family care.

In communicating with different cultures, people use many styles or patterned ways to share their ideas. Figure 7.1 shows some common transcultural communication modes nurses need to consider when conducting assessments or providing daily care (Leininger, 2002a). Nurses who are aware of transcultural communication differences need to be patient when waiting for a reply, especially with members of cultures who communicate through extended families such as Mexicans and Southeast Asians (Leininger, 2002a).

Patterns of Communication

Because transcultural communication is focused on sending and receiving ideas or messages, cultural differences are important to understand; however, one should always realize that cultural differences exist within and among cultures. Hence, it is important to emphasize *patterns of communication* as they are more constant

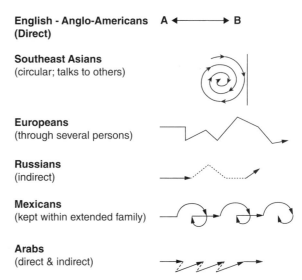

FIGURE 7.1 • Transcultural Communication Modes.

and consistent. There are numerous patterns of communication to consider when caring for diverse cultures. These include kinesics; proxemics; culture, social, and cyclic time; cultural space; and body touching.

Kinesics

Kinesics is the term that "*refers to body movement communication modes which include facial expressions (smile or anger), gestures, eye contact, and other body postures*" (Leininger, 2002a). *Head, face, and hand movements* may have different interpretations for diverse cultures. In New Guinea and some Levant cultures, moving one's head up and down means "no" as opposed to moving it from side to side. For many Arab Muslims, use of the left hand is reserved for unclean or hygiene tasks while the right hand is reserved for clean tasks such as the preparation and consumption of food as well as for shaking hands with others. Therefore, it is preferable to hand Arab Muslim patients their medicines using one's right hand, as opposed to the left one.

Body posture and gestures have different transcultural meanings. For example, shaking hands to greet others may be considered taboo among members of opposite genders in some Asian and Muslim cultures, while Latin Americans shake hands firmly and actively for a somewhat longer period of time than Europeans or Americans (Leininger, 2002a). Although placing the right hand over the heart is a cultural symbol for pledging allegiance to the flag/nation in the U. S., the same gesture is used by some Middle Eastern Muslims when greeting a person of the opposite gender as a sign that they do not shake hands. In many Asian cultures such as Japan and China, greeting a guest or showing respect is exhibited in the form of a forward bow of the head along with deep bow from the waist (Leininger, 2002a). In some Arabian Gulf cultures, men may greet each other by touching nose to nose (Abbadi, 2014). The Maori of New Zealand practice the *Hongi,* a traditional form of greeting also characterized by pressing noses together (Hongi, n.d.).

Slapping Arab Muslims on the back as a form of greeting may be considered offensive and disrespectful and should therefore be avoided (Leininger, 2002a). Crossing one's arms over one's chest may communicate hostility in some cultures but may be viewed as a sign that one is paying attention and showing respect in other cultures. Crossing one's legs and showing the sole of one's shoes when talking to another may be interpreted as showing disrespect in some Middle Eastern cultures.

Facial expressions and *eye contact* vary transculturally and need to be accurately interpreted to avoid miscommunication and misunderstandings. In some cultures [Anglo Americans and Europeans], a broad smile may communicate friendliness while in others [Arabian Gulf], it may be interpreted as flirtation. Most Anglo-Americans tend to maintain direct eye contact whereas some Arabs, Asians, and Native Americans favor avoiding direct or prolonged eye contact. Direct eye focus may be viewed as rude, aggressive, threatening, or a cultural taboo in these and other cultures (Leininger, 2002a).

Proxemics and Cultural Space

Proxemics is another concept essential for understanding transcultural communication. It refers to *"the use and perception of interpersonal or personal space in sociocultural interactions"* (Hall, 1974). *Cultural space* refers to *"the variation of cultures in the use of body, visual, territorial, and interpersonal distance to others"* (Leininger, 2002b). An awareness of how cultures use space and expect others to recognize their territory is essential to prevent conflict, feuds, and violence. To violate the use of another's space can lead to interpersonal stress, anger, and a host of other preventable problems.

Anthropologist Hall (1996) identified and discussed the importance of proxemics and how cultures use space. He stated that diverse cultures had different interpersonal distances or zones that were considered important. He maintained that Western cultures have three primary space dimensions: *the intimate zone* (zero to 18 inches); *the personal zone* (18 inches to three feet); and *the social or public zone* (three to six feet). However, U. S. Americans tend to prefer personal space that ranges from six inches to four feet; social space of four to 13 feet; and public space (for lectures and speeches) greater than 12 feet. Similarly, Germans and Scandinavians desire a lot of personal and public space (Hall, 1996). In contrast, other cultures such as Africans, Latin American, Indonesians, and French favor closeness to better relate to others (Leininger, 2002b). Therefore, sitting behind a desk to interview or assess a client may be considered unacceptable for many non-Western immigrants, minorities, and others who identify with close proxemics.

The use of personal space was also studied by Watson (1980) who found that Canadians, Americans, and British require the most personal space whereas Japanese, Arab Muslims, Latin Americans, and Africans are comfortable with less personal space. Africans seemed to tolerate crowded public spaces but Japanese preferred more open living spaces. Knowledge of personal and public space is important to understanding, interacting with, and providing therapeutic and culturally congruent care to diverse cultures. Personal space has major implications when conducting an assessment and when deciding where one stands or sits when talking or caring for a client in the home, hospital, and other settings (Leininger, 2002b).

Culture, Social, and Cyclic Time

Culture time refers to *"the cultural interpretation of time as it guides an individual or group's thinking, decisions, and actions"* (adapted from Leininger, 2002b). Cultures generally have their own concepts and meanings of time that tend to differ among cultures and often conflicts with the time orientation of health professionals. For example, Anglo-Americans, British, and Australians tend to focus on the immediate and exact present or future times whereas Africans, Hispanics, Latin Americans, and Southeast Asians tend to focus more on past and an extended present time so that noon may mean from 11 a.m. to 1 or 2 p.m. Some clients from diverse cultural backgrounds gauge their activities within *their own* time orientation, may be late for appointments, and not relate to the professional nurses' sense of time.

Because Anglo-Americans tend to live and function by more precise clock time for appointments, cultural conflicts and stresses tend to occur when other cultures do not conform to clock time.

Nurses, physicians, and others who are not familiar with the concept of cultural time may become quite annoyed with clients who are late or cancel appointments at the last minute. Similarly, clients having a different time orientation often become frustrated and upset with precise Western time expectations. Cultural time remains one of the common sources of great tension and conflicts between nurses and clients. However, as clients of diverse cultural backgrounds become more acculturated into the mainstream dominant culture, the gap in time orientation between these two cultures tends to diminish.

Social time refers to "*time for leisurely interactions and activities in which exact time is of less importance*" (Leininger, 2002b). *Cyclic time* refers to "*recurrent daily, nightly, weekly, monthly, annual, or other cultural activities and events that form a rhythm of life*" (adapted from Leininger, 2002b). For example, the Gadsups of New Guinea live by cyclic time defined by structured daily and nightly activities. Most villagers have no watches or clocks and depend on community activities regulated by the sun such as gardening, picking coffee, eating, and hunting to define their concept of time (Leininger, 2002b).

Transcultural and other nurses need to learn about different time orientations to care for or study different cultures. Healthcare providers need to understand cultural time and try to accommodate these time differences to reduce anger, frustration, and nonadherent client responses. Being aware of cultural time orientations facilitates establishing and maintaining favorable and trusting relationships with culturally diverse individuals, families, and groups.

Body Touching

Body touching refers to *culturally appropriate and customary ways of touching as defined by gender, age, religious, social, and other factors*. This varies between and among cultures and is often gender related. Non-Western, *traditionally oriented* women seldomly embrace or shake hands with men in public settings but are usually comfortable *appropriately and selectively* touching social friends, relatives, and acquaintances of the opposite gender in their homes and other similar environments.

However, in several non-Western cultures from places such as Indonesia, Africa, and New Guinea touching and holding hands with members of the same gender is usually interpreted as appropriate behavior (Leininger, 2002b). Westerners may hug, shake hands, or touch friends and relatives of both sexes in diverse customary ways during greetings or farewells. For some Western cultures, same gender touching may not be acceptable and may be viewed as inappropriate behavior; this may be culturally dependent or contextually dependent (e.g., workplace vs. social settings). Body touching as human caring is largely culturally defined and valued as an important mode of communication and human expression for healing and wellbeing (Leininger, 1991b). There is much to be learned about personal and public touching in diverse cultures as it relates to transcultural nursing.

Important Considerations for Transcultural Communication

When Communicating with clients of similar or diverse cultural backgrounds, it is important to keep the following considerations in mind:

- Be aware that similarities and diversities exist within cultural groups and even within the same family unit.
- Introduce yourself and inquire how the client wishes to be addressed so as not to inadvertently offend. Avoid addressing clients with overly familiar terms such as *darling* or *honey* unless permission is obtained from client.
- Speak slowly and clearly and avoid use of slang, medical terminology, or abbreviations (Andrews, 2016). Use of medical terminology may be appropriate when communicating with clients of healthcare backgrounds such as physicians or nurses.
- Be aware of wide cultural variations in the meaning of silence. Silence may indicate agreement [Arabs], respect, need for time to process thinking, or a desire to maintain harmony [Asians] (Andrews, 2016).

Use of Translators to Obtain Accurate Assessments

The following are recommendations for using translators to facilitate accurate assessments:

- Select a professionally trained and certified translator who is knowledgeable about the client's culture and cultural language/dialect (adapted from Leininger, 2002a, p. 128).

- Solicit assistance in translating from a professional colleague who is knowledgeable about the client's culture and/or speaks the client's language/dialect when a professional translator is not available.
- In cases of emergency, when a professional translator or a professional colleague who is knowledgeable about the client's culture and/or speaks the client's language/dialect is unavailable, use of an available family member is justified until a professional translator is secured.
- Seek a translator of relatively the same age for younger clients because when a generational gap exists, translators may miss or misinterpret certain generational knowledge that is unique to children and adolescents (Leininger, 2002a, p. 128).
- Discuss in advance what you are or will be doing during the assessment and the intended purposes of your actions with the client (Leininger, 2002a, p. 128).
- Insist on an exact translation of the client's words, not the translator's views of a desired response (Leininger, 2002a, p. 128).
- Verify terms in writing using both your own and the client's language when you are in doubt about the terms spoken or the translator's translation (Leininger, 2002a, p. 128).
- Try to learn a few words or phrases in the language being translated so as to be able to occasionally verify whether the translator is sharing ideas accurately and completely [sometimes a translator may shorten or omit informant ideas for his or her personal reasons or cultural/personal comfortableness] (Leininger, 2002a, p. 128).
- Always thank the translator afterward, and reverify ideas or observations that remain unclear to you (Leininger, 2002a, p. 128).

■ SUMMARY

Cultural assessments uncover information that guide nurses in providing culturally congruent and competent care while blending professional care with the client's values, beliefs, patterns, expressions, and lifeways. Emic and etic assessments are imperative to ensure quality care and to promote the health and wellbeing of diverse cultures. Nurses prepared in transcultural nursing, as well as other healthcare professionals, will find thecultural assessment guides discussed in this chapter meaningful and easy to use in clinical practice. Assessment data are not only used for client care but also for educational, consultative, and research purposes. Nurses using cultural assessment findings can greatly increase their ways of knowing clients. Discovering culture-specific data and gaining a holistic understanding of cultures can become a most rewarding experience (Leininger, 1999a). Most importantly, conducting cultural assessments enables nurses to learn more about themselves and expand their own worldview as they acquire deeper appreciation of diverse cultures and caring phenomena.

■ DISCUSSION QUESTIONS

1. Why should nurses and other healthcare providers conduct cultural assessments?
2. How can nurses and other healthcare providers conduct cultural assessments?
3. Discuss ways you can apply principles for effective cultural assessments.
4. Discuss important considerations in verbal and nonverbal communication.
5. Discuss important considerations for choosing translators.

■ REFERENCES

Abbadi, F. (2014). *Nose kiss? How the Gulf Arab greet.* Retrieved from http://fatimaabbadi.blogspot.com/2014/10/nose-kiss-how-gulf-arab-greet.html

American Association of Colleges of Nursing. (2015). *Fact sheet: Enhancing diversity in the nursing workforce.* Retrieved from http://www.aacn.nche.edu/media-relations/diversityFS.pdf

Andrews, M. M. (2016). Culturally competent nursing care. In M. M. Andrews & J. S. Boyle (Eds.), *Transcultural concepts in nursing care* (6th ed., pp. 30-54). Philadelphia, PA: Wolters Kluwer Health | Lippincott Williams & Wilkins.

Andrews, M. M., & Boyle, J. S. (2016). *Transcultural concepts in nursing care* (7th ed.). Philadelphia, PA: Wolters Kluwer Health | Lippincott Williams & Wilkins.

Camarota, S., & Zeigler, K. (2014). One in five U.S. residents speaks foreign language at home: Record 61.8 million. Washington, DC: Center For Immigration Studies. Retrieved from http://cis.org//sites/cis.org/files/camarota-language.pdf

Campinha-Bacote, J. (2015). *Transcultural C.A.R.E. assessments.* Retrieved from http://www.transculturalcare.net/

Chrisman, N. (1990). Cultural shock in the operating room: Cultural analysis in transcultural nursing. *Journal of Transcultural Nursing, 1*(2), 33-39.

Giger, J. N., & Davidhizar, R. E. (2004). *Transcultural nursing: Assessment & intervention.* St. Louis, MO: Mosby.

Hall, T. (1996). *The silent language.* Westport, CT: Greenwood Press.

Hall, T. (1974). *Handbook for proxemic research.* Washington, DC: Society for the Ontology of Visual Communication.

Hongi. (n.d.). *Dictionary.com Unabridged.* Retrieved from http://dictionary.reference.com/browse/hongi

Jeffreys, M. R. (2016). *Teaching cultural competence in nursing and health care: Inquiry, action, and innovation.* New York, NY: Springer.

Leininger, M. M. (1970). *Nursing and anthropology: Two worlds to blend.* New York, NY: John Wiley & Sons.

Leininger, M. M. (1977). The phenomenon of caring: The essence and central focus of nursing, *nursing research report. American Nurses' Foundation, 12*(1), 2-14.

Leininger, M. M. (1978). Culturalogical assessment domains for nursing practices. In M. M. Leininger (Ed.), *Transcultural nursing: Concepts, theories, and practices* (pp. 85-106). New York, NY: John Wiley & Sons.

Leininger, M. M. (1988a). *Care discovery and uses in clinical and community nursing.* Detroit, MI: Wayne State Press.

Leininger, M. M. (1988b). Special research report: Dominant culture care (emic) meanings and practice findings from Leininger's theory. *Journal of Transcultural Nursing, 9*(2), 45-48.

Leininger, M. M. (1990). Issues, questions, and concerns related to the nursing diagnosis cultural movement from a transcultural nursing perspective. *Journal of Transcultural Nursing, 2*(1), 23-32. doi: 10.1177/104365969000200104

Leininger, M. M. (1991a). Ethnonursing: A research method with enablers to study the theory of culture care. In M. M. Leininger (Ed.), *Cultural care diversity and universality: A theory of nursing* (pp. 73-118). New York, NY: National League for Nursing Press.

Leininger, M. M. (1991b). Selected culture care findings of diverse cultures using culture care theory and ethnomethods. In M. M. Leininger (Ed.), *Culture care diversity and universality: A theory of nursing* (pp. 345-372). New York, NY: National League for Nursing Press.

Leininger, M. (1991c). The theory of culture care diversity and universality. In M. M. Leininger (Ed.), *Cultural care diversity and universality: A theory of nursing* (pp. 5-72). New York, NY: National League for Nursing Press.

Leininger, M. M. (1994a). The tribes of nursing in the USA culture of nursing. *Journal of Transcultural Nursing, 6*(1), 18-22. doi: 10.1177/104365969400600104

Leininger, M. M. (1994b). *Transcultural nursing: Concepts, theories, and practices.* Columbus, OH: Greyden Press.

Leininger, M. M. (1995). *Transcultural nursing: Concepts, theories, research, and practice.* Blacklick, OH: McGraw-Hill College Custom Series.

Leininger, M. M. (1999a). Transcultural nursing: An imperative nursing practice. *Imprint, 46*(5), 50-52; 61.

Leininger, M. M. (1999b). What is transcultural nursing and culturally competent care? *Journal of Transcultural Nursing, 10*(1), 9.

Leininger, M. M. (2002a). Culture care assessments for congruent competency practices. In M. M. Leininger & M. R. McFarland (Eds.), *Transcultural nursing: Concepts, theories, research, & practice* (3rd ed., pp. 117-144). New York, NY: McGraw-Hill.

Leininger, M. M. (2002b). Essential transcultural nursing care concepts, principles, examples, and policy statements. In M. M. Leininger & M. R. McFarland (Eds.), *Transcultural nursing: Concepts, theories, research, & practice* (3rd ed., pp. 45-70). New York, NY: McGraw-Hill.

Lilley, R. (2010). *The rituals of rest.* Retrieved from http://www.academia.edu/644610/The_Rituals_of_Rest

Purnell, L. (2014). *Guide to culturally competent health care.* Philadelphia, PA: F. A. Davis.

Rukhman, E., Ladizinski, B., & Lee, K. C. (2014). Male circumcision as a religious ritual. *JAMA Dermatology, 150*(1), 103-103. doi: 10.1001/jamadermatol.2013.8367

Schim, S. M., Doorenbos, A. Z., Miller, J., & Benkert, R. (2003). Development of a cultural competence assessment instrument. *Journal of Nursing Measurement, 11*(1), 29-40. doi: 10.1891/jnum.11.1.29.52062.

Spector, R. E. (2016). *Cultural diversity in health and illness.* Upper Saddle River, NJ: Pearson Prentice Hall.

U.S. Department of Commerce, Census Bureau. (2015). *Selected characteristics of the native and foreign-born populations.* Retrieved from http://factfinder.census.gov/faces/tableservices/jsf/pages/productview.xhtml?pid=ACS_13_5YR_S0501&prodType=table

van Gennep, A. (1960). *The rites of passage.* London, UK: Routledge & Kegan Paul.

Watson, M. (1980). *Proxemic behavior: A cross-cultural study.* The Hague, NL: Mouton de Gruyter.

Wehbe-Alamah, H. (2008). Bridging generic and professional care practices for Muslim patients through the use of Leininger's culture care modes. *Contemporary Nurse, 28*(1-2), 83-97.

Wehbe-Alamah, H. B. (2015). Folk care beliefs and practices of traditional Lebanese and Syrian Muslims in the Midwestern United States. In M. R. McFarland & H. B. Wehbe-Alamah (Eds.), *Culture care diversity and universality: A worldwide nursing theory* (3rd ed., pp. 137-182). Burlington, MA: Jones and Bartlett Learning.

Wehbe-Alamah, H. B., & McFarland, M. R. (2015). Transcultural nursing course outline, educational activities, and syllabi using the Culture Care Theory. In M. R. McFarland & H. B. Wehbe-Alamah (Eds.), *Culture care diversity and universality: A worldwide nursing theory* (3rd ed., pp. 553-578). Burlington, MA: Jones and Bartlett Learning.

Wolf, Z. R. (1990). *Nurses' work: The sacred and profane.* Philadelphia, PA: University of Pennsylvania Press.

CHAPTER 8

Integrating Generic and Professional Health Care Practices

Hiba B. Wehbe-Alamah

> *"There remains extremely rich healing, caring, and curing generic traditions of human beings from the distant past that are still limitedly known and await discovery for integration into today's modern professional health services"* (Leininger, 2002, p. 145).

■ INTRODUCTION

According to the World Health Organization (WHO, 2013), complementary medicine and alternative medicine are terms used interchangeably to describe traditional medicine in some countries and refer to "... to a broad set of health care practices that are not part of [a] country's own tradition and are not integrated into the dominant healthcare system" (p. 15). The U.S. National Center for Complementary and Integrative Health (U.S. Department of Health and Human Services [USDHHS], 2015a) defines *complementary* health practices as those that occur together with conventional medicine, whereas *alternative* health practices are those used in place of conventional medicine. *Traditional medicine* as defined by the WHO is "... the sum total of the knowledge, skill, and practices based on the theories, beliefs, and experiences indigenous to different cultures, whether explicable or not, used in the maintenance of health as well as in the prevention, diagnosis, improvement, or treatment of physical and mental illness" (WHO, 2013, p. 15). Leininger used the term *generic care* to refer to lay, indigenous, traditional, emic, or folk care (McFarland and Wehbe-Alamah, 2015).

In the U.S., more than 30% of adults and 12% of children reportedly use nonmainstream practices and often in conjunction with conventional treatments (USDHHS, 2015a). Across health care settings in the United States, there is growing use of integrative healthcare approaches that combine conventional and evidence-based complementary practices (Mayo Clinic, 2014; USDHHS, 2015a). An integrative literature review of 25 articles related to folk medicine and complementary and alternative medicine (CAM) revealed that "... the use of folk medicine and CAM is increasing in the general population and has been growing in popularity over a number of years" (Sackett, Carter, & Stanton, 2014, p. 121). Worldwide, strategies are being developed to facilitate the integration of traditional and complementary medicine/ health approaches into national health systems (WHO, 2013). In the U.K., up to 67% of cancer patients are believed to use CAM (Lorenc, Peace, Vaghela, & Robinson, 2010).

This chapter is not intended to provide a comprehensive review of the diverse types, uses, and techniques of generic (folk, traditional) healing modes or their therapeutic outcomes. The purpose of this chapter is to offer an overview about the rapidly growing interest in generic (traditional) health and healing practices and to offer reflections and comparisons about professional historical viewpoints, trends, and issues. The goal of this chapter is to provide some fresh insights about the nature, development, and importance of generic and professional care from a transcultural nursing perspective to facilitate the provision of integrative culturally congruent, sensitive, and meaningful care to people from diverse cultures. Transcultural nurses have a special interest in providing integrative humanistic, scientific, generic, and professional care in their roles as direct care providers who have special preparation to work with clients from diverse cultures worldwide.

■ DEFINITIONS OF GENERIC (FOLK), PROFESSIONAL, AND INTEGRATIVE CARE

In the early 1960s, Leininger realized two major concepts in the development of the new field of transcultural nursing (Leininger, 2002). She discovered that the nursing profession did not study, teach, or integrate culture and human caring into nursing education and practice regarding folk or indigenous beliefs, values, and practices (Leininger, 2002). Learning about and integrating cultural folk practices into nursing was meager, and there were doubts expressed about the value of folk healing, caring, and curing modalities (Leininger, 2002). As a result, Leininger conceptualized and defined the terms *generic care* and *professional care* drawing from some anthropological viewpoints for generic care and humanistic caring from nursing (Leininger, 1991, 2002). The explication of these two major perspectives was important to discover new knowledge and integrate findings into (what was then) a new body of evolving transcultural nursing knowledge and practices.

Leininger defined generic care as the learned and transmitted lay, indigenous, traditional, or local folk (emic) knowledge and practices to provide assistive, supportive, enabling, and facilitative acts for or toward others with evident or anticipated health needs in order to improve wellbeing or to help with dying or other human conditions (McFarland and Wehbe-Alamah, 2015, p. 14). The word *generic* refers to the original, root sources; the first or earliest knowledge

sources (Leininger, 2002). Anthropologically, humans lived and survived in the world long before professions such as nursing, medicine, and other related fields came into existence. Human beings relied on what was natural biologically, but also on what was familiar to them interpersonally and spiritually within their total cultural ways of knowing and living in different environments. These early cultures had healers, caregivers, curers, medicines, rituals, and indigenous ways of dealing with daily common and recurrent life situations related to birth, living, and dying. Hence, the term generic seemed most appropriate to conceptualize and discover traditional ways of caring, healing, and curing in transcultural nursing, keeping the dominant focus on caring, health, illness, and wellbeing (Leininger, 2002).

Professional care was defined by Leininger as the formal and explicit cognitively learned professional care knowledge and practices obtained generally through educational institutions … [and] are taught to nurses and others to provide assistive, supportive, enabling, or facilitative acts for or to another individual or group in order to improve their health, prevent illnesses, or to help with dying or other human conditions (McFarland & Wehbe-Alamah, 2015, p. 14). According to Leininger (2002), professional care and cure are often viewed as "scientific" knowledge about diagnosing, treating, caring for, or curing people. However, what constitutes scientific and humanistic professional, philosophic, and epistemic knowledge tends to vary among Western and non-Western cultures. Leininger (2002) held that professional or modern nursing caring or curing is not as old as generic care, and the latter holds great importance in many cultures, especially non-Western cultures.

Leininger (2002) maintained that professional care knowledge culturally constituted, learned, and practiced was a relatively new perspective and contrasted with generic care as previously defined. She affirmed that both generic and professional care were crucial for professional nursing and needed to be rigorously studied and used appropriately (Leininger, 2002). The constructs of generic and professional care became an integral part of the Theory of Culture Care Diversity and Universality (also known as the Culture Care Theory or CCT) in the early 1960s (Leininger, 1991, 2002). Since that time, transcultural nurses have used these constructs in research to discover major universalities and diversities between these two types of care. Leininger (2002) held that generic and professional care must continue to be studied worldwide with a focus on their dual relationships and therapeutic values for human caring and wellbeing. Generic care is essentially new knowledge in nursing that is being advocated for and taught by transcultural nurses and others knowledgeable about these phenomena.

In the 1950s, the linguistic terms *emic* and *etic* (Pike, 1954) were of great interest to Leininger to discover culture's insider knowledge, comparing it with outsider knowledge in transcultural nursing (Leininger, 2002). After conferring with Pike and getting his enthusiastic approval, Leininger introduced emic and etic into nursing in the 1960s through her teaching, research, and theory (Leininger, 2002). These two concepts have thus become part of professional nursing discourse and are used to discover embedded and overt culture care phenomena.

The construct of *integrative care* was termed to describe the desired combined approach when generic care and professional care were appropriately and meaningfully used in therapeutic practices. Leininger (2002) defined integrative care as the safe, congruent, and creative ways of blending together holistic, generic, and professional care knowledge and practices so that the client experiences beneficial outcomes for wellbeing or to ameliorate a human condition or lifeway (p. 148). According to Leininger (2002), integrative care was the preferred means to provide culturally congruent care and the desired outcome generated through the Culture Care Theory. It is important to state, however, that sometimes in helping clients, more emphasis needs to be placed on the generic care approaches rather than the professional care ones. However, at other times, it may be necessary or appropriate to place more emphasis on professional care and very little on generic care (Leininger, 2002). Such decisions require knowledge about both generic and professional practices in addition to specific client preferences, values, and beliefs. Most importantly, professional nurses have societal, ethical, moral, and legal obligations to always inform and share relevant professional knowledge with clients without neglecting generic care knowledge in order to empower the client to reach sound and informed individualized decisions. Transcultural nursing practices integrative care thus ensuring that the client benefits from

the best care based on both worlds of knowledge and therapeutics (Leininger, 2002).

There are a number of terms used by different disciplines to refer to lay, folk, or traditional healing practices such as alternative, complementary, traditional, non-Western, indigenous, integrative, and holistic care. In studying and working with many cultures over her scholarly career, Leininger (2002) discovered that most non-Western cultures disliked the term 'alternative' when used by healthcare professionals. She reported that informants were quick to ask: "Alternative to what?" "… Our folk healing ways are not alternatives as they are basic and are the first and oldest ways to heal… They have been important to us for hundreds or even thousands of years" (Leininger, 1997, 2002). Some informants reported that the term 'alternative' was insulting, demeaning, and revealed a lack of appreciation and knowledge of traditional practices (Leininger, 2002). The majority of informants preferred the term *generic care,* which encompassed the native (insider, emic) views, beliefs, and practices that Leininger discovered were often very different from professional ones. They advocated for the constructs of *integrative* care and cure and hoped they would be commonly practiced in the future (Leininger, 2002). For these reasons and others, transcultural nurses use the terms generic, integrative, and professional care and encourage their use by others.

Leininger (2002) believed that blending of *generic* and professional knowledge and practices together through integrative care was best when grounded in rigorous research-based cultural data and knowledge about cultural care and caring practices. She held that biological factors, language, cultural values, and other cultural and social structure dimensions played an important part in providing truly integrative and culturally congruent care and predicted that dominant and specific culturally based caring and healing values and practices would be powerful forces to explain and predict health maintenance and prevention for culturally diverse and similar cultures worldwide (Leininger, 2002). She maintained that generic (emic) and professional (etic) knowledge and practices were essential guides for wellness and especially to prevent illnesses, disabilities, chronic conditions, and destructive health acts (Leininger, 2002).

According to Leininger (2002), knowledge-based integrative professional (etic) and generic (emic) care remained an important goal for transcultural nurses when providing and maintaining culturally congruent care. Figure 8.1 depicts a summary of some major differences between Western etic (column 1) and non-Western emic providers (column 2). The data presented in Figure 8.1 are derived from cultural informants' viewpoints and assessments shared with Leininger (2002) over several decades. Understanding the viewpoints of generic and professional care providers is extremely important for working toward the desired goal of integrative care—culturally congruent care (column 3). The Culture Care Theory can facilitate health professionals to achieve and provide integrative and culturally congruent care. Reflecting on Figure 8.1 will help providers to keep both emic

and etic perspectives in mind as they seek to provide integrative care.

■ FAST-GROWING WESTERN INTEREST IN TRADITIONAL, COMPLEMENTARY, AND ALTERNATIVE HEALTH CARE PRACTICES

One of the fastest growing areas of interest and practice of Western healthcare professionals is complementary and alternative medicine (CAM), which includes traditional folk or indigenous medicines, healers, and naturalistic practices that have survived over thousands of years in many cultures (Johnson, 2013; Lee

1. Western (Etic) professional providers practices	2. Non-Western (Emic) folk provider practices	3. Desired attributes for integrative care
1. Relies mainly on etic biomedical knowledge of diseases, symptoms, and practices.	1. Relies mainly on emic generic (folk) care healing, values, and beliefs.	1. Desires trust and mutual respect in caring, healing, curing, and wellbeing.
2. Uses partial body-mind meanings, practices, and research findings.	2. Seeks holistic culturally based meanings, beliefs, and lifeways for healing.	2. Desires collaborative decision-making using the best of emic and etic practices.
3. Uses actions-oriented modes and largely "scientific" medical facts but *may be* skeptical of folk practices.	3. Uses listening, and watching about professional ideas and practices but often skeptical of them.	3. Seeks etic and emic care-cure practices that are congruent, safe, and meaningful.
4. Defends etic professional knowledge and practices.	4. Uses and defends emic folk lifeways, values, and experiences, especially in home context.	4. Seeks holistic care perspectives to ensure safe and congruent generic practices.
5. Relies heavily on medical, nursing, and other treatment modes as "scientific" and "the best."	5. Relies on folk healers and carers as safe, reliable and trustworthy.	5. Seeks beneficial care or healing practices that incorporate one's values, beliefs, and lifeways within their living environments.
6. Focuses on individual curing and symptom management relief for curing outcomes.	6. Focuses on caring modes and lifeway experiences in community context.	6. Seeks competent, creative, and compassionate practitioners.
↓	↓	↓
Professional etic care	**Generic emic care**	**Integrative etic & emic congruent care**

FIGURE 8.1 • Comparative Western (etic) and non-Western (emic) Cultural Provider Practices With Desired Integrative Congruent Care Attributes.
Adapted from Leininger, M.M. (2002). Part 1. Toward integrative generic and professional care. In M. M. Leininger & M. R. McFarland (Eds.), *Transcultural nursing: Concepts, theories, research, and practice* (3rd ed., p. 150). New York: McGraw-Hill Companies, Inc.

& Cleminson, 2013; Leininger, 2002). Although physicians have become interested in CAM in more recent years (Upsdell & Jaye, 2011), professional nurses working closely with people in homes, hospitals, and community services have long been interested to learn what cultures were using for healing and health maintenance (Leininger, 1994, 2002). Transcultural nurses have stimulated practicing nurses, nursing students, and nurse researchers through education, practice, and research to learn about specific folk practices and how to assimilate them therapeutically into professional care practices.

Despite modern Western technologies and treatments nurses, physicians, and pharmacists have been curious about how non-Western, traditionally oriented cultures heal and cure clients with different herbs, rituals, and practices—often at less cost and with some effective outcomes (Leininger, 2002). Healthcare providers from diverse disciplines were also interested in learning about generic care practices so as to identify and address potential hazardous or harmful practices. In the early 1970s and 1980s, there was general skepticism in the medical community surrounding the use of folk practices; some professionals felt a loss of control and serious interference with scientific medicine largely due to their own lack of knowledge about specific folk practices (Leininger, 1995, 2002).

In the 1970s, transcultural nurses began to learn about and integrate specific folk care modalities in their professional practices. At that time, physicians were greatly immersed in mind and body relationships and the use of new technologies. There was almost no interest in culturally and holistically based care related to healing and wellbeing (Leininger, 2002). Nonetheless, transcultural nurses continued to explore their uses and caring practices using selected folk caring modalities. They were watchful for potential dangers when folk care modes were used with Western medicines and treatments, but remained interested in how cultures used familiar, inexpensive herbs and other folk healing and caring practices. As a result, considerable folk caring and healing knowledge began to emerge and become assimilated into transcultural nursing during the 1970s, 1980s, and 1990s (Leininger, 1991, 1995, 2002).

As medical costs markedly increased, economically poor cultures had limited financial resources to access modern Western medical care and treatments.

Furthermore, some traditional non-Western cultures feared surgical and medical Western interventions based on their beliefs in the risk of soul loss through the use of these "powerful" Western care methods (Leininger, 2002). Transcultural nurses continued to document traditional cultural responses and were keenly aware of what folk medicines and treatments clients preferred to use. Protecting cultural practices was important while still discerning what integrative approaches would be optimally beneficial and fit best with cultural beliefs and lifeways (Leininger, 2002).

With the use of the Culture Care Theory, transcultural nurses became increasingly aware of cultural values and the importance of holistic caring that went beyond the medical focus on mind-body and partial care and cure (Leininger, 2002). The holistic and totality view of cultures emphasized the dynamic role of folk care healing practices as influenced by kinship, religion, specific culture values, and multiple other factors. Emic folk practices and their functions "made sense" as transcultural nurses obtained folk health histories and studied the intergenerational use of these practices over time (Leininger, 2002). Eventually, these holistic care and folk practices transformed the thinking and practices of other nurses. Holistic care became a powerful means to shift nursing practice away from dependence on the medical model of diseases and symptoms to a broad transcultural professional and generic care focus (Leininger, 2002). As managed care came into existence, however, holistic transcultural nursing care with its comprehensive focus became threatened (Leininger, 2002). It was very difficult to maintain a client-centered emic folk and professional focus within the dominance of a managed system that emphasized limited health access, cost reductions, and early discharges (Leininger, 2002). Efforts to maintain the balanced holistic transcultural nursing emic and etic perspective throughout mainstream nursing and to redirect managed care ideology and its long-term sequelae remain ongoing.

Thereafter, for the next few decades, folk healing practices became increasingly studied and recognized by physicians and by other health disciplines and practitioners (Leininger, 2002). The increased interest in traditional, alternative, and complementary care modalities led to the establishment of the National Center for Complementary and Alternative Medicine (NCCAM) in October 1991 after Public Law 102-170 was passed by the U.S. Congress, providing

$2 million in federal funding for the establishment of the NCCAM within the National Institutes of Health (USDHHS, 2015b). In December 2014, the U.S. Congress changed the Center's name from NCCAM to the National Center for Complementary and Integrative Health (NCCIH) (USDHHS, 2015b). Across the globe, numerous centers focus on the discovery of traditional, complementary, and alternative care modalities. One example is the New Zealand Centre for Evidence-based Research into Complementary and Alternative Medicine (ENZCAM) at the University of Canterbury in Christchurch, New Zealand (University of Canterbury, n.d.).

The literature and practice evidence has increased dramatically in the last few decades on alternative medicine and naturalistic healing as presented in the works by Weil (1989, 2004); Pelletier (1997, 2002); Chopra (1989, 2015); and Micozzi (2015). Medical schools in the United States and worldwide have begun to educate students about the practice of CAM and supporting evidence; research is being conducted to document outcomes. Many people around the globe are being attracted to diverse traditional and cultural healing and curing practices and to naturalistic medicines such as herbs and vitamins (Almog, Lev, Schiff, & Linn, 2014; Lorenc, Peace, Vaghela, & Robinson, 2010; Mayberry, Affonso, Shibuya, & Clemmens, 1999; Poss, Jezewski, & Stuart, 2003; Sackett, Carter, & Stranton, 2014; Titus, 2014). Large amounts of money continues to be spent in the United States to advertise "prescriptions for healthy living" that promote dietary pills, foods, and weight loss programs as well as body-building and exercise equipment (Leininger, 2002). Books, articles, and website information about alternative medicine and what is held to "work or not work" are widely available to the general public. Additional research and experiential data continue to be needed to identify or clarify what are the beneficial or potentially harmful outcomes.

In this discussion about the evolutionary development of folk practices, a clear statement is needed that since its beginnings in the 19th century, anthropology has led the way in the discovery, documentation, and interpretation of folk or traditional cultural healing and curing practices (Leininger, 2002). Accordingly, health professionals prepared in anthropology, transcultural nursing, and medical anthropology have studied some of these past and present folk contributions to health care (Kottak, 1991; Leininger, 2002). In addition, anthropological literature has provided several research studies on traditional folk and professional health practices. Amid these rapidly growing trends many critical issues have emerged in the United States related to ethical concerns; costs of treatment; consumer and professional access and usage; and outcome indicators for beneficial and less than beneficial uses of folk practices in conjunction with professional regimes (Leininger, 2002).

■ RATIONALE BEHIND USE OF GENERIC (FOLK) AND CAM

Some nurses who work with immigrants such as Iraqi, Somali, Syrian, Mexican, Vietnamese, Filipino, Chinese, Russian, and Cuban people have observed how families use folk practices in their daily lives to maintain their wellbeing or to treat common illnesses. Military nurses and nurses traveling or working overseas also have become aware of folk or traditional healthcare practices. Almog, Lev, Schiff, and Linn (2014) reported that herbal medicine was highly prevalent in India, China, and the Middle East. Numerous studies have demonstrated that integrating generic (folk) and professional (nursing) care is desired by consumers and considered essential to providing culturally congruent care (Leininger, 2006; Mixer, Fornehed, Varney, & Lindley, 2014).

There are numerous reasons why individuals from diverse cultural backgrounds favor generic or folk care practices. Oleson, Cheute, O'Fallon, and Sherwood (2012) discovered that Burmese refugees in the U.S. sought traditional healers to receive treatment; maintain important spiritual beliefs; and obtain advice about how to acquire prescriptive medications. In addition, Burmese refugees trusted the efficacy of traditional medicine because it was "more natural" and "had fewer side effects" compared to Western medicine (p. 46). Furthermore, they relied on traditional medicine because of its accessibility and lower costs (Oleson, Cheute, O'Fallon, & Sherwood, 2012).

Similarly, Poss, Jezewski, & Stuart (2003) reported that Mexican Americans "… preferred herbal remedies because they were natural" (p. 316). Titus (2014) described how Hispanics relied on traditional medicine, *curenderismo* (a melded holistic practice of traditional medicine associated with spiritual, psychic, and physical healing), and the services of traditional healers (*curanderos* and *curanderas*) to maintain health that reflected their culture. Their reasons for seeking the services of traditional healers included affordability; language use; immigration or undocumented status; cultural appropriateness; and compatibility with Hispanic cultural values, beliefs, and ethnic identity in addition to their general dissatisfaction with Western medicine (Titus, 2014).

Hispanics used traditional healers to treat a wide range of physical, emotional, spiritual, and folk illnesses (Titus, 2014). Accordingly, curanderos/curanderas were sought to heal chronic conditions such as diabetes; obtain relief from pain; engage in prayer services; cure folk illnesses such as *caida de mollera* (sunken fontanel), *susto* (fright sickness), *empacho* (upset stomach), *mal ojo* (evil eye), and *envidia* (envy; Favazza Titus, 2014, p. 197). It is anticipated that by the year 2050, more than 100 million Hispanics would be residing in the U.S. (Titus, 2014). Healthcare providers who are knowledgeable about and understand folk care beliefs, practices, and needs of Hispanics and many other cultural groups will be in a better position to provide their clients with culturally congruent care; earn and maintain their trust; and encourage their use of the Western healthcare system.

■ TRANSCULTURAL GENERIC (FOLK) BELIEFS AND PRACTICES

As worldwide interest about generic or traditional values, beliefs, rituals, and practices has grown, nurses are evermore challenged to study these phenomena in-depth. Many chapters in this text have excellent examples of generic folk healing and caring practices studied using the Culture Care Theory. Sections in other transcultural nursing books (such as Andrews and Boyle, 2015) contain information about traditional generic or folk practices and describe meaningful clinical examples. In addition, many research articles, videos, and magazines about generic folk beliefs, foods, practices, and care-cure rituals showcase the influence of generic folk beliefs and practices within the Culture Care Theory along with some integrative practices (Gunn & Davis, 2011; Strang & Mixer, 2015; Wehbe-Alamah, 2008).

As transcultural nurses, it is important to keep in mind the many different types of generic folk healers (including medicine women and men); caretakers/caregivers; rituals; caring–curing strategies; beliefs; and symbolic material and nonmaterial ways of healing, as well as different ways to integrate generic beliefs into professional practices. Cultural healing and caring studies and obtaining life histories from caretakers/caregivers and healers are valuable data sources (Leininger, 2002). Families often like to share about "their" foods, herbs, medicines, and practices if genuine interest and respect by nurses/healthcare providers is evident (Leininger, 2002). Keeping an open (discovering) mind along with active listening and documenting of what is seen, heard, and done helps the nurse to obtain accurate data (Leininger, 2002). Leininger (2002) strongly advocated for the transcultural principle of learning from others by listening to cultural informants and remaining nonauthoritative.

However, evidence exists that generic/folk care practices are often withheld from healthcare providers, either because patients do not willingly share this information out of fear of being reproached for using traditional folk services, or because healthcare providers fail to elicit such information (Sackett, Carter, & Stanton, 2014; Titus, 2014). The use of the Culture Care Theory with the Sunrise Enabler provides an excellent means to discover generic and professional care for the provision of culturally congruent integrative care (Leininger, 2002). (Refer to Color Insert 1).

It is important to know about the many different types of ancient and current therapies, especially in non-Western cultures. Generic practices include but are not limited to herbs; moxibustion; cupping; acupuncture; coining; massage and manipulation; dance; imagery; aerobic exercises; relaxation; breathing techniques; healing touch; music; Reiki; spiritual meditation; and dry or steam saunas (Leininger, 2002). In addition, internal and external substances and amulets are often used with these therapies in specific ways (Leininger, 2002). Many generic folk therapies or practices are routinely combined with medicines and nursing care practices because these cultural uses were found to be beneficial (Leininger, 2002). It is common for indigenous cultures to integrate several folk practices together into a "regimen." Different cultures have different histories of their "favorite" generic practices or beliefs that they have found through experience to be efficacious ways for obtaining certain health results. One example is the Chinese use of acupuncture and

Qi Gong, an ancient Chinese exercise that integrates breathing, movement, and meditation.

Transcultural nurses and others can learn about different philosophies, schools of thought, and specific generic folk practices to understand and appreciate their usage over time and among diverse cultures. Non-Western philosophies are being studied anew in Western contemporary health systems for their holistic and integrative practices in preserving and promoting optimal health or to help heal selected physical illnesses and chronic cultural conditions. Integrating generic spirituality beliefs and practices with specific exercises and nutrition, sociocultural, and environmental factors are important to many traditional and natural healing practices (Leininger, 2002).

Ayurveda, presented in Chapter 14, is a very ancient non-Western school of thought and practice, especially popular in India and Southeast Asia. Ayurveda is known to be among the oldest systems of natural healing and the origin for many other healing traditions (Leininger, 2002; Maxwell & Morningstar, 2016). Other Chinese and Tibetan non-Western folk care philosophies, medicines, and healing modes include naturopathy, homeopathy, chiropractic, reflexology, meditation, yoga, aromatherapy, Rolfing, shiatsu, among many other therapies and ancient schools of thought (Leininger, 2002). Many lay and professional people use Eastern herbs, exercises, nutritional foods, and several traditional therapies from these ancient schools of thought. Some use them to regulate body weight; prevent illnesses and diseases such as cancer and hypertension; and promote and regulate healthy lifestyles (Leininger, 2002). Western professional institutions now examine generic (folk) therapies as well as natural food supplements for hard "scientific proofs" and confirmable evidence of efficacy (Leininger, 2002). All health professionals, including nurses, need to assess the effectiveness of traditional generic (folk) practices as well as their costs, strengths, and limitations.

New ideas, practices, and discoveries from traditional non-Western cultures have steadily increased in the professional world of nurses, physicians, social workers, pharmacists, and other healthcare disciplines. Some generic practices have entered professional healthcare systems faster than anticipated with nurses often expected to know how to properly integrate them into professional care practices.

Family members bring healing materials into healthcare institutions or use them in their homes for healing or "protection" from the evil eye (*mal de ojo*) or from perceived "dangerous" professional practices, medicines, treatments, and practitioners (Leininger, 1995, 2002). Transcultural nurses with knowledge of and experience in using both generic (folk) and professional practice care modes need to be called on to assess and help other nurses, physicians, and healthcare providers in making collaborative decisions with consumers about the integrative use of generic care and professional care. This is a professional responsibility that carries potential legal implications if omitted or ignored. This responsibility is more easily facilitated when health professionals are educated to integrate traditional generic practices and professional knowledge. The transcultural nurse is often asked to protect clients of non-Western cultures who are unfamiliar with Western medicines and treatments from being demeaned or shunned when using their folk remedies. Establishing mutual and genuine relationships between the healthcare provider and the client or family is critical to promote and practice beneficial integrative care. The following examples of generic and professional situations with different cultures may help the reader to grasp the meaning and importance of these concepts.

■ EXAMPLES OF GENERIC (FOLK) CARE PRACTICES AND PROFESSIONAL RESPONSES

The following real-life clinical examples from different cultures are presented to help raise readers' awareness about common generic care practices and provide a basis for understanding the consequences to patients when clinicians lack cultural knowledge.

Vietnamese Child and Nurse Response Example*

A community health nurse was asked to make a home care visit to a traditionally oriented Vietnamese family, especially to see their sick two-year-old child. When the nurse examined the child, she noted reddened welt areas by the spine and neck and some round reddened areas on the shoulders. She became very alarmed and immediately called the clinic physician to arrange for an x-ray of the child's spine. Because none of the family spoke English, the nurse assumed from her professional studies that the marks resulted from acts of child abuse. The mother's nonverbal communication showed that she was upset that the nurse had called a physician. The mother kept shaking her head as though disapproving the nurse's actions.

The Vietnamese believe that illness (or cold) needs to be drawn out of the body for healing to occur, hence, the generic practice of coining, rubbing, and cupping (Leininger, 2002). Unfortunately, this nurse had not been prepared in transcultural nursing and failed to recognize that Vietnamese family members had used their traditional practice of cupping with warm glasses to promote healing of the child's cold. The coin rubbing (Cao gio) was used near the spine and neck for similar reasons. Although the nurse was very concerned, she did note that the mother was affectionate with her sick child. The nurse felt helpless and left after she took the child's temperature and documented her observations. The visit ended with the mother upset and confused by the nurse's reaction to the mark on her child's back. *(Adapted from Leininger, 2002, p. 152)

Chinese Immigrant and Nurse Example*

A Chinese immigrant who had undergone major surgery was told by the nursing staff to "force fluids." The client refused to drink from the pitcher of ice cold water that had been placed on his bedside stand. The nurses and physicians threatened the client with intravenous fluids if he did not drink more fluids. The staff concluded that the client was uncooperative and noncompliant. When the client's daughter came to visit her father, she told the nursing staff that he would drink warm water or hot herbal tea, but not cold water. Warm water and herbal teas were culturally congruent with the Chinese belief in the use of hot beverages for healing and wellbeing. The theory of hot and cold and belief in the *yin and yang* principles are important to Chinese individuals. Chinese people view many generic herbal teas as healing, use them on a daily basis, and therefore expect teas to be part of their care while in the hospital. *(Adapted from Leininger, 2002, p. 152)

Navajo Folk Birth Expectations Example*

A Navajo woman gave birth to a child in a large urban hospital. The nurses later disposed of the placenta and the child's umbilical cord after inspecting them per hospital protocol. The mother asked for the placenta when she was ready to be discharged and learned about its disposal. She became very upset because could no longer bury the placenta in order to protect her newborn from evil spirits. She had assumed that the staff knew about the importance of this practice and that they would automatically save it for her so she could perform this traditional protective practice. The mother and her family left the hospital in great distress. Because the nurses were not educated about the Navajo culture and the importance of this folk caring practice, they were ineffective in helping the mother to preserve the child's future wellbeing. Lack of knowledge about this important cultural and spiritual practice resulted in cultural negligence and failure to meet the client's needs and expectations. In addition, their lack of integrative culture care knowledge also led to great cultural pain, client dissatisfaction, and lack of trust. As a cumulative result, this mother, child, and family did not receive culturally congruent generic care. *(Adapted from Leininger, 2002, p. 152)

Saudi Arabian Use of Generic Substance Example*

A transcultural nurse came into a hospital room in Saudi Arabia and found a Bedouin mother placing a dark substance into the eye of her sick 10-month-old child. The nurse was knowledgeable about kohl, which is used for cosmetic reasons and to prevent eye infections. This transcultural nurse asked the mother about her reasons for using kohl. The mother replied that she uses kohl "… to make my child beautiful and to prevent diseases." The nurse explained to the mother that the kohl she was using contained lead sulfide as was shown on the container. She advised the mother not to use the kohl because the lead it contained could lead to lead poisoning. The mother had not previously realized what was in the kohl. She thanked the nurse for her caring advice and concerns. This was an example of professional care knowledge shared with a client (parent) and child that prevented a potential negative consequence from a folk practice. It is obligatory for the nurse to inform clients when these situations arise to help them repattern and/or restructure a potentially harmful generic, traditional, folk, or lay care practice. However, the nurse does also keep in mind that the client ultimately has a right to make his (her) own decisions. *(Adapted from Leininger, 2002, pp. 152-153)

■ SUMMARY

To provide culturally congruent, sensitive, meaningful, and beneficial care to individuals, families, and groups from diverse cultural backgrounds nurses and other healthcare providers are encouraged to study generic care beliefs and practices and to reflect on their meaningful uses in professional care practices. During the past six decades, transcultural nurse researchers and practitioners have played a key role in discovering and sharing holding knowledge about different generic (folk) care beliefs and practices and in educating nurses and other healthcare providers about how to creatively integrate generic and professional care practices when caring for people from diverse and similar cultures.

In transcultural nursing, the goal is to discover and identify similarities and differences between generic and professional care practices, and to integrate and appropriately blend or assimilate such knowledge so as to provide culturally congruent, sensitive, and safe care. As a result, generic care practices need to be valued and nurtured for helpful relationships with clients from different cultures to be developed. Nurses prepared in transcultural nursing are encouraged to master knowledge of the generic care beliefs and practices of the people for whom they provide care in the same way nurses working in cardiac care are expected to master cardiovascular knowledge.

Cultures and their generic care beliefs and practices are complex phenomena requiring intensive study. Learning how to provide integrative holistic care can only be achieved through a synthesis of both generic and professional care values and lifeways. It is the philosophy of transcultural nursing to provide culturally competent caring practices that are safe, meaningful, and beneficial to people from diverse and similar cultures worldwide, a process that cannot be achieved by ignoring or avoiding generic (folk) care beliefs and practices.

■ DISCUSSION QUESTIONS

1. Discuss the importance of discovering culturally based generic care practices.
2. Discuss the importance of integrating generic care and professional care practices.
3. Develop a case scenario that depicts the ways healthcare providers could combine generic and professional care beliefs and practices to provide culturally congruent care.
4. Discuss the consequences of ignoring or neglecting generic care beliefs and practices.

■ REFERENCES

Almog, L., Lev, E., Schiff, E., Linn, S., & Ben-Arye, E. (2014). Bridging cross-cultural gaps: Monitoring herbal use during chemotherapy in patients referred to integrative medicine consultation in Israel. *Supportive Care in Cancer*, 22(10), 2793-2804. doi: 10.1007/s00520-014-2261-9

Andrews, M. M., & Boyle, J. S. (2015). *Transcultural concepts in nursing care* (7th ed.). Philadelphia, PA: Wolters Kluwer Health | Lippincott Williams & Wilkins.

Chopra, D. O. (1989). *Healing: Exploring the frontiers of the mind and body medicine.* New York, NY: Bantam Books.

Chopra, D. O. (2015). *Quantum healing (revised and updated): Exploring the frontiers of mind/body medicine.* New York, NY: Bantam Books.

Gunn, J., & Davis, S. (2011). Beliefs, meanings, and practices of healing with botanicals recalled by elder African American women in the Mississippi Delta. *Online Journal of Cultural Care in Nursing and Healthcare*,1(1), 37-49.

Johnson, P. (2013). Global use of complementary and alternative medicine and treatments. In C. Holtz (Ed.), *Global health care issues and policies* (2nd ed., pp. 207-238). Burlington, MA: Jones & Bartlett Learning.

Kottak, C. (1991). *Anthropology: The exploration of diversity.* New York, NY: McGraw-Hill.

Lees, J., & Cleminson, R. (2013). The history and future of psychotherapy and alternative health-related practices: Lessons from the past and from the present. *Psychotherapy and Politics International*, 11(3), 195-209. doi: 10.1002/ppi.1304

Leininger, M. M. (1991). *Culture care diversity and universality: Theory of nursing.* New York, NY: National League for Nursing Press.

Leininger, M. M. (1994). *Transcultural nursing: Concepts, theories, and practices.* Columbus, OH: Greyden Press.

Leininger, M. M. (1995). *Transcultural nursing: Concepts, theories, research and practice* (2nd ed.). Columbus, OH: McGraw Hill College Custom Series.

Leininger, M. M. (1997). Alternative to what?: Generic vs. professional caring, treatments, and healing modes. *Journal of Transcultural Nursing, 19*(1), 37.

Leininger, M. M. (2002). Part I. Toward integrative generic and professional health care. In M. M. Leininger & M. R. McFarland (Eds.), *Transcultural nursing: Concepts, theories, research, & practices* (3rd ed., pp. 145-154). New York, NY: McGraw-Hill.

Lorenc, A., Peace, B., Vaghela, C., & Robinson, N. (2010). The integration of healing into conventional cancer care in the UK. *Complementary Therapies in Clinical Practice, 16*(4), 222-228. doi: 10.1016/j.ctcp.2010.03.001

Mayberry, L. J., Affonso, D. D., Shibuya, J., & Clemmens, D. (1999). Integrating cultural values, beliefs, and customs into pregnancy and postpartum care: Lessons learned from a Hawaiian public health nursing project. *The Journal of Perinatal & Neonatal Nursing, 13*(1), 15-26.

Mayo Clinic. (2014). *Complementary and alternative medicine* [Website]. Rochester, MN: Author. Retrieved from http://www.mayoclinic.org/tests-procedures/complementary-alternative-medicine/basics/definition/prc-20021745

Micozzi, M. (2015). *Fundamentals of complementary and alternative medicine* (5th ed.). Saint Louis, MO: Saunders Elsevier.

Mixer, S., Fornehed, M., Varney, J., & Lindley, L. (2014). Culturally congruent end-of-life care for rural Appalachian people and their families. *Journal of Hospice & Palliative Nursing, 16*(8), 526-535. doi: 10.1097/NJH.0000000000000114

Oleson, H. E., Cheute, S., O'Fallon, A., & Sherwood, N. E. (2012). Health and healing: Traditional medicine and the Karen experience. *Journal of Cultural Diversity, 19*(2), 44-49.

Pelletier, K. R. (1977). *Mind as healer, mind as slayer: A holistic approach to preventing stress disorders.* New York, NY: Delta.

Pelletier, K. (2002). *The best alternative medicine.* New York, NY. Fireside/Simon & Schuster.

Pike, K. (1954). *Language in relation to a unified theory of the structure of human behaviour.* Glendale, CA: Summer Institute Linguistics.

Poss, J. E., Jezewski, M. A., & Stuart, A. G. (2003). Home remedies for type 2 diabetes used by Mexican Americans in El Paso, Texas. *Clinical Nursing Research, 12*(4), 304-323. doi: 10.1177/1054773803256872

Sackett, K., Carter, M., & Stanton, M. (2014). Elders' use of folk medicine and complementary and alternative therapies: An integrative review with implications for case managers. *Professional Case Management, 19*(3), 113-123. doi: 10.1097/NCM.0000000000000025

Strang, C. & Mixer, S. (2015, February 26). Discovery of the meanings, expressions, and practices related to malaria care among the Maasai. *Journal of Transcultural Nursing.* Advance online publication. doi: 10.1177/1043659615573841

Titus, S. K. (2014). Seeking and utilizing a curandero in the United States: A literature review. *Journal of Holistic Nursing, 32*(3), 189-201.

U.S. Department of Health and Human Services, National Institutes of Health, National Center for Complementary and Integrative Health. (2015a). *Complementary, alternative, or integrative health: What's in a name?* [Webpage] Retrieved from https://nccih.nih.gov/sites/nccam.nih.gov/files/CAM_Basics_Whats_In_A_Name_03-26-2015.pdf

U.S. Department of Health and Human Services, National Institutes of Health, National Center for Complementary and Integrative Health. (2015b). *The NIH almanac.* Retrieved from http://www.nih.gov/about/almanac/organization/NCCIH.htm

University of Canturbury, Education, Health, & Human Development, School of Health Sciences. (n.d.). ENZCAM: *New Zealand centre for evidence-based research into complementary and alternative medicine.* Christchurch, NZ: Author. Retrieved from http://www.education.canterbury.ac.nz/healthsciences/enzcam/

Upsdell, M., & Jaye, C. (2011). Engaging with complementary and alternative medicine in general practice. *Journal of Primary Health Care, 3*(1), 29.

Wehbe-Alamah, H. (2008). Bridging generic and professional care practices for Muslim patients through use of Leininger's culture care modes. *Contemporary Nurse: A Journal for the Australian Nursing Profession, 28*(1-2), 83-97.

Weil, A. (1989). A new look at botanical medicine. *Whole Earth Review,* (64), 54.

Weil, A. (2004). *Natural health, natural medicine: A comprehensive manual for wellness and self-care.* Boston, MA: Houghton Mifflin.

World Health Organization. (2013). *WHO traditional medicine strategy 2014-2023.* Retrieved from http://apps.who.int/iris/bitstream/10665/92455/1/9789241506090_eng.pdf?ua=1

Genetics, Genomics, and Transcultural Nursing

Margaret A. Murray-Wright

> *While our behavior is still significantly controlled by our genetic inheritance, we have, through our brains, a much richer opportunity to blaze new behavioral and cultural pathways on short timescales (Sagan, 1977).*
>
> *Humans are born and live within biophysical environments that influence their health and illness factors. Genetic, biocultural, and physical facts influence each other in different ecologies and cultural environments (Leininger, 2002b, p. 53).*

■ INTRODUCTION

Individualized healthcare is the cornerstone of transcultural nursing. Gaining an understanding about the rapidly evolving science of genetics and genomics will help nurses to provide culturally sensitive, holistic, and meaningful care. Initiated in 1989, the Human Genome Project (U. S. Department of Health and Human Services, National Institutes of Health, National Human Genome Research Institute [USDHHS], n. d.-d) unexpectedly found that while human beings have approximately 30,000 genes, any two random individuals can share 99.9% of their total DNA sequence. This means that DNA diversity among individuals only accounts for an approximate 0.1% of their genetic makeup (Porth, 2014). Although people are more alike than different, the growing inventory of human genetic variation nonetheless facilitates having a greater understanding about susceptibilities to common diseases and differing responses to treatments among individuals and populations (Wang, McLeod, & Weinshilbourm, 2011). Leininger (1978, 1991) foreshadowed this paradox when she stated that, *culture care differences and similarities between professional caregiver and client exist in any human culture worldwide.* Embracing individual cultural attributes as both *universal* and *diverse* is pivotal to guiding culture care decisions and actions. Knowledge about genetic variations helps nurses and other healthcare providers to optimize safe medication management; target cancer and immunological treatments; and counsel clients regarding their individual risk factors and personal prevention measures for any given disease (Goodman, Lynm, & Livingston, 2013). However, caution must be exercised when applying genetic information about entire populations or cultural groups using homogenous approaches. Given that our recent ancestral history is complex, group identities such as *race* or *ethnicity* are culturally inappropriate and misleading descriptors to address the full range and spectrum of patterns and variations among and between cultures and individuals (McFarland & Wehbe-Alamah, 2015; Rotimi & Jorde, 2010). According to Leininger (2002b), "...race is generally defined as a biological factor of a discrete group whose members share distinctive genetic, biological, and other factors…. the outward or phenotype appearance such as skin color is not adequate as culture and genetic factors need to be included to understand race" (p. 54). Ethnicity, however, has been defined as an adjective that pertains to "… a social group within a cultural or social system [that has] special status on the basis of complex, often variable traits, including religious, linguistic, ancestral, or physical characteristics" (Davies, 1976 as cited by Spector, 2013, p. 23).

> Within the human gene pool… remains the inheritable characteristics of all our ancestors since the beginning of the human species. Transcultural nursing has a great interest in the inheritance and caring patterns passing from one generation to another. The genetic structure of the culture remains important to study and learn… with current genetic research findings…. Understanding genetics has become more urgent as research about genetics and disease and diversity in [the] human population has increased dramatically. (Glittenberg, 2002, p. 162)

Consideration of culture, ancestry, race, and ethnicity requires a multifaceted and thoughtful approach for the interpretation and application of genetic data. Caution should be used when interpreting or applying genetic data because cultural group identities are not discrete separate entities. *Culture care* in the context of genetics and genomics needs to encompass the uniqueness of individuals while considering their broader and more distinct characteristics.

The exponential rate at which new genetic and genomic information is being generated creates a major challenge for nurses and healthcare providers. Accurate information in this field becomes obsolete within a short time frame and the clinician's knowledge of genetics and genomics needs to be both reliable and up-to-date. Nurses at all levels of practice, administration, consultation, leadership, education, and research need to take ownership of their foundational knowledge related to genomic concepts. The ongoing development of bioinformatics will help to streamline the nursing process. Reliable databases provide access to the ever-expanding informational resources about the human genome, genetic disease, and genetic testing (Jameson & Kopp, 2015). For example, several thousand disorders involving modification of a single gene [monogenic] are summarized

in a large, continually evolving collection referred to as the *Online Mendelian Inheritance in Man* (OMIM) catalogue (U. S. Department of Health and Human Services [USDHHS], n. d.-a). The American College of Medical Genetics and Genomics (n. d.) provides extensive links to other databases relevant to the diagnosis, treatment, and prevention of genetic disease. The National Human Genome Research Institute (USDHHS, n. d.-d) focuses on genomic and genetic research, provides information about the human genome sequence, genomes of other organisms, and genomic research. These and other credible databases permit nurses to access and navigate relevant or needed information (Refer to Table 9.1).

Nursing faculty within academic and healthcare systems are responsible for ensuring that the next generation of nurses understands key genomic concepts so as to provide beneficial culture-specific and congruent care. Read and Ward (2016) discovered that many nurse faculty are not adequately prepared in current fundamental genomic concepts. These gaps need to be eliminated to ensure that curricular content and teaching strategies are updated to prepare nurses who can effectively integrate genetics and genomics into practice. Nurses cannot practice as a solitary discipline in the field of genetics and genomics. Knowledge and education are strengthened through collaboration among practice levels and disciplines when genetic counselors and other key members of the healthcare team remain focused on optimal patient outcomes (Kerber & Ledbetter, 2017a; Seibert, 2014). Ultimately, nurses' comprehension and application of genetics and genomics will help to ensure that clients are educated and empowered to make optimally informed healthcare decisions. Although nurses serve as the cornerstone to care coordination and culturally congruent care, they recognize and respect that *clients as people* are the true center of health care.

■ BACKGROUND

Genetics

In 1863, a monk scientist named Gregor Mendel dabbed borrowed pollen onto other plants and forever changed our understanding about the origins of life (Nirenberg, n. d.). Mendel noted that pea plants inherited their parents' traits in predictable patterns and that some traits were more common than others.

TABLE 9.1. Genetic Resources.

Source	Site	Explanation
American College of Medical Genetics and Genomics	*http://www.acmg.net/*	Provides extensive links to other databases relevant for the diagnosis, treatment, and prevention of genetic disease
Centers for Disease Control National Office of Public Health Genomics	http://www.cdc.gov/genomics/	Public health knowledge base in genomics
Evaluation of Genomic Applications in Practice and Prevention (EGAPP)	https://www.cdc.gov/egappreviews/	Produces evidence-based recommendations for or against specific genomic tests. Nurses can use this information to educate clients about the proper interpretation of test results
Human Genome Epidemiology Network	http://www.cdc.gov/genomics/hugenet/default.htm	Network for sharing population-based human genome epidemiologic information
GeneReviews	http://www.ncbi.nlm.nih.gov/books/NBK1116/	International point-of-care resource for clinicians. Provides clinically relevant and medically actionable information for inherited conditions in a standardized journal-style format, covering diagnosis, management, and genetic counseling for clients and their families
Genetic Alliance	http://www.geneticalliance.org/publications/understandinggenetics	Understanding Genetics: A Guide for Patients and Health Professionals
Genetics and Rare Disease Information Center (GARD)	https://www.genome.gov/10000409/genetic-and-rare-diseases-information-center/	Staffed by experienced information specialists to answer questions in English and Spanish from the general public, including clients and their families, healthcare professionals and biomedical researchers.
Genetics Education Center	http://www.kumc.edu/gec/	For educators interested in human genetics and the Human Genome Project: An informational website sponsored by the University of Kansas Medical Center
G2G2 (Genetics/Genomics Competency Center)	http://g-2-c-2.org/	Provides high quality educational resources for group instruction or self-directed learning in genetics/genomics by healthcare educators and practitioners.
Genetics Home Reference	https://ghr.nlm.nih.gov/	Provides consumer-friendly information about the effects of genetic variation on human health
G3C (Global Genetics and Genomics Community)	http://g-3-c.org/en	Bilingual collection of unfolding case studies for use with students and practicing healthcare providers that helps learners to understand basic genetic/genomic concepts and their application to practice. Includes simulation

(Continued)

TABLE 9.1. Genetic Resources. (Continued)

Source	Site	Explanation
Learn. Genetics Learning Science Learning Center	http://learn.genetics.utah.edu/	Wide range of genetic information sponsored by the University of Utah
Ludwig Cancer Research Center at Johns Hopkins	http://www.ludwigcancer-research.org/location/johns-hopkins-center	Genetic and genomic clinical research with trials
MedGen	http://www.ncbi.nlm.nih.gov/medgen	Organizes information related to human medical genetics, such as attributes of conditions with a genetic contribution
National Cancer Institute	http://www.cancer.gov/about-cancer/causes-prevention/genetics/genetic-testing-fact-sheet	Information on Genetic Testing for Hereditary Cancer Syndromes
National Human Genome Research Institute (NHGRI)	*http://www.genome.gov/*	Focuses on genomic and genetic research providing information about the human genome sequence, genomes of other organisms, and genomic research
NHGRI Talking Glossary	https://www.genome.gov/glossary/	
National Human Genome Research Institute-Specific Genetic Disorders	https://www.genome.gov/10001204/specific-genetic-disorders/	List of selected genetic, orphan and rare diseases
National Newborn Screening and Global Resource Center	http://genes-r-us.uthscsa.edu/	Serves as an independent U. S. national resource center for newborn screening and provides newborn screening information globally
Online Mendelian Inheritance in Man (OMIM) catalogue	https://www.omim.org/	Monogenic disorders are summarized in a large, continuously evolving collection

Where to Locate a Genetics Professional		
ABGC Directory	http://www.abgc.net/ABGC/AmericanBoardofGeneticCounselors.asp	American Board of Genetic Counseling directory of board-certified genetic counselors
ABMGG Directory	http://abmgg.org/	American Board of Medical Genetics and Genomics directory of board-certified geneticists
ACMG Genetics Clinics Database	https://www.acmg.net/	American College of Medical Genetics and Genomics database, with map-based views
NSGC Directory	http://www.nsgc.org/	National Society of Genetic Counselors directory; counseling resource for clients and professionals
NCI Cancer Genetics Services Directory	http://www.cancer.gov/about-cancer/causes-prevention/genetics/directory	National Cancer Institute directory of professionals who provide cancer genetics services

Mendel published his theory of dominant and recessive inheritance in 1866, which countered the then extant belief that offspring were a blended and diluted version of their parents. Although the term *genetics* was not coined until the early 20th century, Mendel is commonly referred to as the *Father of Genetics* (Nirenberg, n. d.). Choosing leukocytes as his source, Swiss physician Friedrich Miescher was the first scientist to identify deoxyribonucleic acid (DNA) as a distinct molecule and has received the distinction as the *Daddy of DNA* (Dahm, 2005). Many other scientists have worked to advance the field of genetics and genomics since these early discoveries.

Genes are comprised of DNA sequences and proteins that cause the DNA to coil into a highly-compressed structure (McCance & Huether, 2014). Before a cell divides, protein and DNA (referred to as chromatin) condense to form microscopically observable threadlike structures called chromosomes (McCance & Huether, 2014). Mendel's work reinforced that chromosomes contain genes, the basic unit of inheritance. An error in one of an individual's 20,000-25,000 genes can lead to an identifiable genetic disease (McCance & Heuther, 2014). Each gene occupies a specific position along the length of a chromosome; this position is known as a *locus* (Porth, 2014). An *allele* is one of multiple forms of a gene at a specific locus that can occur within a population (American Nurses' Association [ANA], 2016, p. 59). Although the term *allele* was originally used to describe variation among genes, it now also refers to variation among noncoding DNA sequences (www.genome.gov/glossary/index.cfm?id=4).

Single nucleotide polymorphisms [variations], frequently called SNPs (pronounced "snips"), are the most common type of genetic variation among individuals. Each SNP represents a difference in a single DNA building block [or nucleotide] (USDHHS, n. d.-h). Approximately one million common SNPs occur in the human genome. While most do not influence protein structure, the common SNPs may serve as valuable biomarkers for determining the effect of genetic variation on complex and common diseases and disorders. Researchers have found SNPs that may help predict an individual's response to certain drugs, susceptibility to environmental factors such as toxins, and risk of developing diseases (USDHHS, n. d.-h). SNPs can also be used to track the inheritance of

disease-specific genes within families. Future studies will seek to identify SNPs associated with complex diseases such as heart disease, diabetes, obesity, and cancer (USDHHS, n. d.-h).

Most common SNPs are shared among populations from different continents, which reflect continued migration and gene flow among humans throughout history. Many studies have shown that 85% to 90% of genetic variations can be found within any human population (Rotimi & Jorde, 2010). For example, geographically distant samples from Great Britain and Ghana have shown genetic similarity (Rotimi & Jorde, 2010). A genetic variation may be relatively common in one population but absent in another due to a recent emergence of the variant that as yet has not had time to spread.

The composition of genes is known as a *genotype*, which refers to the genetic makeup of an organism or complete set of genes. *Phenotype* describes recognizable outward physical or chemical characteristics associated with a specific genotype (Porth, 2014). More than one genotype [set of personal genetics] may have the same phenotype [outward physical trait]. For example, some brown-eyed persons are carriers of the code for blue eyes and other brown-eyed persons are not. The outward appearance of a person is influenced by both genotype and the environment. An infant who is born with phenylketonuria (PKU) has the *PKU genotype*; if the condition is not treated, abnormal metabolites of phenylalanine will accumulate in the infant's brain causing irreversible mental retardation (McCance & Huether, 2014). The cognitive impairment is a feature of the PKU phenotype. With dietary management limiting the intake of food containing phenylalanine, however, retardation can be prevented and produce an outwardly normal phenotype.

Patterns of inheritance vary among individuals and not all persons with a mutant gene are affected by genetic disorders to the same extent. Humans are diploid organisms with each chromosome being represented twice, one each from their father and mother (Porth, 2014). At any given locus, when the genes are identical, the individual is *homozygous*. When the genes are not identical, the individual is *heterozygous* **at that locus**. If the effect of one allele masks those of another, then the effect is observable and *dominant* [brown eye genes dominate in a person with only one blue eye gene/allele, noted by an uppercase letter, e.g., BR]. The term *recessive* is used for the allele whose effects are hidden [blue eye gene/allele in a brown-eyed person, noted by a lowercase letter, e.g., bl). The recessive allele will not be expressed unless it exists in the homozygote form [two blue eye genes/alleles are expressed in a person with blue eyes]. If the individual has a disease-causing allele but is phenotypically normal, they are referred to as a carrier (McCance & Huether, 2014). A *pedigree* is a graphic method for portraying a family history of an inherited trait constructed from a carefully obtained family history and is useful for tracing the pattern of inheritance for that trait.

One of the most important principles of human genetics is that two individuals with the same mutated gene may have different phenotypes. A gene with a dominant mutation is generally expressed by the phenotype in dominance over the trait of the normal gene. That said, not all individuals will necessarily manifest an autosomal dominant condition the same way. Factors that affect the phenotype of an autosomal dominant condition include penetrance and expressivity. *Penetrance* refers to the ability of a gene to express its function (Porth, 2014). This term describes whether or not a dominant gene is expressed at all or remains hidden. A gene with recognizable phenotypic expression in all individuals has 100% penetrance [visibility]. Individuals with the same autosomal dominant trait—even within the same family—may manifest the condition differently. Genes with such variable *expressivity* can produce disease manifestations from mild to very severe. Examples include neurofibromatosis, tuberous sclerosis, and adult polycystic kidney disease (Porth, 2014). Carriers have a 50% chance of passing on an affected gene with each new/subsequent conception.

In the *autosomal dominant* disease known as *type I osteogenesis imperfecta,* the same mutated gene gives rise to a different spectrum of phenotypes with variable expressivity (Barsh, 2014). Blue sclera and short stature may be the only manifestations in one particular individual with type I osteogenesis imperfecta, whereas a sibling who carries the identical mutation may be confined to a wheelchair because of multiple fractures and deformities. The mutation is penetrant (visible) in both individuals, but its expression is variable (dissimilar). Both penetrance and variable expressivity [features] may have a reduced occurrence in individuals who carry the same mutated allele; therefore, phenotypic differences between these individuals must be due to the effects of other "modifier" genes, environmental interactions, or chance (Barsh, 2014). A gene that is expressed in some way in 40% of individuals who have that gene is 40% penetrant. Incomplete penetrance explains why some genetically autosomal dominant diseases appear to "skip" generations.

Autosomal recessive diseases develop only when both gene copies are abnormal. While heterozygous carriers are usually undetectable clinically, they may have biochemical test abnormalities. Many enzyme deficiency diseases display autosomal recessive inheritance, and enzyme activity in the carrier is approximately half of normal (Cunningham, Kramer, & Narayan, 2014). This reduction usually does not cause clinical disease, but does provide a phenotypic alteration that can be used to screen for carriers. Other recessive conditions can be identified only by molecular genetic testing. Carriers are usually recognized only after the birth of an affected child or the diagnosis of an affected family member such as what often occurs with cystic fibrosis. If a couple has a child with an autosomal recessive disease, the recurrence risk is 25% for each subsequent pregnancy. Thus, one-fourth of all offspring will be homozygously normal; two-fourths (or, one half) will be heterozygous carriers; and one-fourth will be homozygously abnormal. In other words, three of four children will be phenotypically normal (Cunningham et al., 2014). Knowledge of carrier status is critical for the client and the nurse to make more fully informed decisions about reproductive choices and prevention of anomalies such as sickle cell disease.

Clinical Exemplars

Hereditary hemochromatosis is an example of a single-nucleotide polymorphism, or SNP, common in Europe but rare elsewhere. Given its more recent emergence, this disease has not yet spread to other populations (Rotimi & Jorde, 2010). Hereditary hemochromatosis is caused by mutations in the *HFE* gene that manifests as a syndrome of iron overload, which can lead to liver disease, skin pigmentation, diabetes mellitus, arthropathy, impotence in males, and cardiac dysfunction (Rotimi & Jorde, 2010). The disorder can be effectively managed with therapeutic phlebotomy if identified early. When the diagnosis of hemochromatosis has been made in the *proband*, it is important to counsel and offer testing to other family members in order to minimize the familial impact of the disorder. The *proband* typically refers to the member of the family seeking medical attention or being studied, even if there are known ancestors who were or are affected and have manifested the disease. The myriad of complex terms and terminology in genetics can be challenging to absorb and understand. The National Human Genome Research Institute (NHGRI) created the *Talking Glossary of Genetic Terms* to help learners at any level better understand genetics terminology (2014a). This site is based on national science standards and input from National Institute of Health (NIH) scientists. In addition to definitions, specialists in the genetics field share their descriptions of terms; many definitions or descriptors include related images, animation, and/or links (USDHHS, n. d.-d).

An example of the coexisting effects of inheritance and culture is the condition known as *hereditary lactase persistence,* prevalent among both European and African pastoral populations where milk consumption beyond childhood has had a selective genetic advantage (Rotimi & Jorde, 2010). *Lactase persistence* is the continued activity of the enzyme lactase into adulthood. Given that the only function of *lactase* is for the digestion of the milk sugar *lactose*, in most mammal species, the activity of the enzyme is dramatically reduced after infant weaning. But in some human populations, lactase persistence has recently evolved as an adaptation to the consumption of nonhuman milk and other dairy products beyond infancy. Over 65% of humans worldwide remain lactase nonpersistent and consequently are affected with varying degrees of lactose intolerance as adults (Labrie, et al., 2016; Swallow, 2003). However, not all genetically lactase nonpersistent individuals are noticeably lactose intolerant, and not all lactose-intolerant individuals have the lactase nonpersistence allele. Recent research has illuminated the complexity of this condition. Because the DNA sequence is stable, more dynamic regulatory systems such as *epigenetics* (Refer to next section) are thought to be involved in producing lactase nonpersistence (Labrie, et al., 2016).

Genomics

Genomics differs from *genetics* in that genetics scrutinizes the functioning and composition of a specific gene, its role and function in disease, and its mode of inheritance. The study or field of genomics addresses all genes and their interrelationships so as to identify their combined influence on the growth and development of the organism (e.g., individual person) and its subsequent health (USDHHS, n. d.-e). Genomics refers to the entire genetic information of an organism (its *genome*), the function and interaction of DNA within the genome, as well as environmental or other nongenetic factors (such as a person's lifestyle). The human genome is divided into 23 different chromosomes: 22 autosomes (numbered 1–22) and the X and Y sex chromosomes. Genomics complements traditional genetics in scientific efforts to clarify the etiology and pathogenesis of disease and to improve therapeutic interventions and outcomes (Jameson & Kopp, 2015).

Traditional human genetics focuses on the ways in which altered DNA sequences can lead to disease. The conventional genetic lens has been viewed through the window of comparatively rare single-gene diseases [monogenic]. Although these disorders account for only 10% of pediatric admissions and childhood mortality (Jameson & Kopp, 2015), it has become apparent that almost every medical condition has a genetic component. Risk assessment and interpretation are therefore integral components of the nurses' role within genetics and genomics practice (ANA, 2016; Seibert, 2014). As is often evident from a patient's family history, many common disorders such as hypertension, heart disease, asthma, diabetes mellitus, and mental illnesses are significantly influenced by a person's genetic background. These *polygenic* (or multifactorial) disorders are complex and involve contributions from many different genes as well as from environmental factors that have the potential to modify disease risk or cause illness.

The Human Genome Project at the National Institutes of Health (NIH; USDHHS, n. d.-d) was initiated when collaborating researchers in laboratories around the globe began to engage in parallel efforts to characterize the entire human genome (USDHHS, n. d.-d). While this effort was initially daunting, technical advances in DNA sequencing and bioinformatics led to a draft of the human sequence in 2000 followed by completion of the human chromosome

DNA sequence in May 2006 (Jameson & Kopp, 2015). Thus far, the locations of more than 25,000 genes have been mapped to a specific chromosome and/or to a specific region on a chromosome (Porth, 2014). *Haplotype maps* (The International HapMap Project) focus on identifying the slight variations in the human genome that affect an individuals' susceptibility to disease and their responses to environmental factors such as microbes, toxins, and drugs (USDHHS, n. d.-c). Genetic mapping continues at a rapid rate and these numbers and associated genetic/genomic discoveries are continually updated. Genome-wide association studies (GWAS) have demonstrated various disease-associated loci and are providing unique insights into the allele architecture of complex traits. The sequencing of whole genomes and genomic substructures is increasingly used in the clinical realm in order to characterize individuals with complex undiagnosed conditions or to characterize the mutational profile of advanced malignancies to better select targeted therapies (McCance & Huether, 2014). A valuable resource for information regarding specific chromosome sequencing in humans is the National Center for Biotechnology Information (NCBI; USDHHS, n. d.-b).

Genetics, Epigenetics, and Genomics

Gosden and Feinberg (2007) described genetics and epigenetics as nature's pen and pencil set. The genetic code is like an indelible ink that is predictably transcribed from cell to cell and from generation to generation with few exceptions. Superimposed on this code, however, lies another layer described as *epigenetics*, which are methyl groups [stable carbon and hydrogen atomic groups or alkyl hydrocarbons] that become added to DNA (Gosden & Feinberg, 2007). These epigenetic changes are inheritable changes in gene expression yet do not involve changes in DNA sequences. This transformation contributes to inheritance of a disease such as alcoholism or obesity without changes to our DNA. *Epigenetics* ("upon genetics") is the study of how genes are influenced by outside forces other than changes in DNA sequences, such as those from the environment, maternal obesity, exercise, food, or medications (Martos, Tang, & Wang, 2015). Epigenetic mechanisms regulate gene expression not by altering the genetic alphabet, but rather by the addition of chemical modifications to proteins associated with the genetic alphabet or

by methyl markers to the alphabet itself. Epigenetic mechanisms of gene regulation are dynamic and serve as an important bridge between environmental stimuli and an individual's genotype (Dias, Maddox, Klengel, & Ressler, 2015). Hence, epigenetic modifications can cause individuals with the same DNA sequences (such as identical twins) to have different disease profiles or other characteristics.

The effects of epigenetics extend to maternal diet during pregnancy. Epigenetic changes play an important role in regulating gene expression, especially during early (fetal and childhood) development (Ma, Tutino, Lillycrop, Hanson, & Tam, 2015). These researchers have identified a number of epigenetic modifications in children that have been associated with gestational exposure to maternal hyperglycemia. Epidemiological studies have identified increased risks for obesity, diabetes (Feil & Fraga, 2011), and cardiovascular disease in offspring exposed to maternal diabetes that then also increases the risk of diabetes in subsequent generations. These consequences create a vicious cycle of propagating the development of diabetes into the future. Animal models of gestational exposure to diabetes or maternal hyperglycemia have highlighted long-term changes in offspring including increased adiposity, insulin resistance, beta cell dysfunction, and hypertension as well as other structural and functional changes (Ma et al., 2015). Several of these changes appear to be transmissible to later generations through the maternal line. Traditionally, prenatal advice has mainly focused on the health of *mothers*. Several epidemiological associations between a *father's* health prior to conceiving and the health of his children have emerged. Epigenetic information can be embedded in sperm in the form of chemical tags that regulate genes or alter microRNA (Abbasi, 2017). Researchers in the Newborn Epigenetics Study (NEST) provided the first molecular evidence that a man's lifestyle may be imprinted onto his child's epigenome (Soubry et al., 2013). This study has provided evidence for the transgenerational effects of paternal obesity that may influence the offspring's future health status. A recent animal model study has also provided evidence that paternal periconceptional body weight may affect daughters' mammary development and breast cancer risk, but warrants further study in other animal models and humans (Fontelles et al., 2016). Fortunately, there are preliminary indications that some paternal lifestyle-associated effects from sperm upon offspring can be reversed through paternal exercise, dietary changes, and weight loss even in the few months leading up to conception (McPherson, Bakos, Owens, Setchell, & Lane, 2013).

The effects of epigenetics are far reaching. Adverse experiences such as stress represent some of the most powerful influences on health and wellbeing. Past research has suggested that stress leaves an epigenetic footprint on cells that alters gene expression (Franklin, Saab, & Mansuy, 2012). The genetic (DNA) programming effects of preconception stress from adversities experienced by parents, grandparents, or earlier generations may exert key influences on the health trajectory across the lifespan of a descendent individual. More recently, it has been found that changes in the regulation of microRNAs (miRNAs) from stress may magnify that person's later vulnerability to certain pathogenic factors (Metz, Ng, Kovalchuk, & Olson, 2015). These researchers suggested that miRNAs are key players linking adverse early environments or ancestral stress with disease risk; thus, these events represent useful predictive disease biomarkers. The hereditary transmission of epigenetic changes to successive generations has been termed *epigenetic transgenerational inheritance* (Martos et al., 2015). Research in this area with humans is ongoing and may shed light on some significant health concerns such as patterns of drug abuse. Genome-wide association studies (GWAS) have identified a number of genes, chromosomal regions, and allelic variants likely to contribute to drug addiction; however, not all inherited information is present in the DNA sequences (Yohn, Bartolomei, & Blendy, 2015). Chemical alterations in the genome have been identified following drug exposures that were not related to DNA sequence variations. These epigenetic modifications may contribute to persons being at risk for drug abuse and dependence across familial generations. Epigenetic modifications could also provide insight into a mechanism underlying the longevity of psychiatric conditions within and across generations (Nielsen, Utrankar, Reyes, Simons, & Kosten, 2010).

Epigenetics can also play a *positive* role in health and wellness. Researchers consider folic acid fortification to be one of the most effective public health interventions in the last several decades (Jacob, 2016). In early 1996, officials from the U. S. Food and Drug

Administration (FDA) crafted the final folic acid fortification federal regulations (U. S. Government Publishing Office, 1996). By January 1, 1998, food manufacturers were required to add 140 micrograms of folic acid to every 100 grams of cereal grain. Cereal grains were chosen because they were already being fortified with other vitamins and minerals, and bread and other foods made from cereal grains are common food staples. The effect from adding folic acid to enriched cereal grain products was remarkable. From October 1998 to December 1999, reported cases of spina bifida decreased 31% and reported cases of anencephaly decreased by 16% (Williams et al., 2015). Fortification now prevents an estimated 1,300 neural tube defects each year in the United States (Williams et al., 2015). While the mechanism of folic acid risk reduction for neural tube defects is not completely understood, researchers believe that it may provide carbon atoms needed for DNA synthesis and play a critical role in DNA methylation. The role of folic acid has significant cultural implications. Research experts from both the Centers for Disease Control and Prevention and the March of Dimes coalition (2012) noted that adequate folic acid intake is particularly important for Hispanic women because they have a 21% greater risk of giving birth to a child with a neural tube defect than non-Hispanic white women (USDHHS, 2010). Hispanic women may be more likely to have a variant of the methylenetetrahydrofolate reductase (*MTHFR*) gene that results in reduced intracellular folate metabolism. In addition, Hispanic women are less likely to consume recommended daily folic acid amounts: Only 17% of Hispanic women reported a daily intake of 400 micrograms or more of folic acid through fortified foods or supplements compared with 30% of non-Hispanic white women (Williams et al., 2015), underscoring the large role diet plays in genetics and genomics as in many other aspects of health and wellness. Hispanic adults tend to eat tortillas and other foods made with unfortified corn masa flour rather than enriched cereal grain products, which is why a coalition led by the March of Dimes and the Spina Bifida Association lobbied the federal government in 2012 to require corn masa flour fortification (March of Dimes, 2012). Their petition was approved on April 14, 2016 by the U. S. Food and Drug Administration, allowing manufacturers to voluntarily add up to 0.7 milligrams of folic acid per pound of corn masa flour, consistent with the levels in certain other enriched cereal grains.

The patient and healthcare provider are crucial partners in this paradigm shift from a genetic to an epigenetic model in health care as they engage in prevention strategies that may precede and potentially reverse genetic mutations (McCance & Huether, 2014). While the main purpose of human genome sequencing was to understand DNA more fully, epigenetics are key aspects for inclusion in patient counseling so that tangible advice can be provided to the person regarding screening and health promotion (McCance & Huether, 2014). The patient can affect the long-term trajectory of their own health by modifying the genetic "hand" they have been dealt through lifestyle modifications and other self-care decisions and actions. For example, epigenetic abnormalities coupled with genetic alterations are the driving forces for the occurrence of cancer (Porth, 2014). Epigenetic processes influence cancer initiation, progression, and treatment. Cancer has a genetic basis because it results from acquired mutations in genes that control growth, apoptosis [planned or normal cell death], and cellular differentiation. In addition, the development of many cancers is associated with a hereditary predisposition. Consider the following two potential epigenetics clinical applications for a person who has several first-order relatives with colon cancer; knowledge of epigenetic forces could influence the client outcomes:

- Use of aspirin and other nonsteroidal anti-inflammatory drugs (NSAIDs) is associated with a lower risk of colorectal cancer. In a genome-wide investigation of genetic versus environmental interactions, use of aspirin and/or NSAIDs was associated with lower risk of colorectal cancer, and this association differed according to genetic variations at two SNPs on chromosomes 12 and 15. Validation of these findings in additional populations may facilitate targeted colorectal cancer prevention strategies. Studies of this type reinforce that certain medications are not one-size-fits-all (Nan et al., 2015). An additional study provided strong evidence that lifestyle modifications are important for the prevention of colorectal polyps especially for advanced cases as well as for multiple adenomas, which have been established as precursors for the development of colorectal cancer (Fu et al., 2012).

The risk of colon polyps increased progressively with increased numbers of adverse lifestyle factors. Six lifestyle factors (cigarette smoking; obesity; lack of regular use of nonsteroidal anti-inflammatory drugs; high intake of red meat; low intake of fiber; and low intake of calcium) were found to be independently associated with the risk of polyps.

- Scientific evidence is rapidly accumulating in support of the primary prevention of cancer through regular physical activity at a moderate or greater intensity level. The evidence for causal-linked physical activity and cancer risk has been found to be strongest for colon cancer prevention (Kruk & Czerniak, 2013). The average risk reductions were reported to be from 20% to 30%. The protective effects of physical activity on cancer risk are thought to occur through multiple interrelated pathways: Decrease in adiposity; decrease in sexual and metabolic hormones; changes in biomarkers and insulin resistance; improvement of immune function; and reduction of inflammation.

A third example involving lifestyle factors illustrates the clinical applicability of *nutrigenomics,* which is the study of nutrition on the phenotypic variability of individuals based on genetic and genomic differences (McCance & Huether, 2014). Research in this field continues to expand as investigators focus on the sequences and functions of genes, single nucleotide polymorphisms (SNPs), and changes within DNA sequences as modifiers of individual metabolic responses to ingested foods and beverages and their components (McCance & Huether, 2014). Food and beverage selection, preparation, and consumption (including alcohol) are uniquely interwoven into the social structure of cultures and may affect individuals epigenetically. Epigenetic modifications can cause individuals who have the same DNA sequences (such as identical twins) to develop different disease profiles (McCance & Huether, 2014). Patient genetic counseling needs to be an integral facet of care so as to reinforce the modifiable and nonmodifiable risk factors that influence health outcomes.

Personalized care and individualized decision-making for each patient rely heavily on genetic information. Significant interindividual variability has been observed in clinical drug response and has led to drug treatment failure or preventable severe adverse drug reactions (Chang, McCarthy, & Shin, 2015). The study of *pharmacogenomics* emerged in the 1950s, stemming from clinical observations that a few rare individuals had unexpected, severe reactions to drugs (O'Donnell, Danahey, & Ratain, 2016). Pharmacogenetics were initially used only to customize treatment for these outlier patients, but currently the pharmacogenetic knowledge base has become more extensive with increased clinical relevance (O'Donnell et al., 2016). *Pharmacogenetics* utilizes a person's genotype to optimize drug therapy selection and dosing by predicting the efficacy, ideal treatment duration, and adverse events for each chosen medication. Pharmacogenetics is the study of how genetic variation can influence a patient's response to specific drugs and/or drug classes (Chang et al., 2015) and uses genomics information to optimize an individual's healthcare and therapy (Sadee, 2017). This evolving field is positioned to play a significant role in the advancement of personalized medicine due to its ability to inform medication choices based on a patient's individual genetic profile (McKillip et al., 2016). These authors also found that privacy, empathy, medical-decision making, and personalized care scores were significantly higher after visits when physicians discussed pharmacogenomic results with their patients (McKillip et al., 2017).

While a large prospective randomized trial examining the effects of pharmacogenomic results on therapeutic parameters for warfarin could not fully support genotype-guided dosing of the anticoagulant (Kimmel et al., 2013), other studies have shown improved patient outcomes and cost-effectiveness. Drugs that could replace warfarin, like dabigatran, have demonstrated compelling pharmacogenomic markers that may be able to recognize a specific genetic subset of patients who have significantly lower bleeding risk— without loss of efficacy—if treated with dabigatran rather than warfarin (O'Donnell et al., 2016; Pare et al., 2013). Subsequent to postoperative deaths in children who were prescribed codeine, several pediatric hospitals removed the drug from their formularies (Gammal et al., 2016). These deaths were attributed to atypical cytochrome P450 2D6 (*CYP2D6*) pharmacogenetics, which is also implicated in poor analgesic response (Gammal et al., 2016). Clinical decision support was integrated into the electronic health record (EHR) to guide the prescribing of codeine with the

goal of preventing its use after tonsillectomy or adenoidectomy in pediatric patients and in *CYP2D6* ultra-rapid and poor metabolizer (high-risk) genotypes through interruptive alerts that warned clinicians against prescribing codeine for these patients. During this evidence-based medication safety study, not one of the patients with an ultra-rapid or poor metabolizer genotype were prescribed codeine. Using genetics to individualize analgesic prescribing also retained an important therapeutic option by limiting codeine use only to patients who could safely receive and benefit from it (Gammal et al., 2016, p. 10).

The emerging field of pharmacogenomics is positioned to play a significant role in the advancement of personalized medicine due to its capacity to better-inform providers when recommending medication options based on a patient's individual genetic profile (McKillip et al., 2016). This knowledge facilitates the identification of biomarkers that can help the advanced practice nurse and other healthcare providers safely prescribe and administer medications. Although current EHR systems do provide clinicians with useful triggers and prompts regarding drug-drug and drug-food interactions, drug-genome information is not always readily available. Clinical decision support and pharmacy consultation services will be a useful tool for use in the future.

While bioinformaticists strive to meet the need for readily available drug-genome information, the Pharmacogenomics Knowledgebase (PharmGKB) is a resource that catalogs and disseminates comprehensive information about the effects of human genetic variations on drug responses (USDHHS, n. d.-g). This site provides clinically relevant information, including dosing guidelines, annotated drug labels, and potentially actionable gene-drug associations and genotype-phenotype relationships (Whirl-Carrillo et al., 2012). The database curators assign levels of evidence to variant gene-drug associations using well-defined criteria based on careful literature review (USDHHS, n. d.-g). These dosing guidelines take into consideration patient genotype and have been published by the Clinical Pharmacogenetics Implementation Consortium (CPIC; USDHHS, n. d.-i) to support *personalized medicine* practices and implementation projects. The PharmGKB website also has links to the U. S. Food and Drug Administration (FDA) recommendations for modified drug labels, actionable prescribing information, and warnings about pharmacogenomic variations related to drug responses. Drug labels may contain information on genomic biomarkers; drug exposure and clinical response variability; risk for adverse events; genotype-specific dosing; and mechanisms of drug action. This FDA database contains a list of approximately 200 medications with accompanying guidelines and evidence-based practice applications and is regularly updated.

The Microbiome and Metagenomics

A novel and evolving aspect that merits assessment by the nurse is the advent and development of *metagenomics*. Metagenomics is defined as the direct genetic analysis of genomes contained within an environmental sample (Thomas, Gilbert, & Meyer, 2012). The study and field of genetics has provided opportunities to explain the *human microbiome,* which comprises diverse microbiologic ecosystems and is composed of the variety of bacteria, viruses, and parasites that coexist on and within humans and other animals (Gordon & Knight, 2015; Hollister, Gao, & Versalovic, 2014). Each human being encounters a unique environment during the course of his or her lifetime. This personally experienced environment becomes integrated into their genes and resultant functional capabilities of our microbial communities (Gordon & Knight, 2015). Breastfeeding, birth mode (vaginal delivery or C-section), vitamin D levels in cord blood, and race/ethnicity have all been associated with alterations in the infant gut microbiome (Sordillo et al., 2017). As the most densely populated and diverse of the microbial communities, the intestinal microbiome has a fundamental role in maintaining physiological homeostasis; resident microbes in the human gut discourage invasion by pathogens, process viral nutrients, and harvest energy otherwise inaccessible from within human cells (Hollister et al., 2014). Having a greater richness and diversity of bacterial species in the human intestine may be an indicator of better health. Reduced bacterial gastrointestinal diversity has been associated with an increased risk of necrotizing enterocolitis in preterm infants as well as the development of allergic diseases later in life (Hollister et al., 2014). The infant gut microbiome may set the stage for the composition of gut flora by three years of age as well as onward into adulthood, with potential health implications for both early and later life. Sordillo et al. (2016) noted that a reduction in potentially protective bacteria (such as

Bacteroides species) in the microbiome of minority children could partially explain the increased incidence of asthma among these population groups. These relationships are complex given that gut microbiota [bacteria] may vary by race because of differences in dietary patterns, personal care product use, or host genetics (Sordillo et al., 2016). Nurse researchers at Emory University in Atlanta, GA, have embarked on a five-year longitudinal study, *Biobehavioral Determinants of the Microbiome and Preterm Birth in Black Women*, as an intra-race study to enable the investigation of risk and protective factors within this group (Corwin et al., 2017). Their goal is to improve adverse birth and neonatal outcomes that disproportionately affect African American women and infants compared to birth outcomes in other races/ethnicities.

■ ANCESTRY, RACE, DISEASE, AND GENOMICS

Disease Occurrence

Renal disease

Reliance on ancestry and population categories must be balanced with an understanding of specific genetic variants with individuals. The use of general ancestry as a referent illustrates how genomic science may inform our understanding of kidney disease and prostate cancer. Americans of African ancestry have a significantly greater risk of chronic kidney disease and kidney failure than do European Americans (Freedman, 2003). After adjusting for socioeconomic factors and diseases such as hypertension and diabetes, substantial risk remains, suggesting a genetic influence. A two to four times increased risk for focal segmental glomerulosclerosis and end-stage renal disease has been noted in the African American population (Rao & Balakrishnan, 2009). These authors proposed that a genetic variation in *MYH9* accounted for a large proportion of the increased risk for kidney disease that was observed among African Americans compared with European Americans.

Prostate cancer

Prostate cancer is a second example of a disease that varies significantly among diverse populations. While disparities in treatment and access to adequate health care may contribute to the high prevalence of prostate cancer among African American males, evidence has shown genetic variation as a significant contributor (Haiman et al., 2007; Tan, Mok, & Rebbeck, 2016). Several independent studies have identified and replicated a locus on *chromosome 8q24* that was shown to be associated with prostate cancer in men from diverse ancestral backgrounds (Haiman et al., 2007). The population-attributable risk, defined as the proportion of cases that would not occur if the risk factor were eliminated, varied significantly according to ancestry. Attributable risks ranged from 32% among European Americans to 46% among Hispanic Americans and 68% among African Americans (Haiman et al., 2007).

Cardiac dysfunction

Cardiac dysfunction is a significant and independent risk factor for the eventual development of clinical heart failure (Kane et al., 2011). Early recognition and treatment of stage B heart failure (HF), defined by the American College of Cardiology Foundation/American Heart Association (Hunt et al., 2009) as cardiac dysfunction without signs or symptoms of HF, is a potentially powerful strategy to prevent disease progression to later stages that are clinically symptomatic (Hunt et al., 2009). Unfortunately, current population-based estimates of cardiac dysfunction are based on studies that did not include Hispanics/Latinos (Rodriguez et al., 2014). In a recent large scale echocardiographic study of Hispanics, researchers noted that the prevalence of cardiac dysfunction was high among the Hispanic/Latino populations (Mehta et al., 2016). Among this population, which included persons from Mexico and Central America, most cardiac dysfunction was either subclinical or unrecognized (Mehta et al., 2016). The researchers found a high prevalence of HF risk factors among the study participants, half of whom had obesity or hypertension and another two-thirds who had either diabetes or prediabetes. Cardiac dysfunction was identified in almost half of the study cohort and was predominantly a diastolic dysfunction [heart failure with preserved ejection fraction] with 95% being unrecognized or subclinical. The study by Mehta et al. (2016) substantiated the need for aggressive risk factor modification in this at-risk population to prevent further cardiac remodeling and subsequent progression to clinical heart failure, as recommended in the American Heart Association guidelines. This study identified a specific ethnic population at-risk for the development of clinical heart failure that has further implications for nursing practice.

Medication sensitivity

Identifying individuals who are at an increased risk for adverse drug reactions prior to initiation of treatment is an important element of prescribing medications. Among minority populations, Asian clients have demonstrated significant hypersensitivity to seizure medications with the potential for developing severe mucocutaneous diseases such as toxic epidermal necrolysis or Steven-Johnson Syndrome (TEN/SJS; Chung et al., 2014). Both disorders are rare but carry a mortality rate of 10% to 50%, a fact that should be considered *whenever* carbamazepine or phenytoin are prescribed, especially for Asians. Carbamazepine is routinely prescribed for the treatment of seizure disorders as well as neuropathic pain and bipolar mental illness (Grover & Kukreti, 2014). The *HLA-B* 1502* and *HLA-A*3101* alleles are the most commonly reported genetic polymorphisms identified as predictors for cutaneous adverse drug reactions to carbamazepine (Grover & Kukreti, 2014; McCormack et al., 2011). Strong associations between the *HLA B* 1502* allele and carbamazepine-induced SJS and TEN was demonstrated among the Han Chinese (Lim, Kwan, & Tan, 2008). However, these studies from Europe revealed the *HLA B* 1502* allele not as a universal marker for SJS/TEN, but as ethnicity-specific for some Asians. Reports across Asia have shown a higher prevalence of *HLA B* 1502* allele among Han Chinese (5% -15%); Malaysians (12% -15%); and Thais (8% - 27%), but lower among Japanese, Koreans, Sri Lankans, and most ethnic groups in India (Lim et al., 2008). In contrast, the *HLA-A*3101* allele was prevalent among 2% to 5% of Northern European populations and showed a strong association to the SJS/TEN hypersensitivity syndromes, with an increased risk from 5% to 26% (McCormack et al., 2011). These findings underscore the importance of following FDA recommendations for genetic testing for carbamazepine among these populations.

Phenytoin (Dilantin) is also a commonly prescribed antiepileptic drug and remains the most frequently used first-line anti-seizure drug in hospitalized patients (Chung, et al., 2014). While the strength of association is much weaker than that found for carbamazepine-related TEN/SJS, the FDA has suggested that providers should avoid prescribing phenytoin as an alternative to carbamazepine for patients who carry the *HLA-B*1502* allele (Chung, et al., 2014). Allopurinol dosages should also be carefully considered during the care of Asian groups as a significant dose-related TEN/SJS association with allopurinol was found to exist among Japanese clients (Tohkin et al., 2013). The biomarker *rs9263726* is easily identified making it useful for monitoring allopurinol-related TEN/SJS among Japanese clients (Tohkin et al., 2013). The 2012 American College of Rheumatology Guidelines for the Management of Gout recommended testing for the *HLA-B*58:01* allele in selected subpopulations who are at increased risk for allopurinol hypersensitivity syndrome, such as individuals of Korean descent with stage 3 or worse chronic kidney disease and those of Han-Chinese or Thai descent, prior to initiation of the drug (Khanna et al., 2012). Asian Americans are the fastest growing racial/ethnic group in the United States, yet problems exist with the collection and interpretation of Asian American health data (Holland & Palaniappan, 2012). Much of our knowledge about Asian American health has been from studies in which researchers have either statistically grouped all Asian Americans together or studied only one subgroup (e.g., Indian, Chinese, Filipino, Japanese, Korean, or Vietnamese). Clinicians and healthcare teams need to remain cognizant about the significant heterogeneity among Asian American subgroups when collecting and interpreting health data (Holland & Palaniappan, 2012).

Prostate cancer, kidney disease, drug hypersensitivity, and heart failure all provide compelling reasons to utilize information about individual and group ancestry during the nursing assessment process. However, identification by continental ancestry [African, Asian, European]; race [brown, white, black, yellow]; and ethnic group [Hispanic, Jewish, Eskimo] are usually inadequate and limited descriptors in the nurse's assessment. Direct genetic testing may offer a more accurate alternative than using such broad—and often erroneously stereotypical—categories.

About 4% to 8% of clients with human immunodeficiency virus (HIV) infection who are treated with abacavir have serious, potentially life-threatening abacavir hypersensitivity syndrome (AHS; Hetherington et al., 2002). While genetic testing was initially recommended only for high-risk populations in an effort to save costs, further research has since illustrated why this approach can be problematic. A double-blind, prospective, randomized study involving 1,956 clients from 19 countries demonstrated that screening for the *HLA-B*5701* allele substantially reduced the incidence of AHS (Hetherington et al., 2002). Considerable interpopulation variation in the frequency of this allele was evidenced, ranging from zero to approximately 20%. The highest prevalence of *HLA-B*5701* (17.6%) was seen not among Americans of European ancestry but among Gujarati Indians in Houston, Texas (Hetherington et al., 2002). Sampling from a cohort of persons from India revealed a similarly estimated result (Nolan, Gaudieri, & Mallal, 2003). In addition, substantial differences in allele prevalence were also shown in two distinct African populations. The prevalence in the Kenyan Maasai group was 13.6%, while the frequency of the allele was zero among the Yoruba in Nigeria (Nolan et al., 2003).

Caution should be used when using labels to identify individuals or groups, as this practice may easily obscure biomedically relevant variations and could lead to diminished vigilance among healthcare practitioners for AHS in susceptible clients (Rotimi & Jorde, 2010). Because of the risk for interpopulation variability, the U. S. Food and Drug Administration made the prudent recommendation to screen all groups for *HLA-B*5701* before abacavir administration, regardless of ancestral, ethnic, or cultural identity (USDHHS, 2008). Cultural or ethnic stereotypes may hinder the nursing assessment for other conditions as well. Consider the elevated prevalence of Tay-Sachs disease among persons with Ashkenazi Jewish ancestry. Tay-Sachs, a devastating neuromuscular disease affecting infants is also observed in non-Jewish populations, such as its relatively high prevalence in parts of French-speaking Canada (Jewish Genetic Disease Consortium, n. d.).

Human genetic variations contribute significantly to the physical diversities that occur among individuals. The nurse should balance ancestry information with the identification of individual traits when conducting a nursing assessment. For example, persons who self-report as African Americans can have significantly different levels of African or European ancestry (Mersha & Abebe, 2015). Genetic analysis of individual ancestry demonstrates that some self-identified African Americans have up to 99% of

European ancestry, while some self-identified European Americans have substantial admixture from African ancestry (Mersha & Abebe, 2015). Interestingly, African ancestry variability in the Latino population varies between 3% in Mexican Americans to 16% in Puerto Ricans, which stands as an indicator that self-reported and ancestry may not be as accurate as a direct assessment of individual genomic information in predicting treatment outcomes (Mersha & Abebe, 2015). However, when the *HLA-B* 1502* genotype was quantified in approximately 50,000 Asian patients to establish who should not receive carbamazepine for seizure control, the frequency of life threatening Stevens-Johns Syndrome and toxic epidermal necrolysis decreased to 0% (Chen et al., 2011). Predictors of disease risk, expression, and responses to treatment, such as specific genotypes, biomarkers, or phenotypes will become more precise and better developed, and consequently surpass the current use of conventional racial/ethnic/geographic ancestry descriptors (Rotimi & Jorde, 2010). The nurse is in an ideal position to be the steward of this information and an advocate for the patient. The careful balance of culture, race, and ancestry information is key to sound genetic and genomic nursing.

■ PERSONALIZED GENETICS AND GENOMICS: HOW DNA SHAPES CARE

Precision or personalized medicine, the individualization of health care based on unique patient-specific characteristics, is not new (Diouf et al., 2015) and has traditionally included consideration of family history and environmental influences. As the science of genetics and genomics has progressed, this new information is becoming more integrated into mainstream clinical practice influencing risk assessment, diagnosis, prognosis, and treatment decisions and actions. Since 2007, there has been increasing interest in the use of genomic data to more precisely diagnose cancer, predict outcomes, and prescribe "targeted" therapies (Schnepp, Bosse, & Maris, 2015). These authors proposed that considerable progress has been made but many challenges remain before it is scientifically confirmed that personalized genomic medicine can substantively improve outcomes for clients with cancer. Recent reports reflect the following progress:

- **Tamoxifen *CYP2D6*; genotype-guided therapy.** Tamoxifen is a selective estrogen-receptor modulator (SERM) that is commonly utilized in the treatment and prevention of estrogen receptor-positive breast cancer. Ultimate conversion of the parent drug by the enzyme *CYP2D6* into the active metabolite, endoxifen, is required for tamoxifen to exert its anticancer effects. *CYP2D6* exists in varying concentrations across individuals due, in part, to genetic variation. *CYP2D6 genotype* can be used to classify clients into metabolizer phenotypes that include *ultra-rapid metabolizers* (UM); *extensive metabolizers* (EM); *intermediate metabolizers* (IM); or *poor metabolizers* (PM; Walko & McLeod, 2012). Endoxifen concentrations vary with respect to *CYP2D6 genotype* within homozygous PM client groups. Variability in response can affect ultimate disease outcomes and is of special concern among premenopausal women for whom drug therapy options are more limited or involve higher morbidity. Therefore, efforts to minimize this variability are needed to optimize disease outcomes (Walko & McLeod, 2012). In the future, investigations of this type will be conducted to direct the clinical benefit of genotype-guided therapy and identify the optimal dose needed for specific clients.

- With cure rates of childhood lymphoblastic leukemia (ALL) exceeding 85%, a need was identified to reduce treatment toxicities that could compromise life, such as peripheral neuropathy from vincristine treatment. Diouf et al. (2015) identified germline [gamete cell] variants associated with the occurrence or severity of vincristine-induced peripheral neuropathy among children with ALL. During the researchers' preliminary study, an inherited polymorphism in the promoter region of *CEP72* was associated with increased risk for and severity of vincristine-induced peripheral neuropathy (Diouf et al., 2015, p. 822). Other researchers subsequently identified the *CEP72 polymorphism* as a strategy to recognize adults at increased risk for vincristine-induced peripheral neuropathy (Stock et al, 2017). These findings may provide the foundation for safer treatment dosing in the future as well as improved patient comfort and quality of life.

TABLE 9.2. Genetic Implications for Specific Groups, Cultures, Ethnicities, or Ancestries.

Disease or Condition	Affected Population	Clinical Considerations
Alpha α_1 antitrypsin deficiency(AAT) Autosomal recessive disorder resulting in early onset emphysema and liver disease	Northern European, Scandinavian, and Iberian ancestry Rare in Jewish, black, and Japanese populations AAT deficiency affects 1% -2% of clients with chronic obstructive pulmonary disease	**Consider diagnosis for:** • Adults with emphysema with onset at ≤ 40 years old and without risk factors (no history of smoking or occupational dust exposure) **Diagnosis made by:** • Serum Alpha α_1 antitrypsin levels and confirmed with genetic testing
Breast Cancer **BRCA1 1 and BRCA1 2** Autosomal dominant; accounting for approximately 5% of cases in U.S.	Ashkenazi Jewish women	**Counseling** U. S. Preventive Services Task Force recommends genetic counseling and evaluation for BRCA testing for: • Ashkenazi Jewish women with any first-degree relative with breast or ovarian cancer or second-degree or relatives on same side of family with breast or ovarian cancer
G6PD Deficiency (Glucose-6-phosphate dehydrogenase deficiency) X-linked genetic defect with clinical manifestations of neonatal jaundice and/or acute or chronic hemolytic anemia triggered by medications, infections, and fava beans	Highest frequency found in: Africa, southern Europe (Mediterranean region), Middle East, southeast Asia, central and southern Pacific islands: • Deficiency is found in 10% of Blacks; can occur in Sephardic Jews, Greeks, Iranians, Chinese, Filipinos, and Indonesians with a frequency ranging from 5% to 40% • Kurdish Jews 50% of males reported to be affected. • Most common human enzyme defect worldwide	**Relevant history** Ask about family history of G6PD deficiency and hemolytic factors that can be transmitted to infants via mother's milk, such as after ingestion of fava beans; certain drugs; or herbal remedies (hemolytic anemia occurs about 24 hours after ingestion of fava beans) **Medication history** Ask about recent history of medications that may have precipitated hemolytic anemia such as antimalarials, nitrofurantoin (urinary tract infections); phenazopyridine (for dysuria); and topical application of henna
Leiden V The most common hereditary abnormality of hemostasis predisposing to thrombosis Autosomal dominant inheritance single mutation causes mild hypercoagulable state	Highest in Caucasian Americans and European populations Prevalence may be higher in some Middle Eastern countries including Jordanians (12.3%) and Lebanese (14.4%)	**Relevant Assessment** May have no clinical symptoms. Mutation is present in about 15% to 20% clients with first deep vein thrombosis and up to 50% of clients with recurrent venous thromboembolism **Medication history** Risk for thromboembolism increased with oral contraceptives, hormonal replacement therapy (HRT); and selective estrogen receptor modulators (SERMs)

TABLE 9.2. Genetic Implications for Specific Groups, Cultures, Ethnicities, or Ancestries. (Continued)

Disease or Condition	Affected Population	Clinical Considerations
Sickle Cell Disease Autosomal recessive genetic disorder; patients with same genotype may have highly variable phenotypes, ranging from asymptomatic to life-threatening complications; interaction of environmental factors with genetic polymorphisms may explain disease variation Chronic inflammation, ischemia, and vaso-occlusion contribute to chronic organ damage	African, Mediterranean, Middle Eastern, Indian ancestry, Caribbean and parts of Central and South America: • most prevalent disease detected by neonatal blood screening • alpha-thalassemia and beta-thalassemia may be coinherited	**Relevant Assessment** Affected infants not identified through neonatal screening usually present clinically during infancy/early childhood with: • painful swelling of hands and feet (dactylitis) • pneumococcal sepsis or meningitis • severe anemia and acute splenic enlargement (splenic sequestration) • acute chest syndrome • jaundice • pallor **Counseling** Many adolescents and young adults are unaware of their sickle cell trait status-higher risk for rhabdomyolysis during rigorous sports: • prenatal diagnosis may be made in first and second trimester • preimplantation genetic diagnosis is available during in vitro fertilization. (Embryos not affected with sickle cell disease may be selected)
Tay-Sachs Disease Neurodegenerative disorder caused by inborn error of metabolism; genetic mutation results in central nervous system degeneration and loss of organ function	Ashkenazi Jews • incidence of 1 out of every 3,600 births among Ashkenazi Jews • carrier rate of 1 out of every 30 persons among Jewish Americans of Ashkenazi descent • additional risk factors include: French Canadians living in Eastern Quebec or New England; selected Cajun communities in Louisiana; and Pennsylvania Dutch (semi-isolated)	**Relevant Assessment** Classic or acute infantile is the most common type: • infants appear normal at birth • rapidly progressive neuro-degenerative disorder characterized by progressive motor weakness beginning at 3-6 months old; loss of developmental milestones and death within first few years of life

(Continued)

TABLE 9.2. Genetic Implications for Specific Groups, Cultures, Ethnicities, or Ancestries. (Continued)

Disease or Condition	Affected Population	Clinical Considerations
Alpha Thalassemia Hereditary anemia caused by defect during hemoglobin production; various clinical phenotypes from silent carrier to more severe	Inhabitants or descendants of Southeast Asia, Middle Eastern, and Mediterranean countries: • 80%–90% may be carriers of alpha-thalassemia in tropical and subtropical regions • about 30% of African Americans	**Relevant Assessment** Patients can be asymptomatic or have mild symptoms of anemia including fatigue and dyspnea, poor growth in children, and jaundice: • Abnormal physical findings occur with more severe phenotypes
Beta Thalassemia Autosomal recessive inherited anemia caused by absent or decreased beta globin chain synthesis during hemoglobin production. Also referred to as Cooley's or Mediterranean anemia	Inhabitants or descendants of Mediterranean countries; Middle East; Central Asia; India; Southern China; Far East; South America; and African north coast **Incidence/Prevalence** Estimated annual incidence of symptomatic individuals: • 1 in 100,000 people globally • 1 in 10,000 people in European communities	**Relevant Assessment** Symptoms emerge at 6-12 months: failure to thrive, feeding problems, diarrhea, fever, and progressive enlargement of abdomen due to hepatosplenomegaly Symptoms in patients who have not been treated or who have received inadequate transfusion treatments may include growth retardation, jaundice, and craniofacial changes
von Willebrand Disease Bleeding disorder resulting in platelet and clotting defect Vary from mild to more severe forms Three types exist most commonly autosomal dominant	Type three may be more prevalent in Swedish communities • 7:3 female: male ratio • racial characteristics of all patients • 75.1% of European descendants • 10.9% Hispanic descendants • 7.5% of African descendants • 2.6% Asian/Pacific Islander descendants • 0.4% American Indian/ Alaskan Native descendants	**Preoperative Assessment** May be asymptomatic All patients having major surgery should have a personal and family history of bleeding to determine if laboratory diagnostic tests for von Willebrand's are indicated: • symptoms typical of bleeding disorder, most commonly mucosal bleeding such as nosebleed; gingival bleeding; easy bruising; or menorrhagia (most common bleeding disorder in women who present with menorrhagia 12% -20%)

© M. M. Wright (2017)

Cancer disease management can now be customized with a *precision* approach. An understanding of the genome has led to fundamentally unique insights into cancer biology and demonstrated that the genomic profile of mutations is in many cases more essential for determining the appropriate chemotherapy than the organ in which the tumor originated (Schnepp et al., 2015). Malignancies are profiled so as to optimize the choice of targeted therapies and thereby improve outcomes.

Identification of genotype may contribute to the cancer treatment for clients along the continuum of care from diagnosis to rehabilitation. The role of apolipoprotein E (APOE) in the cognitive function of postmenopausal women with early-stage breast cancer prior to initiation of adjuvant therapy as well as during the period of treatment was examined by nurse researchers in a longitudinal, genetic association study (Koleck et al., 2014). This research demonstrated that changes in the performance for tasks of executive function, attention, verbal learning and memory, and visual learning and memory were found to be influenced by *APOE genotype* (Koleck et al., 2014). In the future, the *APOE genotype* along with other biomarkers may be used to assist nurses to identify women with breast cancer who may be most at risk for cognitive decline (Koleck et al, 2014). This is another example of nurses using genetic knowledge to improve patient outcomes. Researchers Kerber and Ledbetter (2017a, 2017b) provided a comprehensive framework for applying genetics and genomics resources to both basic and advanced practice roles in oncology nursing. The previous examples reflected that nurses should be able to apply genetic nursing standards to specific patient situations (Kerber & Ledbetter, 2017b). Additional competencies are expected of the advanced practitioner specifically related to test selection, interpretation, and coordination of care for genetic evaluation and testing.

Selection of the optimal pharmacologic agent for heart failure and hypertension have been undergoing increased scientific review. Analyses of heart failure (HF) trials comparing persons of African descent with those of European descent revealed significant ethnic differences in responses to treatment. The African American Heart Failure Trial (A-HeFT) demonstrated that fixed-dose combined isosorbide dinitrate/hydralazine therapy added to customary treatment significantly improved survival in self-identified African American men and women with symptomatic advanced heart failure (Ferdinand et al., 2014). Investigators have been focusing on genetic variations among populations, which may yield more complete characterizations of risk and permit specifically focused treatment for HF clients (Anwar et al., 2015). Anecdotally observed poor outcomes associated with ACE-inhibitor-based therapy among hypertensive persons of African descent compared with those of European descent has been confirmed by clinical trial evidence (Ogedegbe et al., 2015). In a large cohort of hypertensive African-Americans, angiotensin-converting enzyme inhibitors were associated with a greater risk of cardiovascular events compared with calcium channel blockers or thiazide diuretics (Bangalore et al., 2015). In the future, more precisely selected therapies for heart failure and hypertension based on genotype may be superior to selecting therapy based on a patient's ethnicity [or phenotype](Anwar et al., 2015). Collins et al. (2010) also determined that being of African descent was an independent predictor of stent thrombosis after stent placement for coronary revascularization. Adherence to their clopidogrel (antiplatelet medication) regimen at the time of the stenosis was higher among African-descended adult males, yet their rate of stent stenosis was greater than in the non-African-descended population.

Recent developments in genomic research have created opportunities to expand and improve our understanding of how genetic variability affects response to prescribed medications. The definitive goal of pharmacogenomic research is to offer individually focused care to improve the efficacy of medications as well as enhance patient safety by helping to predict the risk of adverse outcomes (Li-Wan-Po, 2012). Phenotypic variations of *CYP450* enzymes influence how clients metabolize medications and contribute to the varying responses among individuals (DeFeo, Sykora, Eley, & Vincent, 2014). There are six significant *CYP450* enzymes that metabolize: *CYP1A2*; *CYP2C9*; *CYP2C19*; *CYP2D6*; *CYP3A4*; and *CYP3A5*. These enzymes play significant roles in the metabolism of 90% of the most commonly prescribed medications (Li-Wan-Po, 2012). Both pain medications and psychotropic medications are frequently affected by these enzymes and individuals may have unpredictable interindividual variability in their responses to medications from either class. Approximately 7% to 10% of persons of European descent have well-characterized genetic polymorphisms in the liver enzyme *CYP2D6* that leads to their inability to catalyze the conversion of codeine into its active metabolite, morphine (Li-Wan-Po, 2012). The discovery of genetic polymorphisms among drug metabolizing enzymes provided an explanation as to why some clients do not obtain the expected drug effects or show exaggerated drug response and/or serious toxicity after consuming the standard and safe dose of a drug (Eichelbaum & Evert, 1996). Other polymorphisms (e.g., the *CYP2D6*2x2 genotype*) can lead to *ultra-rapid* metabolism and thus *increased* sensitivity to effects of codeine due to higher than expected serum morphine levels in approximately 5% of the United States population and 16% to 28% of North African, Ethiopian, and Arabic cultural groups (Eichelbaum & Evert, 1996).

Other genetic variations affecting metabolic efficiency among ethnic groups are also scientifically known. Chinese people produce less morphine from codeine; exhibit reduced sensitivity to morphine; and may experience reduced analgesic effects in response to codeine in comparison to persons of European descent (Caraco, Sheller, & Wood, 1999). These researchers proposed that this reduced sensitivity to morphine may be due to decreased production of morphine-6-glucuronide. Persons with red hair also have genetic variations affecting their responses to both pain and anesthesia (Deutsh, 2002; Gradwohl et al., 2015; Liem et al., 2004). The dysfunctional melanocortin 1 receptor on certain cells that gives people their red hair also increases production of a hormone that causes heightened pain sensitivity (Deutsh, 2002). While genetic testing in routine clinical situations is not recommended, nurses should anticipate these responses without conducting formal testing. Nurses should also consider the possibility of metabolic genetic variations in any patient who experiences a medication toxicity or who does not receive adequate analgesia from codeine or other opioid drugs (e.g., hydrocodone or oxycodone). In these examples of genetic variations, it is essential for nurses to be prudent in utilizing the information (Vuilleumier, Stamer, & Landau, 2012). There are clear limitations in addition to known benefits with the applications of genetics and genomics that nurses should carefully consider for each individual patient. Refer to Table 9.3 for additional information regarding FDA genetic testing requirements.

Readily accessible genetic research studies explicate the safety and efficacy of therapeutic medications providing information about a wide variety of disease conditions far beyond better-known inherited diseases such as sickle cell disease or cystic fibrosis. This growing informational inventory about genetic human variations facilitates understanding about the reasons susceptibilities to common diseases vary among individuals and diverse cultural groups (Rotimi & Jorde, 2010). Nurses need to help individuals navigate through this vast amount of research data so as to enable them to make fully informed decisions.

■ LEGAL AND ETHICAL ASPECTS OF GENETIC TESTING

Many ethical and legal issues surround the identification of genetic defects in the presence of disease, comprehensive collection of individual genome data, and research studies about genetic variations. Protection of genetic privacy is a valid concern; this information should not be made readily accessible without explicit consent. The Genetic Information Nondiscrimination Act (GINA) took effect in November 2009, which prevents health insurers and employers from discriminating against an individual based on his or her genetic information (U. S. Equal Employment Opportunity Commission [EEOC], 2009a). The law was designed to protect *asymptomatic* individuals against the misuse of genetic information by health insurers and employers, and was intended to allow Americans to undergo genetic testing without fear of losing their health insurance or their jobs. This legislation prohibited health insurers from requesting or requiring genetic information from or about an individual or their family members, or using it for decisions regarding coverage, rates, or pre-existing conditions (USEEOC, 2009a). In addition, the GINA prevented employers from using genetic information regarding hiring, firing, promotion, or any other employment purpose including health or other benefits. The law specifically addressed individual genetic information obtained through participation in research that encompassed a range of genetic services including genetic testing, counseling, or education. The GINA *does not* provide protections for *symptomatic* individuals–those with signs and symptoms of a genetically-determined disease (USEEOC, 2009a). Provisions of the U. S. Patient Protection and Affordable Care Act (2014) fill this gap and prohibit exclusion from or termination of health insurance based on personal health status (USDHHS, 2014b).

Protections provided by the American Disabilities Act (ADA) remain relevant to help narrow other gaps in genetic privacy protection (Klitzman, 2010). The circumstances surrounding Terri Sergeant and her potential genetic discrimination suit illustrates the importance of genetic privacy to protect *presymptomatic* individuals (Klitzman, 2010). Sergeant is an individual with a family history of alpha-1-antitrypsin, a serious chronic obstructive lung disease. When

TABLE 9.3. Drugs with FDA Recommended or Required Genetic Testing. Adapted from Clinical Pharmacogenetics Implementation Consortium (CPIC) Level Evidence A and PharmGKB Level 1A.

Gene	Drug	Use	FDA Label
HLA-B	abacavir (Ziiagen)	HIV treatment	Genetic testing recommended
CYP2D6 and CYP2C19	amitriptyline (Elavil)	Depression, Insomnia, Chronic Pain	Actionable prescribing information
TPMT	azathioprine (Imuran)	Immunosuppressive	Genetic testing recommended
HLA-A	carbamazepine (Tegretol)	Seizures	Actionable prescribing information
HLA-B	carbamazepine (Tegretol)	Seizures	Genetic testing **required**
CYP2C19	clopidogrel (Plavix)	Antiplatelet	Actionable prescribing information
CYP2D6	codeine	Analgesia	Actionable prescribing information
CFTR	ivacaftor	Cystic fibrosis	Genetic testing **required**
TPMT	mercaptopurine	Immunosuppressive	Genetic testing recommended
CYP2D6	nortriptyline (Pamelor, Aventyl)	Depression, Insomnia, Chronic Pain	Actionable prescribing information
G6PD	rasburicase	Uric acid control	Genetic testing **required**
ERBB2 ESR1	palbociclib (Ibrance)	Breast cancer	Genetic testing **required**
G6PD	rasburicase (Elitek)	Uric acid control	Genetic testing **required**

Data from U.S. Department of Health and Human Services, Stanford University & St. Jude's Children's Medical Center, Clinical Pharmacogenetics Implementation Consortium of the Pharmacogenomics Research Network. Drugs with FDA Recommended or Required Genetic Testing [Table, partial listing]. Accessible at https://cpicpgx.org/genes-drugs/

asymptomatic, she tested positive for the genetic disposition for the disease that had killed her brother at 37 years of age. Based on her positive test result, her physician initiated preventative therapy to deter disease development and protect against lung infection. The treatment cost exceeded $45,000 annually but permitted her to work and engage in her life activities without limitation. Sergeant worked for a firm that self-funded its employees' health insurance; her employment was terminated only one month following an excellent performance review that had generated her a merit increase. Subsequently, Terri Sergeant's testimony before the Senate Health, Education, Labor, and Pension Committee helped pave the way for enactment of the GINA regulation (Silvers & Stein, 2003). Sergeant was not alone. When the late social scientist Dorothy

C. Wertz, PhD, from the University of Massachusetts Medical Center in Worcester, surveyed U. S. genetics professionals in 1999, she found 693 reported cases where either clients or their family members had been refused life insurance or employment based on their genetic status, even when they showed no symptoms of disease (Wertz, 1999).

More recently, a federal genetic discrimination lawsuit raised broader concerns about testing and privacy. The case involved a middle school student affected by results from a genetic screening test conducted when he was a newborn (Levenson, 2016). The parents of Colman Chadam alleged that in 2012 the Palo Alto Unified School District (PAUSD) violated two federal laws that protected people with disabilities, the Americans with Disabilities Act (ADA) and

Section 504 of the Rehabilitation Act. The parents further alleged that their son's First Amendment right to privacy had been breached when his middle school teacher allegedly divulged to the parents of two other students at the school that the boy carried "genetic markers" for cystic fibrosis (CF), information that had been shared with the school when he had first enrolled (Levenson, 2016). Colman's physician noted that the student did not have active disease, according to court documents (Levenson, 2016). The suit alleged that the school district improperly ordered Colman to change schools after the parents of two other students with CF complained about the risk of cross-infection from particular bacteria that are especially harmful to people with CF. The Cystic Fibrosis Foundation (n. d.) recommended that people with the disease maintain a distance of at least six feet from other CF sufferers to reduce this risk. Following a brief absence, Colman was allowed to return to school after his parents registered their complaint. In this case, the Genetic Information Nondiscrimination Act (GINA) was not helpful because the law is applicable only to situations involving either employment and health insurance. Legal experts at the intersection of law and genetics say the Chadams' case underscored the need to protect children's privacy concerning genetic information as well as highlighting how little attention the issue has been given in federal law (Levenson, 2016). Lack of privacy protections could make parents reluctant to have their children undergo genetic testing even when medically indicated (Levinson, 2016).

Exclusion of genetic information from standard health records has been proposed to ensure appropriate use of this data and nondisclosure to insurance companies (Klitzman, 2010). However, shadow or secondary records would prove cumbersome in actual clinical use, especially within the context of an electronic health record (EHR). All practice sites or settings and their staff should be aware of the importance of safeguarding genetic information that may be contained in any patient's health or medical record, and the implications to all concerned if divulged (USEEOC, 2009b).

A guiding principle derived from the United Nations Educational, Scientific and Cultural Organisation (1997) *Universal Declaration on the Human Genome and Human Rights* was that benefits from advances in biology, genetics, and medicine concerning the human genome shall be made available to all, with due regard for the dignity and human rights of each individual (Article 12). Genetic health care based on new genomic knowledge has the potential to both expand and reduce disparities among populations (Badzek, Henaghan, Turner, & Monsen, 2013). Currently, few individuals of childbearing age born in the United States are aware of their sickle cell trait (SCT) status; the most recent community-based survey revealed that only 16% of respondents knew this information even though it is collected as part of standardized newborn laboratory blood screening procedures (Taylor, Kavanagh, & Zuckerman, 2014).

Parents *are* routinely notified by newborn screening programs if their child has sickle cell *disease* (SCD), but only 37% are notified if their child has sickle cell *trait* (Taylor et al., 2014). If the parents do receive SCT screening results, it is not known whether they understand the ramifications and/or share them with the affected child during adolescence so as to enable informed future reproductive decisions. This gap is a missed opportunity to provide appropriate health care and prenatal counseling and testing. Preimplantation genetic diagnosis (PGD) provides these future parents an opportunity to choose whether to implant an embryo that has been screened for serious genetic disorders, yet this service is not universally covered by insurances or in all countries (Badzek et al., 2013). In 2013, the United Kingdom's National Health Service approved coverage for three cycles of *in vitro* fertilization and preimplantation genetic diagnosis for fertile couples meeting age and basic health requirements when both prospective parents have SCT and they do not have an unaffected child (Taylor et al., 2014). These researchers advocated for reducing the burden of SCD—a common, clearly delineated, and easily identified genetic disease—through the implementation of similar testing programs in other countries (Taylor et al., 2014). Such programs could enable individuals to better understand the implications of their genetic data within the modern healthcare system. Providing culturally sensitive information could complement information provided by healthcare practitioners, including hematologists and primary care providers, and help address the stigma associated with genetic conditions found in minority communities (Taylor et al., 2014). These authors suggested that by working together, the healthcare system, school systems, and relevant community organizations may be able to improve knowledge and awareness about SCT so that affected individuals are able to become informed and have increased access to reproductive options.

Direct-to-Consumer Genetic Testing (DTC-GT)

Genetic information is embedded in the human genome, which is composed of 23 pairs of chromosomes (Porth, 2014). In 2007, some biotechnology firms altered the healthcare environment by making personal genetics tests accessible to individual consumers at an affordable cost. Previously, this type of testing had been available only with an order from a healthcare provider. Subsequent research analysis revealed that the results from these personal genetic tests were neither consistent nor reliable (Delaney & Christman, 2016). Direct-to-consumer genetic testing was interrupted in November 2013 when the U. S. Food and Drug Administration (FDA) instructed "23andMe" to discontinue marketing and sales of their personal genetic testing service until 2015 when the company received FDA approval to market a limited number of genetic carrier tests (Delaney & Christman, 2016). The FDA regulates companies that provide genetic testing and has expressed concern about how consumers might use the information obtained from these tests. Consumer groups/agencies have argued that genetic information belongs to the individual and that the right to access this information supersedes concerns held by regulatory agencies (Delaney & Christman, 2016). The pendulum has moved steadily toward the acceptance of direct-to-consumer genetic testing (DTC-GT) among the regulatory agencies and medical communities, as shown by the FDA reclassification of carrier tests to Class II medical devices in 2015. Further, the National Society of Genetic Counselors (NSGC) also revised their position to reflect that people have every right to pursue DTC-GT (2015). The NSGC added a caveat recommending that DTC companies be required to offer consumers easy access and/or referral to appropriate resources and qualified professionals in the field of clinical genetics and genomics (National Society of Genetic Counselors, 2015).

Precision medicine has enabled the development of drugs that can target individual-specific diseases by focusing on their unique (genetic) characteristics.

Consumers and their healthcare providers need access to this type of information, but genetic tests and diagnostics tools must first be accurate and reliable. Critical decisions may need to be made and consumers deserve correct, accurate, and reliable information comprehensively presented in a compassionate and culturally-supportive environment. In 2015, the American College of Medical Genetics and Genomics (ACMGG) Board of Directors approved their revised position statement on direct-to-consumer genetic testing (ACMGG, 2016). These recommendations were designed primarily as an educational resource for medical geneticists and other healthcare providers to help them provide quality medical genetics services (ACMGG, 2016). The recommendations emphasize that it is critical for the public to realize that genetic testing is only one part of a complex process that includes genetic risk assessment, diagnosis, and disease management (ACMGG, 2016). The ACMGG affirmed that the results of DTC genetic testing can have important health implications for individuals and their family members.

The odds for developing most diseases do not depend solely on genetic influences but also on a variety of other factors such as environment, diet, and activity level (McCance & Huether, 2014). Being at an increased risk does not confer certainty for the development of any given disease or condition because expressions or manifestations are difficult to predict (Domchek, Jameson, & Miesfeldt, 2015). An additional ethical consideration in regard to genetic testing is that there may not be any advantage to the individual knowing whether he or she carries a specific genetic variation for conditions such as Alzheimer's disease. The key question is whether the personal genetic information demonstrates value; that is, will the knowledge lead to better health? Child psychologists caution that despite assertions that predictive genomic testing can be a tool for use in primary disease prevention, little discussion has focused on its application with children (Tarini, Tercyak, & Wilfond, 2011). These authors raised ethical concerns, including the potential for psychological and behavioral harm for children as a result of positive predictive genetic tests for diseases with genetically-determined Mendelian characteristics.

Direct-to-consumer genetic testing will soon become more readily available and nurses need to be prepared and in position to act as knowledgeable patient advocates. Providing individualized genetic information to clients with an informed and balanced discussion that encompasses the spectrum of arguments from patient harm to patient ownership has been recommended (Delaney & Christman, 2015).

■ TRANSCULTURAL NURSING IMPLICATIONS

Differing healthcare outcomes among diverse cultural groups or populations (whether identified by ethnicity, heritage, or geographic ancestry) are important challenges for nurses to address. These differences include biologic, genetic, environmental, and social structure factors that are complexly and holistically interrelated (Glittenberg, 2002). Transcultural nursing focuses on cultural values, beliefs, expressions, and patterns based on observed behaviors and practices, but more attention needs to be paid to the observed as well as genetically-inherited characteristics being carried forward from one generation to the next (Glittenberg, 2002; McFarland & Wehbe-Alamah, 2015). Transcultural nursing theorists have addressed genetics and genomics care decisions and actions with individuals from diverse cultural groups in their theoretical precepts, research, and publications.

Locsin, Purnell, Tanioka, and Osaka (2016) described the transition of care from *home* ("usually by the women of the family, herbalists, midwives, or neighbors") to *hospital* that occurred as early as the 19th century, stating:

> …the layers in development and adoption of highly sophisticated technologies for medical use [and] the trajectory of modern medical technology…evolved amid great intellectual, social, and political upheavals [that] provided deep foundations for the present hegemony [dominance or authority over others] in healthcare…spurred worldwide development of technological development [and] changed the way in which human care was provided. (p. 347)

As multidisciplinary research and interprofessional clinical practice evolves and discovered data adds new insights into pathophysiologic and genetic variations in disease mechanisms, nurses will be able to conduct more focused and evidence-based client assessments and coparticipatively engage in better-informed

culture-specific and culturally congruent care decisions and actions (McFarland & Wehbe-Alamah, 2015). *Racialized ethnicity* leads to issues in health care and nursing situations where by thought and action, nurses stereotype people who are from a diverse race or blend of races and cultures into a *specific ethnic group with specific traits* (Ray, 2016, p. 111). "Nursing care may then be inappropriate unless persons are asked their cultural preferences and what has meaning for them" (p. 111). Conducting a cultural interview and assessment, therefore, remains paramount to avoiding stereotypes, biases, cultural imposition practices, and cultural pain (Leininger, 2002a, pp. 117-120).

The collection of health status data among diverse cultural groups; assessment of differences in culture-specific or culture-bound disease patterns; and individually-focused designs of clinical drug and treatment trials are key aspects of applied genetic research. Table 9.2 (Genetic Implications for Specific Groups) provides an introduction to diseases that may vary significantly among diverse cultural groups. Conducting the nursing assessment within the framework of this knowledge will facilitate earlier detection, identify triggers for ongoing assessment, and serve as a catalyst for more individualized care (USDHHS, n. d.-f). Nurses are better able to provide optimal and beneficial culture-specific care through their knowledge and application of genetics and genomics principles. The 16 American Nurses' Association (ANA) Standards of Practice for Genetics/Genomics Nursing (2016) provide a firm foundation for and describe competency levels of genetics and genomics nursing using the demonstrated critical thinking model extantly embedded in the nursing process (ANA, 2016). Opportunities to address genetics and genomics in the provision of culturally congruent and competent nursing care exist at key intervals across the continuum of care such as with nursing assessment; genetic counseling; genetic education; therapeutic drug monitoring; and research study participant recruitment.

Nursing Assessment

Genetic assessment begins with a family history and should be recorded in the form of a pedigree (Refer to Figure 9.1). First, the nurse obtains health-related data about first- and second-degree relatives, then expands the inquiry to include additional family members if the pedigree suggests any inherited disease

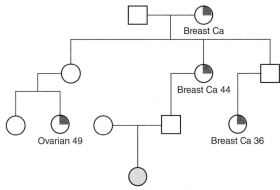

34-year-old patient questioning need for genetic testing

1) Genetic testing for BRCA1 and BRCA2 mutations should be offered to individuals with a personal history suspicious for hereditary breast and cancer syndrome (pink circle). Cancer diagnosed before age 50, multiple primary cancers or bilateral cancers in one individual should serve as triggers.

2) Testing should be offered in the setting of appropriate genetic counseling to ensure individuals are provided relevant information regarding the risks, benefits, and limitations of genetic testing. Counseling should also include consideration of how the results of such testing might impact other family members including children.

3) When possible, genetic testing should be performed on an individual who has been diagnosed with breast or ovarian cancer because this strategy provides the most information for other members of the family (purple triangles).

4) Genetic testing can lead to varied outcomes; a positive (mutation found), true negative, or a variant of uncertain significance (VUS) (ANA, 2016; Kerber & Ledbetter, 2017b; McReynolds & Lewis, 2017).

FIGURE 9.1 • A Stepwise Approach to Genetic Counseling. © M. M. Wright (2017).

(McReynolds & Lewis, 2017). Family history collection is dynamic and should not be a one-time event; it should be revisited whenever significant changes have occurred (McReynolds & Lewis, 2017). When assessing an asymptomatic individual, the determination of risk will vary depending on ages at disease onset, types of diagnoses, and the historical depth and breadth required for the pedigree. For example, if two or more first-degree relatives are affected with asthma, cardiovascular disease, type 2 diabetes, breast cancer, colon cancer, or melanoma, the relative risk for disease among close relatives ranges from two- to fivefold for these prevalent diseases (Domchek et al., 2015). Factors such as adoption and limited numbers of women in a family should be taken into consideration when analyzing the pedigree. Specific attention should be paid to note any young age at disease onset (e.g., 36-year-old nonsmoking woman with emphysema); atypical diseases (e.g., male breast cancer); and the finding of multiple potentially related diseases in the same patient (e.g., woman with both colon and endometrial cancer).

It is essential to equally consider the pedigree in light of the individual's ancestry, culture, and ethnicity. Three specific mutations account for approximately 85% of the mutations found in the *BRCA1* and *BRCA2* genes among the Ashkenazi Jewish population. The prevalence of these three mutations is approximately 10 times that of all *BRCA1* and *BRCA2* mutations among the general U. S. population. The risk of developing breast and ovarian cancer is significantly increased in Ashkenazi Jewish women who carry one (or more) of these three founder mutations (McClain, Nathanson, Palomaki, & Haddow, 2005). This autosomally-dominant inherited mutation is associated with a high penetrance and a lifetime cancer risk ranging between 35% and 65% (McClain et al., 2005). A focused genetic assessment is relevant when therapeutic decisions could be influenced by ancestry. Nurses must strike a balance between practicing reasonable follow-through regarding observable ethnic and racial characteristics while at the same time avoiding stereotyping individuals based on their ancestry. Identification of known genetic triggers should be routinely addressed as part of the baseline nursing assessment. For example, astute assessment could prevent unnecessary post-operative bleeding for a patient with a previously undiagnosed von Willebrand Disease (vWSD)—if atypical bleeding in the individual or family is identified in the history—or avert exertional rhabdomyolysis for a young athlete with sickle cell trait but without any heretofore disease expression (Ferrari, Parker, Grubs, & Krishnamurti, 2015; Porth, 2014).

The nurse should explore further genetic risk variables including nonhereditary risk factors among persons exhibiting or diagnosed with disease—, such as cigarette smoking history or exposures for persons with cardiovascular disease; asbestos exposures among persons with lung disease; and previous radiation exposures among persons with cancer (Domchek et al., 2015). Extensive personal or family history associated—with venous thromboembolic disease in the absence of medical risk factors such as orthostasis or injury could be a harbinger of a hypercoagulable disorder such as Leiden V (Porth, 2014). The physical examination will complement the history and may identify risk factor signs for an inherited disorder. A young adult patient presenting with periorbital or facial xanthomas should prompt evaluation for familial hypercholesterolemia (Domchek et al., 2015).

The nurse should consider both family history and clinical manifestations when considering to advice for the patient and their family to pursue genetic counseling and testing. General triggers would include:

- Personal or family history of known or suspected genetic disorder or congenital abnormality
- Multiple family members with similar or related disorders
- Ethnic predisposition
- Earlier than expected age of disease onset
- Consanguinity-marriage between related individuals, from the Latin root "with blood" *
- Previous history of a child with birth defects or genetic disorder
- Personal or family history of hereditary cancers

Preconceptual/Prenatal	Child	Adult
• Previous history of a child with birth defects or a genetic disorder • Advanced maternal age (>35 years) at time of delivery • Two or more pregnancy losses • Unexplained infertility • Ultrasound or prenatal testing suggesting a genetic disorder • Abnormal maternal serum screening • Exposure to teratogen • Maternal condition impacting fetal development	• One or more major malformations or dysmorphic features • Abnormal newborn screening • Abnormal development • Congenital hearing loss or blindness • Features suggestive of genetic disorder or chromosome abnormality • Development of degenerative neurologic disorder or unexplained seizures	• Early onset disorder, especially if multiple family members are affected (e.g., emphysema or heart disease under age 40) • Unusual manifestation of disease (e.g., male breast cancer, multiple primary cancers) • Extreme lab values (e.g., hypercholesterolemia)

* **Consanguinity:** Marriage between related individuals is referred to as consanguinity and may be a factor in producing children with recessive genetic diseases such as cystic fibrosis (McCance & Huether, 2014). Related individuals are more likely to share the same recessive genes, which then have a greater probability of interacting with each other. Cultures that accept or practice consanguinity may be at greater risk for such genetic disorders.

FIGURE 9.2 • Clues for Genetic Testing. © M. M. Wright (2017).
Compiled from Domchek, Jameson, & Miesfeldt, 2015; McCance & Huether, 2014; National Society of Genetic Counselors (http://about-geneticcounselors.com/Genetic-Testing); Porth, 2014.

Adult-onset hereditary diseases follow multiple patterns of inheritance and the nurse should be vigilant during the processes of assessment and evaluation to identify historical risk factors and physical signs, which are opportunities to improve patient outcomes. Standard 1 of the Scope and Standards of Genetic/Genomics Nursing reinforces that the nurse should recognize the influence of personal attitudes, values, beliefs, and culture during the client assessment (ANA, 2016, p. 26).

Genetic Counseling

Genetic counseling can be beneficial for a wide range of clinical or health situations. The National Society of Genetic Counselors has defined *genetic counseling* as "…the process of helping people understand and adapt to the medical, psychological, and familial implications of genetic contributions to disease" (2015). Genetic counseling should include interpretation of family and medical histories to assess the chance of disease occurrence or recurrence; education about inheritance, testing, management, prevention, resources, and research; and counseling to promote informed choice and adaptation to the risk or condition (Resta, 2006). More importantly, Domchek, Jameson, and Miesfeldt (2015) described genetic counseling as a communication *process* that deals with human problems associated with the occurrence of risk for a genetic disorder in a family. This strategy requires a holistic approach, which is crucially important; genetic risk assessment can be intricately complex and often involves elements of uncertainty. The ANA 2016 Genetics and Genomics Standards for Nurses lists *genetic education* as well as *psychosocial counseling* as key components of the genetic counseling process.

The Genetics and Genomics Nursing Standards and Scope of Practice were revised in 2016 by the ANA and International Society of Nurses in Genetics (ISONG) as a copublication that reflected updates in nursing and genetics and genomics practices. The revision specified integrated *basic* registered nurse (RN) and *advanced practice* (APRN) roles and responsibilities as well as certification in genetics and genomics by the American Nurses' Credentialing Center (ANCC). Each standard or substandard has competencies delineated for each level of practice. The standards are presented below; a broad overview of the Levels of Genetics Nursing Practice from the Standards is provided in the chapter Appendix.

The Standards of *Practice* are:
- Standard 1. Assessment
  The genetics nurse collects comprehensive data pertinent to the client's health and/or the situation.

- Standard 2. Diagnosis
  The genetics nurse analyzes the assessment data to determine the diagnoses or the issues.

- Standard 3. Outcomes Identification
  The genetics nurse identifies expected outcomes for a plan individualized to the client or the situation.

- Standard 4. Planning
  The genetics nurse develops a plan that prescribes strategies and alternatives to attain expected outcomes.

- Standard 5. Implementation
  The genetics nurse implements the identified plan.
- Standard 5A. Coordination of Care
  The genetics nurse coordinates care delivery.

- Standard 5B. Health Teaching and Health Promotion
  The genetics nurse employs strategies to promote health and a safe environment.

- Standard 5C. Consultation
  The graduate-level prepared genetics nurse or advanced practice registered nurse provides consultation to influence the identified plan, enhance the abilities of others, and effect change.

- Standard 5D. Prescriptive Authority and Treatment
  The APRN uses prescriptive authority, procedures, referrals, treatments, and therapies in accordance with state and federal laws and regulations.

- Standard 6. Evaluation
  The registered nurse evaluates progress toward attainment of outcomes.

The Standards of *Professional Performance* are:
- Standard 7. Ethics
  The genetics nurse practices ethically. (*Code of Ethics for Nurses with Interpretive Statements*)

- Standard 8. Education
  The genetics nurse attains knowledge and competence that reflects current nursing practice.

- Standard 9. Evidence-Based Practice and Research
- The genetics nurse integrates evidence and research findings into practice.

- Standard 10. Quality of Practice
  The genetics nurse contributes to quality genetics nursing practice.

- Standard 11. Communication
  The genetics nurse communicates effectively in a variety of formats in all areas of practice.

- Standard 12. Leadership
  The genetics nurse demonstrates leadership in the professional practice setting and the profession.

- Standard 13. Collaboration
  The genetics nurse collaborates with client, family, and others in the conduct of nursing practice.

- Standard 14. Professional Practice Evaluation
  The genetics nurse evaluates her or his own nursing practice in relation to professional practice standards and guidelines, relevant statutes, rules, and regulations.

- Standard 15. Resource Utilization
  The genetics nurse utilizes appropriate resources to plan and provide nursing services that are safe, effective, and financially responsible.

- Standard 16. Environmental Health
  The genetics nurse practices in an environmentally safe and healthy manner. (ANA, 2016)

Genetic Education

Client education is central to a person's ability to make informed decisions regarding genetic testing and treatment options. Adequate knowledge about inheritance patterns will allow individuals to more readily comprehend the probability of disease risk for themselves and other family members. It is especially important to understandably impart the concepts of *disease penetrance* and *disease expression* for informed decision-making to occur. For most complex adult-onset genetic disorders, asymptomatic clients should be advised that a positive test result does not always translate into future disease development. For example, advances in sequencing analysis have made multigene testing or "panel testing" a practical option when searching for genetic variants that may be associated with a risk of breast cancer (Easton et al., 2015). After a June 2013 Supreme Court decision, multiple companies immediately began to offer panel tests for breast cancer genes that included *BRCA1*

and *BRCA2*. While the presence of the BRCA 1 and BRCA 2 genes confer a high risk of breast cancer, other genes may be predictive of moderate to lower risk. *Panel testing* provides a useful contribution to the prediction of a woman's risk of breast cancer, but end-users need to be aware of their limitations (Easton et al., 2015). In addition, the role of nongenetic factors such as environmental exposures and lifestyle must be discussed in the context of an overall multifactorial disease risk and potential amelioration through disease prevention efforts. Importantly, clients should understand the natural history of the disease in question as well as the potential options for intervention including screening, prevention, and—in certain circumstances—pharmacologic treatment or prophylactic surgery. Many lay and professional resources are shown in Table 9.1 with specific sites that provide extensive information for educators such as teaching tools and simulation scenarios.

Therapeutic Drug Monitoring

Research findings have revealed that genetics and genomics fingerprints may influence either a patient's exaggerated or subtherapeutic response to medications (Wang et al., 2015). The effects from analgesic, psychotropic, oncologic, immunosuppressive, antiseizure, antiplatelet, anticoagulant, and cardiovascular medications have been found to vary significantly based on a person's genetic makeup (USDHHS, n. d.-h). Individualized drug therapy is especially desirable when the therapeutic index is narrow and the consequences of drug toxicity are life-threatening such as with antineoplastics and anticoagulants (Wilke & Dolan, 2011). Because drug prescribing is based on population averages, as many as one-third of drug-exposed patients may develop an unacceptable toxicity and a significant proportion of patients will not experience a drug response (Wilke & Dolan, 2011). This places an economic burden on the healthcare system and negatively affects the patient. An unanswered question remains: Will therapeutic drug monitoring solve this problem or add further healthcare costs with only a relatively small outcome benefit? As additional pharmacogenomic studies are conducted, more individualized approaches to medication selection and therapeutic drug monitoring will be discovered. The nurse should be able to utilize current research to identify at-risk clients and develop effective identification and monitoring strategies for clinical practice.

Medication selection must be tailored to the individual. Clopidogrel is an important platelet aggregation inhibitor used for the prevention of myocardial infarction and stroke. The effects from metabolized clopidogrel on the prevalence and recurrence rates of cerebrovascular events in a multiethnic population has reinforced the importance of precision medications and pharmacogenomics (Spokoyny et al., 2014). Reduced clopidogrel efficacy among multiethnic populations may occur because of genetic variations in cytochrome P450 and polypeptide 19 [*CYP2C19*] (Spokoyny et al., 2014). A 'Black Box Warning' from the U. S. Food and Drug Administration now recommends that all prospective clopidogrel clients be tested for these genetic enzyme variations prior to initiation of the drug (USDHHS, 2010). While previous studies have explored the effect of this metabolic variation on heart disease treatment outcomes, Spokoyny et al. (2014) found that only an approximate one-fourth of White patients were intermediate or poor metabolizers compared to nearly half of non-Whites. Poor/intermediate clopidogrel metabolizers have an increased risk of recurrent cerebrovascular events (Spokoyny et al., 2014). These findings are comparable with those from other cardiovascular studies (Mega et al., 2009) and provided indications that routine clinical testing for *CYP2C19* may be warranted. These results emphasized the value of genetic and cultural implications in clinical practice; aided in the identification of the medication's enzymatic metabolic pathway; and provided practitioners with clearer guideposts for making more culturally congruent, effective, and meaningful care decisions and actions toward optimal cardiovascular outcomes.

Research Recruitment

As the science of genomics continues to be translated into healthcare practice, research regarding therapeutic options (including drug efficacy and safety) relies on involving participants and cohorts from culturally diverse groups. Phenotypic variations in drug responses have the potential to create augmented or super-therapeutic responses; exacerbated disease and/or symptoms due to decreased efficacy; and/or life-threatening situations that cause plasma drug level variations despite identically-calculated doses for individuals with similar body weight (Fishbain et al., 2004). Historically, research studies have been conducted predominately with Caucasian males. Past medical experimentation and poor medical treatment fortified mistrust in the medical system by African-Americans and other ethnic and cultural minority groups that greatly contributed to their reluctance to participate in research activities (Coakley et al., 2012). These authors described major barriers to African American participation in clinical trials that included lack of awareness about trials; low socioeconomic status; mistrust; poor communication skills; and a lack of disease education (Coakley et al., 2012). Successful recruitment and retention of African American participants in clinical trials could be facilitated by having clinical and translational research teams who are culturally competent (Otado et al., 2015). Utilizing multiethnic investigators and coordinators who actively engage with minority communities; authentically demonstrating trust and respect to participants and potential participants; and providing culturally relevant and meaningful education about the research endeavor and its potential benefits could also improve participation (Otado et al., 2015). In addition, this study revealed that the best strategy to reduce identified and nonidentified cultural barriers and retain participants was associated with the ability to maintain continual contact and open communication with participants using a caring and respectful approach.

Maintaining a structured focus on the unique healthcare and social structure needs and values held by diverse minority groups will help to define optimal evidence-based therapeutic strategies. Nurses need to play a role in the recruitment and inclusion of adequate numbers of diverse ethnic and cultural groups so as to enable scientific investigation about any differences in pathophysiology and potential response variabilities. Continued collection of data about health status among diverse ethnic and cultural groups; assessment of differences in culture-specific disease patterns; and focused designs of clinical drug and treatment trials are key to effective recruitment of minority group participants. In addition, researchers need to increase their collaboration with interdisciplinary *clinical* teams to enroll greater numbers of diverse ethnic, cultural, and gender participants into ongoing research studies toward reaching conclusions that may benefit all.

■ DISCUSSION: MORAL CONUNDRUMS

Is it acceptable for patients/clients to decline genetic testing?

Nurses need to maintain respect for the individual who elects not to participate in genetic testing for the detection of genetically based illnesses such as Alzheimer's disease when a family member develops the early form of the disorder (or at any time). Personal choice is an ethical right. Increasing patient autonomy in healthcare decisions continues to grow and the tenets of *autonomy* and *self-determination* in health care are central to genomic counseling (Hawkins & Ho, 2012). Testing for mutations associated with genetic health may reveal unexpected findings such as nonpaternity or an incidental finding of a genetic variant that could have health implications for the individual or family but were not the primary reason for the test (Badzek et al., 2013). Cultural sensitivity and awareness are essential as well; genetic and genomic nursing needs to be mindful about providing culturally congruent, meaningful, and beneficial care that respects the values, beliefs, patterns, and expressions of the individual and (if appropriate) their family (Wehbe-Alamah, 2015).

Are mandatory testing programs ethical?

In 2010, the National Collegiate Athletic Association (NCAA) required all student-athletes to have their sickle cell trait (SCT) status confirmed prior to athletic participation (Bonham, Dover, & Brody, 2010). The mandated screening program evolved from the death of a 19-year-old college football player. The cause of death was attributable to acute exertional rhabdomyolysis associated with sickle cell trait. The family took legal action in hopes of preventing future deaths. The NCAA approved the screening program in 2010 for institutions participating in Division I athletics and extended it in subsequent years to institutions at Division II and III levels. Bonham, Dover, and Brody (2010) posed legitimate questions about unintended consequences of this mandate as follows:

- *Would the athlete's privacy be protected?*
- *Would the program lead to stigmatization?*
- *Would the athlete's self-image be affected?*
- *Would the carrier status affect their potential participation and career progression in sports?*

Ethical concerns continue to be raised at this writing about the mandatory nature of the ruling and potential effects on student-athletes, particularly through stigmatization of and discrimination against those with SCT. The American Society of Hematology (ASH) opposed "…the imposition of SCT testing and instead recommended …universal precautions such as gradual buildup of performance [to] prevent exercise-related illnesses [that] would benefit the entire student-athlete population and avoid violating the privacy of [students] with SCT" (Ferrari et al., 2015, p. 876). These researchers have proposed that implementation of universal precautions would help to ensure that the most ethically sound practices are afforded to every student-athlete (Ferrari et al., 2015).

What are the ethics related to disclosing (or not disclosing) non-actionable yet serious genomic risks discovered incidentally during other testing?

The healthcare team needs to balance a patient's right to autonomy and information with the moral duty of nonmaleficence (do no harm). Certain genetic/genomic test results can have profound implications for clients and could create severe psychological distress, particularly if not accompanied by proper pre- and post-test counseling (Offit, 2011). Information revealed by genomic testing is not always clinically actionable, such as an individual's risk for developing Huntington's Chorea or Alzheimer disease (AD). Presymptomatic tests for AD are under development and pose serious ethical concerns. A survey was conducted to explore the self-expressed desire for, envisioned reaction to, and basic understanding of presymptomatic Alzheimer disease-related genetic and biomarker tests (Caselli et al., 2014). A total of 80.2% of the 4,036 respondents desired biomarker testing; another 90.5% confirmed that they would "pursue a healthier lifestyle" if found to be at high risk for AD, but 11.6% seriously considered suicide (Caselli et al., 2014). These researchers suggested that greater education of the public was indicated and recommended that interested clients should probably undergo psychological screening to identify those at high risk for adverse psychological outcomes upon disclosure of positive findings from presymptomatic test results. Pre-test screening should be anchored to tangible, constructive action plans such as healthy lifestyle changes, long-term care planning, and participation in research trials when available and appropriate (Caselli et al., 2014). In this clinical scenario, the nurse again maintains a vital and significant role as client advocate throughout the informed consent, genetic testing, and pre/post test counseling processes.

■ SUMMARY

Nurses serve as authentic patient advocates when they engage in a comprehensive and multifaceted assessment that includes genetics and genomics. The addition of genetics and genomics to the traditional nursing assessment will inform and engage the patient when making key decisions about their personal healthcare plan. Based on their ethnicity and race, clients are sometimes identified as at-risk for specific diseases such as diabetes mellitus among Native Americans; breast cancer among Ashkenazi Jews; and prostate cancer among African Americans (Herman & Cohen, 2012; Porth, 2014). Particular forms of treatment are also more (or less) effective among certain racial/ethnic groups compared with others. Among African Americans, angiotensin-converting enzyme (ACE) inhibitors have been shown to be less effective for essential hypertension, and therapeutic responses to selective serotonin reuptake inhibitor (SSRI) antidepressants occur at lower doses in comparison to persons of European descent (Ferdinand et al., 2014; Narasimhan & Lohoff, 2012). Patient safety related to drug dosing, targeted treatment, and personalized medicine has the potential to be markedly improved by applying sound principles of genetics and genomics (Chung, et al., 2014; Diouf et al., 2015; Walko & McLeod, 2012). Pain management, a key tool in the nurse's arsenal of effective therapeutic interventions, cannot be accomplished without specific knowledge about the patient's genetic/genomic responses. Both poor metabolizers and ultra-rapid metabolizers are at risk for suboptimal or marginal therapeutic outcomes (Rahim-Williams, Riley, Williams, & Fillingim, 2012).

Nurses should avoid oversimplifying genetic relationships and outcomes when communicating with individuals and their families. These discussions can be polarizing given the complex interactions among culture, ethnicity, ancestry, genetics, and socioeconomic factors. Knowledge about ethnicity might prompt genetic testing or detailed family history taking in particular instances (e.g., with Ashkenazi Jews). The issues are too complex for nurses to make unqualified assertions to clients that they are *at-risk for a particular illness* or that they may be *unlikely to respond to therapies* solely on the basis of their racial/ethnic background (Rotimi & Jorde, 2010). As previously discussed, inheritance is multifaceted; disease penetrance and disease expressivity vary considerably. Believing that one is vulnerable may needlessly increase stress, fear, and feelings of stigma, uncertainty, and worthlessness. For example, one must consider whether the athlete who has been apprised regarding his carrier status for sickle cell trait is an informed, empowered, or stigmatized person as a result of having this knowledge. The nurse is in an ideal position to ensure that culturally congruent genetic-genomic care is provided through a genuine process of communication and an ongoing commitment to the patient. Nurses must exercise caution and use sound judgment when applying genetics and genomics knowledge in transcultural nursing practice. It is essential to integrate critical thinking and sensitivity along with truth-telling throughout these crucial conversations to ensure optimal care outcomes. Nurses will play an important stewardship role with the implementation of genetic and genomics into practice. The unique contributions made by nurses as client advocates and educators will remain pivotal in this evolving healthcare transformation.

■ DEDICATION

To the genetics and genomics clients we serve: You are strong, tenacious, resilient, determined, and stalwart. As nurses we remain constant, persevering, diligent, and steadfast in our efforts to be your advocates through critical thinking, care, and caring.

■ APPENDIX

Levels of Genetics Nursing Practice

The scope of genetics specialty nursing practice comprises two levels—basic and advanced. Both include application of genetics and genomics knowledge in risk assessment, outcome identification, intervention, and evaluation. What distinguishes them is their level of formal education, and the depth and breadth of knowledge and skills.

Basic Level

- Basic level genetics nurses routinely provide genetics services to clients.
- They are expected to have either formal genetics clinical experiences from their basic nursing preparatory programs or on-the-job training from professionals trained in genetics, such as graduate nursing or medical faculty with genetics expertise, advanced practice registered nurses in a genetics healthcare setting, appropriately credentialed genetics professionals, or other clinicians who provide genetics-based clinical services or conduct genetic research within their specialty. The genetics nurse's knowledge and skill base is maintained through participation in genetics and nursing continuing education. Credentialing in genetics is strongly encouraged (p. 13).

Advanced Level

- The characteristics that distinguish advanced from basic level genetics nursing practice are expanded practice skills and knowledge in nursing and genetics, increased complexity of decision-making, leadership, and the ability to negotiate complex organizations.
- A nurse with a graduate degree in nursing who practices in genetics at the advanced practice level will be referred to as a *genetics nurse in advanced practice.* Genetics nurses in advanced practice are nurses who have successfully completed an accredited graduate (master's or doctoral) program in nursing and routinely provide genetics services to clients. They are expected to have completed a genetics curriculum that includes human, molecular, biochemical, and population genetics, technological applications, therapeutic modalities, and ethical, legal, and social implications of genetics information and technology. They are also expected to have either formal genetics clinical experiences or on-the-job training in their specified advanced practice role under the supervision of a professional trained in genetics.
- The genetics nurse in advanced practice is expected to maintain their knowledge and skill base through ongoing participation in genetics and nursing continued education. This knowledge can be acquired through completion of didactic and clinical courses

in a formal program of study leading to a master's or doctoral degree in nursing with a concentration in advanced practice in genetics nursing. Didactic or clinical courses can also be obtained through postgraduate degree certification programs. Nurses may elect to achieve a Ph.D. in Nursing or a related discipline, or a practice doctorate that includes academic courses focused on specific clinical or research genetics content. Credentialing in genetics at the advanced practice level is strongly encouraged.

- These traditional roles for genetics nurses in advanced practice have evolved to include research, education, and administration in a wide variety of clinical arenas. At the same time genetics nurses with advanced nursing degrees are using their advanced practice skills in ways that affect the genomic health of individuals, families, communities, and populations through research, education, policy, administration, and other activities. Technological advances have also expanded clinical nursing practice to include healthcare provided through telemedicine, computerized patient education, and interactive technology. As a result, contemporary genetics/genomics nursing practice is broad and diverse. The scope and standards of genetics and genomics nursing practice uses the term *genetics nurses in advanced practice,* which is intended to include the broad range of genetics nurse advanced practice roles. Advanced level genetics nurses in the United States may also have completed advanced graduate or doctoral educational preparation and certification for recognition as advanced practice registered nurses (APRNs) in the roles of certified nurse midwife, certified nurse practitioner, certified registered nurse anesthetist, or clinical nurse specialist (pp. 13-14).

■ DISCUSSION QUESTIONS

1. Analyze your personal genetic risk for disease after completing a pedigree of first- and second-degree relatives. Discuss the implications of genetic and non-genetic factors with one family member using the pedigree.

Chapter 9: Genetics, Genomics, and Transcultural Nursing 175

2. Identify key moral, ethical, and legal principles when applying genetics and genomics to vulnerable populations including pediatric and minority patients. For example, when should an individual be told that they have sickle cell trait? Should counseling occur at predictable intervals? Prior to exertional sports? Prior to reproductive decisions? Will genetics and genomics expand or reduce healthcare disparities?

3. Should direct-to-consumer genetic testing be made available commercially? What are the unintended consequences? If you elect to have genetic testing completed by your healthcare provider, should you inform your parents, siblings, or children of the results? Cousins or other genetically-descendant relatives?

4. Develop a case study or simulation using tools found on the reference list websites for use in your practice setting.

■ REFERENCES

Abbasi, J. (2017). The paternal epigenome makes its mark. *Journal of the American Medical Association, 317*(20), 2049-2051.

American College of Medical Genetics and Genomics. (n. d.). *Medical genetics: Translating genes to health* [Website]. Bethesda, MD: Author. Retrieved from www.acmg.net

American College of Medical Genetics and Genomics Board of Directors. (2016). Direct-to-consumer genetic testing: A revised position statement of the American College of Medical Genetics and Genomics. *Genetics in Medicine: Official Journal of the American College of Medical Genetics, 18*(2), 207-208.

American Nurses' Association & International Society of Nurses in Genetics. (2016). *Genetics/Genomics Nursing: Scope and Standards of Practice* (2nd ed.). Silver Spring, MD: Author.

Anwar, M. S., Iskandar, M. Z., Parry, H. M., Doney, A. S., Palmer, C. N., & Lang, C. C. (2015). The future of pharmacogenetics in the treatment of heart failure. *Pharmacogenomics, 16*(16), 1817-1827.

Badzek, L., Henaghan, M., Turner, M., & Monsen, R. (2013). Ethical, legal, and social issues in the translation of genomics into health care. *Journal of Nursing Scholarship: An Official Publication of Sigma Theta Tau International Honor Society of Nursing, 45*(1), 15-24.

Bangalore, S., Ogedegbe, G., Gyamfi, J., Guo, Y., Roy, J., Goldfeld, K., ... Shah, N. R. (2015). Outcomes with angiotensin-converting enzyme inhibitors vs. other antihypertensive agents in hypertensive Blacks. *The American Journal of Medicine, 128*(11), 1195-1203.

Barsh, G. (2014). Genetic disease. In G. Hammer and S. McPhee (Eds.), *Pathophysiology of disease: An introduction to clinical medicine* (7th ed.) Chicago, IL: McGraw Hill.

Bonham, V. L., Dover, G. J., & Brody, L. C. (2010, September 9). Screening student athletes for sickle cell trait: A social and clinical experiment. *New England Journal of Medicine, 363*(11), 997-999. doi: 10.1056/NEJMp1007639

Caraco, Y., Sheller, J., & Wood, A. J. (1999). Impact of ethnic origin and quinidine coadministration on codeine's disposition and pharmacodynamic effects. *The Journal of Pharmacology and Experimental Therapeutics, 290*(1), 413-422.

Caselli, R. J., Langbaum, J., Marchant, G. E., Lindor, R. A., Hunt, K. S., Henslin, B. R., ... Robert, J. S. (2014). Public perceptions of presymptomatic testing for Alzheimer disease. *Mayo Clinic Proceedings, 89*(10), 1389-1396.

Chang, M. T., McCarthy, J. J., & Shin, J. (2015). Clinical application of pharmacogenetics: Focusing on practical issues. *Pharmacogenomics, 16*(15), 1733-1741.

Chen, P., Lin, J. J., Lu, C. S., Ong, C. T., Hsieh, P. F., Yang, C. C., ... Shen, C. Y. (2011). Carbamazepine-induced toxic effects and HLA-B*1502 screening in Taiwan. *The New England Journal of Medicine, 364*(12), 1126-1133.

Chung, W.-H., Chang, W.-C., Lee, Y.-S., Wu, Y.-Y., Yang, C-H., Ho, H-C., ... Hung, S-I. (2014). Genetic variants associated with phenytoin-related severe cutaneous adverse reactions. *Journal of the American Medical Association, 312*(5), 525-534. doi: 10.1001/jama.2014.7859

Coakley, M., Fadiran, E. O., Parrish, L. J., Griffith, R. A., Weiss, E., & Carter, C. (2012). Dialogues on diversifying clinical trials: Successful strategies for engaging women and minorities in clinical trials. *Journal of Women's Health, 21*(7), 713-716.

Collins, S. D., Torguson, R., Gaglia, M. A., Lemesle, G., Syed, A. I., Ben-Dor, I., ... Waksman, R. (2010). Does Black ethnicity influence the development of stent thrombosis in the drug-eluting stent era? *Circulation, 122*(11), 1085-1090.

Corwin, E. J., Hogue, C. J., Pearce, B., Hill, C. C., Read, T. D., Mulle, J., ... Dunlop, A. L. (2017). Protocol for the Emory University African American vaginal, oral, and gut microbiome in pregnancy cohort study. *BMC Pregnancy and Childbirth, 17*(1), 161. doi: 10.1186/s12884-017-1357-x.

Cunningham, S. A., Kramer, M. R., & Narayan, K. M. V. (2014). Incidence of childhood obesity in the United States. *New England Journal of Medicine, 370*(5), 403-411. doi: 10.1056/NEJMoa1309753

Cystic Fibrosis Foundation. (n. d.). *8 ways to guard against germs in everyday life* [Webpage]. Bethesda, MD: Author. Retrieved from https://www.cff.org/Life-With-CF/Daily-Life/Germs-and-Staying-Healthy/How-Can-You-Avoid-Germs/8-Ways-to-Guard-Against-Germs-in-Everyday-Life/

Dahm, R. (2005). Friedrich Miescher and the discovery of DNA. *Developmental Biology, 278*(2), 274-288.

DeFeo, K., Sykora, K., Eley, S., & Vincent, D. (2014). How does pharmacogenetic testing alter the treatment course and patient response for chronic-pain patients in comparison with the current "trial-and-error" standard of care? *Journal of the American Association of Nurse Practitioners, 26*(10), 530-536.

Delaney, S. K., & Christman, M. F. (2016). Direct-to-consumer genetic testing: Perspectives on its value in healthcare. *Clinical Pharmacology and Therapeutics, 99*(2), 146-148.

Dias, B. G., Maddox, S. A., Klengel, T., & Ressler, K. J. (2015). Epigenetic mechanisms underlying learning and the inheritance of learned behaviors. *Trends in Neurosciences, 38*(2), 96-107.

Diouf, B., Crews, K. R., Lew, G., Pei, D., Cheng, C., Bao, J., … Evans, W. E. (2015). Association of an inherited genetic variant with vincristine-related peripheral neuropathy in children with acute lymphoblastic leukemia. *Journal of the American Medical Association, 313*(8), 815-823.

Domchek, S. M., Jameson, J. L., & Miesfeldt, S. (2015). The practice of genetics in clinical medicine. In D. Kasper, A. Fauci, S. Jauser, D. L. Long, J. L. Jameson, and J. Loscalzo (Eds.), *Harrison's Principles of Internal Medicine* (19th ed.). Chicago, IL: McGraw Hill.

Easton, D. F., Pharoah, P. D., Antoniou, A. C., Tischkowitz, M., Tavtigian, S. V., Nathanson, K. L., … Foulkes, W. D. (2015). Gene-panel sequencing and the prediction of breast-cancer risk. *The New England Journal of Medicine, 372*(23), 2243-2257.

Eichelbaum, M., & Evert, B. (1996). Influence of pharmacogenetics on drug disposition and response. *Clinical and Experimental Pharmacology & Physiology, 23*(10-11), 983-985.

Feil, R., & Fraga, M. F. (2011). Epigenetics and the environment: Emerging patterns and implications. *Nature Reviews Genetics, 13*(2), 97-109.

Ferdinand, K. C., Elkayam, U., Mancini, D., Ofili, E., Pina, I., Anand, I., … Leggett, C. (2014). Use of isosorbide, dinitrate, and hydralazine in African-Americans with heart failure 9 years after the African-American Heart Failure Trial. *The American Journal of Cardiology, 114*(1), 151-159.

Holland, A. T., & Palaniappan, L. P. (2012). Problems with the collection and interpretation of Asian-American health data: Omission, aggregation, and extrapolation. *Annals of Epidemiology, 22*(6), 397-405.

Ferrari, R., Parker, L. S., Grubs, R. E., & Krishnamurti, L. (2015). Sickle cell trait screening of collegiate athletes: Ethical reasons for program reform. *Journal of Genetic Counseling, 24*(6), 873-877.

Fishbain, D. A., Fishbain, D., Lewis, J., Cutler, R. B., Cole, B., Rosemoff, H. L., & Rosomoff, R. S. (2004). Genetic testing for enzymes of drug metabolism: Does it have clinical utility for pain medicine at the present time? A structured review. *American Academy of Pain Medicine, 5*(1), 81-93.

Fontelles, C. C., Carney, E., Clarke, J., Nguyen, N. M., Yin, C., Jin, L., … de Assis, S. (2016). Paternal overweight is associated with increased breast cancer risk in daughters in a mouse model. *Scientific Reports, 6*, 28602. doi: 10.1038/srep28602

Franklin, T. B., Saab, B. J., Mansuy, I. M. (2012). Neural mechanisms of stress resilience and vulnerability. *Neuron, 75*(5), 747-761.

Freedman, B. I. (2003). Susceptibility genes for hypertension and renal failure. *Journal of the American Society of Nephrologists, 14*(7), Supplement 2, S192-S194.

Fu, Z., Shrubsole, M. J., Smalley, W. E., Wu, H., Chen, Z., Shyr, Y., … Zheng, W. (2012). Lifestyle factors and their combined impact on the risk of colorectal polyps. *American Journal of Epidemiology, 176*(9), 766-776.

Gammal, R. S., Crews, K. R., Haidar, C. E., Hoffman, J. M., Baker, D. K.,. Barker, P. J., … Hankins, J. (2016, July). Pharmacogenetics for safe codeine use in sickle cell disease. *Pediatrics, 138*(1), e20153479.

Glittenberg (Hinrichs), J. (2002). The biocultural basis of transcultural nursing. In M. M. Leininger and M. R. McFarland (Eds.), *Transcultural nursing: Concepts, theories, research, & practice* (3rd ed., p. 162). New York, NY: McGraw Hill.

Goodman, D. M., Lynm, C., & Livingston, E. H. (2013). Genomic medicine. *Journal of the American Medical Association, 309*(14), 1544. doi:10.1001/jama.2013.1927

Gordon, J. I., & Knight, R. (2015). The human microbiome. In D. L. Kasper, A. S. Fauci, S. L. Hauser, D. L. Longo, J. L. Jameson, & J. Loscalzo (Eds.), *Harrison's principles of internal medicine* (19th ed.). New York, NY: McGraw Hill.

Jacob, J. A. (2016). Twenty years after folic acid fortification: FDA ponders expansion to corn masa flour. *Journal of the American Medical Association, 315*(17), 1821-1822.

Gosden, R. G., & Feinberg, A. P. (2007). Genetics and epigenetics—nature's pen-and-pencil set. *The New England Journal of Medicine, 356*(7), 731-733.

Gradwohl, S. C., Aranake, A., Abdallah, A. B., McNair, P., Lin, N., Fritz, B. A., … Avidan, M. S. (2015). Intraoperative awareness risk, anesthetic sensitivity, and anesthetic management for patients with natural red hair: A matched cohort study. *Canadian Journal of Anaesthesia/ Journal Canadien D'anesthesie, 62*(4), 345-355.

Grover, S., & Kukreti, R. (2014). HLA alleles and hypersensitivity to carbamazepine: An updated systematic review with meta-analysis. *Pharmacogenetics and Genomics, 24*(2), 94-112.

Haiman, C. A., Patterson, N., Freedman, M. L., Myers, S. R., Pike, M. C., Waliszewska, A., ... Reich, D. (2007). Multiple regions within 8q24 independently affect risk for prostate cancer. *Nature Genetics, 39*(5), 638-644.

Hawkins, A. K., & Ho, A. (2012). Genetic counseling and the ethical issues around direct to consumer genetic testing. *Journal of Genetic Counseling, 21*(3), 367-373. doi: 10.1007/s10897-012-9488-8.

Herman, W. H., & Cohen, R. M. (2012). Racial and ethnic differences in the relationship between HgbA1C and blood glucose: Implications for the diagnosis of diabetes. *The Journal of Clinical Endocrinology & Metabolism, 97*(4), 1067-1072.

Hetherington, S., Hughes, A. R., Mosteller, M., Shortino, D., Baker, K. L., Spreen, W., ... Roses, A. D. (2002). Genetic variations in HLA-B region and hypersensitivity reactions to abacavir. *The Lancet, 359*(9312), 1121-1122.

Hollister, E. B., Gao, C., & Versalovic, J. (2014). Compositional and functional features of the gastrointestinal microbiome and their effects on human health. *Gastroenterology, 146*(6), 1449-1458.

Hunt, S. A., Abraham, W. T., Chin, M. H., Feldman, A. M., Francis, G. S., Ganiats, T. G., ... Yancy, C. W. (2009). Focused update incorporated into the ACC/AHA 2005 Guidelines for the Diagnosis and Management of Heart Failure in Adults. *Journal of the American College of Cardiology, 53*(15), e1-e90.

Jameson, J., & Kopp, P. (2015). Genes, the environment, and disease. In D. L. Kasper, A. S. Fauci, S. L. Hauser, D. L. Longo, J. L. Jameson, & J. Loscalzo (Eds.), *Harrison's principles of internal medicine* (19th ed.). New York, NY: McGraw Hill.

Jewish Genetic Disease Consortium. (n. d.). *Tay-Sachs Disease.* Retrieved from http://www.jewishgeneticdiseases.org/jewish-genetic-diseases/

Kane, G. C., Karon, B. L., Mahoney, D. W., Redfield, M. M., Roger, V. L., Burnett, J. C., ... Rodeheffer, R. J. (2011). Progression of left ventricular diastolic dysfunction and risk of heart failure. *Journal of the American Medical Association, 306*(8), 856-863.

Khanna, D., FitzGerald, J. D., Khanna, P. P., Bae, S., Singh, M., Neogi, T., ... Terkeltaub, R. (2012). 2012 American College of Rheumatology Guidelines for Management of Gout Part I: Systematic Non-pharmacologic and Pharmacologic Therapeutic Approaches to Hyperuricemia. *Arthritis Care & Research, 64*(10), 1431-1446. doi.org/10.1002/acr.21772

Kerber, A. S., & Ledbetter, N. J. (2017a). Standards of practice: Applying genetics and genomics resources to oncology. *Clinical Journal of Oncology Nursing, 21*(2), 169-173.

Kerber, A. S., & Ledbetter, N. J. (2017b). Scope and standards: Defining the advanced practice role in genetics. *Clinical Journal of Oncology Nursing, 21*(3), 309-313.

Kimmel, S. E., French, B., Kasner, S. E., Johnson, J. A., Anderson, J. L., Gage, B. F., ... Ellenberg, J. H. (2013). A pharmacogenetic versus a clinical algorithm for warfarin dosing. *The New England Journal of Medicine, 369*(24), 2283-2293.

Klitzman, R. (2010). Views of discrimination among individuals confronting genetic disease. *Journal of Genetic Counseling, 19*(1), 68-83.

Koleck, T. A., Bender, C. M., Sereka, S. M., Ahrendt, G., Jankowetz, R. C., McGuire, K. P.,... Conley, Y. P. (2014). Apolipoprotein e genotype and cognitive function in postmenopausal women with early-stage breast cancer. *Oncology Nursing Forum, 41*(6), 313-325.

Kruk, J., & Czerniak, U. (2013). Physical activity and its relation to cancer risk: Updating the evidence. *Asian Pacific Journal of Cancer Prevention (APJCP), 14*(7), 3993-4003.

Labrie, V., Buske, O. J., Oh, E., Jeremian, R., Ptak, C., Gasiunas, G. (June 2016). Lactase nonpersistence is directed by DNA-variation-dependent epigenetic aging. *Nature Structural & Molecular Biology, 23*(6), 566-573. doi: http://dx.doi.org/10.1038/nsmb.3227

Leininger, M. M. (Ed.). (1978). *Transcultural nursing: Concepts, theories, & practices.* New York, NY: Wiley & Sons.

Leininger, M. M. (Ed.). (1991). *Culture care diversity and universality: Theory of nursing.* New York, NY: National League for Nursing.

Leininger, M. M. (2002a). Culture care assessments for congruent competency practices. In M. M. Leininger and M. R. McFarland (Eds.), *Transcultural nursing: Concepts, theories, research, & practice* (3rd ed., pp. 117-120). New York, NY: McGraw Hill.

Leininger, M. M. (2002b). Essential transcultural nursing concepts, principles, examples, and policy statements. In M. M. Leininger and M. R. McFarland (Eds.), *Transcultural nursing: Concepts, theories, research, & practice* (3rd ed., pp. 53-54). New York, NY: McGraw Hill.

Levenson, D. (2016). Genetic discrimination lawsuit raises broader concerns about testing, privacy: Case involves middle school student impacted by results of genetic screening test as newborn. *American Journal of Medical Genetics, Part A, 170*(5), 1111-1112.

Liem, E. B., Lin, C. M., Suleman, M. I., Doufas, A. G., Gregg RG, Veauthier, J. M., ... Sessler DI. (2004). Anesthetic requirement is increased in redheads. *Anesthesiology, 101*(2), 279-283.

Lim, K. S., Kwan, P., & Tan, C.T. (2008). Association of HLA-B*1502 allele and carbamazepine-induced severe adverse cutaneous drug reaction among Asians: A review. *Neurology Asia, 13*, 15-21.

Li-Wan-Po, A. (2012). Pharmacogenetics and personalized medicine. *Journal of Clinical Pharmacy and Therapeutics, 37*(6), 617-619.

Locsin, R., Purnell, M., Tanioka, T., & Osaka, K. (2016). Human rights and humanoid relationships in nursing and complexity science. In A. W. Davidson, M. A. Ray, and M. C. Turkel (Eds.), *Nursing, caring, and complexity science: For human-environment wellbeing* (1st ed., p. 347). New York, NY: Springer.

McCance, K. L., & Huether, S. E. (2014). *Pathophysiology: The biologic basis for disease in adults and children* (7th ed.). St. Louis, MO: Elsevier.

McCormack, M., Alfirevic, A., Bourgeois, S., Farrell, J., Kasperaviciute, D., Carrington, … Permohamed, M. (2011). HLA-A*3101 and carbamazepine-induced hypersensitivity reactions in Europeans. *New England Journal of Medicine, 364*(12), 1134-1143.

McClain, M. R., Nathanson, K. L., Palomaki, G. E., & Haddow, J. E. (2005). An evaluation of BRCA1 and BRCA2 founder mutations penetrance estimates for breast cancer among Ashkenazi Jewish women. *Genetics in Medicine: Official Journal of the American College of Medical Genetics, 7*(1), 34-39.

McPherson, N. O., Bakos, H. W., Owens, J. A., Setchell, B. P., & Lane, M. (2013). Improving metabolic health in obese male mice via diet and exercise restores embryo development and fetal growth. *PloS One, 8*(8), e71459.

McReynolds, K., & Lewis, S. (2017) Genetic counseling for hereditary cancer: A primer for NPs. *The Nurse Practitioner, 42*(7), 28-29.

Ma, R. C., Tutino, G. E., Lillycrop, K. A., Hanson, M. A., & Tam, W. H. (2015). Maternal diabetes, gestational diabetes and the role of epigenetics in their long term effects on offspring. *Progress in Biophysics and Molecular Biology, 118*(1-2), 55-68.

March of Dimes, & Spina Bifida Association. (2012). *Coalition petitions FDA to fortify corn masa flour with folic acid* [Webpage]. White Plains, NY: Authors. Retrieved from http://www.marchofdimes.org/news/coalition-petitions-fda-to-fortify-corn-masa-flour-with-folic-acid.aspx

Martos, S. N., Tang W-Y., & Wang, Z. (2015). Elusive inheritance: Transgenerational effects and epigenetic inheritance in human environmental disease. *Progress in Biophysics and Molecular Biology, 118*(1-2), 44-54.

McFarland, M. R., & Wehbe-Alamah, H. B. (2015). The theory of culture care diversity and universality. In M. R. McFarland and H. B. Wehbe-Alamah (Eds.), *Leininger's culture care diversity and universality: A worldwide nursing theory* (3rd ed., pp. 1-34). Burlington, MA: Jones & Bartlett Learning.

McKillip, R. P., Borden, B. A., Galecki, P., Ham, S. A., Patrick-Miller, L., Hall, J. P., … O'Donnell, P. H. (2016). Patient perceptions of care as influenced by a large institutional pharmacogenomic implementation program. *Clinical Pharmacology and Therapeutics, 102*(1),106-114.

Mega, J. L., Close, S. L., Wiviott, S. D., Shen, L., Hockett, R. D., Brandt, J. T., … Sabatine, M. S. (2009). Cytochrome p-450 polymorphisms and response to clopidogrel. *The New England Journal of Medicine, 360*(4), 354-362.

Mehta, H., Armstrong, A., Swett, K., Shah, S. J., Allison, M. A., Hurwitz, B., … Rodriguez, C. J. (2016). Burden of systolic and diastolic left ventricular dysfunction among Hispanics in the United States: Insights From the echocardiographic study of Latinos. *Circulation: Heart Failure, 9*(4), e002733 1-11. doi: 10.1161/CIRCHEARTFAILURE.115.002733

Mersha, T. B., & Abebe, T. (2015). Self-reported race/ethnicity in the age of genomic research: Its potential impact on understanding health disparities. *BMC Human Genomics, 9*, 1-15. doi 10.1186/s40246-014-0023-x

Metz, G. A. S., Ng, J. W. Y., Kovalchuk, I., & Olson, D. M. (2015). Ancestral experience as a game changer in stress vulnerability and disease outcomes. *BioEssays: News and Reviews in Molecular, Cellular, and Developmental Biology, 37*(6), 602-611.

Nan, H., Hutter, C. M., Lin, Y., Jacobs, E. J., Ulrich, C. M., White, E., …. Chan, A. T. for the Colon Cancer Family Registry and the Genetics and Epidemiology of Colorectal Cancer Consortium. (2015). Association of aspirin and NSAID use with risk of colorectal cancer according to genetic variants. *Journal of the American Medical Association, 313*(11), 1133-1142. doi: 10.1001/jama.2015.1815

Narasimhan, S., & Lohoff, F. W. (2012). Pharmacogenetics of antidepressant drugs: Current clinical practice and future directions. *Pharmacogenomics, 13*(4), 441-464.

National Society of Genetic Counselors. (2015, June 19). *National Society of Genetic Counselors position statement: Direct access to genetic testing.* Chicago, IL: Author. Retrieved from http://www.nsgc.org/

Nielsen, D., Utrankar, A., Reyes, J. A., Simons, D. D., & Kosten, T. (2012). Epigenetics of drug abuse: Predisposition or response. *Pharmacogenomics, 13*(10), 1149-1160.

Nirenberg, M. (n. d.). *Deciphering the genetic code: Gregor Mendel: The father of modern genetics* [Webpage]. Bethesda, MD: U. S. Department of Health and Human Services, National Institutes of Health, Office of NIH History. Retrieved from https://history.nih.gov/exhibits/nirenberg/HS1_mendel.htm

Nolan, D., Gaudieri, S., & Mallal, S. (2003). Pharmacogenetics: A practical role in predicting antiretroviral drug toxicity? *Journal of HIV Therapy, 8*(2), 36-41.

O'Donnell, P. H., Danahey, K., & Ratain, M. J. (2016). The outlier in all of us: Why implementing pharmacogenomics could matter for everyone. *Clinical Pharmacology and Therapeutics, 99*(4), 401-404. doi: 10.1002/cpt.333

Offit, K. (2011). Personalized medicine: New genomics, old lessons. *Human Genetics, 130*(1), 3-14.

Ogedegbe, G., Shah, N. R., Phillips, C., Goldfeld, K., Roy, J., Guo Y., ... Bangalore, S. (2015). Comparative effectiveness of angiotensin-converting enzyme inhibitor-based treatment on cardiovascular outcomes in hypertensive Blacks versus Whites. *Journal of the American College of Cardiology, 66*(11), 1224-1233.

Otado, J., Kwagyan, J., Edwards, D., Ukaegbu, A., Rockcliffe, F., & Osafo, N. (2015). Culturally competent strategies for recruitment and retention of African American populations into clinical trials. *Clinical and Translational Science, 8*(5), 460-466.

Pare, G., Eriksson, N., Lehr, T., Connolly, S., Eikelboom, J., Ezekowitz, M. D., ... Wallentin, L. (2013). Genetic determinants of dabigatran plasma levels and their relation to bleeding. *Circulation, 127*(13), 1404-1412.

Porth, C. M. (2014). *Essentials of pathophysiology: Concepts of altered health states* (4th ed.). Philadelphia, PA: Lippincott | Wolters Kluwer.

Rahim-Williams, B., Riley, J., Williams, A. K., & Fillingim, R. B. (2012). A quantitative review of ethnic group differences in experimental pain response: Do biology, psychology, and culture matter? *Pain Medicine, 13*(4), 522-540.

Rao, M., & Balakrishnan, V. S. (2009). The genetic basis of kidney disease risk in African Americans: MYH9 as a new candidate gene. *American Journal of Kidney Diseases, 53*(4), 579-583.

Ray, M. A. (2016). *Transcultural caring dynamics in nursing and health care* (2nd ed., p. 111). Philadelphia, PA: F. A. Davis.

Read, C. Y., & Ward, L. D. (2016). Faculty performance on the Genomic Nursing Concept Inventory. *Journal of Nursing Scholarship, 48*(1), 5-13.

Resta, R. G. (2006). Defining and redefining the scope and goals of genetic counseling. *American Journal of Medical Genetics, Part C: Seminars in Medical Genetics, 142C*(4), 269-275.

Rodriguez, C. J., Allison, M., Daviglus, M. L., Isasi, C. R., Keller, C., Leira, E. C., ... Sims, M. and the American Heart Association Council on Epidemiology and Prevention; American Heart Association Council on Clinical Cardiology; American Heart Association Council on Cardiovascular and Stroke Nursing. (2014). Status of cardiovascular disease and stroke in Hispanics/Latinos in the United States: A science advisory from the American Heart Association. *Circulation, 130*(7), 593-625.

Rotimi, C. N., & Jorde, L. B. (2010). Ancestry and disease in the age of genomic medicine. *The New England Journal of Medicine, 363*(16), 1551-1558.

Sadee, W. (2017). Personalized therapeutics and pharmacogenomics: Integral to personalized health care. *Pharmaceutical Research, 34*(8), 1535-1538.

Sagan, C. (1977). *Dragons of Eden: Speculations on the evolution of human intelligence.* New York, NY: Random House.

Schnepp, R. W., Bosse, K. R., & Maris, J. M. (2015). Improving patient outcomes with cancer genomics: Unique opportunities and challenges in pediatric oncology. *Journal of the American Medical Association, 314*(9), 881-883.

Seibert, D. C. (2014). Genomics and nurse practitioner practice. *The Nurse Practitioner, 39*(10), 18-28.

Silvers, A., & Stein, M. A. (2003). Human rights and genetic discrimination: Protecting genomics' promise for public health. *The Journal of Law, Medicine & Ethics: A Journal of the American Society of Law, Medicine & Ethics, 31*(3), 377-389.

Sordillo, J. E., Zhou, Y., McGeachie, M. J., Ziniti, J., Lange, N., Laranjo, N., ... Litonjua, A. A. (2017). Factors influencing the infant gut microbiome at age 3-6 months: Findings from the ethnically diverse Vitamin D Antenatal Asthma Reduction Trial (VDAART). *The Journal of Allergy and Clinical Immunology, 139*(2), 482-491.

Soubry, A., Schildkraut, J. M., Murtha, A., Wang, F., Huang, Z., Bernal, A., ... Hoyo, C. (2013). Paternal obesity is associated with IGF2 hypomethylation in newborns: Results from a Newborn Epigenetics Study (NEST) cohort. *BMC Medicine, 11*, 29. doi.org/10.1186/1741-7015-11-29

Spector, R. E. (2013). *Cultural diversity in health and illness* (8th ed., p. 23). Boston, MA: Pearson.

Spokoyny, L., Barazangi, N., Jaramillo, B., Rose, J., Chen, C., & Tong, D. (2014). Reduced clopidogrel metabolism in a multiethnic population: Prevalence and rates of recurrent cerebrovascular events. *Journal of Stroke and Cerebrovascular Diseases, 23*(4), 694-698.

Swallow, D. M. (2003). Genetics of lactase persistence and lactose intolerance. *Annual Review of Genetics, 37*(1), 197-219.

Tan, D. S., Mok, T. S., & Rebbeck, T. R. (2016). Cancer genomics: Diversity and disparity across ethnicity and geography. *Journal of Clinical Oncology: Official Journal of the American Society of Clinical Oncology, 34*(1), 91-101.

Tarini, B. A., Tercyak, K. P., & Wilfond, B. S. (2011). Commentary: Children and predictive genomic testing: disease prevention, research protection, and our future. *Journal of Pediatric Psychology, 36*(10), 1113-1121.

Thomas, T., Gilbert, J., & Meyer, F. (2012). Metagenomics—a guide from sampling to data analysis. *Microbial Informatics and Experimentation, 2*, 3. http://doi.org/10.1186/2042-5783-2-3

Taylor, C., Kavanagh, P., & Zuckerman, B. (2014). Sickle cell trait: Neglected opportunities in the era of genomic medicine. *Journal of the American Medical Association, 311*(15), 1495-1496.

Tohkin, M., Kaniwa, N., Saito, Y., Sugiyama, E., Kurose, K., Nishikawa, J., ... Ikezawa, Z. (2013). A whole-genome association study of major determinants for allopurinol-related Stevens-Johnson syndrome and toxic epidermal necrolysis in Japanese patients. *The Pharmacogenomics Journal, 13*(1), 60-69.

United Nations Educational, Scientific and Cultural Organisation. (1997). *Universal declaration on the human genome and human rights*. Retrieved from http://www.unesco.org/new/en/social-and-human-sciences/themes/bioethics/human-genome-and-human-rights/

U. S. Department of Health and Human Services, National Institutes of Health, National Center for Biotechnology Information, U. S. National Library of Medicine. (n. d.-a). *Online Mendelian Inheritance in Man* (OMIM) [Catalogue]. Bethesda, MD: Author. Accessible at ncbi.nlm.nih.gov/omim

U. S. Department of Health and Human Services, National Institutes of Health, National Center for Biotechnology Information, U. S. National Library of Medicine. (n. d.-b). [Website]. Bethesda, MD: Author. Accessible at http://www.ncbi.nlm.nih.gov/

U. S. Department of Health and Human Services, National Institutes of Health, National Center for Biotechnology Information [Website]. (n. d.-c). *The International HapMap Project*. Bethesda, MD: Author. Accessible at https://www.ncbi.nlm.nih.gov/variation/news/NCBI_retiring_HapMap/

U. S. Department of Health and Human Services, National Institutes of Health, National Human Genome Research Institute. (n. d.-d). [Website]. Bethesda, MD: Author. Accessible at www.nih.gov/about-nih/what-we-do/nih-almanac/national-human-genome-research-institute-nhgri

U. S. Department of Health and Human Services, National Institutes of Health, National Human Genome Research Institute. (n. d.-e). *Health* [Website]. Bethesda, MD: Author. Accessible at https://www.genome.gov/health/

U. S. Department of Health and Human Services, National Institutes of Health, National Human Genome Research Institute. (n. d.-f). *Specific genetic disorders* [Website]. Bethesda, MD: Author. Accessible at https://www.genome.gov/10001204/specific-genetic-disorders/

U. S. Department of Health and Human Services, National Institutes of Health, National Institute of General Medical Sciences and Stanford University. (n. d.-g). *Pharmacogenomics Knowledgebase (PharmGKB)*. Stanford, CA: Authors. Accessible at www.pharmgkb.org

U. S. Department of Health and Human Services, National Institutes of Health, National Library of Medicine, Genetics Home Reference. (n. d.-h). *What are single polymorphisms (SNPs)?* Bethesda, MD: Author. Retrieved from https://ghr.nlm.nih.gov/primer/genomicresearch/snp

U. S. Department of Health and Human Services, Stanford University & St. Jude's Children's Medical Center, Clinical Pharmacogenetics Implementation Consortium of the Pharmacogenomics Research Network. (n. d.-i). *Drugs with FDA Recommended or Required Genetic Testing* [Table]. Stanford, CA/Memphis, TN: Authors. Accessible at https://cpicpgx.org/genes-drugs/

U. S. Department of Health and Human Services, Food and Drug Administration, Drugs. (2008). *Information for healthcare professionals: Abacavir (marketed as Ziagen) and Abacavir-containing medications*. Silver Spring, MD: Author. Retrieved from http://www.fda.gov/Drugs/DrugSafety/PostmarketDrugSafetyInformationforPatientsandProviders/ucm123927.htm

U. S. Department of Health and Human Services, Food and Drug Administration, Drugs. (2010). *FDA Drug Safety Communication: Reduced effectiveness of Plavix (clopidogrel) in patients who are poor metabolizers of the drug*. Silver Spring, MD: Author. Retrieved from https://www.fda.gov/drugs/drugsafety/postmarketdrugsafetyinformationforpatientsandproviders/ucm203888.htm

U. S. Department of Health and Human Services, The Centers for Disease Control and Prevention. (2010). CDC Grand Rounds: Additional opportunities to prevent neural tube defects with folic acid fortification. *Morbidity and Mortality Weekly Report*, (2010, August 13), *59*(31), 980-984. Accessible at http://1.usa.gov/1S4pw3f

U. S. Department of Health and Human Services, National Institutes of Health, National Human Genome Research Institute. (2014). *Talking Glossary of Genetic Terms*. Bethesda, MD: Author.

U. S. Department of Health and Human Services, Office of Population Affairs. (2014). *Affordable care act collaborative* [Webpage]. Washington, DC: Author. Accessible at https://www.hhs.gov/opa/title-x-family-planning/affordable-care-act/initiatives/aca-collaborative/index.html

U. S. Equal Employment Opportunity Commission. (2009a). *The Genetic Information Nondiscrimination Act of 2008* [Webpage]. Washington, DC: Author. Accessible at https://www.eeoc.gov/laws/statutes/gina.cfm

U. S. Equal Employment Opportunity Commission. (2009b). *Genetic Information Discrimination* [Webpage]. Washington, DC: Author. Accessible at http://www.eeoc.gov/laws/types/genetic.cfm

U. S. Government Publishing Office, Office of the Federal Register, National Archives and Records Administration, Rules and Regulation Section. (1996, March 5). Food standards: Amendment of standards of identity for enriched grain products to require addition of folic acid. *Federal Register*, *61*(44), 8781-8797. Accessible at https://www.federalregister.gov/documents/1996/03/05/96-5013/food-labeling-health-claims-and-label-statements-folate-and-neural-tube-defects

Vuilleumier, P. H., Stamer, U. M., & Landau, R. (2012). Pharmacogenomic considerations in opioid analgesia. *Pharmacogenomics and Personalized Medicine, 5*(2012 Annual), 73-87.

Walko, C. M., & McLeod, H. (2012). Use of CYP2D6 genotyping in practice: Tamoxifen dose adjustment. *Pharmacogenomics, 13*(6), 691-697.

Wang, L., McLeod, H. L., & Weinshilbourm, R. M. (2011). Genomics and drug response. *New England Journal of Medicine, 364*(12), 1144-1153.

Wang, H., Park, S. L., Stram, D. O., Haiman, C. A., Wilkens, L. R., Hecht, S. S., … Le Marchand, L. (2015). Associations between genetic ancestries and nicotine metabolism biomarkers in the multiethnic cohort study. *American Journal of Epidemiology, 182*(11), 945-951.

Wehbe-Alamah, H. B. (2015). Folk care beliefs and practices of traditional Lebanese and Syrian Muslims in the Midwestern United States. In M. R. McFarland and H. B. Wehbe-Alamah (Eds.), *Leininger's culture care diversity and universality: A worldwide nursing theory* (3rd ed., p. 140). Burlington, MA: Jones & Bartlett Learning.

Wertz, D. (1999). Genetic discrimination: Results of a survey of genetics professionals, primary care physicians, patients, and public. *Health Law Review, 7*(3), 7-8.

Whirl-Carrillo, M., McDonagh, E. M., Hebert, J. M., Gong, L., Sangkuhl, K., Thorn, C. F., … Klein, T. E. (2012). Pharmacogenomics knowledge for personalized medicine. *Clinical Pharmacology and Therapeutics, 92*(4), 414-417.

Wilke, R. A., & Dolan, M. E. (2011). Genetics and variable drug response. *Journal of the American Medical Association (JAMA), 306*(3), 306-307.

Williams, J., Mai, C. T., Mulinare, J., Isenburg, J., Flood, T. J., Ethen, M., … Kirby, R. S. (2015). Updated estimates of neural tube defects prevented by mandatory folic acid fortification - United States, 1995-2011. *Morbidity and Mortality Weekly Report, 64*(1), 1-5.

Yohn, N. L., Bartolomei, M. S., & Blendy, J. A. (2015). Multigenerational and transgenerational inheritance of drug exposure: The effects of alcohol, opiates, cocaine, marijuana, and nicotine. *Progress in Biophysics and Molecular Biology, 118*(1-2), 21-33.

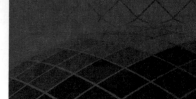

10

Transcultural Food Functions, Beliefs, and Practices

Hiba B. Wehbe-Alamah

> *"Food plays a significant role in the biological, social, political, cultural as well as the very personal spheres of our everyday lives.... Food is an integral part of all cultures around the world, thus having a universal significance. However, food is associated with a variety of practices and endowed with diverse meanings across cultures, and therefore it has a potential to represent cultural specificities and differences"* *(Hinnerová, 2007, p. 92).*

■ INTRODUCTION

Food beliefs and practices are closely intertwined with the social fabric of everyday life (Fernandez, Rolley, Rajaratnam, Everett, & Davidson, 2015). The topic of food is popular and infiltrates people's lives at home, the workplace, social gatherings, health care settings, and virtually every place where people live or interact with each other (Leininger, 2002). From an anthropological perspective, food is more than a biological source of nutrition and has social, economic, political, religious, and cultural meanings and uses (Leininger, 2002). *Food as one of the most fundamental manifestations of culture can become a transcultural device. But its sole ingesting is not enough. It is only a step, though important, towards different forms of communication. However, the potential of food to establish awareness of diversity, challenge exclusionary attitudes and stimulate cross-cultural exchanges and interaction should not be underestimated* (Hinnerová, 2007, pp. 87-88).

Food beliefs and lifeways are often associated with cultural identity (Koening, Dutta, Kandula, & Palaniappan, 2012; Momin, Chung, & Olson, 2014; Vue, Wolff, & Goto, 2011) and function as an indicator of social status (Johnson, White, Boyd, & Cohen, 2011). Food customs embody symbolic meaning and values (Shatenstein & Ghadirian, 1998; Wright St-Clair, Pierce, Bunrayong, Rattakorn, Vittayakorn, Shordike, & Hocking, 2013). From a transcultural nursing view, food remains essential for human growth, health, and cultural survival (Leininger, 2002). The literature is rich with studies that illustrate how food impacts social relationships and cohesion, nurtures intergenerational bonds, fosters cultural unity and community solidarity, and marks group boundaries (Fernandez et al., 2015; Johnson et al., 2011; Koening et al., 2012; Wright St-Clair et al., 2013).

Dietary habits vary from culture to culture. Cultural dietary norms affect health, illness, and nutrition (Farahmand, Tehrani, Amiri, & Azizi, 2012; James,

2004; Lee, Yang, & Yang, 2013; Leung, 2013). Dietary choices are sometimes manifestations of faith and reflect adherence to religious rules and taboos (Johnson et al., 2011; Nath, 2010; Shatenstein & Ghadrian, 1998). Culture-specific food choices and lifeways are influenced by acculturation and perceptions of what is culturally acceptable, prohibited, and needed (James, 2004; Shatenstein & Ghardian, 1998; Vue et al., 2011). Knowledge of food beliefs, practices, and lifeways, as well as facilitators and barriers to healthy eating practices is extremely important for nurses and other health care providers to learn so they can provide culturally meaningful, congruent, and beneficial integrative care (Chen, Juon, & Lee, 2012; Fernandez et al., 2015; Leininger, 2002; Shatenstein & Ghadirian, 1998).

In this chapter, the relevance of food beliefs, meanings, uses, symbols, practices, and functions is highlighted from a transcultural nursing perspective to help nurses and other healthcare professionals understand the role of food in keeping people well and in aiding recovery from illness. Differences and similarities related to food functions and uses among Western and non-Western cultures are discussed. Since culture strongly influences food beliefs and uses in health and wellness, nurses and other healthcare providers need to recognize the significant part cultural food factors play in the care of clients from diverse cultures. Conducting a cultural food assessment to gain an understanding of culture-specific transcultural food beliefs, functions, and practices, will assist in the formulation and delivery of integrative culturally sensitive and congruent care practices.

■ CULTURAL FOOD MEANINGS AND SYMBOLS

Cultural beliefs, practices, lifeways, and customs have long influenced food choices and habits (Amarasekara, Fongkaew, Turale, Wimalasekara, & Chanprasit, 2014). However, traditional dietary selections are often not recognized as an important aspect of culture that impacts overall health (Koenig et al., 2012). In order to provide culturally meaningful and congruent care to people of diverse cultural backgrounds, it is important to understand the cultural meanings of food and what they symbolize.

A Marker of Cultural and/or Ethnic Identity

Food attitudes and behaviors are often established early in life and are shaped by cultural, psychosocial, and socioeconomic factors (James, 2004). Food selection, preparation, and timing and manner of serving are often recognized as socially organized behavior that symbolizes and reflects ethnic identity (Koenig et al., 2012). Members of a cultural group may consciously or unconsciously participate in food behaviors to "preserve traditions and maintain group identity" (James, 2004, p. 351). Traditional foods are integral to the development and maintenance or retaining of ethnic identity (Momin et al., 2013; Vue et al., 2011). Food-related activities signify cultural unity, cultural stability, and continuance and handing on of cultural heritage and traditions (Wright-St Clair et al., 2013). They may hold similar meanings or unique expressions across cultures (Wright-St Clair et al., 2013).

A Marker of Social Identity

Food behaviors define social meanings and interpersonal and nonpersonal relationships (Koenig et al., 2012; Wright-St Clair et al., 2013). Food choices that are influenced by cultural, religious, and social norms help to create and maintain social identities and solidify group membership (Koenig et al., 2012; Wright-St Clair et al., 2013). Diet plays an important role in culture and self-identity and provides the basis for group bonding, socialization, and the development of a social support systems (Vue et al., 2011). For example, many Thai women view preparation of traditional foods as an action that is imbued with the symbolic meaning of helping to create a strong, intergenerational society and use special ingredients to instill traditional meanings into their dishes. Accordingly, long glass noodles are used to symbolize having long lives and cooking *khanom jok* (a dessert) signifies togetherness (Wright-St Clair et al., 2013).

Social relationships and lived experiences, as well as life trajectories, environmental, and cultural contexts affect food choices and behaviors (Koenig et al., 2012). Social status may also be determined by food choices. Dietary selections and habits, such as type of food consumed and order of food serving, may indicate higher or lower position within the same group or relative to another (Johnson et al., 2011). Food habits may promote social cohesion and dietary intimacy, equality, solidarity, and harmony among group members (Fernandez et al., 2015; Koenig et al., 2012; Wright-St Clair et al., 2013). Traditional foods propagate a sense of belonging and a connection to a social group (James, 2004). On the other hand, food habits may also lead to increased dietary fragmentation, distance, and inequality among group members (Koenig et al., 2012).

Another symbolic food use that indicates social status is associated with lifecycle initiation rites (Leininger, 2002). Traditional foods may be used in ceremonies to recognize that an individual has moved from one lifecycle period to another with changes in social status (Leininger, 2002). For example, in many Papua New Guinea villages, lifecycle rituals are important for the transition from a young boy to becoming a man (Leininger, 1988 & 2002). For Mexican girls turning 15 years of age, *Quinceañera* is a celebration that marks passage from childhood to adulthood. A reception is typically held following a mass, featuring traditional food, music, and dancing (Quinceañera, 2013).

A Marker of Religious, Spiritual, or Moral Identity

Food selection, preparation, and/or consumption is a daily occurrence that may take on substantial religious, spiritual, or moral meanings. Religions and cultures may be deeply intertwined and may influence cultural or religious food practices (Johnson et al., 2011). *Food and faith are highly interdependent....* Any doctrines or practices representative of human attachment to a higher level of existence are grounded through the physical act of eating certain foods and abstaining from others...and nutritional choices... become a literal manifestation of faith (Nath, 2010, p. 357). Religious dietary laws or rules directly impact and influence food choices and eating habits (Shatenstein & Ghadirian, 1998), especially for ethnic minorities (Leung, 2013). Nath (2010) maintains that "the ritual significance and symbolic history of food in mainstream religions is well-established" (p. 357) and that food, worship, and health are often intertwined. Food needs and restrictions may signal a religious cultural identity and are a means of marking group identity (Johnson et al., 2011).

Diet is essential to maintain health and shape morality (Johnson et al., 2011; Nath, 2010). Many groups base their food choices on religious need, a moral commitment to preserving health and abstaining from harm (vegetarianism), and spiritual presence associated with certain foods (Johnson et al., 2011). Dietary prescriptions and restrictions often reinforce religious beliefs and ethnic identity, and foster a sense of security (Shatenstein & Ghadirian, 1998). They convey cultural constructions of class, gender, religion, health, social order, and morality (Johnson et al., 2011). Certain faiths require fasting from food or food and drink as a religious observance to increase introspection, pay homage to the hungry, remember a historical religious event, bring oneself closer to God, and/or gain spiritual merit. Such fasting symbolizes religious piety, shared identity, and a bond to a community (Shatenstein & Ghadirian, 1998) and is considered an identifier of social and moral commitment (Johnson et al., 2011).

■ RELIGIOCULTURE SPECIFIC DIETARY BELIEFS, PRACTICES, NEEDS AND RESTRICTIONS

In the following paragraphs, a presentation of some essential dietary religious and spiritual beliefs, practices, prescriptions, and restrictions or taboos to select groups are provided. Readers are encouraged to remember that similarities and differences exist within and among groups and that individuals adhere to the teachings of religions in varying degrees. Some people claim allegiance to a faith and practice a few or none of its tenants. It is therefore important to avoid generalizations and assumptions that may lead to stereotyping. It is equally essential to conduct cultural food assessments to discover what applies to individuals, families, groups, and organizations and to develop culturally sensitive, meaningful, and congruent collaborative integrative plans of care.

Judaism

Observant Jewish individuals follow *kosher* laws when purchasing and preparing food (Johnson et al., 2011). Kosher laws refer to rules that govern which foods or animals are deemed fit for ingestion, how animals are slaughtered, how food is prepared, and how different dietary ingredients are mixed (or not mixed) together (Eliasi & Dwyer, 2002; Kosher, 2016). Pork is considered taboo (Johnson et al., 2001), or *treif* (unclean), as are nondomesticated birds, insects, birds of prey, and animals who die of natural causes (Eliasi & Dwyer, 2002; Kosher, 2016). Foods containing blood are forbidden and even eggs that contain a small amount of blood may need to be discarded (Elias & Dwyer, 2002). Fruits, vegetables, flour, sugar, coffee, tea, and pure juices are considered kosher. Fish with lifelong fins and scales and animals that chew the cud and have cloven or split hoofs are considered kosher (Eliasi & Dwyer, 2002; Kosher, 2016). Kosher laws dictate that animals may not be stunned before slaughter (Kosher, 2016); instead, following a specific religious ritual, a specially trained *shochet* (religious butcher) slaughters the animals in a manner that causes minimal pain and facilitates draining of the blood (Eliasi & Dwyer, 2002; Kosher, 2016).

Many Jewish people follow the laws of *Kashrut* that discourage the consumption of dairy and meat in the same meal (Cassar, 2006). Accordingly, one must not consume or mix together meat, milk, or their byproducts. As a result, some Jewish people use distinct sets of dishes, utensils, and cookware for milk (*milchig*) and meat (*fleishing*) preparation and consumption, and may space food containing meat or dairy by one to six hours, depending on their custom (Elias & Dwyer, 2002). Judaism encourages individuals to wash their hands and to say special prayers before eating (Cassar, 2006). Devotees may start each meal with grace recitation and end it with a prayer. No meals are supposed to be cooked on the Sabbath (Elias & Dwyer, 2002). There are a total of six fast days per year and the timing of these days is based on a lunar calendar and changes from year to year. Typically, religious fasting begins at sundown (of previous day) or sunrise (of same day) and ends at sundown (Elias & Dwyer, 2002).

Islam

In Islam, the body is viewed as a gift from God. It is therefore the responsibility of humans to keep the body healthy by avoiding ingesting foods that are considered harmful to the body and therefore *haram* (unlawful/forbidden) (Wehbe-Alamah, 2008), washing hands before consuming food, and eating only foods that is considered *halal* (lawful/licit/permissible) (Cassar, 2006; Elias & Dwyer, 2002; Mukherjee, 2014). Muslims are encouraged to say short prayers or supplications before and after eating and/or drinking to remember God and thank Him for his blessings (Wehbe-Alamah, 2015). Many Muslims will say

Bismillah (In the name of Allah/God) and *Alhamdulliah* (Thanks to Allah/God) before and after each meal (Wehbe-Alamah, 2015).

Examples of haram dietary items include intoxicants such as alcohol and alcohol-based medications (cough syrup) and mind-altering drugs such as cocaine and marijuana (Wehbe-Alamah, 2008). Other unlawful foods include pork and pork-derivatives such as lard, ham, bacon, insulin, and gelatin (Cassar, 2006; Wehbe-Alamah, 2008). The meat of animals that die from disease or a natural death, blood, as well as the flesh of wild, nondomesticated animals and birds that kill their prey are also forbidden (Elias & Dwyer, 2002; Wehbe-Alamah, 2008). Medications containing alcohol or pork derivatives (porcine insulin or gelatin) are permitted when there are no alternatives (Wehbe-Alamah, 2008).

Halal refers to Muslim law as it relates to dietary as well as other aspects of daily life (Mukherjee, 2014). The rules of halal pertaining to diet consist of reciting "In the name of Allah" before slaughtering the animal in a manner that minimizes suffering and allows for complete draining of the blood (Elias & Dwyer, 2002; Wehbe-Alamah, 2008). Fish is considered inherently halal (Elias & Dwyer, 2002). Meat prepared according to Muslim law is also known as *zabihah* (Elias & Dwyer, 2002). While Muslim law considers halal/ zabiha principles as primary, it is permissible to eat food prepared by *the People of the Book*, mainly Christians and Jews (Elias & Dwyer, 2002; Wehbe-Alamah, 2008). Muslims living in geographical areas where they constitute a minority rely on reading food labels to identify and avoid haram ingredients (Elias & Dwyer, 2002).

It is mandatory in Islam for Muslims who are mentally and physically fit and have reached puberty to fast during the month of Ramadan (El-Ashi, n.d.). Fasting is optional on any other days and the dates of fasting change from year to year as Muslims, like Jewish individuals, follow a lunar as opposed to Gregorian calendar (Wehbe-Alamah, 2008). Individuals who are ill, children, elders, pregnant or breastfeeding women, travelers, and menstruating women are exempt from fasting (El- Ashi, n.d.). When fasting, Muslims abstain from eating, drinking, and sexual intercourse from sunrise to sunset (Elias & Dwyer, 2002; Wehbe-Alamah, 2008).

Hinduism and Hare Krishna

The theology of Hinduism is based on the sacred *Vedas* literature, which recommend nonviolence and vegetarianism (Kang, 2010; Shanmugasundaram, O'Connor, & Sellick, 2010). A major premise in Hindu philosophy is following the principle of *ahimsa* (do no harm) (Shanmugasundaram et al., 2010). Adopting a vegetarian diet is believed to support this principle, although not all Hindus are universal in this belief (Shanmugasundaram et al., 2010). In Hinduism, souls of humans as well as animals are to be respected, and many birds and animals such as apes, cobras, and peacocks are worshiped (Shanmugasundaram et al., 2010).

Cows are believed to have been created by *Brahma* (the creator) (Shatenstein & Ghadirian, 1998) and are therefore considered sacred (Shanmugasundaram et al., 2010) or taboo (ReligionFacts, 2015b); as a result, it is generally forbidden to consume anything derived from cows or other animals and birds (Shanmugasundaram et al., 2010). Consequently, most (but not all) Hindus will not partake in beef, milk, cheese, or eggs (Shanmugasundaram et al., 2010). On the other hand, when food is prepared and before it is consumed, it is usually offered to God along with a prayer of thanks. It is believed that this practice will result in the sanctification of food (*prasad*) (Kang, 2010). Furthermore, many Hindus believe that fasting results in cleansing the physiological system of the human body. For end of life patients, this belief may impact nutritional status, hydration, and drug administration process (Shanmugasundaram et al., 2010).

Hare Krishna is a religious movement based in Hinduism (ReligionFacts, 2015a). Devotees believe that God (Krishna) is vegetarian and that dietary choices can have varying influences on human health and worship. They typically abstain from consumption of meat, alcohol, gambling, and sexual intercourse outside of marriage or for nonprocreation purposes (Nath, 2010). Faith is expressed by eating food that is acceptable and pleasing to God, by offering food to God to be sanctified before consumption, and by avoiding dietary items deemed unacceptable, such as meat, fish, eggs, and mushrooms (Nath, 2010). Hare Krishna devotees believe that consuming meat promotes a cycle of violence between humans and animals; on the other hand, eating food that has been sanctified advances spirituality and protects from karmic reactions (Nath, 2010).

Food choices are linked to the emotional states of ignorance (lowest mode), passion (lower mode), and goodness (higher mode) and drive social actions and interactions. Dietary ingredients that promote a desired state of goodness include butter, cheese, yogurt, sugar, honey, herbs, spices, fruits, nuts, grains, beans, and most vegetables; those that lead to unacceptable passionate demeanors include onions, garlic, leeks, shallots, chives, and caffeinated beverages; foods that are likewise undesirable and linked to a state of ignorance include mushrooms, eggs, and meat (Nath, 2010). Moreover, adopting dietary habits that promote desired nutritional choices and eliminate or reduce objectionable selections helps to maintain optimal health and determine the nature of relationship with God (Krishna) (Nath, 2010).

Buddhism

"Buddhist doctrine stipulates that it is forbidden to kill living beings" (Shatenstein & Ghadirian, 1998, p. 226), that humans and animals are equal biological entities, and that one is to adhere to the principle of *ahimsa* or nonviolence (Nath, 2010). However, while the precept of no killing governs faith and social life, vegetarianism is not mandatory; instead, it is a choice that is typically adopted by devout Buddhists who are interested in achieving a particular level of consciousness (Nath, 2010). Therefore, one should not assume that all Buddhists are vegetarians. In fact, some Buddhists will not consume meat, but will eat fish (Elias & Dwyer, 2002). In Buddhism, food is viewed as an essential component of biospirituality (Nath, 2010). Dietary quality and quantity is believed to assist with the maintenance of focus and balance for spiritual meditations and social actions and interactions (Nath, 2010).

Seventh-Day Adventist Church & Church of the Latter Day Saints

Seventh-Day Adventists ideology is immersed in the belief that a healthy mind and a healthy body are crucial for faith and worship (Nath, 2010). Vegetarianism and avoidance of meat are viewed as means to maintain health and enhance a spiritual relationship with God (Nath, 2010). Adventists range from strict to less rigid lacto-ovo-vegetarians (Nath, 2010; Shatenstein & Ghadirian, 1998). Most Adventists abstain from alcohol, tobacco, and caffeine and embrace a strict lacto-ovo-vegetarian diet that is rich in whole grains, fruits, vegetables, and legumes (Elias & Dwyer, 2002; Shatenstein & Ghadirian, 1998). Food choices usually exclude meat, fish and poultry (Elias & Dwyer, 2002). However, meat consumption is becoming more accepted (Nath, 2010). Due to lower consumption of meat, tobacco, and alcohol, and adherence to low-fat, high fiber diets that are rich in vitamins A and C, Adventists experience lower mortality rate associated with cancer and cardiovascular disease (Nath, 2010).

Members of the Church of the Latter Day Saints, also known as Mormons, believe that *the human body is the temple of God* (Shatenstein & Ghadirian, 1998, p. 227). Therefore, to preserve the body in fit condition, Mormons abstain from caffeine, tobacco, alcohol, and espouse diets that include whole grains, plant proteins, vegetables, and fruits (Elias & Dwyer, 2002; Shatenstein & Ghadirian, 1998). Eating meat is not prohibited, although moderation is encouraged (Elias & Dwyer, 2002). Adherents to this faith experience lower mortality rates associated with *diseases of affluence* (Shatenstein & Ghadirian, 1998, pp. 226-227) such as obesity, cardiovascular disease, and various forms of cancer.

■ FOOD HABITS, HEALTH, AND ILLNESS

Studies have supported a link between unhealthy dietary lifestyles and noncommunicable diseases including, but not limited to, obesity, coronary heart disease, cancer, and diabetes mellitus (Farahmand et al., 2012; Leung, 2013; Shatenstein & Ghadirian, 1998; Vue et al., 2011). Cultural dietary patterns contribute to nutritional etiology that underlines most chronic illnesses (Shatenstein & Ghadirian, 1998). Unhealthful food choices may increase the risk for developing chronic diseases, impact quality of life, and even result in premature death (Vue et al., 2011). Food beliefs and practices may affect individuals' state of health or illness (Johnson et al., 2011). Similarly, food choices and habits may be influenced by health or religious beliefs (Kara, 2014; Leung, 2014).

As discussed earlier, the dietary lifestyle of some religious groups has been found to positively impact disease status and mortality rate (Nath, 2010; Shatenstein & Ghadirian, 1998). Some cultures use culinary spices that have antimicrobial property to

avoid disease, while others rely on the religiocultural practices of cleansing food ingredients, sterilizing surfaces and utensils used for food preparation, and other food rules and laws to promote health and circumvent the threat of disease (Johnson et al., 2011). Avoidance of certain food items due to religiocultural beliefs may also affect health status. For example, the Hua of Papua New Guinea have been known to suffer from high rates of malnutrition associated with avoidance of certain foods (Johnson et al., 2011); likewise, dietary restrictions have also been associated with low iron status in some minority ethnic groups (Leung, 2013).

Food practices are very much related to or affected by cultural perceptions. *Soul food* is a 400-year-old African-American cuisine that evolved from a history of slavery, persecution, and segregation in an effort to *nourish the body, nurture the spirit, and comfort the soul* (James, 2004, p. 361). Soul food diet favors greens, corn, sweet potatoes, pork fat, spices, salt meats, pork and chicken, fried foods, cobblers, and one-pot meals (Beagan & Chapman, 2012). African Americans view soul food as an affirmation of their ethnic identity (Beagan & Chapman, 2012). Many consider having to conform to a mainstream culture's definition of healthy eating as giving up their own cultural heritage (James, 2004). In the African-American community, offering others large amounts of food conveys love and caring while eating what is offered communicates good hospitality, appreciation, and respect (Beagan & Chapman, 2012; James, 2004). Another cultural perception held by African Americans is that it is acceptable for women with children to be heavier than their childless counterparts (James, 2004).

Moreover, many other cultures associate plumpness/chubbiness, or obesity with health or affluence (Leung, 2013). Vue et al. (2011) reported that Hmong culture views *being big and bulky as a good thing* (p. 202), and American food as unhealthful and less filling. Beagan and Chapman (2012) discovered that some African Nova Scotians correlate low-fat, low-sugar diets with ill-health and view mainstream food guidelines as based on White culture (and therefore discounted Black cultural dietary practices). Fernandez et al. (2015) related that Asian Indians in Australia did not identify being overweight as a health-negative issue.

■ FOOD HABITS INFLUENCERS

In addition to cultural, religious, spiritual, and moral beliefs, practices, and customs, numerous other factors influence food habits. Barriers and facilitators to healthy eating include, but are not limited to:

- Time: Preparation of healthy meals may be viewed as a time consuming process that requires advanced planning and preparation, especially for working women (Farahmand et al., 2012; James, 2004; Momin et al., 2013).
- Cost: Higher cost of healthy foods may create a barrier for those who cannot afford it, leading to health disparities (Farahmand et al., 2012; Fernandez et al., 2015; Momin et al., 2013; Shatenstein & Ghadirian, 1998). In addition, inappropriate prioritization of family budgets may result in limited resources allocated for the purchase of quality food (Farahmand et al., 2012). Furthermore, lack of knowledge on how to prepare healthy food choices with limited budgets may impact dietary habits (James, 2004).
- Lack of access: In the absence of availability or proximity of local grocery stores that offer healthy food options, preparing healthy food selections may prove to be challenging (James, 2004). Fast foods and frozen meals are often used as substitutes to traditional home-cooked meals due to convenience and easy availability (Farahmand et al., 2012; James, 2004).
- Misconception/lack of knowledge: Lack of knowledge or misconception about nutritional value of food may lead to the inability to identify healthy food choices; similarly, lack of awareness of proper food preparation techniques may lead to loss of nutritional value (Farahmand et al., 2012; James, 2004). In addition, traditional ways of food preparation is usually passed on from generation to generation, resulting in lack of knowledge of contemporary healthy food preparation strategies (Farahmand et al., 2012; James, 2004).
- Lack of social support: In cultures where traditional foods are associated with ethnic or cultural identity, adopting a different (albeit healthier) dietary lifestyle may be faced with resistance or lack of support from family members and friends (James, 2004; Vue et al., 2011). For immigrants, lack of social support, resulting from absence of extended family members, may affect adherence to healthy traditional food habits (Fernandez et al., 2015).

- Food security: Some immigrants from countries with a history of food insecurity, such as Thailand and Laos, may experience dietary changes, such as overeating, when faced with food security and abundance (Vue et al., 2012).
- Lack of food cultural sensitivity: Many studies revealed that people from diverse cultural backgrounds view food guides and/or professional educational counseling as reflective of the dominant White culture and devoid of culture-specific knowledge and food examples (Beagan & Chapman, 2012; Fernandez et al., 2015; James, 2004; Shatenstein & Ghadirian, 1998). They exposed a need for culturally sensitive dietary counseling and guidance that integrates generic dietary beliefs, practices, needs, and taboos, along with professional interventions to effect positive dietary change (Beagan & Chapman, 2012; Crogan & Evans, 2010; Fernandez et al., 2015; James, 2004; Shatenstein & Ghadirian, 1998).

■ THE NURSE'S ROLE IN NUTRITION USES

One of the most important functions of the nurse is to take an active role in helping clients maintain a favorable nutritional status within their culture. The client's daily wellbeing and nutritional needs in illness depend considerably on the nurse's knowledge, decisions, and actions to provide appropriate nutrients to clients (Leininger, 2002). Helping the client recover from illnesses through appropriate food uses that are acceptable in the culture is an important role for nurses and other healthcare providers.

As stated previously, to be effective in maintaining the health of clients and preventing illnesses, nurses and others need to be knowledgeable about different cultural foods, needs, prohibitions, and the cultural context in which food is prepared, served, and eaten (Leininger, 2002). An understanding of how food is used for ceremonial purposes at birth, marriage, death, and religious events, is also needed to better communicate with and provide diverse individuals, families, and groups with culturally sensitive and meaningful care. In general, the nurse needs to know that cultural foods are a powerful means to facilitate family relationships, communication, and wellbeing (Leininger, 2002). Becoming aware of different traditional foods, cultural eating patterns, and the ways foods are used to help individuals either stay well or fight the threat of illness is essential.

■ UNIVERSAL FUNCTIONS AND USES OF FOODS

Food for Biophysical Needs/Physical Wellbeing

First, food is universally used *to provide essential nutrition and energy needed for physical wellbeing, survival, and maintenance of biophysical needs* (Leininger, 2002). Food provides energy and strength necessary to perform daily activities and body functions, keep well, grow, work, and socialize with others (Beagan & Chapman, 2012; Leininger, 2002). Basic or essential nutritional needs differ from culture to culture and in different ecological settings (Leininger, 2002). In addition, cultural diversity exists in how nutrients are used, and how foods are produced, processed, and prepared for consumption (Leininger, 2002). These factors are important to consider while working with clients of different cultures in their homes, inpatient or outpatient healthcare settings, or other places.

Nutritionists and anthropologists have discovered that biological, genetic, social, cultural, and ecological factors play a role in determining cultural food needs (Leininger, 2002). Every culture has developed over time essential and preferred traditional food choices and habits (Leininger, 2002). When basic food needs are not met, signs of nutritional deficiencies, illnesses, inability to function, and even death may occur (Leininger, 2002). For example, *kwashiorkor*, a nutritional disorder caused by a diet that is deficient in protein and energy-producing foods, is commonly seen in children of certain African tribes, between the ages of one to three years (Kwashiorkor, 2015). *Marasmus* is another condition caused by dietary deficiency of proteins and calories, affecting mostly infants, and resulting in a body weight that is 60% below the norm (Marasmus, 2015).

Food for Human Relationships/Social Wellbeing

A *second* universal function of food is *establishing and maintaining social and cultural relationships with friends, kinfolk, strangers, and others* (Leininger, 2002).

Food plays an important role in cultivating and maintaining social wellbeing (Beagan & Chapman, 2012). Many social friendships and professional ties have been initiated and sustained with the sharing of food. Food rituals unite people and preserve cultural beliefs and values (Leininger, 2002). Relationships with strangers that are tense and questionable are often eased and improved through social food offerings (Leininger, 2002).

Food to Assess Interpersonal Distance

A *third* function of *food is to assess interpersonal closeness or distance between people* (Leininger, 2002). Universally, foods are often used to determine the extent of friendship or distrust between individuals, families, or groups. How food is used reflects cultural stranger-to-trusted friend interpersonal relationships (Leininger, 2002). Leininger (1991, 2002) explained this function by sharing her food experiences with the Gadsup of New Guinea when she was conducting her first ethnonursing research study. Accordingly, when she first entered the world of the Gadsup as a complete stranger, she was initially perceived as a potentially harmful white sorcerer, and was served withered, dry, and scrubby-looking sweet potatoes, fruits, and greens. Six weeks later, as the villagers got to know her, they began to bring her *better quality fruits and vegetables and, occasionally, fresh foods from distant places* (Leininger, 2002, p. 209). By the end of the first year, the Gadsup brought her *lots of fresh pineapple, vegetables, and even rare foods that they had obtained by walking nearly 20 miles* (Leininger, 2002, p. 209). Leininger (2002) reflected that as she became accepted and viewed as a friend, the quality and quantity of food served to her markedly improved.

Transculturally and universally, food use often reflects the social stratification of society and indicates which persons are to be respected or held in positions of higher authority or status (Leininger, 2002). Often, stratified cultures with castes, classes, gender, and hierarchies determine who gets what foods and how the foods can be used by people of particular statuses. In some stratified societies such as India certain foods are highly restricted for certain castes, and food is regulated by the rules of the caste system (Leininger, 2002). People in higher castes such as the Brahmins often are given high-quality food. Food also becomes a powerful means for regulating social and political controls and maintaining cultural norms and rules of behavior (Leininger, 2002).

Food to Cope with Stress and Conflict

A *fourth universal function and symbolic use of food is to cope with emotional stresses, conflicts, and traumatic life events* (Leininger, 2002). In many cultures, food is used to relieve anxiety, tensions, and interpersonal conflicts or frustrations (Leininger, 2002). The way diverse cultures deal with emotional stresses and conflicts varies considerably in Western and non-Western cultures. Western cultures such as Anglo-Americans, Europeans, Canadians, and Australians often consciously or unconsciously rely on eating to relieve their stresses, a process that may lead to weight gain (Leininger, 2002). Some people tend to almost constantly eat or nibble on food or drink to relieve their anger, frustrations, or anxieties. Compulsive eating and hoarding of food to relieve tensions or anxieties are largely learned and patterned lifeways influenced by cultural practices (Leininger, 2002). Compulsive eating to relieve tension tends to occur more frequently in Western cultures where food is more readily available. In many non-Western cultures and cultures where food is often scarce, people relieve their anxieties by activities such as running, hunting, or fighting (Leininger, 2002). In these cultures one seldom finds obesity or overweight problems, although other nutritional problems, such as malnourishment may be prevalent (Leininger, 2002).

On the other hand, in some Western American and European cultures, individuals may handle their anxieties and tensions by avoiding eating (Leininger, 2002). In Western cultures, eating disorders such as anorexia nervosa and bulimia are prevalent, especially in teenagers (Leininger, 2002). Anorexia nervosa is an eating disorder that affects one in 100-200 girls in the United States, resulting in at least 15% loss in ideal body weight and even leading to starvation (Harvard Health Publications, 2015). Individuals with anorexia nervosa usually refuse to eat anything or engage in binge-purging by gorging on food and then vomiting it (Leininger, 2002; Outten, 2015). They use dieting as a means to cope with environmental pressures, cultural influences, and difficult family or other relationships. They view diet restriction as a source of power and control over others (Harvard Health Publications, 2015). While nutritional disorders are prevalent in Western cultures, they are limitedly found in non-Western cultures,

thus reflecting global differences (Leininger, 2002). Nurses with transcultural preparation are alert to such variations related to cultural patterns of over-eating or under-eating and can observe, listen to, and counsel their clients, and help them and their families work toward resolving their problems within their cultural lifeways and values (Leininger, 2002).

Most cultures have prescribed food ways to relieve feelings of boredom, disappointments, dissatisfactions, and depression (Leininger, 2002). Foods such as sweets and drinks are commonly used in the United States by adults and children to handle anger, emotional frustrations, and disappointments, whereas vegetables and daily outside activities are generally used in non-Western cultures (Leininger, 2002). Nurses prepared in transcultural nursing can assess cultural food beliefs and lifeways and work collaboratively with their clients to provide them with culturally congruent and meaningful care.

Food for Rewards and Punishments

A *fifth* universal function of food transculturally, but with some cultural variations, *is the use of food to reward, punish, and influence the behavior of others* (Leininger, 2002). In most cultures, there are norms and practices of the ways children and adults are rewarded, punished, or receive positive or negative sanctions with food (Leininger, 2002). Foods have long been used by humans to regulate, reward, maintain, or curtail cultural and social behaviors. Moreover, cultures know which foods are viewed as favorable rewards and which ones communicate dislikes or negative rewards (Leininger, 2002). For example, Anglo-American children are often rewarded for good behavior with sweets such as candy, sugared cereals and drinks, and cookies (Leininger, 2002). Asian Indian mothers reward their children with sweets to encourage them to eat fruits and vegetables or to finish an entire meal (Momin et al., 2013). In contrast, Gadsup children are rewarded for desired cultural behavior with nonrefined foods such as vegetables, nuts, taro, fruits, or fish (Leininger, 2002).

Food to Influence Status

A *sixth* universal function of food is *to influence the political and economic status of an individual or a group* (Leininger, 2002). Transculturally, food has great economic importance and political uses, and these two aspects are closely interrelated. Food has been used to build political alliances and foster economic gains (Leininger, 2002). Politically and economically, food can reaffirm, and sustain traditional power ties and establish new power alliances. Serving food before, during, and after political meetings often leads to friendly and congenial outcomes, and tempers political group behavior (Leininger, 2002). Historically, food has been a means to build and maintain smooth relationships, gain votes, and foster desired political and economic alliances and support (Leininger, 2002).

Economically, food is important in exchanges to maintain basic food supplies and to provide diversity in the people's diets (Leininger, 2002). Food is of great concern worldwide as it plays a considerable role in economic production, accumulation, and distribution of goods and services (Leininger, 2002). Cultures learn what food other groups need or desire. They try to increase the demand in trade exchange patterns for economic benefits (Leininger, 2002). For hundreds of years people have made food exchanges to support political ties, provide essential foods, and to strengthen financial positions (Leininger, 2002).

Essential food imports and exports are central to the development, maintenance, and survival of cultures worldwide. Periods of drought, floods, earthquakes, tornadoes, and other environmental conditions also have a devastating impact on the production and distribution of foods all around the world (Leininger, 2002). An imbalance in the production and distribution of foods can cause serious problems in any society and can ultimately influence the health status of people (Leininger, 2002). Historically, thousands of people in many countries have died of hunger as a result of war, political feuds, economic greed, and poor distribution of foods (Leininger, 2002). Even food taken to international food distribution points may never reach intended destinations because of political groups taking the food (Leininger, 2002). In fact, there are numerous reports denouncing the thieving of international food aid resources in countries such as Somalia and Syria and the resulting catastrophic effects on human lives (Houreld, 2011; Pandey, 2015).

Food to maintain Health and Prevent and/or Treat Illness

A *seventh* and major universal function of food is *to maintain health and prevent and/or treat illness.* Anthropologists have long observed and studied how food is used as a means to diagnose, treat, and deal with illnesses and stresses in different cultures (Leininger, 2002). People from diverse cultures have and continue to rely on both generic (folk) and professional practices to preserve health and cure illnesses (Leininger, 2002). Some cultures prefer the use of traditional foods and herbs and seek traditional skilled folk healers such as the Curandero, yerbero, shaman, and others (Andrews & Boyle, 2015) before considering professional services.

In many cultures, food remains important to maintain health and prevent or cure certain illnesses such as hypertension, diabetes mellitus, peptic ulcers, coronary diseases, and other conditions or disorders (Leininger, 2002). A Middle Eastern folk food practice used by Lebanese and Syrians to maintain health and boost the immune system is the early morning consumption of a spoon of honey mixed with black seeds (Wehbe-Alamah, 2015). Sri Lankans use herbs such as *thebu* (Crape Ginger) and vegetables such as *bitter melon* and *karawila* to control their blood glucose and treat diabetes mellitus (Amarasekara et al., 2014).

■ FOOD CHOICES FOR YIN YANG BALANCE

Fundamental to Taoism and Traditional Chinese Medicine (TCM) philosophy, is the belief that in terms of health functionality, there are four natures of foods, mainly cold, cool, warm, and hot (Liu et al., 2012). The natures of cold and cool are typically referred to as *yin* while *yang* designates warm and hot natures (Liu et al., 2012). Additionally, yin signifies the cold, female, and darkness element, whereas yang signifies the hot, male, and light element (Leininger, 2002). For nearly 3,000 years, Chinese and other cultures have been attentive to the yin and yang elements to maintain harmony and balance in the universe (Leininger, 2002; Manderson, 1987). Yin-yang equilibrium is viewed as the foundation for health and wellbeing (Lee, Yang, & Yang, 2013).

Yin foods typically moisturize and cool down body heat and tension while yang foods warm the body, create tension, and have a drying effect (Liu et al., 2012; Prout, 2016). Excesses or imbalances of either yin or yang foods can lead to illnesses, diseases, or unfavorable conditions (Leininger, 2002). Food choices that create a state of balance are therefore important in maintaining an optimal state of health (Prout, 2016). Diseases and health conditions are also classified as hot or cold and require food of opposite classification. Yin (cold) conditions such as cancer, pregnancy, and postpartum are therefore treated with yang (hot) foods such as ginger, beef, eggs, and chicken. Yang (hot) conditions such as venereal diseases, hypertension, and infections are treated with yin (cold) foods like fish, pork, bland foods, and fresh fruits and vegetables (Lee, Yang, & Yang, 2013).

Some clients may be labeled as noncompliant by nurses and other healthcare providers because they refuse to take medicine with cold or icy water, or because they refuse certain treatments that they view as inconsistent with their yin-yang beliefs. The transcultural nurse knows that noncompliance or refusal of professional care practices may be related to cultural fears, clashes, or taboos (Leininger, 2002). To provide culturally congruent and competent care, nurses need to be knowledgeable about the diverse cultural meanings of food beliefs, classifications, and practices, including the hot and cold or yin-yang theory.

■ CULTURAL FOOD ASSESSMENT

Considering the universalities and diversities in food meanings, beliefs, and practices, acculturation process, dynamic and fluid nature of cultures, and the relationship between food, health, and illness, it is extremely important for nurses, physicians, nutritionists, and other healthcare providers caring for people of different cultural backgrounds, to examine the relationship between food and cultural and social structure dimensions as delineated in the Sunrise Enabler (Refer to Color Insert 1). "Cultural, ethnic, and religious dietary habits are in constant evolution from their place of origin, incorporating environmental adaptation and changes in societal mores, while forming an integral part of the individual's self-perception" (Shatenstein & Ghadirian, 1998, p. 228).

Conducting a cultural food assessment leads to the discovery of individualized culture-specific beliefs and practices from an emic perspective, helps to avoid stereotypical assumptions, and assists in the formulation of a culturally sensitive integrative plan of care that is developed in collaboration with the client. Suggested

questions (adapted from Leininger, 2002, pp. 205-206) include:

- What is the meaning of food in your culture?
- What role does food play in your culture?
- How do worldview, technological, religious/spiritual, kinship/social, cultural, political, economic, and/or educational factors influence food preparation, use, and consumption in your culture?
- What are the basic nutritional needs and concerns of people from your culture?
- What common traditional foods tend to be eaten or avoided in your culture when well or sick? When celebrating? After special events or milestones?
- What foods tend to support wellness patterns over time in your culture?
- What foods are held to be most beneficial throughout the lifecycle for infants, children, women, men, and elders?
- What are facilitators or barriers to healthy food habits?
- What is the role of nurses and other healthcare providers in preserving and/or maintaining, accommodating and/or negotiating, and repatterning and/or restructuring the food beliefs and practices of people from your culture?

The transcultural nurse who studies the cultural differences in the uses of foods and conducts a cultural assessment will be attentive to food preferences that promote health and prevent or cause illnesses. Since cultures have specific food preferences and dislikes, which can make a difference in caring for clients of different cultures, the nurse assesses these foods and their nutritional values within the client's health needs to facilitate recovery from illness, maintain health status, prevent illness, and provide culturally congruent care (Leininger, 2002).

Eating culturally desired foods, especially during times of illness, can lead to a quicker recovery from illness and to greater client satisfaction (Leininger, 2002). Many clients may refuse hospital foods that they view as culturally taboo or inappropriate. Transcultural nurses accommodate the need for cultural foods when no harm can be caused as a result. It is therefore important that hospital dietary staff are educated about cultural food likes and dislikes. For example, the nurse who understands that Vietnamese people like fish, rice, fresh vegetables, and herbal teas would try to accommodate such dietary practices when hospitalized. The transcultural nurse is aware that unless acculturated, Vietnamese patients may refuse hamburgers, potatoes, carbonated beverages or other Western foods (Leininger, 2002). Similarly, observant Muslim or Jewish patients may require *halal* or *kosher* diets to accommodate their religious beliefs (Johnson et al., 2011; Wehbe-Alamah, 2008).

■ CONCLUSION

Leininger (2002) predicted that demands for culture-specific foods to maintain and enhance health, prevent or treat illness, and improve overall healthcare will increase with time. Numerous studies have confirmed that people want professional interventions that are based on an understanding of cultural food beliefs and lifeways and that integrate culture-specific tailored integrative care practices (Beagan & Chapman, 2012; Chen et al., 2012; Fernandez et al., 2015; James, 2005). Transcultural nursing insights about general aspects of food culture is essential to delivering culturally meaningful and congruent care. A cultural food assessment helps the nurse identify food beliefs, practices, needs, preferences, and taboos. It increases professional (etic) awareness of important emic concepts. Such knowledge will help nurses avoid imposing Western cultural food values and lifeways on people of diverse cultural backgrounds. Nurses who engage in cultural ethnocentrism with imposition practices may unknowingly cause cultural pain (Leininger, 2002). On the other hand, seeking input from individuals, families, and groups about their food likes and dislikes, habits and lifeways, encourages collaboration, compliance, and satisfaction.

In an ever-changing multicultural world, nurses with transcultural knowledge about food uses and functions are invaluable to promote client wellbeing, daily functioning, and recovery from illness (Leininger, 2002). The use of the three modes of culture care decisions and actions can help the nurse work collaboratively with the client to develop a professional plan of care that preserves and/or maintains, accommodates and/or negotiates, and restructures and/or repatterns culture-specific food beliefs and habits. Transcultural nurses desiring to provide holistic care should keep this message in mind: *Culture defines food uses, functions, and benefits over time and in different places in the world. The nurse's challenge is to discover this reality and to use foods congruently with cultures and therapeutic modes of care* (Leininger, 2002, p. 215).

■ DISCUSSION QUESTIONS

1. Discuss the various food symbols and meanings and implication to clinical practice.
2. Discuss how nurses can preserve and accommodate specific religiocultural needs and taboos.
3. Discuss the various functions and uses of food and implication to clinical practice
4. Discuss how doing a food cultural assessment can enhance development of culturally congruent professional plans of care.

■ REFERENCES

Amarasekara, D., Fongkaew, W., Turale, S., Wimalasekara, W., & Chanprasit, C. (2014). An ethnographic study of diabetes health beliefs and practices in Sri Lankan adults. *International Nursing Review, 61*(4), 507-514. doi: 10.1111/inr.12136

Andrews, M. & Boyle, J. (2015). *Transcultural concepts in nursing care* (7th ed.). Philadelphia: Wolters Kluwer Health|Lippincott Williams & Wilkins.

Beagan, L., & Chapman, E. (2012). Meanings of food, eating and health among African Nova Scotians: 'Certain things aren't meant for black folk.' *Ethnicity & Health, 17*(5), 513-529. doi: 10.1080/13557858.2012.661844

Cassar, L. (2006). Cultural expectations of Muslims and orthodox Jews in regard to pregnancy and the postpartum period: A study in comparison and contrast. *International Journal of Childbirth Education, 21*(2), 27-41. Retrieved from http://libproxy.umflint.edu:2067/login.aspx?direct=true&db=ccm&AN=106333332&site=ehost-live&scope=site

Chen, L., Juon, H., & Lee, S. (2012). Acculturation and BMI among Chinese, Korean and Vietnamese adults. *Journal of Community Health, 37*(3), 539-546. doi: 10.1007/s10900-011-9476-1

Crogan, L., & Evans, C. (2010). Food expectations-long term care Spanish questionnaire: Pilot testing with older Mexican American nursing home residents. *Research in Gerontological Nursing, 3*(4), 282-290. doi: 10.3928/19404921-20100330-02

El-Ashi, A. (n.d.). *Fasting in Islam*. Islamic Society of Rutgers University. Retrieved from http://www.eden.rutgers.edu/~muslims/fasting.htm

Eliasi, R., & Dwyer, T. (2002). Kosher and Halal: Religious observances affecting dietary intakes. *Journal of the American Dietetic Association, 102*(7), 911-913. doi: 10.1016/S0002-8223(02)90203-8

Farahmand, M., Tehrani, R., Amiri, P., & Azizi, F. (2012). Barriers to healthy nutrition: Perceptions and experiences of Iranian women. *BMC Public Health, 12*(1), 1064-1064. doi: 10.1186/1471-2458-12-1064

Fernandez, R., Rolley, X., Rajaratnam, R., Everett, B., & Davidson, M. (2015). Reducing the risk of heart disease among Indian Australians: Knowledge, attitudes, and beliefs regarding food practices—a focus group study. *Food & Nutrition Research, 59*, 1-7. doi: 10.3402/fnr.v59.25770

Harvard Health Publications. (2015). *Health Topics A-Z: Anorexia Nervosa*. Retrieved from http://www.health.harvard.edu/diseases-and-conditions/anorexia

Hinnerová, K. (2007). *Food as a transcultural metaphor food imagery and ethnocultural identities in contemporary multicultural women writing in Canada*. Retrieved from http://is.muni.cz/th/74496/ff_m/food_as_transcultural_metaphor.pdf?lang=en

Houreld, K. (2011). Somalia famine: Food Aid Stolen. *The World Post*. Retrieved from http://www.huffingtonpost.com/2011/08/15/somalia-famine-aid-stolen_n_927126.html

James, D. (2004). Factors influencing food choices, dietary intake, and nutrition-related attitudes among African Americans: Application of a culturally sensitive model. *Ethnicity & Health, 9*(4), 349-367. doi: 10.1080/1355785042000285375

Johnson, A., White, E., Boyd, M., & Cohen, B. (2011). Matzah, meat, milk, and mana: Psychological influences on religiocultural food practices. *Journal of Cross-Cultural Psychology, 42*(8), 1421-1436. doi: 10.1177/0022022111412528

Kang, C. (2010). Hinduism and mental health: Engaging British Hindus. *Mental Health, Religion & Culture, 13*(6), 587-593. doi: 10.1080/13674676.2010.488427

Kara, B. (2014). Health beliefs related to salt-restricted diet in patients on hemodialysis: Psychometric evaluation of the Turkish version of the beliefs about dietary compliance scale. *Journal of Transcultural Nursing, 25*(3), 256-264. doi: 10.1177/1043659613514114

Koenig, J., Dutta, J., Kandula, N., & Palaniappan, L. (2012). "All of those things we don't eat": A culture-centered approach to dietary health meanings for Asian Indians living in the United States. *Health Communication, 27*(8), 818-828. doi: 10.1080/10410236.2011.651708

Kosher (2016). *Fowler's Concise Dictionary of Modern English Usage*. Oxford University Press.

Kwashiorkor (2015). *Concise Medical Dictionary*. Oxford University Press.

Lee, S., Yang, S., & Yang, Y. (2013). Doing-in-month ritual among Chinese and Chinese-American. *Journal of Cultural Diversity, 20*(2), 94-99.

Leininger, M. (1988). Transcultural eating patterns and nutrition: Transcultural nursing and anthropological perspectives. *Holistic Nursing Practice, 3*(1), 12-26.

Leininger, M. (1991). Culture Care of the Gadsup Akuna of the Eastern Highlands of New Guinea. In M. Leininger (Ed.), *Culture care diversity and universality: A theory of nursing,* (pp. 231-280). New York, NY: National League for Nursing.

Leininger, M. (2002). Transcultural food functions, beliefs, and practices. In M. Leininger & M. McFarland (Eds.)., *Transcultural nursing concepts, theories, research & practice,* (pp. 205-216). New York, NY: McGraw-Hill.

Leung, G. (2013). Health impact of diet in minority ethnic groups. *Practice Nurse, 43*(12), 26-29.

Liu, C., Sun, Y., Li, Y., Yang, W., Zhang, M., Xiong, C., & Yang, Y. (2012). The relationship between cold-hot nature and nutrient contents of foods. *Nutrition & Dietetics, 69*(1), 64-68. doi:10.1111/j.1747-0080.2011.01565.x

Manderson, L., (1987). Hot-cold food and medical theories: Cross cultural perspectives. *Introduction to Social Science and Medicine, 25*(4), 329-420.

Marasmus (2015). *Concise Medical Dictionary*. Oxford University Press.

Momin, R., Chung, R., & Olson, H. (2014; 2013). A qualitative study to understand positive and negative child feeding behaviors of immigrant Asian Indian mothers in the US. *Maternal and Child Health Journal, 18*(7), 1699-1710. doi:10.1007/s10995-013-1412-9

Mukherjee, R. (2014). Global halal: Meat, money, and religion. *Religions, 5*(1), 22-75. doi: 10.3390/rel5010022

Nath, J. (2010). "God is a vegetarian": The food, health and bio-spirituality of Hare Krishna, Buddhist and Seventh-Day Adventist devotees. *Health Sociology Review, 19*(3), 356-368. doi: 10.5172/hesr.2010.19.3.356

Outten, E. (2015). Anorexia nervosa. *Journal of the American Academy of Physician Assistants, 28*(2), 43-44. doi: 10.1097/01.JAA.0000459819.47779.b8

Pandey, A. (2015). UN "Deeply Concerned" over reports of ISIS stealing, relabeling syrian food aid. *International Business Times*. Retrieved from http://www.ibtimes.com/un-deeply-concerned-over-reports-isis-stealing-relabeling-syrian-food-aid-1803524

Prout, L. (2016). *Yin-Yang balance and food choice*. ACUFINDER.COM. Retrieved from https://www.acufinder.com/Acupuncture+Information/Detail/Yin-Yang+Balance+and+Food+Choice

Quinceañera (2013). Encyclopaedia Britannica Inc.

ReligionFacts (2015a). *Hare Krishna.* Retrieved from http://www.religionfacts.com/hare-krishna

ReligionFacts (2015b). *Hindu cow taboo.* Retrieved from www.religionfacts.com/cow-taboo

Shanmugasundaram, S., O'Connor, M., & Sellick, K. (2010). Culturally competent care at the end of life: A Hindu perspective. *End of Life Care Journal, 4*(1), 26-31.

Shatenstein, B. & Ghadirian, P. (1998). Influences on diet, health behaviours and their outcome in select ethno-cultural and religious groups. *Nutrition, 14*(2), 223-230. doi: 10.1016/S0899-9007(97)00425-5

Vue, W., Wolff, C., & Goto, K. (2011). Hmong food helps us remember who we are: Perspectives of food culture and health among Hmong women with young children. *Journal of Nutrition Education and Behavior, 43*(3), 199-204. doi: 10.1016/j.jneb.2009.10.011

Wehbe-Alamah, H. (2008). Bridging generic and professional care practices for Muslim patients through use of Leininger's culture care modes. *Contemporary Nurse, 28*(1), 83-97. doi: 10.5172/conu.673.28.1-2.83

Wehbe-Alamah, H. (2015). Folk Care Beliefs and Practices of Traditional Lebanese and Syrian Muslims in the Midwestern United States. In M. McFarland, & H. Wehbe-Alamah (Eds.), *Culture Care Diversity and Universality: A Worldwide Nursing Theory,* 137-182. Sudbury, MA: Jones and Bartlett Publishers, Inc.

Wright-St Clair, A., Pierce, D., Bunrayong, W., Rattakorn, P., Vittayakorn, S., Shordike, A., & Hocking, C. (2013). Cross-cultural understandings of festival food-related activities for older women in Chiang Mai, Thailand, Eastern Kentucky, USA and Auckland, New Zealand. *Journal of Cross-Cultural Gerontology, 28*(2), 103-119. doi: 10.1007/s10823-013-9194-5

Special Topics in Transcultural Nursing Using the Culture Care Theory

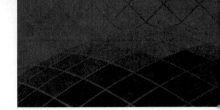

Using a Culturally Congruent Approach in Mental Health Care

Helene B. Vossos and Hiba B. Wehbe-Alamah

> *"Without the inclusion of explicit cultural and care-health research-based knowledge, mental health nursing will have limited meanings and beneficial therapy outcomes"* (Leininger, 2002e, p. 239).

■ INTRODUCTION

Many individuals across the wide multicultural world of diversity have labelled unexplained behaviors (including cultural-bound syndromes) as *mental illness* based on the complexities and potential misinterpretations found within and among cultural relationships (Townsend, 2014). The National Institute of Mental Health (NIMH) reported that the life expectancy rate in the United States (U.S.) improved for adults ranging from age 47 to 78 during the 20th century, having gained one year in longevity for every six years from 1900 to 2000, and that the rate of mental illness occurrence paralleled this increased life expectancy (NIMH, 2013a). The American Psychological Association (APA) reported that 20% of Americans over the age of 55 and 37% of adults residing in nursing homes suffer with some type of mental condition and significant symptoms such as depression that are often overlooked (APA, 2015). According to the Centers for Disease Control and Prevention (CDCP) "…

the prevalence of depression in 20 year and older individuals is at increased risk for reduced social productivity, poorer quality of life, morbidity, and premature mortality" (CDCP, 2011a, p. 38).

Stereotyping, prejudice, and discrimination are invisible walls that create barriers to mental healthcare (Leininger, 2002e). Cultural imposition and ethnocentrism are deeply ingrained throughout society. Nurses and other healthcare providers who ignore transcultural aspects of care and rely solely on traditional psychoanalytic or other models of care may compartmentalize mental health solely as a mental psychobiological pathology (Ehrmin, 2012). Providing holistic culturally congruent care may reduce stigma and improve access to mental health care (Ehrmin, 2012). Educational outreach and delivery of culturally congruent mental health care may support mental health wellbeing (Knecht & Sabatine, 2015). To address the social stigma and disparities in accessing mental health care, the National Institutes of Mental Health (NIMH) and the World Health Organization (WHO) have developed new initiatives entitled, *Transforming the Understanding and Treatment of Mental Illnesses*, that include educational community outreach programs and plans for future research (NIMH, 2015) and the "Comprehensive Mental Health Action Plan 2013-2020" (WHO, 2015).

The community outreach program designed by the NIMH (2015) through their Office of Constituency Relations and Liaisons is a public education program that encourages efforts to reach diverse cultural groups with mental health issues. The outreach goals focus on facilitating science-based education and research in collaboration with community-based organizations with the goal of increasing mental health awareness as well as care and treatment opportunities for vulnerable cultural groups with mental health conditions (NIMH, 2015). In an effort to reduce the stigma and stereotypes surrounding mental health and promote widespread education about mental health disorders including information about attitudes, behaviors, and brain function, the NIMH developed 80 interprofessional collaborations with social workers, mental health service-related professionals, and interested clients and their family members (NIMH, 2015).

The Comprehensive Mental Health Action Plan developed by the WHO focuses on a new initiative titled "Mental Health Gap Action Programme" (mhGAP, 2015). This program provides a free guide and education modules for healthcare professionals and the public about such topics as acute stress disorder, depression, suicide, psychosis, harmful use of drugs and alcohol, dementia, and other mental health disorders (WHO, 2015). The mhGAP program provides mental health training for mental health professionals, referral for mental health clients to community services, and promotes awareness—specializing in marginalized culturally diverse persons worldwide (WHO, 2015). Healthcare professionals serve as the local and global care and referral linkages for diverse clients and needed mental health services. It is, therefore, crucial that they familiarize themselves with existing resources needed to provide comprehensive and culturally inclusive care.

Leininger (2002a) predicted that nurses, psychiatric mental health nurse practitioners, primary care nurse practitioners, physicians, physician assistants, and other healthcare professionals providing culturally congruent and sensitive care to individuals with mental health diagnoses would enable improved access to care and treatment. She maintained that culturally congruent care would reduce the risk of cultural pain and lead to the discovery of multiple influencers for the promotion of safe care, health, and wellbeing (Leininger, 2002e). In addition, Leininger (2002d) held that the provision of meaningful and beneficial culturally congruent care would not only improve health and wellbeing, but also result in optimal outcomes for diverse cultural groups. Leininger's Theory of Culture Care Diversity and Universality (also known as the Culture Care Theory or CCT) and the Sunrise Enabler, which support the discovery and application of beneficial and culturally meaningful mental health care practices (Leininger, 2002b), were used as the theoretical framework for this chapter and guided the review of the literature.

Cultural assessments that integrate Leininger's foundational concepts into transcultural mental health nursing principles will facilitate the provision of culturally congruent mental health care, without which many at-risk individuals may remain untreated, continue to suffer needlessly, and possibly be at risk for misdiagnosis or self-harm (Leininger, 2002e). Healthcare providers need to integrate mental health cultural assessments into their professional care to evaluate for cultural bound syndromes, provide accurate and time-sensitive diagnoses, avoid misdiagnosis, and collaboratively develop a mutually acceptable plan of care with clients.

■ PURPOSE

The purpose of this chapter is to provide orientational definitions of concepts that are important and relevant in mental health care and to examine how Leininger's CCT and Sunrise Enabler can be used to conduct a review of the literature and acquire holding knowledge that may influence cultural assessments and formulation of culturally congruent professional decisions and actions. Resources such as the Cultural Formulation Interview Guide (CFI; Diagnostic and Statistical Manual [DSM-5], 2013, p. 752-757) are presented to guide healthcare providers in their clinical practice as they gather relevant and much needed cultural information for accurate diagnosis and the co-development of integrative, culturally congruent, sensitive plans of care with clients.

■ ORIENTATIONAL DEFINITIONS

The following key terms are the orientational definitions used for mental health throughout this chapter:

- *Cultural awareness in mental health* refers to the deliberate self-assessment and in-depth exploration of one's own cultural background, beliefs, and self-awareness of personal prejudice and stereotypes directed at diverse cultures (Sagar, 2012).
- *Cultural bound syndromes* refer to disorders restricted to a particular culture or group of cultures related to certain psychosocial characteristics of those cultures. These syndromes are often referred to as *folk illnesses or folk diseases in which* altered behaviors or life experiences are prominent features (Andrews, 2012, p. 41).
- *Cultural competence in mental health* refers to values, principles, and beneficial behaviors of nurses, advance practice nurse practitioners, physician assistants, physicians, and other healthcare workers comprising a complex integration of skills that enhance cross-cultural communications and interactions and help to reduce disparities for mental health clients (who have health care beliefs, practices and linguistic needs) to bring about positive health outcomes (Andrews, 2012, p. 18).
- *Culturally congruent mental health care* refers to culturally-based knowledge, decisions, and actions used in culturally sensitive ways along with meaningful actions developed to provide care for diverse mental health clients that integrates their expressed cultural beliefs, values, and lifeways to promote health, wellbeing, or face disabilities or death (adapted from McFarland & Wehbe-Alamah, 2015, p. 14).
- *Cultural explanation* refers to the etiology for a pattern of behavior discovered or identified within a cultural or religious group (DSM-5, 2013, p. 758).
- *Cultural formulation interview (CFI)* refers to an evidence-based field-tested interviewing framework for assessing cultural information as it relates to an individual's mental health problem, social context, and history (and is intended) for use among clinicians to prevent misdiagnosis (DSM-5, 2013, p. 749).
- *Cultural idiom of distress* refers to the suffering reported by individuals within a cultural or religious group (DSM-5, 2013, p. 758).
- *Cultural imposition* refers to tendencies of a group or individual to impose their beliefs and values onto another individual or group [such as mental health clients] for various reasons (Leininger, 2002b, p. 51).
- *Cultural syndromes* refer to a cluster of co-occurring symptoms found in a specific culture (DSM-5, 2013, p. 14).
- *Diagnostic and Statistical Manual of Mental Disorders (DSM-5)* refers to a publication from the American Psychiatric Association used as an evidence-based diagnostic textbook that has classification criteria and descriptions of pathological processes for mental health disorders (DSM-5, 2013, p. xli, *Preface*).
- *Discrimination* refers to an overt or covert action that limits opportunities or life experiences or imposes racial biases based on faulty feelings (Leininger, 2002b).
- *Ethnocentrism* refers to the belief that one's own lifeways and/or beliefs are the best or most superior way to believe or behave (Leininger, 2002b, p. 50).
- *Major depressive episode (MDE)* is defined as [a person] experiencing at least five of the nine symptoms of depression during the same two-week period or longer over the previous 12 months, of which one symptom must be depressed mood or loss of interest or pleasure in daily activities, in addition to other [listed] depressive symptoms (The Substance Abuse and Mental Health Administration [SAMHSA], 2013a).
- *Mental health* refers to the emotional and psychological wellness with the successful capacity to interact with others, deal with ordinary stress according to cultural norms, and the ability to perceive one's surroundings realistically (American Nurses' Association, 2014, p. 89).
- *Mental illness* refers to a maladaptive response to stressors from external or internal environments as evidenced by feelings, thoughts, and behaviors that are incongruent with local and cultural norms and interfere with the individual's social, occupational, and/or physical functioning (Townsend, 2014, p. 4).
- *Prejudice* refers to a preconceived belief or opinion about an individual or cultural group that limits the full and accurate understanding of the individual, culture, gender, event, or situation (Leininger, 2002b, p. 55).

- *Recovery* refers to the process of change during which individuals are able to improve their mental health and wellness, live a self-directed life, and strive to reach to their full potential (SAMHSA as cited by Townsend, 2014, p. 205).
- *Remission* refers to the state of being wherein an individual exhibits the lack of significant signs or symptoms of mental disturbance (DSM-5, 2013, p. 188).
- *Serious mental illness* refers to serious and persistent [emotional, psychological, and physical] functional impairment that substantially interferes or limits one or more of life's major activities (NIMH, 2013a).
- *Stereotyping* refers to a snap judgment that classifies a person or group without understanding the cultural differences of that individual or group (Leininger, 2002b, p. 55).
- *Stigma in mental health* refers to the stereotype, prejudice, and discrimination against individuals with mental illness (SAMHSA, 2006).
- *Worldview* refers to the way individuals view their world or universe and hold values or broad perspectives about their orientation to life, including groups or other individuals of diverse or similar cultures which influence care, decisions, or actions toward health, wellbeing, or illness (McFarland & Wehbe-Alamah, 2015, p. 15).

■ THEORETICAL FRAMEWORK

The Culture Care Theory (CCT) is a rich holistic approach for the provision of culturally congruent care for people who experience mental health disorders and provides for the discovery and application of beneficial and culturally meaningful practices in mental health care (Leininger, 2006b). It was chosen as the theoretical framework for this chapter so as to disseminate meaningful and evidence-based holding knowledge and to guide mental health care providers when conducting cultural assessments.

Two main theoretical assumptions the CCT that underpin this chapter are that "care is the essence of nursing and humanistic and scientific care is essential for human growth, wellbeing, health, survival, and to face death or disabilities" (McFarland & Wehbe-Alamah, 2015, p. 8). Another adapted assumptive premise of importance to this chapter is that "transcultural care is essential for the provision of culturally congruent mental health care" (Leininger, 2002f) and

mental health recovery and remission. Transcultural mental health care plays an important role in reducing prejudice, stigma, and health disparities as well as in facilitating access to care (Leininger, 2002e).

Ethnonursing research studies guided by the CCT have discovered that diverse and similar cultural groups preferred professional care practices that are inclusive of generic folk beliefs and healing practices. Leininger's three modes of culture care decisions and actions can guide the delivery of culturally congruent and therapeutic care for mental health clients of diverse and similar cultures (Leininger, 2006b). The culture care modes encompass preservation and/or maintenance; accommodation and/or negotiation, and repatterning and/or restructuring (McFarland & Wehbe-Alamah, 2015, p. 16). These modes may be used in various healthcare settings to assist healthcare providers in planning culturally congruent approaches for mental health care. Healthcare providers will need to assess, be sensitive to, and account for diverse mental health beliefs, traditions, and generic/folk healing practices when developing a plan of care for their clients. For example, Lebanese and Syrian Muslim informants reported associating health with the wellbeing of mind, body, and soul. They believed illness to be related to the evil eye or God's will. "… If the Lord of the universe wills to cure this person, she/he will be cured without a doctor" (Wehbe-Alamah, 2015, p. 147). These informants wanted nurses to assist with accommodations for prayers and other rituals when hospitalized and indicated that such activities enhance mental and spiritual as well as physical wellbeing (Wehbe-Alamah, 2015).

■ REVIEW OF THE LITERATURE USING THE SUNRISE ENABLER

Ethnodemograpics

The number of individuals with mental illness is rising worldwide with approximately 400 million individuals experiencing significant depression (WHO, 2014). The burden of mental illness affects health, social interactions, human rights, and access to care (WHO, 2014). In low to middle income countries, 76% to 85% of people with mental illness do not receive care in comparison to 35% to 50% in higher-income countries (WHO, 2014). Mental illness has become epidemic, not only in the U.S. but globally.

Adults

During 2012, 43.7 million adults in the U.S. aged 18 years and older (approximately 18.6% of the adult population) experienced some form of mental illness (NIMH, 2013b) with an additional 9.6 million adults (4.1% of the adult population) experiencing a *serious* mental illness. Sixteen million adults (6.9% of the adult population) reported experiencing at least one major depressive episode *that year* (NIMH, 2013a). In addition, 3.3 million individuals or 28.5% of adults with depression comorbidly experienced substance abuse (CDCP, 2011b; NIMH, 2013b). However, approximately 54% of young Americans aged 18 to 24 years with mental illness lead normal lives (NIMH, 2013b).

Surveys of prisoners in U.S. state and federal correctional facilities in 2002 and 2004 revealed that 56% of state prisoners and 45% of federal prisoners had mental illnesses such as mania (43%), depression (24%), and psychotic disorders (15%; Bonczar, 2008). According to statistics in 2006 from the Bureau of Justice approximately 300,000 adults in the U.S. aged 18 years and older who were conditionally released from jail or prison (on probation or parole) were diagnosed with or had a history of mental illness; of these, 16% were considered at high risk for reincarceration related to their history of substance abuse (Bonczar, 2008). Between 1986 and 1997, 13.4% of prisoners were reincarcerated on charges related to their substance abuse (Sabol, Adams, Parthasarathy, & Yuan, 2000). In 2011, 9.6% of all U.S. military personal reported experiencing depression; 25.6% perceived the need for mental health services; and 24.9% received counseling (NIMH, 2013a). An estimated 26% of homeless U.S. citizens living in shelters have mental illness; many suffer untreated (Mental Health America [MHA], 2015).

Among U.S. adults, the prevalence by age for depressive symptoms was reported by the NIMH in 2013b as 8.7% for ages 18-27; 7.6% for ages 26-49; and 5.5% for ages 50 and older. More women (8.4%) than men (5.2%) experienced a major depressive episode (MDE; SAMHSA, 2013b; NIMH, 2013b). MDE rates also vary among ethnic groups as follows: Native Hawaiians and Pacific Islanders (1.6%); Asians (4%); African Americans (4.6%); Hispanics (5.8%); Caucasians (7.3%); American Indians or Alaska Natives (8.9%); and mixed heritage persons (11.4%; SAMHSA, p. 14).

Children

Children in the U.S. between the ages of 12 and 17 years living with a major depressive episode reportedly increased from 17% in 2011 to 19% in 2012 (NIMH, 2013b). Two out of five children in the U.S. who need mental health care do not receive it (MHA, 2015). The SAMHSA reports reflect that among adolescents aged 12 to 17 years, more than three million sought out mental healthcare services at educationally based clinical settings and more than half a million (686,000) youths at medical clinic settings *annually* (2013b, p. 32). The most commonly reported reasons for these visits were depression (40%); "acting out" behaviors (22%); anxiety (18%); interpersonal relationship problems (17.7%); and family concerns (16%) (SAMHSA, 2013b, p. 42).

These statistics emphasize the prevalence of mental illness across all demographic groups in the U.S. They reveal the potential for significant societal consequences, including loss of life from untreated or inadequately treated mental illness and related conditions. According to the NIMH (2013a), approximately 100 billion wage dollars are lost annually because of untreated mental illness. The Affordable Care Act has increased the number of insured individuals in the U.S. However, 3.9% or 8.1 million of American adults who reported having a mental illness remained uninsured and only 41.4% of adults with mental illness received mental health treatment (MHA, 2015, p. 25).

As stated earlier, the World Health Organization (2015) initiated a *Mental Health Gap Action Programme* (mhGAP) in 2010 to address the lack of care for individuals suffering worldwide from mental, neurological, and substance abuse conditions and in 2015 released the mhGAP Intervention Guide for general or primary care providers working in nonspecialized healthcare settings about mental, neurological, and substance abuse disorders. This program initially focused its efforts in Syria, Yemen, and Nepal but will be expanded to other regions (WHO, 2015). Potentially tens of thousands of individuals are estimated to need mental health care; the mhGAP initiative is predicted to facilitate the availability of mental health services to individuals with depression, schizophrenia, substance abuse conditions, and other neurological disorders in locations with scarce mental health resources (WHO, 2015).

Worldview

Mental health clients who experience paranoia, psychotic symptoms, or depressive thoughts are often uncomfortable talking to healthcare professionals because their *worldview* of nurses, psychiatrists, or therapists identifies these professionals as *strangers* who "… do not understand [their] lifeways and often misdiagnose [them]" (Leininger, 2002, p. 382). Stigma and attitude toward individuals with mental illness are shaped by one's personal beliefs, knowledge or previous experiences (CDCP, 2009, p. 4). *Stigma* in relation to mental health has been defined as the stereotype, prejudice, and discrimination against individuals with mental illness (WHO, 2015).

Stigma affects the worldview of how individuals perceive mental illness. According to the WHO (n.d.), misunderstandings and stigma surround mental illness and are widespread. Examples of misunderstandings include the beliefs that mental illness is difficult to treat and individuals with mental disorders are difficult, unintelligent, and incapable of decision-making. Such stigma has led to abuse, rejection, isolation, and exclusion from mental healthcare access and treatment (WHO, n.d.). Additionally, different types of abuse, wars, and disasters have doubled the need for mental health services worldwide (WHO, n.d.).

Unfortunately, there is global inequity in the distribution of skilled human resources for professional mental healthcare characterized by a shortage in psychiatrists, psychiatric nurse practitioners, mental health nurses, social workers, and psychologists in low and middle income countries compared to high income countries (WHO, n.d.). In addition, individuals with mental and psychosocial disabilities experience more human rights violations across most countries such as being physically restrained, quarantined into seclusion, and denied having basic needs met including privacy (WHO, n.d.). Fortunately, emerging programs that focus on increasing access to care by providing local and global care services for maternal-child health, human immunodeficiency virus, and noncommunicable diseases in addition to integrating mental health care services into communities are being led by researchers, clinicians, and diverse organizations such as the National Institutes of Mental Health (2013a) Office of Research on Disparities and Global Mental Health (Collins, Insel, Chockalingam, Daar, & Maddox, 2013). Leininger (2009) encouraged

psychiatric nurses to share their stories and skills to discover mental health clients' preferred lifeways, beliefs, and values to assist nurses to understand their worldview and consequently, to provide them with culturally congruent and meaningful mental health-care using the three modes of culture care decisions and actions. George (as cited in Leininger, 2002e) reported that mental health clients preferred being accommodated by having later medication administration times which in turn increased medication adherence. Practicing mental health Muslim patients who fast during the month of Ramadan may need to be accommodated by having their meals and medications offered after sunset or prior to dawn so as to respect and help them maintain their religious practices and to improve adherence with the professional plan of care (Wehbe-Alamah, 2015). The integration of the Culture Care Theory into mental health clinical care may guide clinicians to discover their clients' worldviews and provide culturally congruent professional health care that is devoid of cultural imposition, stereotypes, prejudices, or discrimination.

Cultural Values, Beliefs, and Lifeways

Cultural values, beliefs, and lifeways regarding specific mental health symptoms vary among diverse cultural groups (Ehrmin, 2012). Some cultural values and beliefs associated with mental health include stigma, stereotypes, prejudice, and discrimination (Ehrmin, 2012). Stigma associated with mental health leads to feelings of isolation because of embarrassment, disgrace, or disconnection from society for being different from others because of a mental disorder diagnosis. Stereotyping, prejudice, and discrimination have contributed to disparities and barriers to mental health care. In addition, stigma associated with mental illness causes individuals and families to avoid seeking treatment because of encountered prejudices, stereotypes, discrimination, and social-cognitive dynamics (SAMHSA, 2006). Proper identification of the cultural beliefs, values, and practices of mental health clients is essential for the early diagnosis and treatment of mental illness, including differentiation between mental illness, cultural norms, and cultural bound syndromes.

Kinship and Social Factors

Global perspectives and migratory trends have illuminated the diverse kinship and social factors that affect mental health care. Ehrmin (2012) discovered that African-American families relied on substance abuse as a means to "… tune out physical and emotional pain" that was related to racism and oppression. Ehrmin also discovered in her ethnonursing transcultural study that African-American families have strong matriarchal kinship-family structures, but that substance dependent African-American women felt they needed respect, care, and being listened to in a nonjudgmental manner to resolve past cultural pain experiences (p. 259).

Hispanic immigrants from Mexico, Spain, Cuba, and Southern and Central America that traditionally have large extended families are the fastest growing cultural group in the Unites States (Ehrmin, 2012). Hispanic extended family members rely on each other; offer each other emotional support; and use cultural folk medicine, folk healers, and naturalist doctors for treating illnesses (Ehrmin). The Hispanic social structure encompasses a strong father or male dominant role and value system based on the premise that trust must be earned (Ehrmin). Culturally sensitive mental health care providers assess for and incorporate kinship and social factors in their plans of care.

Spiritual, Religious, and Philosophical Factors

Coping mechanisms and/or spiritual or religious beliefs and values may differ from one cultural group to another or from individual to individual, especially in relation to mental health. Magico-religious beliefs vary among diverse populations and have been found to be especially meaningful for individuals with mental health illness, as stated by Ehrmin (2012): "… African American church leaders have reported fighting off demons with prayer" (p. 270). Some of the author's African-American clients have presented to her psychiatric practice wearing a "warding off bone" on a necklace, carrying a favorite Bible, or wearing a cross adorned necklace for "warding off evil spirits" and auditory or visual hallucinations. Some members of Mediterranean, Hispanic, and Jewish cultures believe the "evil eye" gaze will project a "malicious evil spirit," termed *Mishnah* in Judaism, and *mal de ojo* in Hispanic cultures (Ehrmin, 2012, p. 254; Jacobs, n.d.). It is important for nurses and other healthcare providers to identify, understand, and overcome any personal biases or prejudices related to culturally diverse mental health religious and folk care beliefs and practices

(Ehrmin, 2012) and to incorporate such findings in a culturally congruent plan of care.

Economic, Political, and Legal Factors

Mental illness and psychosocial disabilities account for up to 90% of unemployment worldwide (WHO, 2013). Many individuals with mental health illness who attend vocational training programs may be able to reach their full potential and become productive members of society (WHO, 2013). The Comprehensive Mental Health Action Plan 2013-2020 developed by the WHO (2013) was designed to empower mental health clients; integrate and improve access to mental health care; implement health promotion/prevention strategies; strengthen information systems, research, and leadership; and disseminate evidence for the expansion of mental health care services. One initiative for suicide prevention was implemented as an integral component to access to care for mental health clients (WHO, 2013). This global initiative includes support, education, awareness, advocacy, and research that will guide nurses and other healthcare providers toward meeting the needs of mental health clients (WHO, 2013).

One of the goals of Mental Health Action Plan 2013/2020 is for 50% of the United States to have developed or updated their mental health regulations to be aligned with international and regional policy provisions for human rights by 2020 (Stavert, 2015). Further, the integration of mental health disorders into the United Nations Convention on the Rights of Persons with Disabilities (CRPD) is expected to facilitate the development of mental health policies in many countries around the globe (Sachan, 2013).

Approximately 50% of mental health clients in the U.S. avoid seeking care due to multifactorial disparities and barriers to access to care (NIMH, 2013b). To address this problem, institutionally-based mental healthcare services are being transitioned to outpatient clinics, primary care settings, and community-based mental health clinics (NIMH, 2013b). In 2015, the State of Michigan announced the planned merger of the Department of Community Health with the Department of Human Services (public health departments) to improve the delivery of publically funded primary care and mental health care (State of Michigan, Department of Community Health, n.d.). This is a futuristic endeavor that will meet the needs of mental health clients through improved access in an interprofessionally collaborative continuum-of-care in the clinical setting (State of Michigan, Department of Community Health, n.d.). Healthcare providers including nurses are positioned to engage in advocacy, education, awareness, and support for mental health clients.

Cultural Bound Syndromes

Mental health behavior is influenced by cultural values, beliefs, and practices. Cultural bound syndromes may be thought of as a type of "culture-specific illness" (Ehrmin, 2012, p. 243). Cultural bound syndromes (also termed folk illnesses or culture-specific syndromes) are influenced by trends within a community (Ehrmin, 2012, p. 253). "It is essential that healthcare providers recognize and accurately diagnose individuals with cultural bound syndromes in order to avoid misdiagnosis and/or delay treatment" (Leininger, 2002e, p. 240). The caveat is that a cultural bound syndrome may in fact be a mental illness (Ehrmin, 2012). "If the cultural symptoms or behaviors are persistent; negatively affect social interactions; impair the client's functional ability in their environment, workplace, or close relationships; or lead to maladaptation in the environment, then this cluster of symptoms once analyzed may be most likely classified as a mental illness/disorder" (DSM-5, 2013, p. 14). The healthcare provider needs to perform a cultural assessment to determine whether the client is displaying culturally accepted behaviors, a cultural bound syndrome, or an acute or persistent mental illness (DSM-5, 2013, p. 14). Mental health clinicians and primary care providers may encounter clients with cultural bound syndromes (Refer to Figure 11.1) in their professional practices and will need to have holding knowledge about frequently encountered cultures and their culture specific beliefs, values, and practices to provide accurate and timely diagnosis, referral, and/or treatment.

■ CULTURAL ASSESSMENT

It is important for mental health nurses and healthcare providers to draw from the body of transcultural knowledge and use the Culture Care Theory to guide them in assessing mental health clients. Clinicians who wish to provide culturally congruent care to mental health patients should first become knowledgeable about concepts such as *cultural imposition, ethnocentrism,* and *cultural explanation,* then complete a cultural self-assessment before performing a cultural assessment of others (Andrews & Boyle, 2012). "The purpose of a self-assessment is for the clinician to discover his/her own cultural beliefs, values, practices, lifeways, as well as own cultural biases and prejudices, with the goal of improving his/her *cultural sensitivity and cultural competence* when working with mental health clients from diverse cultural groups" (Leininger, 2002b, p. 122). This process is known as *know thyself* and is critical for identifying misconceptions, ethnocentric tendencies, and predetermined views that may otherwise greatly limit the accuracy of cultural assessments of others (Leininger, 2002b).

When clinicians plan to conduct a cultural assessment of mental health clients, it is important to remain mindful about existing holding knowledge, evidence-based study findings, and the fact that many cultures do not report, explain, or define mental illness (Leininger, 2002e). "Clinicians should familiarize themselves with the diverse populations' cultural beliefs and values in order to devise collaboratively with their patients plans of care that respect, preserve, accommodate, negotiate, or restructure the patients' lifeways and practices." Because most cultures have generic (folk or indigenous) lifeways to help people cope with emotional or mental conditions, healthcare providers should assess such indigenous cultural care modalities and rituals for their therapeutic healing properties (Leininger, 2002b). A culturally congruent mental healthcare approach will facilitate client willingness to access care and improve outcomes for culturally diverse mental health clients.

The DSM-5 Cultural Formulation Interview

Mental health clients experience economic inequities, discrimination, stereotyping, prejudice, and disparities (Diagnostic and Statistical Manual of Mental Disorders [DSM-5], 2013, p. 749). To promote "… assessing a client's mental health problem and how it relates to social, cultural context, and history" the DSM-5 published a cultural formulation interview (CFI). The DSM-5 (2013) CFI has been field tested for diagnostic use by health care providers" (p. 749) and consists of 16 main questions that clinicians can ask clients to discover whether the influence of culture may be key in the mental health clinical, behavioral, and/or symptomatic presentations (p. 750). The provision of culturally congruent and therapeutic mental healthcare is thereby enhanced by "… avoiding misdiagnosis, obtaining pertinent

Culture	Syndrome	Symptoms
Chinese	Qi-jong psychotic reaction	Dissociation and paranoia
Haiti, West Africa	Boufee Delirate	Outbursts of agitation, aggression, and confusion
Inuit	Arctic Hysteria	Depressive silences, fatigue, confusion following a loss
Japan	Taijin Kyofusho	Intense fear one's body odor or appearance offends others
Korea	Hwa-Byung	Insomnia, suicide ideation, sadness, guilt, fearfulness. May occur middle-aged/elderly women
Korean	Shin-Byung	Anxiety, fear, weakness, gastro-intestinal, and sleep disturbances
Latin America, Latinos in United States	Susto, Soul Loss (Espantro, Pasmo)	Fright, low self-esteem, sadness, lack of motivation, gastrointestinal disturbances, muscle aches, headaches
Latino Cultures	Mal-Puesto "voodoo-death"	Afraid of being poisoned or killed; anxiety
Malaysia, China	Koro	Fear that penis or vulva/nipples will retract possibly causing death
Malaysia, Siberia	Latah	Exaggerated startle response, laughing with echopraxia/ echolalia; cursing
Mediterranean	Mal-de-ojo, "evil-eye"	Sleep disturbance, diarrhea, vomiting, crying
Navajo	Ghost Sickness	Preoccupation with death, pending thoughts of doom, loss of appetite, weakness, hallucinations
North Africa, Middle East	Zar "feeling possessed by a spirit"	Dissociation, hurting self, laughing, singing, crying, withdrawal, self-neglect
Polynesia	Amok	Brooding with subsequent aggression followed by amnesia
Portuguese, Cape Verde Island	Sangue Dormido	Pain, numbness, paralysis, convulsions
Southern U.S. Caribbean	Rootwork "Witchcraft, Vodoo"	Evil influences are responsible for illnesses
Southern United States	Spell	Trance-like state, communication with dead spirits. May be mistaken for psychosis
West Africa	Brain fog/Brain fag "Brain fatigue"	Difficulty concentrating; depression. Mostly seen high school or college students

FIGURE 11.1 • Cultural Bound Syndromes.

Adapted, with permission, from Ehrmin, J. T. (2016). Transcultural perspectives in mental health care. In M. M. Andrews, & J. S. Boyle (Eds.), *Transcultural concepts in nursing care* (7th ed., pp. 288-290). Philadelphia: Wolters Kluwer/Lippincott.

clinical/cultural information, cultivating clinical rapport and engagement, improving therapeutic efficacy, guiding clinical research, and clarifying cultural epidemiology" (DSM-5, 2013, p. 759). The APA offers free online access to the CFI (http://www.multiculturalmental-health.ca/wp-content/uploads/2013/10/2013_DSM5_CFI.pdf) for researchers and clinicians to use with their study participants and patients in clinical practice.

Cultural assessments should not be overgeneralized or rushed; adequate time is needed for reciprocal communication that facilitates building rapport and earning trust and respect (DSM-5, 2013). Cultural assessments [interviews] should be an open process to allow for the free discovery of culturally defined problems and expressions of causation as well as the identification of context, supportive networks, stressors, and cultural, spiritual, and/or religious values, beliefs, and expressions. In addition, the cultural assessment interview will allow for documentation of self-coping mechanisms, caregiver (kinship) support, historical method of seeking help, barriers to care, and clarification of cultural factors and preferences which may lead to psychological, interpersonal, and intergenerational conflicts or adaptations that may or may not enhance resilience (DSM-5, 2013).

The CFI was developed as a resource for clinicians to guide their assessment, diagnosis, and plan for the provision of holistic cultural mental health care and can be used to discern whether a mental condition or cultural bound syndrome exists (DSM-5, 2013). The integration of cultural mental health assessment assists the healthcare provider to reach an accurate client diagnosis and treatment plan in a time effective manner (DSM-5, 2013, p. 759).

Leininger's Transcultural Principles in Mental Health Care

In the 1950s, Leininger (2002f) advocated for education about cultural diversity in anticipation of possible "cultural crises" as globalization trends rose (p. 3). She maintained that psychiatric nurses and other healthcare providers must develop new ways to analyze cultural behavior, consider new "lenses" to diagnose, explain, and interpret client behavior, beliefs, values, and lifeways (Leininger, 2002d, p. 3). Leininger's theoretical framework encouraged psychiatric nurses and other healthcare providers to re-examine traditional psychoanalytical approaches, and apply anthropological and transcultural nursing concepts, principles, and research in the clinical setting (Leininger, 2002d). Leininger conducted many ethnonursing studies over the span of her career, collecting, analyzing, and interpreting findings related to Western and non-Western cultural ethnocentric and "strange behaviors" related to mental health beliefs, expressions, and lifeways (Leininger, 2002e,

p. 240). In the process, she discovered and reported the following mental health concerns:

- Mental pathologies in the Western world do not universally exist in non-Western cultures.
- Western diagnostic categories, symptoms, and treatment outcomes are difficult to use or fit in a number of cultures, but Western healthcare providers often try to impose these categories on diverse cultures.
- Some cultures do not explain, define, and know mental illnesses as identified by Western healthcare providers.
- What is "normal or abnormal" is usually very difficult to define in dualistic terms because of cultural influences and variabilities.
- Many cultures do not use psychological language terms to explain cultural phenomena.
- Culture-bound conditions exist and may be described and explained with nonpsychological and nonbiological terms.
- The Western dualistic mind-body focus is often most difficult to use in non-Western cultures that rely on holistic data.
- Most cultures have generic (folk or indigenous) ways to help their people with emotional concerns or conditions.
- Indigenous cultural care modalities for therapeutic healing outcomes are generally the least known and understood by mental healthcare providers.
- In-depth study of cultures from a holistic social structure, worldview, gender, class, language use, and in environmental cultural contexts are essential to grasp accurate expressions of mental illness, health or another human conditions, and to develop effective therapies. (Leininger, 2002e, p. 240).

In order to assist mental healthcare providers to reduce stigma, remove barriers, and facilitate the provision of holistic culturally congruent mental health care, Leininger (2002e) developed six transcultural mental health principles (Refer to Figure 11.2) integrating constructs of the Culture Care Theory.

Three Modes of Culture Care Decisions and Actions

Leininger's Sunrise Enabler (Refer to Color Insert 1) provides a visual map of the CCT that guides the transcultural clinician in developing a culturally congruent plan of care by integrating the three culture care modes

	Transcultural Principles for Mental Healthcare Providers	Clinical Application
1	Understand and respect mental health clients' cultural differences and care for them as human beings.	Recognize meanings in cultural differences and variabilities and similarities in mental expressions.
2	Understand own cultural values, beliefs, and lifeways to obtain accurate client assessments and interpretations.	Misinterpretations may result in insensitive decisions or actions with associated poor client outcomes.
3	Identify and work with a transcultural mentor to become effective in therapy.	Mentors may help novices consider the context of clients' behaviors, learn about verbal and nonverbal cues, and develop meaningful and appropriate culture care decisions and actions that assist mentally ill clients and/or their families.
4	Learn about the clients' cultural lifeways, multiple social structure factors, worldview, and environmental context as influencers of mental health behaviors.	Specific knowledge and assessment data will guide the clinician in grasping the totality of the clients' environments or situations and in providing culturally congruent care.
5	Allow time and be patient when working with clients whose language and behaviors are different in beliefs, values, and lifeways.	Verbal and nonverbal communication requires paying attention, active listening, patience, reflective thinking, periodic assessment, and being aware of the cultural situation.
6	Learn about cultural bound illnesses/syndromes and wellness states and respond in a culturally sensitive and appropriate way.	Cultural variability exists and presents with different expressions. The healthcare provider would need to recognize diverse cultural expressions as normal or abnormal as defined by the culture itself.

FIGURE 11.2 • Leininger's Fundamental Principles for Transcultural Mental Health Care.
Adapted from Leininger, M.M. (2002). Transcultural mental health nursing. In M. M. Leininger, & M. R. McFarland (Eds.), *Transcultural Nursing: Concepts, theories, research, and practice* (3rd ed., pp. 241-244). New York: McGraw-Hill Companies, Inc.

of decisions and actions (McFarland & Wehbe-Alamah, 2015, p. 25). The three culture care modes are *culture care preservation and/or maintenance*; *culture care accommodation and/or negotiation*; and *culture care repatterning and/or restructuring* (McFarland & Wehbe-Alamah, 2015, p. 16). The modes guide the mental healthcare provider to collaboratively develop with the client a plan of care that leads to optimal health and wellbeing outcomes or adapts to or copes with illness and sometimes death (McFarland & Wehbe-Alamah, 2015, p. 16).

Culture care preservation and/or maintenance refers to supporting, facilitating, or enabling culture care decisions and actions toward helping people of a particular culture preserve or maintain beneficial indigenous lifeways for their health and wellbeing and/or to recover from mental health illness (McFarland & Wehbe-Alamah, 2015, p. 16). George (1998) conducted a study with the chronically mentally ill that revealed the care construct *survival care* whereby the clients were able to maintain their usual patterns of daily living outside the

mental institution while continuing their mental health care regimes. Clients living in transition homes were able to come and go independently largely due to the involvement of nurse case managers who were available to assist them with maintaining their community-based Alcoholic Anonymous and Narcotic Anonymous meetings (George, 1998). This facilitative care assisted the mental health clients toward meeting their sobriety and mental health goals.

Culture care accommodation and/or negotiation refers to those accommodating, assisting, and/or facilitating culture care decisions and actions with people of a particular culture that help them adapt to or negotiate with the healthcare system and providers for beneficial, culturally congruent, and meaningful safe care (McFarland & Wehbe-Alamah, 2015, p. 16). An example of accommodation and/or negotiation is modifying medication administration times based on the preferences of mental health clients' to facilitate consistent acceptance of their medication regimen

(Leininger, 2006b). For example, some mental health clients report staying up late at night and waking later in the morning. Healthcare professionals can accommodate this lifeway pattern by administering some morning medications at noon-time and evening/supper medications at bedtime (Leininger, 2002e).

Culture care repatterning and/or restructuring refers to assistive, supportive, facilitative, or enabling professional actions and mutual decisions that would help people to reorder, change, modify, or restructure their lifeways and institutions for better (or beneficial) healthcare patterns, practices, or outcomes (McFarland & Wehbe-Alamah, 2015, p. 16). Examples of repatterning and/or restructuring actions for chronically mental ill clients include providing living arrangements in alternative community settings that improve lifeways, healthcare patterns, and outcomes (George, 1998, p. 73). Another example is restructuring mental health clients' self-cutting/self-injurious behaviors by substituting red ink pens that are not harmful in place of the sharp tools customarily used during skin cutting behaviors.

■ THEORY APPLICATION FOR MENTAL HEALTH CARE PRACTICES

Chronically mentally ill people prefer culturally congruent modalities that help them meet their needs, support their potential growth, and work toward health and wellbeing (George, cited by Leininger, 2002e, p. 250). The constructs of the Culture Care Theory and the cultural and social structure dimensions of the Sunrise Enabler can be adapted by mental health providers for client assessment and the provision of holistic culturally congruent mental health care in diverse environmental contexts. The goal of the Culture Care Theory is to assist people from diverse cultures for their general health and wellbeing or to help them face disabilities or death (Leininger, 2002c). The three modes of culture care decisions and actions focus on providing holistic and culturally sensitive care based on mutually agreed upon goals. Strategies for providing culturally congruent care for mental health clients include integrating the concepts and principles of Culture Care Theory into clinical practice (Leininger, 2002e).

The provision of holistic mental health care is facilitated when providers are respectful and sensitive to cultural values, diversities, needs, and taboos; aware of their own beliefs, practices, cultural bias and prejudices; willing to take the time to learn about their patients' cultural beliefs, practices, expressions, and lifeways by conducting a cultural assessment; open to seeking guidance from transcultural mentors or interpreters as needed; and keen to learn about cultural bound syndromes to avoid mental health misdiagnosis (Leininger, 2002e).

■ SUMMARY

The importance of developing a culturally congruent plan of care for diverse mental health clients based on a holistic assessment has been discussed within the framework of the Culture Care Theory. Establishing a trusting therapeutic relationship with clients improves their health and wellbeing and leads to optimal care outcomes. Without strategies to facilitate culturally congruent mental health care, many at-risk individuals may remain untreated and continue to suffer needlessly. Many diverse cultures do not use or have psychiatric mental health terminology to explain cultural phenomena (Leininger, 2002e). Healthcare clinicians are encouraged to integrate mental health cultural assessments into their routine assessments/care to rule out cultural bound syndromes and to collaboratively develop mutually agreed upon plans of care with their clients.

Culturally sensitive and competent healthcare clinicians are essential for the provision of culturally congruent mental health care for diverse and vulnerable clients. The Sunrise Enabler depicts the cultural and social structure dimensions that influence people and their mental health care. Both *culture care* and *mental health care* are influenced by cultural lifeways, values, and beliefs. Culturally congruent mental health care may reduce prejudice, stigma, and health disparities as well as facilitate access to mental health care (Leininger, 2002e).

Transcultural mental health assessment using the Culture Care Theory and the DSM-5 Cultural Formulation Interview may assist the clinician in identifying what is and what is not a mental illness. Cultural bound syndromes exist within and among diverse and similar cultures. It is critical that clinicians acquire the ability to accurately identify these syndromes and how to alleviate their clients' emotional distress. A holistic transcultural approach empowers both the healthcare clinician and mental health client toward achieving optimal outcomes for health and wellbeing, recovery, and/or remission.

■ DEDICATION

This chapter is dedicated to Dr. Madeleine Leininger, transcultural theorist, anthropologist, psychiatric nurse, and influential author, and to Dr. Margaret Andrews, Dr. Marilyn McFarland, and Dr. Hiba Wehbe-Alamah who are transcultural scholars, colleagues, teachers, and my mentors. They have inspired me to critically analyze the Theory of Culture Care Diversity and Universality and apply it in my mental health clinical practice. I thank you for helping me meet Dr. Leininger in person, which was a pinnacle event in my scholarly journey. It is my hope that mental health care continues to evolve toward being culturally congruent. *Helene Vossos*

This chapter is dedicated to health care providers interested in providing culturally congruent and sensitive mental health care to their patients. It is also dedicated to Dr. Madeleine Leininger who earned her Masters of Science in psychiatric and mental health nursing in 1954 from the Catholic University of America in Washington, D.C. It is thanks to her observations while working at a child guidance home, and decades of hard work and struggles, that transcultural nursing emerged and was established as a discipline. She was indeed instrumental in raising awareness and reinforcing the importance of and need for delivering culturally congruent and competent health care. *Hiba Wehbe-Alamah*

■ DISCUSSION QUESTIONS

1. Discuss the value of integrating cultural assessments into mental health evaluations/care.
2. Discuss how providing culturally congruent care for mental health clients may help to reduce stigma.
3. Discuss ways that the Culture Care Theory facilitates the provision of culturally congruent care in mental health.
4. Discuss how to differentiate mental illness from a culture-bound syndrome in a client from a diverse cultural group.

■ REFERENCES

American Nurses' Association. (2014). *Scope and standards of practice: Psychiatric-mental health nursing* (2nd ed.). Silver Springs, MD.

American Psychiatric Association. (2013). Diagnostic and statistical manual of mental disorders [DSM-5] (5th ed., pp. 752-757). Washington, DC: Author.

Andrews, M. M. (2012). Cultural competence in the health history and physical examination. In M. M. Andrews & J. S. Boyle (Eds.), *Transcultural concepts in nursing care*, (6th ed., p. 41). Philadelphia, PA: Wolters Kluwer | Lippincott.

Andrews, M. M., & Boyle, J. S. (2012). Theoretical foundations of transcultural Nursing. In M. M. Andrews & J. S. Boyle (Eds.), *Transcultural concepts in nursing care* (6th ed., pp. 3-16). Philadelphia, PA: Wolters Kluwer | Lippincott.

Bonczar, T. P. (2008). Characteristics of state parole supervising agencies, 2006. *Bureau of Justice Statistics*. Retrieved from http://www.bjs.gov/index.cfm?ty=pbdetail&iid=549

Centers for Disease Control and Prevention. (2009). Attitudes toward mental illness: Results from the behavioral risk factor surveillance system. Retrieved from http://www.cdc.gov/hrqol/Mental_Health_Reports/pdf/BRFSS_Full%20Report.pdf

Centers for Disease Control and Prevention. (2011a). Health, United States, 2011, with special feature on socioeconomic status and health. Retrieved from http://www.cdc.gov/nchs/data/hus/hus11.pdf#fig32

Centers for Disease Control and Prevention. (2011b). Life expectancy and fast facts. Retrieved from http://www.cdc.gov/nchs/fastats/life-expectancy.htm

Collins, P., Insel, T., Chockalingam, A., Daar, A. & Maddox, Y. (2013). Grand challenges in global mental health: Integration and implementation in research, policy and practice. *PLoS Med, 10*(4), e1001434. doi: 10.1371/journal.pmed.1001434. Retrieved from http://journals.plos.org/plosmedicine/article?id=10.1371/journal.pmed.1001434

Ehrmin, J. T. (2012). Transcultural perspectives in mental health care. In M. M. Andrews & J. S. Boyle (Eds.), *Transcultural concepts in nursing care* (6th ed., pp. 243-276). Philadelphia, PA: Wolters Kluwer | Lippincott.

George, T. B. (1998). *Meanings, expressions, and experiences of care of chronically mentally ill in a day treatment center, using Leininger's culture care theory* [Doctoral dissertation]. Retrieved from UMI database (Accession No. 9915656)

Jacobs, L. (n.d.). *Evil eye in Judaism*. New York, NY: MyJewishLearning.com. [Reprinted from *The Jewish religion: A companion* (1st ed.) by L. Jacobs, Ed., 1995, New York, NY: Oxford University Press.] Retrieved from http://www.myjewishlearning.com/article/evil-eye-in-judaism/

Knecht, L., & Sabatine, C. (2015). Application of culture care theory to international service-learning experiences in Kenya. In M. R. McFarland & H. B. Wehbe-Alamah (Eds.), *Leininger's culture care diversity and universality: A worldwide nursing theory* (3rd ed., pp. 475-499). Burlington, MA: Jones and Bartlett Learning.

Leininger, M. M. (2002a). Culture care assessments for congruent competency practices. In M. M. Leininger & M. R. McFarland (Eds.), *Transcultural nursing: Concepts, theories, research, & practice* (3rd ed., p. 122). New York, NY: McGraw-Hill.

Leininger, M. M. (2002b). Essential transcultural nursing care concepts, principles, examples and policy statements. In M. M. Leininger & M. R. McFarland (Eds.), *Transcultural nursing: Concepts, theories, research, & practice* (3rd ed., pp. 48-55). New York, NY: McGraw-Hill.

Leininger, M. M. (2002c). Part I. The theory of culture care and the ethnonursing research method. In M. M. Leininger & M. R. McFarland (Eds.), *Transcultural nursing: Concepts, theories, research, & practice* (3rd ed., pp. 78, 79.) New York, NY: McGraw-Hill.

Leininger, M. M. (2002d). Philippine Americans and culture care. In M. M. Leininger & M. R. McFarland (Eds.), *Transcultural nursing: Concepts, theories, research, & practice* (3rd ed., p. 380). New York, NY: McGraw-Hill.

Leininger, M. M. (2002e). Transcultural mental health nursing. In M. M. Leininger & M. R. McFarland (Eds.), *Transcultural nursing: Concepts, theories, research, & practice* (3rd ed., pp. 239-252). New York, NY: McGraw-Hill.

Leininger, M. M. (2002f). Transcultural nursing and globalization of health care: Importance, focus and historical aspects. In M. M. Leininger & M. R. McFarland (Eds.), *Transcultural nursing: Concepts, theories, research, & practice* (3rd ed., pp. 3-43). New York, NY: McGraw-Hill.

Leininger, M. M. (2006a). Culture care diversity and universality theory and evolution of the ethnonursing research method. In M. M. Leininger & M. R. McFarland (Eds.), *Culture care diversity and universality: A worldwide nursing theory* (2nd ed., p. 35). Burlington, MA: Jones and Bartlett Learning.

Leininger, M. M. (2006b). Culture care theory with Sudanese of Africa. In M. M. Leininger & M. R. McFarland (Eds.), *Culture care diversity and universality: A worldwide nursing theory* (2nd ed., pp. 267-272). Burlington, MA: Jones and Bartlett Learning.

Leininger, M. M. (1992). Psychiatric nursing and transculturalism: Quo vadis? *Perspectives in Psychiatric Care, 28*(1), 3-4. doi: 10.1111/j.1744-6163.1992.tb00353.x

McFarland, M. R., & Wehbe-Alamah, H. B. (2015). The theory of culture care diversity and universality. In M. R. McFarland & H. B. Wehbe-Alamah (Eds.), *Leininger's culture care diversity and universality: A worldwide nursing theory* (3rd ed., pp. 15-17). Burlington, MA: Jones and Bartlett Learning.

Mental Health America. (2015). *Parity or disparity: The state of mental health in America*. Retrieved from http://www.mentalhealthamerica.net/sites/default/files/Parity%20or%20Disparity%20Report%20FINAL.pdf

Mental Health in Multicultural Australia. (2013). Framework for mental health in multicultural Australia: Towards culturally inclusive service delivery. Retrieved from http://framework.mhima.org.au/framework/index.htm

National Institutes for Health, National Institutes for Mental Health. (2013a). *Serious mental illness (SMI) among U.S. adults: Data from the 2013 National Survey on Drug Use and Health*. Retrieved from http://www.nimh.nih.gov/health/statistics/prevalence/serious-mental-illness-smi-among-us-adults.shtml

National Institutes for Health, National Institutes for Mental Health. (2013b). *Any mental illness among adults: Data from the 2013 National Survey on Drug Use and Health*. Retrieved from http://www.nimh.nih.gov/health/statistics/prevalence/any-mental-illness-ami-among-adults.shtml

National Institutes for Health, National Institutes for Mental Health. (2015). *NIMH Outreach Partnership Program*. Retrieved from http://www.nimh.nih.gov/outreach/partnership-program/index.shtml

Sabol, W., Adams, W., Parthasarathy, B., & Yuan, Y. (2000, September). *Bureau of Justice Statistics special report: Offenders returning to federal prison 1986-1997*. Washington, DC: U.S. Department of Justice, Office of Justice Programs. Retrieved from http://www.bjs.gov/content/pub/pdf/orfp97.pdf

Sachan, D. (2013, July 27). Mental health bill set to revolutionise care in India. *The Lancet, 382* (9889), 296. doi: 10.1016./SO140-6736 (13)61620-7

Sagar, P. L. (2012). *Transcultural nursing theory and models: Application in nursing education, practice, and administration* (p. 41). New York, NY. Springer.

State of Michigan, Department of Health and Human Services. (n.d.). *Behavioral health and developmental disabilities* [webpage]. Retrieved from http://www.michigan.gov/mdch/0,4612,7-132-2941---,00.html

Stavert, J. (2015). The exercise of legal capacity, supported decision-making and Scotland's mental health and incapacity legislation: Working with CRPD challenges. *Laws 2015, 4*(2), 296-313. doi: 10.3390/laws4020296. Retrieved from http://www.mdpi.com/search?q=&journal=laws&volume=&authors=Stavert%2C+J&section=issue=&article_type=&special_issue=&page=&search=Search

Townsend, M. C. (2014). *Essentials of psychiatric mental health nursing: Concepts of care in evidence-based practice* (6th ed., pp. 205-206). Philadelphia, PA: FA Davis.

U.S. Department of Health and Human Services, Substance Abuse and Mental Health Services Administration, Center for Behavioral Health Statistics and Quality Review. (2006). *National mental health anti-stigma campaign: What a difference a friend makes.* Retrieved from https://store.samhsa.gov/shin/content/SMA07-4257/SMA07-4257.pdf

U.S. Department of Health and Human Services, Substance Abuse and Mental Health Administration Center for Behavioral Health Statistics and Quality Review. (2012). *Results from the 2012 National Survey on Drug Use and Health: Survey of inmates in state and federal correctional facilities.* Rockville, MD: Author. Retrieved from http://archive.samhsa.gov/data/NSDUH/2k12MH_FindingsandDetTables/2K12MHF/NSDUHmhfr2012.htm#tabb-1

U.S. Department of Health and Human Services, Substance Abuse and Mental Health Administration Center for Behavioral Health Statistics and Quality Review. (2013a). *Results from the 2013 National Survey on Drug Use AND Health: Mental health findings.* Rockville, MD: Author. Retrieved from http://www.samhsa.gov/data/sites/default/files/NSDUHmhfr2013/NSDUHmhfr2013.pdf

U.S. Department of Health and Human Services, Substance Abuse and Mental Health Services Administration, Center for Behavioral Health Statistics and Quality Review. (2013b, December). Results from the 2012 National survey on drug use and health: Mental health findings. Rockville, MD: Author. Retrieved from http://archive.samhsa.gov/data/NSDUH/2k12MH_FindingsandDetTables/2K12MHF/NSDUHmhfr2012.htm

Wehbe-Alamah, H. (2015). Folk care beliefs and practices of traditional Lebanese and Syrian Muslims in the Midwestern United States. In M. R. McFarland and H. B. Wehbe-Alamah (Eds.), *Leininger's culture care diversity and universality: A worldwide nursing theory* (3rd ed., pp. 137-181). Burlington, MA: Jones and Bartlett Learning.

World Health Organization. (n.d.). *Ten facts on mental health* [slide set]. Geneva, SUI: Author. Retrieved from http://www.who.int/features/factfiles/mental_health/mental_health_facts/en/

World Health Organization. (2013). *Comprehensive mental health action plan 2013-2020* [webpage]. Geneva, SUI: Author. Retrieved from http://www.who.int/mental_health/action_plan_2013/en/

World Health Organization. (2014, October). *Mental disorders: Fact sheet N*396* [webpage]. Geneva, SUI: Author. Retrieved from http://www.who.int/mediacentre/factsheets/fs396/en/

World Health Organization. (2015). *Mental health: WHO mental health Gap Action Programme (mhGAP)* [webpage]. Geneva, SUI: Author. Retrieved from http://www.who.int/mental_health/mhgap/en/

CHAPTER 12

Care, Caring, and Nursing Practice

Marilyn K. Eipperle

> *"Caring is nursing; caring is the heart and soul of nursing; caring is power; caring is healing; caring is the distinctive feature that makes nursing what is or should be as a profession and discipline"* (Leininger, 2002c, p. 11).

■ INTRODUCTION

Nurses have long been perceived by the public as caring and trustworthy. This historical aspect of their role has remained essentially unchanged for decades. In 2016, it was reported for the 15th consecutive year that nurses, "… ranked [as] the most trusted out of a wide spectrum of professions" with the highest honesty and ethical standards (American Nurses' Association, 2016) and were listed as the largest group of healthcare professionals, numbering 3,328,771 (Kaiser Family Foundation, 2017). Sagar (2017) further emphasized that:

> …Nurses must use such honor and trust in safeguarding the public welfare. As nurses it is imperative that we harness this power and capitalize on this trust and our strength in numbers to effect changes in health care that would contribute to improved health and wellbeing for all. (p. 220)

Several key factors have increasingly converged to impede and constrain nurses' execution of their inherent, central, and core role: *care* and *caring*. Most challenging among these factors is the emphasis on cost containment, which has led to shifts in staffing composition/ratios; systems-thinking and system-based provider practices; and the prioritization of technology uses (Baumann, 2012; Flynn, 1988; Leininger, 1988a). Mandated shorter hospital stays; increased medical specialization; increased needs for community-based care; and widening healthcare inequities have also become barriers to nurses' ability to spend necessary, quality, and meaningful time with patients. With increased focus on the needs of *systems* (data-driven practice outcomes, targets, or goals), *patients as individuals* are getting lost in the healthcare system (Ackerman, 2016, p. 108). Nonetheless, individualized caring approaches are still needed.

Although some of these system-focused or data-based changes have resulted in documented improvements in health outcomes, it is also true that the quality and context of the time nurses have or do spend with patients has been reduced as an outgrowth of these changes (Fitzpatrick, 2015). Clinical encounters between nurses and patients are less interactive and more rushed/time pressured, focused on tasks to be accomplished, teaching to perform, documentation to be completed, and boxes to mark (Raferty & O'Connell, 2016). As a further consequence, nurses are quite often perceived as too busy to really listen, hear, *care* (Baumann, 2012; Latham, 1996; Leininger, 1988a).

■ LITERATURE REVIEW

Concepts of Care and Caring in Transcultural Nursing

A review of the literature revealed nursing educational program theoretical or construct foci are mainly limited to simulation, research, outcomes analysis, and specific care settings or diseases. Most nursing educational curricula in the United States lack an organizing theoretical framework for teaching transcultural nursing and culture care, relying instead on anecdotal experience (Labrague, McEnroe-Petitte, Papathanasiou, Edet, & Arulappan, 2015; Mixer, 2011). Garneau and Pepin (2015) emphasized the need for using critical reflection teaching-learning methods to build bridges between newly acquired informational learning, sociopolitical influences in the practice environment, and life experiences of students when teaching transcultural care in nursing education (p. 14). "If nursing …claims to be a caring profession, then care should be reflected in nurses' actions. Sensitivity and other appropriate care behaviors should be evident in daily lifeways. …Evidence of care being central to nursing [in] curricula is still negligible" (Leininger, 1988a, p. 25). It is important to emphasize that while nursing theory frameworks are not in strong evidentiary use as the foundational structure for nursing educational programs feasible, applicable, and workable frameworks are extant in many transcultural nursing and caring science theories and models. Integrating care and caring into nursing as a valued, essential, and necessary element of holistic practice should begin at entry-level and continue across all levels and forms of nursing education (Gillespie, Kelly, Duggan, & Dornan, 2017).

Let us begin with some basic questions:

- What is care or caring?
- What does it mean to care?
- How do we know when someone cares or is caring?

Nursing as a profession and discipline has a societal mandate to serve and provide care to people, to anticipate or respond to their known and unknown care needs. Leininger (2002a) conceptualized *human care and caring* as "…the central, distinct, and dominant foci to explain, interpret, and predict nursing as a discipline and profession. Human *care* refers to a specific *phenomenon* that is characterized to assist, support, or enable another human being or group to achieve one's desired goals or obtain assistance with certain human needs. In contrast, human *caring* is focused on the action aspect or activities" (p. 46).

Increased focus on the importance of care and caring has occurred in the arena of healthcare policy as well as in nursing. In 2015, the American Nurses' Association (ANA) issued an updated *Nursing Scope and Standards of Practice* that included culturally congruent practice as a standard of performance (ANA, pp. 15; 69-70), listing 13 basic, five graduate, and two advanced practice competencies (Marion et al., 2016). Although the performance parameters for this standard did not specify *care* per se, using language for competencies such as "…respect, equity, and empathy in actions and interactions" with clients and "…respects consumer decisions" (p. 69), care and caring were described under the section entitled, *Scope of Nursing Practice* (p. 11). Under the subheading of *Care and Caring in Nursing Practice*, the ANA cited Watson (2012) and her *Theory of Human Caring Science*, to underscore "…the personal relationship between patient and nurse [because]…Human caring is not just an emotion, concern, attitude, or benevolent desire" (ANA, 2015, p. 11). Moreover, citing Finfgeld-Connett (2008), the ANA affirmed that, "Interventions that reflect a caring consciousness may require creativity and daring, but can also be demonstrated in simple gestures of interpersonal connection such as attentive listening, touching, and making eye contact; and [in] sensitivity to cultural meanings associated with caring behaviors (ANA, 2015, p. 12). Finfgeld-Connett emphasized that "Expert nursing practice is a critical attribute of the caring process" (2008, p. 199). The ANA further strengthened the connection between *caring* and *culture* in nursing practice by citing Leininger (1988c) and stating, "Transcultural literacy has deepened nursing's holistic approach by providing a guiding framework to better understand and provide care to culturally diverse individuals, groups, and communities" (ANA, 2015, p. 13).

The United States Institute of Medicine (2011) also stated that "…care must meet patient preferences, needs, and values and that patient values guide all clinical decisions" (p. 3). However, much of this document focused on driving the systems of health care and technological sharing of patient data, including health outcomes and billing information, across systems so as to reduce costs and save time. These two foci, *meeting patient needs and preferences* and *reducing costs while saving time*, have not quite come together as idealized. "The perceptions and ratings of the recipients of care remain largely overlooked in contemporary measures of quality of care" (Edvardsson, Watt, & Pearce, 2016, p. 219).

Care and Person-Centeredness

Person-centeredness is a contemporary concept stemming from psychotherapy and the consumer-participant movement (Edvardsson et al., 2016, p. 219). Citing Edvardsson (2015), these authors added:

> The focus of nursing care explicitly includes the relational aspects of health and illness as much as biological aspects and strives toward integrating the relational 'being with' together with the task-based 'doing for' in nursing. ... Person-centered care has been described as bringing back the *person* [emphasis added] into care and by that [act] reinforcing the ethical demand of nursing to safeguard patient dignity and autonomy, as well as inviting and respecting shared decision-making, choice, and control. (p. 219)

Just as 'help is not *help* if it is not helpful' it follows that 'care is not *care* if it is not perceived as caring'. Care and caring must be more than an internal reflection or intention held by the nurse; they must be perceived by the person/intended recipient to be meaningful, valued/valuable, or beneficial. Genuine care or caring must be *conveyed* and be in support of the values of the person, engender perceptions of support, and also empower the recipient as an autonomous, self-determining individual. *Patient*-centered care is not *person*-centered if the individual involved (or their delegate) is not an equally active participant in the decision-making process. Holding the *patient* in the center of a team conversation is not *person*-centered care. Establishing medically-focused goals on behalf of the patient congruent solely or mainly with those of the clinician is not person-centered care and often results in care dissatisfaction and grievances (Potter & Oehlert, 2015), as Leininger previously had predicted (2002b).

Daly (2012) described person-centered care as a *design of care delivery* that ensures patient/family engagement and identification of their goals that are prioritized in the plan of care, and would require multi-level, system-wide healthcare change based on an "honest appraisal" to redesign provider processes and resources to focus care on a person's priorities and needs, "rather than simply on how the system defines its own needs, priorities of care, and successful health outcomes" (para. 3). Milton (2012) proposed the metaphoric idea of the *nurse as a guest* in the care experiences of patients or clients, and

posited that healthcare clinicians need to enter into the lives and care of clients from an other-servedness and coparticipative viewpoint (p. 138). This author advocated stepping away from the consumeristic and reductionistic foci on quality improvement, safety initiatives, and teaching-learning practices as the main priorities, goals, and standards for the nursing profession (Milton, 2012, p. 138). Similarly, Bartol (2016) editorialized that enhancing the patient experience entails more than reactive attempts to address issues identified in client satisfaction surveys (p. 14), stating that an *enhanced patient experience*:

> ...redefines the measure of a successful day, the culture of our practice, from seeing a certain number of patients or achieving a percentage of quality measures, to connecting with an individual to helping create positive life changes. This takes into account the needs, values, and choices of a patient, finding out not just "what is the matter" but "what matters most." (p. 14)

Having *caring feelings* without demonstrable *caring behaviors* is not meaningful to intended recipients: Caring must be visible, shown, perceived, and felt by clients (Gillespie et al., 2017). Across time, numerous research studies have discovered recurrent concepts of care and caring that bridge age, gender, setting, and reason or purpose for receiving care (Dewar & Nolan, 2013; Gillespie et al., 2017; Merrill, Hayes, Clukey, & Curtis, 2012). Genuine *caring* is *person-centered* (Edvardsson et al., 2016; Ferguson, Ward, Card, Sheppard, & McMurtry, 2013), requiring an encompassed integration of mindfulness; empathy; compassion (Dewar & Nolan, 2013; Papadopoulos & Ali, 2016; Papadopoulos et al., 2017); enablement (Frost, Currie, Cruickshank, & Northam, 2017); engagement; self-determination; benevolence (Davidhizar, 2005); ethics (Gardner, 2008, as cited by Baumann, 2012; Leininger, 2002b; Ray, 2016); recognition; individualization; collaboration (McFarland & Eipperle, 2008; Potter, 2012; Tyler & Horner, 2008); mutuality (Leininger 2002b; 2015; Eipperle, 2015); trust (Lundgren & Berg, 2011); and respect (Fergusen, Ward, Card, Sheppard, & McMurtry, 2013). Caring may be enacted through listening; advocacy; physical care; presencing; counseling; and/or sharing (Merrill et al., 2012). Caring enhances quality of life, health, wellbeing, and healing (Edvardsson et al., 2016; Leininger, 1994;

Oh, Cho, Kim, Y. Y., Park, & Kim, H. K. , 2015). Brown (1991) described care congruent with cultural values, lifeways, or worldviews as:

> …authentic caring …expressed in part through empowering others to act on behalf of themselves… The central theme of authentic caring is allowing freedom, freedom to be, become, to actualize one's self as well as the freedom to exercise self-control over individual actions and being. Promotion of self-actualization, both for self and other, is a further expression of caring through empowerment in relationships…. Authentic caring is empowering of the other and is characterized by trust in and respect for the other." (p. 127)

Papadopoulos et al. (2017) shared the National Health Service (U. K.) definition of compassion as, "…how care is given through relationships based on empathy, respect, and dignity; it can also be described as intelligent kindness, and is central to how people perceive their care" (p. 287). These authors, in part, depict care provided through *conscious and intentional compassion* as having five key components: *time*; *being there*; *going the extra mile*; *defending and advocating*; and *personalization* (Papadopoulos et al., 2017, p. 289). For care and caring to occur, the action elements for *time* (to listen; to talk; to hold someone's hand; to support someone; to develop a therapeutic relationship), and the latter component, *personalization*, which requires consideration of culture and vulnerability, must be embraced and integrated into daily nursing actions and decisions. "Caring relationships involve unique interactions between individuals that can either be supported or undermined by environmental, cultural, or systemic conditions" (Seager, 2014, as cited by Papadopoulos et al., 2017, p. 292). Themes of compassion identified by Papadopoulos and Ali (2016) included *being empathetic*; *being caring*; *recognizing and ending suffering*; *communicating with patients*; *connecting to and relating with patients*; *being competent*; *attending to patients' needs/going the extra mile*; and *involving the patient* (pp. 136-137). These findings underscore the need for and value of compassion as an element care and caring across all levels of nursing practice.

Enablement, engagement, and self-determination/autonomy are key elements in the provision of client-centered care and caring. Client-centered care values the perspectives, meanings, and values of the person. Thus, client satisfaction is the individual's own subjective rating of healthcare experiences. Client engagement, on the other hand, as defined by Christenson (2017), refers to *actions people take for their own health* and as a *means to benefit from provisions of care*, spanning the continuum of experiences across healthcare settings, including the community and the home. What Leininger (2002b) referred to as *mutually coparticipative care* decisions and actions, Christenson called *co-designed care* within the medical model as described throughout the Institute for Healthcare Improvement website (2017).

Self-determination and autonomy are inherently held client rights, but are often presented as empowerment strategies that clinicians afford clients toward motivating plan of care adherence and perceptions of self-competence (Podlog & Brown, 2016). In contrast, authentic, mindful, and empathetic care and caring approached through the three modes of decisions and actions is based on a collaboration that fosters development of a genuine mutuality and shared connectivity with the client. "The central theme in authentic caring is freedom to exercise control over individual actions and being" (Brown, 1991, p. 127).

■ CARE AND CARING REQUIREMENTS: COMPARISON OF NURSE AND PATIENT PERCEPTIONS

Nurses and clients have differing perceptions about phenomenon of care and the acceptance of care and caring acts. Merrill, Hayes, Clukey, and Curtis (2012) described the *Theory of Nursing as Caring* (Boykin & Schoenhofer, 1993), wherein caring is seen as a dynamic process focused on personhood and altruistic love shared by the nurse and the patient (p. 13). These authors described nurse behaviors that males and females valued most, finding both similarities and differences. Citing Rieman (1986), they explicated *being physically present; feeling valued by the nurse entering the room without being called*; and *being assisted to be comfortable before tasks were initiated* as important to males, whereas females sought *listening; feeling valued as a unique human being (not a diagnosis or a number); providing care that helped them feel comforted, relaxed, and secure;* and *wanting to reciprocate* (p. 33). Merrill et al. (2012) concluded that

"Caring is the heart and artistry of nursing so understanding what actions, attitudes, and behaviors convey caring is essential to good practice" (p. 36).

Nursing care actions frequently involve procedural and nonprocedural touch as explicated by Marchetti, Piredda, and De Marinis (2016) who found that "...body and embodiment are rooted in nursing practice and generate more holistic and complex ways of understanding patients" (p. 36) and practicing nursing. The shared intimacy that occurs during physical care acts creates a different relational dynamic between the client and the nurse and can bridge "...the meanings given to body and embodiment [that] are linked to social rules and cultural beliefs" (p. 32). Patients' need for care and caring is universal and transcends cultures and professional disciplines, notably with a desire for increased amount and quality of time with clinicians (Gillespie et al., 2017). Findings from this qualitative study revealed themes and sub-themes: *Competence*; *positive attitudes*; *effective communication* (talking; listening; non-verbal behavior; sharing; explaining/listening); *relationships* (trust and respect; patients as individuals); *help with navigating clinical services* (caring internally motivated; caring was continuing; caring included patients); and *emotional engagement* (supportiveness; guidance; careful explanations; p. 1631). Clients also valued *remembrance* and *inclusion* as well as careful explanations that meant being informed of "everything there is to know, not just what the doctors think you should know" (p. 1631). *Humility, being fully present*, and *demonstrating fallibility* by the admission of errors or wrong-doing fostered development of *mutual trust, respect*, and a *sense of safety* (p. 1632). *Reciprocity* as caring was experienced by having independence and choice to the degree desired and needed to navigate systems of care was a valued behavior. "Caring was listening and conversing *with* rather than communicating *to*...sharing control called for genuine respect towards others" [by clinicians] (p. 1632). The authors noted that their study "...challenges the dichotomy between competence and caring. Both are important but neither alone is sufficient" and called these interprofessional differences "a false dichotomy" (p. 1632). The differing capacities for *clinical competency skills* and *caring skills* may not be discernable by clients and may therefore be perceived as a single capacity, *care and caring*.

■ NURSING THEORIES TO GUIDE CARE

The Theory of Culture Care Diversity and Universality

Beginning her work with the philosophical belief that "...the nursing profession had a moral and ethical responsibility to discover, know, and use culturally-based caring modalities as one of our unique and distinct contributions to humanity" (p. 76), Leininger (2002b) conceptualized the Theory of Culture Care Diversity and Universality from the synthesized concepts of *care/caring* and *culture*. These were integral to the four major theory tenets that stated *care diversities (differences) and universalities (commonalities) exist among and between cultures in the world; worldview and the social structure factors influence cultural care meanings, expressions, and patterns in diverse cultures; diverse generic [emic] and professional [etic] care practices significantly influence health, illness, and wellness outcomes;* and *the three culture care modes of decisions and actions are necessary to provide safe, effective, meaningful, and culturally congruent care* (Leininger, 1991, 2002b, 2006). Care and caring are dynamically interwoven throughout the theory, creating a conceptualized thread that provides internal consistency and unifies the theory constructs in the Sunrise Enabler and Ethnonursing Research method (McFarland & Wehbe-Alamah, 2015).

A key Assumptive Premise of the theory posited *care* as the essence and central dominant, distinct, and unifying focus of nursing (McFarland & Wehbe-Alamah, 2015, p. 8). Leininger (2002c) described care as both an abstract and/or concrete phenomenon (p. 12), wherein "...*care is those assistive, supportive, and enabling experiences or ideas toward others with evident or anticipated needs to ameliorate or improve a human condition or lifeway*" (p. 12). Care meanings can have cultural and symbolic linkages; these are essential for the provision of culture-specific care. *Caring refers to decisions, actions, attitudes, and practices (including advocacy) that assist or guide others* in their quest for health or wellness (Leininger, 1991, 2002b, 2006; McFarland & Wehbe-Alamah, 2015).

Culture is the second and equally major and independent construct of Leininger's Culture Care Theory, and as such does not adverbially or adjectively modify the construct word, *care* (2006, p. 23), and is described as *the intergenerationally known learned, shared, and transmitted values, beliefs, norms, and lifeways of a particular people group that guides thinking, decisions, and actions in patterned ways.* Thus, Leininger (2006) conceptualized *culture care* as the *synthesis of two closely linked phenomena with interrelated ideas* (p. 13). Culture care is both humanistic and holistic in its goal and purpose, and seeks to find care values, beliefs, practices, and expressions in all cultures and cultural lifeways, embracing both non-Western and Western domains, groups, or peoples.

Care can be an individual, familial, tribal, communal, organizational, or institutional value or expression; it can be held as a single value or a system of beliefs. It can be a blend or integration of various approaches and beliefs, such as shamanism, Buddhism, Taoism, herbalism, chiropractic, Ayurvedic, Hinduism, Sikhism, or Islamic care practices, with Western healthcare practices. Authentic care and caring strives to preserve and/or maintain quality of life as envisioned or valued by the individual and/or their family as a main focus of professional care provided through coparticipatively established decisions and/or actions.

The modes (*culture care preservation and/or maintenance*; *culture care accommodation and/or negotiation*; and, *culture care repatterning and/or restructuring*) are used to apply the theory across all levels of nursing practice, education, endeavor, or setting and serve as the holistic starting point from which to approach care. With every client, whether individual, family, group, community, organization, or institution, use of the modes focuses on retaining current or extant approaches that are functional, useful, or non-harmful. Modifications are approached through mutual compromise; changes are co-developed to promote safety or mitigate harm. All people are diverse in overt and subtle ways and unique in the expression of their needs, values, beliefs, lifeways, and worldviews that reflect cultural identities and ethnohistories as well as personal experiences. Leininger (2002b) identified this phenomenon as *comparative care* that needed to be explicated using culture-specific constructs and meanings so as to provide individualized culturally congruent care (p. 85).

McFarland, Wehbe-Alamah, Vossos, and Wilson (2015) provided confirmation in their metasynthesis for the credibility of culture care findings from 23 doctoral dissertations based on Leininger's Theory of Culture Care Diversity and Universality (pp. 287-288). The domain of inquiry focused on three main research questions to discover the influences of the social structure factors on the care expressions, beliefs, and practices of people from diverse and similar cultures and ways that application of the theory through the modes could facilitate the provision of culturally congruent care (pp. 288-289). The authors concluded the metasynthesis resulted in theory building and a higher level of abstraction of findings beyond the themes from the original dissertations, and that through the discovery of meta-themes, meta-patterns, and meta-modes their study made a significant contribution to support the practice of nursing and the provision of culturally congruent care (p. 307). The 2008 Fingeld-Connett meta-analysis found 49 qualitative reports and six concept analyses of caring. These meta-analysis findings affirmed that the outcomes of caring for the recipient included improved physical and mental wellbeing for patients as well as improved mental health and an elevated sense of professional satisfaction by nurses. *"Caring is essential to healing for there can be no curing without caring, but caring can exist without curing – there is a high predictive value to the power of caring"* (Leininger, 1991, p. 38).

Other Care Theories in Nursing

Rosenbaum (1986) conducted a comparison of care and caring as conceptualized by Leininger (1978) and Orem (1983). Although these early theorists embraced the concepts of care and caring, they envisioned them differently within the discipline of nursing. Orem placed great emphasis on the *individual* and the value of *self-care*, whereas Leininger believed these foci to be Western values not ubiquitously held among other cultures of the world, differentiating the constructs under the taxonomies of *attitude* and *taking responsibility*.

In 1988, Leininger reiterated her earlier observation that:

> One of the most essential, promising, and important areas of study in nursing is the concept of caring, and yet is has been one of the most neglected areas of systematic research. Although nurses are a professional group who repeatedly use the expression nursing care, care, and caring in everyday parlance, the linguistic, sematic, and professional usages of these terms are still limitedly understood and studied. (Leininger, 1974, as cited by Leininger, 1988b, p. 48)

However, since Leininger first made this observation, care and caring have been studied extensively within various other nursing contexts, theories, and paradigms but remain elusively difficult to define (Gillespie et al., 2017). Ray developed three theories of caring in transcultural nursing: *The Theory of Bureaucratic Caring* (Ray, 1989); *The Theory of Relational Caring Complexity* (Davidson, Ray, & Turkel, 2011); and *The Theory of Caring Dynamics in Nursing and Health Care* (Ray, 2016). The *Caring Dynamics Theory* was appraised in the foreword by Dr. Leininger as a "...breakthrough not only to understand the caring dynamics of human caring, but to understand how local and global cultural and organizational processes and contexts influence and shape care meanings and expressions that affect choices for health, healing, and wellbeing" (2016, p. xii). Watson (1985) developed the *Theory of Human Caring Science*, founded on the evolving conceptualization of transpersonal caring relationships between the nurse and the client, wherein the nurse seeks to 'see' the spirit of the person beyond their disease or other presentation (Watson, 2015, pp. 326-327). In this sense, transpersonal caring requires an "...authenticity of being and becoming, an ability to be present to self and others in a reflective frame" with a centered "consciousness and intentionality on caring, healing, and wholeness..." (p. 327). Subsequent models of care and caring have emerged from other scholars in transcultural nursing in publications by Andrews and Boyle (*Transcultural Concepts in Nursing Care*, 2016); Basuray (*Culture and Health: Concept and Practice*, 2014); Campinha-Bacote (*The Process of Cultural Competence in the Delivery of Healthcare Services*, 2007); and Giger and Davidhizar (*Transcultural Nursing: Assessment and Intervention*, 2008) who have acknowledged Leininger's theory largely or in part as the basis of their work.

■ NURSING CARE VALUES AND PRACTICES

"The discipline of nursing needs to focus more on care/caring to explain health and wellbeing in different or similar cultures" (Leininger, 2002a, p. 46). Gillespie, Kelly, Duggan, and Dornan (2017) acknowledged that healthcare workers reasonably cannot be expected to provide ideal care at all times and under all circumstances (p. 1632). Instead, the authors advocate

striving to enact one or two of the valued aspects, such as being pleasant, to offset having less time within the constraints of a fast-paced or under-resourced clinical environment (p. 1632). However, nurses can alter their routines to engage clients by lessening time spent in front of computer and increasing eye-contact with clients. Given the ubiquitous nature of documentation technologies, the need to assess the individual permeants all client-nurse encounters and settings rather than primarily focusing on the electronic health record. Care and caring need to be interwoven in and among all nursing practice behaviors, practice activities, interactions, tasks, processes, procedures, and policies. How can nurses do this? It takes awareness. It takes refocusing. Care and caring integration requires actively directing the nurse's focus, attention, and efforts on the person. ...Being mindful of what is being said, how it is being said, why it is being said; consciously focusing the nurse's thoughts on the person and their needs and concerns as they see them and convey them. ...Setting aside the nurse's own perceptions, ideas, or wishes and being open to 'the other' is what care and caring is about. This builds trust and sharing. "...Caring [is] a significant universal human capacity as well as an intentioned, proficient, professional service in nursing" (Leininger, 1988b, p. 72).

Nurses need to place greater emphasis and attention on developing a genuine, authentic relationship with each client, albeit if only briefly. This is differentiated from the 'professional interaction' or 'team building' skills that systems encourage as part of their 'consumer of health services' approach. A sincere form of bonding connectivity is required that enables the patient to truly know the nurse sees, hears, and understands her or him as a holistic individual. Davidhizar (2005) offered that a *relationship* with a patient provides the opportunity for "...a real, caring, respectful encounter with someone who is safe" adding later that the therapeutic value of any patient care encounter involves *communicating commitment* and *concern* (p. 8). This was well-explicated by Sister Roach as the *Five Cs of Caring: Compassion, Competence, Confidence, Conscience,* and *Commitment* (Roach, 1991, p. 9). "Nursing is no more and no less than the professionalization of the human capacity to care through acquisition and application of the knowledge, attitudes, and skills appropriate to nursing's ...roles" (p. 9). *Compassionate caring* has been identified as a fundamental aspect of quality nursing care that also requires self-care and regenerative skills to prevent emotional disconnection or "energetic withdrawal" by the nurse that results in activities focused on tasks and *doing for* rather than *being with* clients (Joseph, 1991, p. 57). According to Edvardsson et al. (2016), "Caring or the cost of not caring in nursing practice has been linked to financial outcomes for the health system, as well as physical and emotional patient outcomes. ....However, some questions remain regarding the congruence between perceptions of patients and nurses as to which nursing attributes and behaviours are considered caring" (p. 219). Nonetheless, Joseph asserted that nurses' self-awareness and centeredness borne through reflection enables *conscious caring* (p. 59), that courage and devotion are required to be fully present with patients for the provision of energetically open and compassionate care and caring (p. 57).

Individualized caring approaches are still needed; nursing care is not formulaic, one approach does not fit all. Evidence-based practice (EBP) does not entail mandated approaches. Although research findings are regarded as either generalizable (quantitative) or transferrable (qualitative), they need to be used within the context of the individual in a manner that recognizes and is acceptable and meaningful to that person in order to be beneficial and effect positive outcomes. Healthcare decisions and actions that do not integrate the person's own values, beliefs, patterns, lifeways, or worldview will not be accepted or maintained. A tall order, definitely, but necessary. Using *evidence-informed* practice guidelines (Moore, Titler, Low, Dalton, & Sampselle, 2015; refer to Figure 12.1) to reach coparticipative and mutually agreed-upon decisions wherein client knowledge, meanings, and preferences are fully/equally considered constitutes genuinely person-centered care and caring, and can be approached by application of the three modes of culture care decisions and actions (Eipperle, 2015; Leininger, 2002b, 2006; McFarland & Wehbe-Alamah, 2015). Milton (2012) explicated this differently through the *nurse as guest* metaphor, emphasizing approaches that include appropriate client engagement; deferred judgments; and care foci on health, quality of life, and client/community preferences (p. 138). Appropriate client engagement in the community setting entailed waiting for host (client) invitations to participate; exhibiting non-demanding

behaviors; acceptance of host-offered courtesies; and mutually participative and other-serving interactions (p. 138). The metaphor closely parallels the spirit and intent of the three culture care modes of decisions and actions of Leininger's theory (Eipperle, 2015; Leininger, 2002b, 2006; McFarland & Wehbe-Alamah, 2015). Exhibiting respectful, courteous, and non-judgmental *bedside manners* is a care/caring essential. Mindfulness and being fully present through culturally-appropriate acknowledgements (eye-contact, touch, smiling, body language) when clients are speaking or exhibiting symptoms or behaviors of discomfort or unease; and protecting physical, auditory, and emotional privacy — especially in the company of others regardless of relationship or profession — by minimizing exposures and/or enacting facilitative advocacy measures are key to developing and sustaining client trust and engagement (Anonymous, 2016). Avoiding paternalistic imposition practices during care and care coordination by engaging clients and/or families from the outset of care provision and care planning or decision-making ensures the provision of culturally congruent, meaningful, and beneficial person-centered care (Ackerman, 2016; Brach, 2014; Dewar & Nolan, 2013; Eipperle, 2015; Powell, Mabry, & Mixer, 2015). Such care endeavors may require creative efforts to overcome organizational and other policy barriers to find acceptable solutions (Baumann, 2012; Eipperle, 2015; McFarland & Wehbe-Alamah, 2015; Mixer, 2015; Powell et al., 2015). The ethical and moral intentions of the nurse to fulfill the mandates of person-centered care may *lurk in the shadows* between these values and challenging contextual conditions or praxis standards as described by Anderson, Sjöström-Strand, Willman, and Borglin (2015, p. 3489). Leininger (2002b, 2006) long-espoused the premise of client acceptance as an outcome or measure of care, more recently echoed by Moore, Titler, Low, Dalton, and Sampselle (2015) who discussed the framing effect of informational sharing and stated, "...the outcomes that measure client-centered care must also be client-centered" (p. 281). These authors added that the success measures for client-centered care *do not rest solely on evaluative measures* but on the experience and evaluation of the individual, "...starting with whether or not patient activation or engagement occurred" (p. 281). When a person does not feel recognized, respected, or valued in receiving

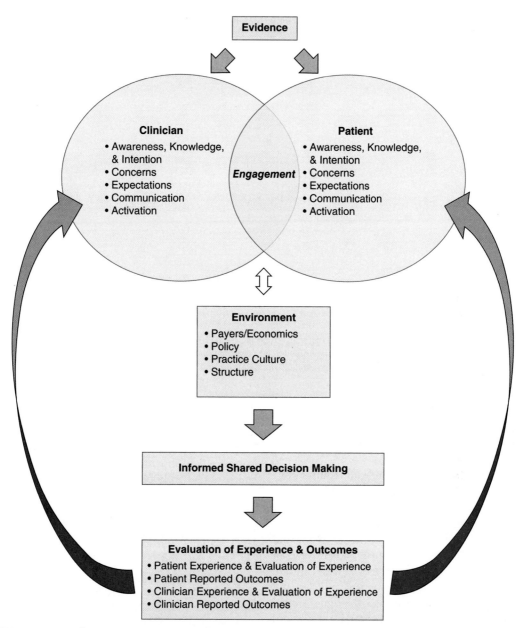

FIGURE 12.1 • Transforming patient-centered care: Development of the evidence-informed decision-making through engagement model. © Jennifer E. Moore (2014).

Moore, J., Titler, M. G., Low, L. K., Dalton, V. K., & Sampselle, C. M. (2014). Transforming patient-centered care: Development of the evidence-informed decision-making through engagement model [Figure]. *Women's Health Issues, 25*(3), 278.

health care they may opt out of the system, which may result negative health outcomes and higher costs as well as in more frequent encounters — all at a higher financial cost and use of resources. By integrating care and caring through the application of the three culture care modes of decisions and actions, these negative outcomes are preventable (Eipperle, 2015; McFarland & Eipperle, 2008).

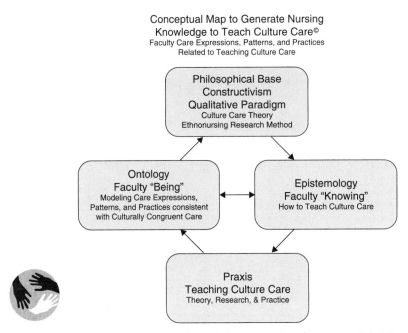

FIGURE 12.2 • Conceptual map to generate nursing knowledge to teach culture care. © S. Mixer (2004).

Mixer, S. J. (2015). Conceptual map to generate nursing knowledge to teach culture care [Figure]. In M. R. McFarland and H. B. Wehbe-Alamah (Eds.), *Leininger's culture care diversity and universality: A worldwide nursing theory* (3rd ed., p. 372). Burlington, MA: Jones & Bartlett Learning.

■ CARING FRAMEWORKS IN NURSING EDUCATION

Changing nursing practice is not easy; it requires evaluation and re-evaluation of values and beliefs through sharp critical reflection regarding stereotypes and biases, a process that may be uncomfortable, unsettling, or painful to experience. For the discipline and profession of nursing to grow, mature, and evolve as an equal partner in the healthcare system, and for care and caring to be central to nursing practices, policies, and procedures requires refocusing the thoughts, words, and actions of current and future nurses. Care and caring needs to be fully integrated as an essential component of the clinical evaluation process at all levels of student learning to ensure the vital provision of *meaningful, beneficial, acceptable, and culturally congruent care by culturally competent nurses* (Mixer, 2011). This will require changing how nurses are educated as well as regaining a nursing leadership stronghold throughout all dimensions of the healthcare system.

Integrating transcultural learning in nursing education begins by requiring transcultural nursing courses that emphasize theory constructs, ethics, and social disparities as well as enmeshed transcultural or culture care objectives and outcomes for each nursing program course across all levels of nursing education. This can be approached by using the three modes of culture care decisions and actions as a care/caring framework from the very outset of nurse education (Refer to Figure 12.2). Understanding and applying the modes can begin simply, yet grow and evolve greater depth and breadth as the knowledge, experience, and expertise of the nurse matures (Mixer, 2011, 2015; Mixer, McFarland, Andrews, & Strang, 2013). The three modes of culture care decisions and actions as tenets of the Theory of Culture Care Diversity and Universality were explicated by Leininger (1991, 2002b, 2006) as follows:

• Culture care preservation and/or maintenance refers to those assistive, supportive, facilitative, or enabling professional acts or decisions that help cultures to retain, preserve, or maintain beneficial care beliefs and values or to face handicaps and death;

• Culture care accommodation and/or negotiation refers to those assistive, accommodating, facilitative, or enabling creative provider care actions or decisions that help cultures adapt to or negotiate with others for culturally congruent, safe, and effective care for their health, wellbeing, or to deal with illness or dying; and

- Culture care repatterning and/or restructuring refers to those assistive, supportive, facilitative, or enabling professional actions and mutual decisions that would help people to reorder, change, modify, or restructure their lifeways and institutions for better (or beneficial) health care patterns, practices, or outcomes.

Nursing students ought to learn the value and need for care and caring as they enter into professional education. These concepts should be taught beyond the theoretical focus; they need to be exemplified through role modeling, expected behaviors, and clinical practicum performance measures. Didactic learning and clinical experiences are insufficient in time and depth for students to internally assimilate the meanings of care and caring as core values of nursing as a profession without explicit teaching and observed and experienced role modeling (Halldórsdóttir, 1990; Mixer, 2011; Mixer et al., 2013; Powell et al., 2015). Academic rigor, scholarship requirements, and clinical standards need to be balanced with respectful engagement of students as future professional peers while functioning within an environment of mutual civility and interactive boundaries (Mixer, 2011). Promoting self-care, honoring cultural traditions, and accommodating family needs for students as well as faculty fosters a healthy and caring learning environment where students observe positive peer relationships and feel valued and respected (Halldórsdóttir, 1990; Mixer, 2011; Mixer et al., 2013).

■ DISCUSSION

Challenges Encountered Within the Healthcare System

The healthcare system remains fiscally-driven and medicolegally structured with physicians holding greater hierarchal power or authority with, among, or over 'team' members regarding decisions about individuals, policies, practices, and organizations as well as the healthcare system overall (André, Nøst, Frigstad, & Sjøvold, 2016). The American Medical Association is one of the top 50 most powerful lobbies in the United States, wielding significant influence

among its membership as well as legislators (Wilson, 2017). Insurers have been slow to accept clinicians other than physicians as decision-making providers for purposes of reimbursement or authorization of care. Physicians, nurses, and other health disciplines have differing values, priorities, and communication styles; lack of interdisciplinary respect and civility compromise communication and patient outcomes (André, et al., 2016; Forunda, McWilliams, & McArthur, 2016). Within this environment, one wonders whether the concept of *patient/person-centered care* is effecting any change in client participation or perception, or in nursing practice. "Observations of medical practice revealed a discipline that has been oriented toward curing with focus on physical diagnoses, internal pathology, and treatments aimed at cure. In contrast, nursing was directed toward caring acts and processes focusing on multiple factors influencing illness and wellness" (Leininger, 1988b, p. 48).

At this writing, ANA president Patrician Cipriano has responded in an open letter to the American Medical Association (AMA) regarding their opposition to "...continual, nationwide efforts to grant independent practice . . . to non-physician practitioners" (as cited by Japson, 2017) including advanced practice registered nurses (APRNs). Cipriano noted that the AMA House of Delegates interim meeting moved to design an intensified lobbying agenda through model legislation in Washington and state capitals "...to initiate creation of a consistent national strategy" and further accused the AMA of perpetuating "...the dangerous and erroneous narrative that APRNs are trying to 'act' as physicians and are unqualified to provide timely, effective and efficient care" (Cipriano, 2017 as cited by Japson, 2017). Several nursing organizations along with the ANA and American Association of Nurse Practitioners (AANP) have stated that updated state and federal laws are intended to facilitate direct client access to care and lessen bureaucratic red tape (Japson, 2017). These legislative updates are congruent with movements across the U. S. health system toward value-based models of care (Japson, 2017).

Envisioning the Future: How Nurses can Overcome

The Australian Nursing and Midwifery Council and Nursing Council of New Zealand (2004) *Nurse Practitioner Competency Framework* established

"...therapeutic links with the client that recognize and respect cultural identity and lifestyle choices" as a standard of care in advanced practice nursing (p. 4). Finding ways to demonstrate care and caring in the course of a busy office day, hospital shift, or homecare schedule can be challenging. The old saying *little things mean a lot* still holds true and is applicable in nursing. Studies have demonstrated that presencing, culturally appropriate eye contact or touch, attentiveness, respect, sensitivity, and acknowledgement during clinical encounters are recognized by and meaningful to clients (ANA, 2015; Eipperle, 2015; Marchetti et al., 2016). McFarland and Eipperle (2008) described application of the three modes of culture care through diverse ways of knowing for nurse practitioners in primary care settings to provide holistic culturally congruent care. In addition to shared decision-making, Hull (2015) advocated for learning and sharing the stories (ethnohistory) of clients, their families, and caregivers. Sharing a bit of one's own story with clients can also help to establish a shared humanity and foster connectivity.

Client/patient advocacy is one of nurses' most essential roles (ANA, 2015b). Nursing and nurses are repeatedly cited as the most trusted profession (Advisory Board, 2017) predicated on the credibility, reliability, and trustworthiness of nurses and the nursing profession. These factors add complexity when nurses participate in the process of interdisciplinary communication and collaboration. Clients and nurses can learn from each other (Mixer et al., 2013). Care decisions and actions should be coparticipatory and collaborative to achieve health outcomes meaningful, acceptable, and beneficial to clients" (Eipperle, 2015). Patient/person-centered care can only occur in a patient-led health care environment where clients are fully self-determining participants and nurses are recognized and valued for their knowledge, skills, and client advocacy and with equitable decision-making authority and power. "Since the 1800s...caring has been a dominant feature in the language of nursing. The nurse-patient interaction.... remains the essential, and potentially most rewarding, aspect of nursing" (Sherwood, 1991, p. 80).

Nursing as a profession can change health care and the system to evolve to where health and wellness based on care and caring are the central foci, and where healthcare professionals view patients not as entities to receive services, but as persons who seek or require care. We must reclaim our historic role as leaders in the forefront of all health care, to ensure that culturally congruent, holistic, humanistic care and caring are provided by transculturally aware and prepared nurses in all settings and across all levels of professional education. The future of health care requires a return to the idea of professional nursing as a calling with dedication to high ideals based on care and caring and not simply a job with growth potential and market security. Nurses must "...help the public to understand nursing as a caring profession and demonstrate the power and effectiveness of care to help people recover from illnesses and disabilities and maintain wellness. The culture of nursing needs to separate itself from medicine's public cure-image to establish a distinct care model with health-promoting outcomes" (Leininger, 1988a, p. 26).

Everyone [emphasis added] involved must understand what it takes to create an environment that fosters full expression of the essence of nursing. Healthcare organizations must learn and replicate best practices that validate, appreciate, and recognize the essence of nursing. This, in turn, helps raise the standard of patient care while nurturing nursing staff and making their work more satisfying.

The art of nursing must coexist with today's technology-driven, evidence-based science of nursing. To ensure such coexistence, nurses must manifest the essence of nursing in every patient and family encounter. To a large degree, the future of healthcare delivery hinges on our ability to optimize the work of nurses and enable them to practice the essence of nursing. (Fitzpatrick, 2015, p. 3S)

Nurses can role-model care and caring behaviors not just for patients and their families but also for colleagues and interdisciplinary clinicians and staff as well as students and new employees and other members or participants in healthcare provision (Labrague, et al., 2015; Mixer, 2011).

■ SUMMARY

The healthcare system can evolve through active integration of care and caring practices. It is imperative that the *discipline* of nursing refocus the *culture* of nursing to whole-heartedly embrace cultural competence and fully integrate culturally congruent care based on the transcultural concepts of care and caring. A transcultural nursing model of health care requires that nursing as a profession holds an equal place of power and position in a medically- and financially-driven system that on many levels still views nurses as secondary players. Placing the *patient* as a culturally defined or identified *person* at the center of care requires that nurses have an equal voice with equal power among healthcare disciplines. The value of care and caring to the healthcare system and associated stakeholders can be evidenced through improved client engagement with their own health and chosen healthcare system; improved health behaviors, health outcomes, and wellbeing and quality of life; and subsequent reductions in personal and system-wide health costs (Powell et al., 2015, p. 348).

Transcultural nurses stand poised and ready to provide coparticipative client-centered culturally congruent care locally, regionally, nationally, and globally. The discipline of nursing must do more than discuss and educate; we must act. We must act to reclaim and revamp the healthcare system to be both client-focused and client-centered to provide culture-specific, meaningful, and beneficial care for optimal health and wellness outcomes. Mutually coparticipative care decisions and actions that equitably integrate client preferences, values, beliefs, and expressions must become the system-wide norm across all disciplines, settings, and levels of care provision.

A ripple effect connects past to present to future with an intersection and dynamic mutuality of events linking people across time and relationships. Culture is the historically unifying thread that globally connects people with one another through similarities as well as differences. Our shared humanity binds us together as we seek expression and recognition for individual or group uniquenesses. The human need for care and caring is universal; the values, beliefs, patterns, and expressions that are meaningful and beneficial can be both diversely and universally held. Moreover, Leininger (2006) posited *care as the essence and central, unifying focus of nursing* (p. 18). *Culture care* is thus coparticipatively approached by nurses through a mutually agreed-upon plan using the modes of decisions and actions. Placing the client at the center of each healthcare relationship and encounter as a self-directing, self-determining autonomous being will enable all levels of nursing practice to be facilitative and client-promoting to the degree desired and/or capable by that individual. Care and caring is provided through various nursing acts or actions including (but not limited to) advocacy, communication, presencing, listening, sharing, education, and physical care.

There is no better way to end this chapter than with the words of Dr. Leininger:

> Nursing has the potential strength and leverage to help realign many of the prevailing distorted values in our society, but first we have to stop abandoning our values as…nurses. Our task to bring about change is difficult because the questions nursing needs to ask are not the usual and more acceptable questions…. Although we desperately need theory and research, we also desperately need caring and human kindness. (1988b, p. 25)

◼ DEDICATION

This chapter is dedicated in memory of my Mother and Best Friend, Billie J. Eipperle.

◼ ACKNOWLEDGEMENTS

I wish to acknowledge the caring support of my friends and colleagues, Dr. Marilyn R. McFarland, Dr. Hiba Wehbe-Alamah, and Dr. Marilyn S. Filter.

◼ DISCUSSION QUESTIONS

1. Discuss the meaning of care and caring to you personally. Professionally? How are they different or the same?
2. Discuss how you may change your approach to caring for clients or patients after reading this chapter.
3. Discuss the care and caring challenges encountered within the healthcare system overall.
4. Discuss the specific or unique challenges encountered in the setting where you work in striving to meet the care and caring needs of clients.
5. Discuss how care and caring theories can guide your care actions and decisions in providing culturally congruent care to diverse people.

◼ REFERENCES

Ackerman, M. (2016). Keep the care in care coordination [Commentary]. *Clinical Advisor, 19*(3), p. 108.

Advisory Board. (2017, January 3). *Nursing is America's most trusted profession yet again, Gallup finds.* Retrieved from https://www.advisory.com/daily-briefing/2017/01/03/nurse-trusted-profession

American Nurses' Association. (2015). *Nursing scope and standards of practice* (3rd ed.). Silver Spring, MD: Author.

American Nurses' Association. (2016, December 19). *Nurses rank #1 most trusted profession for 15th year in a row*. Retrieved from http://www.nursingworld.org/FunctionalMenuCategories/MediaResources/Press Releases/2016-News-Releases/Nurses-Rank-1-Most-Trusted-Profession-2.pdf

Anderson, E. K., Sjöström-Strand, A., Willman, A., & Borglin, G. (2015). Registered nurses' views of caring in coronary care — A deductive and inductive content analysis. *Journal of Clinical Nursing*, 24(23-24), 3481-3493.

André, B., Nøst, T. H., Frigstad, S., & Sjøvold, E. (2016). Differences in communication within the nursing group and with other professions at a hospital unit. *Journal of Clinical Nursing*, 26(7-8), 956-963.

Andrews, M. M., & Boyle, J. S. (2016). *Transcultural concepts in nursing care* (7th ed.). Philadelphia, PA: Wolters Kluwer.

Anonymous. (2016, January 6). *Behind nurses' eyes: Going from bad to bedside manners*. Retrieved from http://scrubsmag.com/behind-nurses-eyes-going-from-bad-to-bedside-manners/

Australian Nursing and Midwifery Council and Nursing Council of New Zealand. (2004). *National competency standards for the nurse practitioner*. Retrieved from www.anmc.org.au

Bartol, T. (2016). Enhancing the patient experience [Editorial]. *The Nurse Practitioner*, 41(8), 14-15.

Basuray (Maxwell), J. (2014). *Culture and health: Concept and practice* (2nd ed.). Ronkonkoma, NY: Linus.

Baumann, S. L. (2012). Making a meaningful contribution to nursing theory. *Nursing Science Quarterly*, 25(2), 155-159.

Brach, C. (2014). A daughter's frustration with the dearth of patient- and family-centered care. *Patient Experience Journal*, 1(1), 7. Retrieved from http://pxjournal.org/journal/vol1/iss1/7/

Brown, C. L. (1991). Caring in nursing administration: Healing through empowering. In D. A. Gaut and M. M. Leininger (Eds.), *Caring: The compassionate healer* (pp. 123-133). New York, NY: National League for Nursing Press.

Campinha-Bacote, J. (2007). *The process of cultural competence in the delivery of healthcare services: The journey continues*. Cincinnati, OH: Transcultural C.A.R.E. Associates.

Christensen, T. (2017, September 14). *The evolution of patient-centered care and the meaning of co-design*. Retrieved from http://www.ihi.org/communities/blogs/_layouts/15/ihi/community/blog/itemview.aspx?List=7d1126ec-8f63-4a3b-9926-c44ea3036813&ID=431

Daly, K. A. (2012, December 3). Person-centered care – What does it actually mean [Editorial]. *The American Nurse*. Retrieved from http://www.theamericannurse.org/2012/12/03/person-centered-care-what-does-it-actually-mean/

Davidhizar, R. E. (2005). Benevolent power. *Journal of Practical Nursing*, 55(4), 4-9.

Davidson, A. W., Ray, M. A., & Turkel, M. C. (2011). *Nursing caring and complexity science: For human-environment wellbeing*. New York, NY: Springer.

Dewar, B., & Nolan, M. (2013). Caring about caring: Developing a model to implement relationship centered care in an older people care setting. *International Journal of Nursing Studies*, 50(9), 1247-1248.

Edvardsson, D., Watt, E., & Pearce, F. (2016). Patient experiences of caring and person-centeredness are associated with perceived nursing care quality. *Journal of Advanced Nursing*, 73(1), 217-227.

Eipperle, M. K. (2015). Application of the three modes of decisions and actions in advanced practice primary care. In M. R. McFarland and H. B. Wehbe-Alamah (Eds.), *Leininger's culture care diversity and universality: A worldwide nursing theory* (3rd ed., pp. 317-344). Burlington, MA: Jones & Bartlett.

Ferguson, L. M., Ward, H., Card, S., Sheppard, S., & McMurtry, J. (2013). Putting the 'patient' back into patient-centered care: An education perspective. *Nurse Education in Practice*, 13(4), 283-287.

Finfgeld-Connett, D. (2008). Metasynthesis of caring in nursing. *Journal of Clinical Nursing*, 17(2), 196-204.

Fitzpatrick, M. A. (2015, May). The essence of nursing: It's time to put basic nursing care back in the spotlight. *American Nurse Today: Essence of Nursing* (Supplement), 2S-3S. Retrieved from www.AmericanNurseToday.com

Flynn, B. C. (1988). The caring community: Health care and nursing in England and the United States. In M. M. Leininger (Ed.), *Care: Discovery and uses in clinical and community nursing* (pp. 29-38).

Forunda, C., MacWilliams, B., & McArthur, E. (2016). Interprofessional communication in healthcare: An integrative review. *Nurse Education in Practice*, 19, 36-40. Retrieved from http://dx.doi.org/10.1016/j.nepr.2016.04.005 1471-5953/

Frost, J. S., Currie, M. J., Cruickshank, M., & Northam, H. L. (2017). Viewing nurse practitioner perceptions of patient care through the lens of enablement. *Journal of Nurse Practitioners*, 13(8), 570-576.

Garneau, A. B., & Pepin, J. (2015). Cultural competence: A constructivist definition. *Journal of Transcultural Nursing*, 26(1), 9-15.

Giger, J. N., & Davidhizar, R. E. (2008). *Transcultural nursing: Assessment and intervention* (5th ed.). St. Louis, MO: Mosby Elsevier.

Gillespie, H., Kelly, M., Duggan, S., & Dornan, T. (2017). How do patients experience caring? Scoping review. *Patient Education and Counseling, 100*(9), 1622-1633.

Halldórsdóttir, S. (1990). The essential structure of a caring and an uncaring encounter with a teacher: The perspective of the nursing student. In M. M. Leininger and J. Watson (Eds.), *The caring imperative in education* (pp. 95-106). New York, NY: National League for Nursing.

Hull, S. C. (2015, May). Enhance patient engagement through sharing. *American Nurse Today: Essence of Nursing* (Supplement), 6S-7S. Retrieved from www.AmericanNurseToday.com

Japson, B. (2017, November 20). *Nurses say AMA launching 'turf war' over direct patient access*. Retrieved from https://www.forbes.com/sites/brucejapsen/2017/11/20/nurses-say-ama-launching-turf-war-over-direct-patient-access/#478547bd1168

Joseph, L. (1991). The energetics of conscious caring for the compassionate healer. In D. A. Gaut and M. M. Leininger (Eds.), *Caring: The compassionate healer* (pp. 56-59). New York, NY: National League for Nursing Press.

Labrague, L. J., McEnroe-Petitte, D. M., Papathanasiou, I. V., Edet, O. B., & Arulappan, J. (2015). Impact of instructors' caring on students' perceptions of their own caring behaviors. *Journal of Nursing Scholarship, 47*(4), 338-346.

Latham, C. P. (1996). Predictors of patient outcomes following interactions with nurses. *Western Journal of Nursing Research, 18*(5), 548-564.

Leininger, M. M. (1978). *Transcultural nursing: Concepts, theories, and practices*. New York, NY: John Wiley & Sons.

Leininger, M. M. (1988a). *Care: Discovery and uses in clinical and community nursing*. Detroit, MI: Wayne State University Press.

Leininger, M. M. (1988b). *Care: The essence of nursing and health*. Detroit, MI: Wayne State University Press.

Leininger, M. M. (1988c). Leininger's theory of nursing: Culture care diversity and universality. *Nursing Science Quarterly, 1*(4), 152-160.

Leininger, M. M. (1991). *Culture care diversity and universality: A theory of nursing*. Washington, DC: National League for Nursing Press.

Leininger, M. M. (1994). Quality of life from a transcultural nursing perspective. *Nursing Science Quarterly, 7*(1), 22-28.

Leininger, M. M. (2002a). Essential transcultural nursing care concepts, principles, examples, and policy statements. In M. M. Leininger and M. R. McFarland (Eds.), *Transcultural nursing: Concepts, theories, research, and practice* (3rd ed., pp. 45-69).

Leininger, M. M. (2002b). Part I: The theory of culture care and the ethnonursing method. In M. M. Leininger and M. R. McFarland (Eds.), *Transcultural nursing: Concepts, theories, research, and practice* (3rd ed., pp. 71-98).

Leininger, M. M. (2002c). Transcultural nursing and globalization of health care: Importance, focus, and historical aspects. In M. M. Leininger and M. R. McFarland (Eds.), *Transcultural nursing: Concepts, theories, research, and practice* (3rd ed., pp. 3-43).

Leininger, M. M. (2006). Culture care diversity and universality theory and evolution of the ethnonursing method. In M. M. Leininger and M. R. McFarland (Eds.), *Culture care diversity and universality: A worldwide nursing theory* (2nd ed., pp. 1-41). Sudbury, MA: Jones and Bartlett.

Leininger, M. M. (2015). The benefits of the culture care theory and a look to the future of transcultural nursing. In M. R. McFarland and H. B. Wehbe-Alamah (Eds.), *Leininger's culture care diversity and universality: A worldwide nursing theory* (3rd ed., pp. 101-118). Burlington, MA: Jones & Bartlett Learning.

Lundgren, S. M., & Berg, L. (2011). The meanings and implications of receiving care. *Scandinavian Journal of Caring Sciences, 25*(2), 235-242.

Marchetti, A., Piredda, M., & deMarinis, M. G. (2016). Centrality of body and embodiment in nursing care: A scoping study of the Italian literature. *Journal of Nursing Scholarship, 48*(1), 31-38.

Marion, L., Douglas, M., Lavin, M. A., Barr, N., Gazaway, S., Thomas, E., & Bickford, C. (2016). *Implementing the new ANA standard 8: Culturally congruent practice. The Online Journal of Issues in Nursing, 22*(1). Retrieved from http://www.nursingworld.org/MainMenuCategories/ANAMarketplace/ANAPeriodicals/OJIN/TableofContents/Vol-22-2017/No1-Jan-2017/Articles-Previous-Topics/Implementing-the-New-ANA-Standard-8.html

McFarland, M. R., & Eipperle, M. K. (2008). Culture care theory: A proposed practice theory guide for nurse practitioners in primary care settings. *Contemporary Nurse* [Australia], *28*(1-2), 48-63.

McFarland, M. R., & Wehbe-Alamah, H. B. (2015). The theory of culture care diversity and universality. In M. R. McFarland and H. B. Wehbe-Alamah (Eds.), *Leininger's culture care diversity and universality: A worldwide nursing theory* (3rd ed., pp. 1-34). Burlington, MA: Jones & Bartlett.

McFarland, M. R., Wehbe-Alamah, H. B., Vossos, H. B., & Wilson, M. (2015). Synopsis of findings discovered within a descriptive metasynthesis of doctoral dissertations guided by the culture care theory with use of the ethnonursing research method. In M. R. McFarland and H. B. Wehbe-Alamah (Eds.), *Leininger's culture care diversity and universality: A worldwide nursing theory* (3rd ed., pp. 287-315). Burlington, MA: Jones & Bartlett.

Merrill, A. S., Hayes, J. S., Clukey, L., & Curtis, D. (2012). Do they really care? How trauma patients perceive nurses' caring behaviors. *Journal of Trauma Nursing, 19*(1), 33-37.

Milton, C. L. (2012). Teaching-learning in community: The metaphor of nurse as guest. *Nursing Science Quarterly*, 25(2), 137-139.

Mixer, S. J. (2011). Use of the culture care theory to discover nursing faculty care expressions, patterns, and practices related to teaching culture care. *The Online Journal of Cultural Competence in Nursing and Healthcare*, 1(1), 3-14.

Mixer, S. J. (2015). Application of the culture care theory in teaching cultural competence and culturally congruent care. In M. R. McFarland and H. B. Wehbe-Alamah (Eds.), *Leininger's culture care diversity and universality: A worldwide nursing theory* (3rd ed., p. 372). Burlington, MA: Jones & Bartlett.

Mixer, S. J., McFarland, M. R., Andrews, M. M., & Strang, C. W. (2013). Exploring faculty health and wellbeing: Creating a scholarly community. *Nurse Education Today*, 33(12), 1471-1476. Retrieved from http://dx.doi.org/10.1016/j.nedt.2013.05.019

Moore, J., Titler, M. G., Low, L. K., Dalton, V. K., & Sampselle, C. M. (2014). Transforming patient-centered care: Development of the evidence-informed decision-making through engagement model. *Women's Health Issues*, 25(3), 276-282.

Oh, J., Cho, H., Kim, Y. Y., Park, H. J., & Kim, H. K. (2015). An integrative review on development of "QUality Of care Through the patients' Eyes" (QUOTE) Instruments. *Journal of Nursing Care Quality*, 30(4), e26-e31. doi: 10.1097/NCQ.0000000000000127

Orem, D. (1983). The self-care deficit theory of nursing: A general theory. In I. Clements and F. Roberts (Eds.), *Family health: A theoretical approach in nursing care*. New York, NY: Wiley.

Papadopoulos, I., & Ali, S. (2016). Measuring compassion in nurses and other healthcare professionals: An integrative review. *Nurse Education in Practice*, 16(1), 133-139. Retrieved from http://dx.doi.org/10.1016/j.nepr.2015.08.001

Papadopoulos, I., Taylor, G., Ali, S., Aagard, M., Akman, O., Alpers, L-M., ... Zorba, A. (2017). Exploring nurses' meaning and experiences of compassion: An international online survey involving 15 countries. *Journal of Transcultural Nursing*, 28(3), 286-295.

Podlog, L. W., & Brown, W. J. (2016). Self-determination theory: A framework for enhancing patient-centered care. *Journal for Nurse Practitioners*, 12(8), e359-e362.

Potter, T. M. (2012). Partnership nursing: Recovering lost threads of the nursing story. *Creative Nursing*, 18(2), 50-56.

Potter, T., & Oehlert, J. K. (2015). To move health care to health caring: A conversation with Julie Kennedy Oehlert. *Creative Nursing*, 21(1), 30-37.

Powell, K. R., Mabry, J. L., & Mixer, S. J. (2015). Emotional intelligence: A critical evaluation of the literature with implications for mental health nursing leadership. *Issues in Mental Health Nursing*, 36(5), 346-356.

Raferty, C., & O'Connell, J. (2016). Care versus process [Editorial]. *Journal for Nurse Practitioners*, 12(1), 60.

Ray, M. A. (1989). The theory of bureaucratic caring for nursing practice in the organizational culture. *Nursing Science Quarterly*, 13(2), 31-42.

Ray, M. A. (2016). *The theory of caring dynamics in nursing and health care* (2nd ed.). Philadelphia, PA: F. A. Davis.

Roach, Sr. M S. (1991). The call to consciousness: Compassion in today's health world. In D. A. Gaut and M. M. Leininger (Eds.), *Caring: The compassionate healer* (pp. 7-17). New York, NY: National League for Nursing Press.

Rosenbaum, J. N. (1986). Comparison of two theorists: Orem and Leininger. *Journal of Advanced Nursing*, 11(4), 409-419.

Sagar, P. L. (2017). The public trust and our strength in numbers: Harnessing the power of nursing [Commentary]. *Journal of Transcultural Nursing*, 28(2), 220.

Sherwood, G. (1991). Expressions of nurse's caring: The role of the compassionate healer. In D. A. Gaut and M. M. Leininger (Eds.), *Caring: The compassionate healer* (pp. 79-88). New York, NY: National League for Nursing Press.

The Henry J. Kaiser Family Foundation. (2017, October). *Total number of professionally active nurses_Registered nurse (RN)* [Webpage]. Retrieved from https://www.kff.org/other/state-indicator/total-registered-nurses/?currentTimeframe=0&sortModel=%7B%22colId%22:%22Location%22,%22sort%22:%22asc%22%7D

Tyler, D. O., & Horner, S. D. (2008). Family-centered collaborative negotiation: A model for facilitating behavior change in primary care. *Journal of the American Academy of Nurse Practitioners*, 20(4), 194-203.

United States Institute of Medicine of the National Academies, & Robert Wood Johnson Foundation Initiative on the Future of Nursing. (2011). *The future of nursing: Leading change, advancing health*. Washington, DC: National Academies Press.

Watson, J. (1985). *Human science and human care: A theory of nursing*. Norwalk, CT: Appleton-Century-Crofts.

Watson, J. (2015). Jean Watson's theory of human caring. In M. C. Smith and M. E. Parker (Eds.), *Nursing theories and nursing practice* (4th ed., pp. 321-339).

CHAPTER 13

Providing Culturally Congruent Care to Haitians Using Leininger's Culture Care Theory

Robert H. Kelch and Hiba B. Wehbe-Alamah

> *Senye, Si n'ap viv jodi a malgre siklon, grangou, ak maladi, nou dwe di, "Mesi, Senye. Nou genle la pou yon bi."*
> *Lord, if we are alive today in spite of hurricanes, hunger, and sickness, we should say, "Thank you, Lord. We must be here for a reason."*
>
> Traditional Haitian Prayer

■ INTRODUCTION

It is vitally important for health care providers to develop a transcultural understanding of the people for whom they provide care. Awareness of the worldview, traditions, values, beliefs, and practices of people from different cultures is essential for the provision of culturally congruent and holistic care (McFarland & Wehbe-Alamah, 2015). We live in an increasingly multicultural world due to immigration and resettlement trends, frequent international volunteer opportunities, and global work assignments. Healthcare providers from Western or developed countries caring for people from developing nations such as Haiti need to acquire some holding knowledge about the people's cultural and social structure dimensions, as described in the Culture Care Theory and depicted in the Sunrise Enabler, to provide culturally congruent and sensitive care (Wehbe-Alamah & McFarland, 2015b).

The purpose of this chapter is to present an overview of Haitian cultural characteristics derived from an intensive review of the literature, personal observations acquired during 15 short-term volunteer medical mission trips to Haiti over the past seven years, and a translational research study conducted with Haitian staff members from a nonprofit relief organization (Kelch, Wehbe-Alamah, & McFarland, 2015. The holding knowledge presented in this chapter influencing Haitians and encountered by those who work with Haitians may not apply to all people of Haitian descent, however, healthcare providers may use this information to assist them in conducting a cultural assessment or providing culturally congruent care for Haitians.

■ THEORETICAL FRAMEWORK

Madeleine Leininger was the first nursing theorist to focus on culturally congruent care. Over the span of six decades beginning in the 1950s, she used her study of anthropology and nursing background to understand the cultural aspects of different people groups so as to provide optimum health care (McFarland & Wehbe-Alamah, 2015). Traditional Western medical practices, standards, procedures, and norms are often inappropriate or insufficient when caring for patients and families from diverse cultures. The Theory of Culture Care Diversity and Universality (also known as Culture Care Theory or CCT) was developed to help healthcare professionals understand and appropriately care for patients from different cultural backgrounds (McFarland & Wehbe-Alamah, 2015). One of the premises of Leininger's Culture Care Theory is that healthcare professionals need to develop relationships with the people to understand their values, beliefs, patterns, and expressions more fully (McFarland & Wehbe-Alamah, 2015; Wehbe-Alamah & McFarland, 2015b). Although it is not practical for all healthcare providers to live with different cultures to gain a deeper understanding of them, it is nonetheless important for caregivers to have a basic knowledge (known as *holding knowledge*) about cultures they commonly encounter so as to understand how to assess for and integrate cultural beliefs, norms, lifeways, decisions, and actions into their professional practices (Eipperle, 2015; McFarland & Wehbe-Alamah, 2015; Wehbe-Alamah & McFarland, 2015b) and thus provide culturally competent and congruent care that is meaningful and beneficial to clients.

The provision of *culturally congruent care* is essential for all healthcare providers (physicians, nurses, mental health counselors, technologists, etc.) to integrate into their practices (McFarland & Wehbe-Alamah, 2015). Culturally congruent care can be defined as "… culturally-based care knowledge, acts, and decisions used in sensitive and knowledgeable ways to appropriately and meaningfully fit the cultural values, beliefs, and lifeways of clients for their health and wellbeing" (McFarland & Wehbe-Alamah, 2015, p. 14). It is the predicted outcome from the clinical application of the theory constructs.

One construct central to Leininger's theory is the differentiation between emic and etic cultural knowledge (McFarland & Wehbe-Alamah, 2015). *Emic* knowledge is the generic or local, indigenous knowledge and practices that are learned and transmitted within the people group of interest. It is considered "insider" knowledge whereas *etic* knowledge is held by "outsiders" and is professionally learned (McFarland & Wehbe-Alamah, 2015). In the context of this chapter, the understandings, experiences, traditions, and cultural practices of Haitians shall be considered as their *emic* knowledge. Healthcare providers educated and trained in Western medical care who prescribe modern pharmaceuticals and utilize peer-reviewed and/or standardized treatment approaches have *etic* knowledge that may or may not be practiced, accepted, or suitable by persons or groups from diverse cultures or in different environmental settings. Thus, healthcare providers with *etic* knowledge need to understand and be sensitive to the cultural diverse individual, families, communities, or groups and their *emic* knowledge, beliefs, and experiences in order to provide culturally acceptable and beneficial care (McFarland & Wehbe-Alamah, 2015).

Leininger developed the *Stranger-to-Trusted-Friend Enabler* to help direct and guide CCT researchers and healthcare providers as they interact with people from a different culture to gather accurate and meaningful information and understanding about the culture (Wehbe-Alamah & McFarland, 2015b). In a foreign culture, healthcare providers need to gain the trust and friendship of new people. As an "outsider" with *etic* knowledge, developing *emic* knowledge and understanding comes after the native people learn to accept and trust the new person as a friend. The use of Stranger-to-Trusted-Friend Enabler can assist clinicians toward providing culturally congruent care.

The Sunrise Enabler

The Sunrise Enabler (Refer to Color Insert 1) is a cognitive map of the theory developed by Leininger to help nurses and other healthcare professionals to better understand the multiple cultural influences upon culturally congruent care (Wehbe-Alamah & McFarland, 2015a, p. 75). The Sunrise Enabler comprises various interrelated cultural and social structure dimensions that influence the overall cultural beliefs and practices of the people group of interest. These numerous factors are linked by dual-directional arrows that indicate the interconnectedness and interrelatedness of their influences care (Wehbe-Alamah & McFarland, 2015a). Political, economic, educational, spiritual, religious, philosophical, ethnohistorical, cultural, and social factors are all equally considered within the context of the people's worldview, which ultimately affects their expressions, patterns, and practices related to health, wellbeing, disability, illness, and dying (Wehbe-Alamah & McFarland, 2015a). These culture-specific and culturally based care practices are part of a client assessment completed by the transcultural healthcare practitioner. The transcultural nurse, advanced practice nurse, medical provider, or other healthcare professional needs to collaborate with the client to co-participatively determine a culturally appropriate plan of care (Eipperle, 2015).

Western healthcare professionals working in Haiti or other developing nations, or with Haitian immigrants, can utilize the CCT and the Sunrise Enabler to enhance their understanding about environmental and cultural contexts. Both the theory and the Sunrise Enabler can serve as a guiding framework in providing holistic care to Haitians or other culturally diverse people. The various factors specific to Haitian life, culture, beliefs, and practices discovered through the authors' use of the Sunrise Enabler and that can help the transcultural nurse or provider to collaboratively develop culturally congruent decisions and actions are presented in the following sections.

■ WORLDVIEW

Haitians' worldview has been shaped by a national history of revolution, political instability, and governmental corruption and ineffectiveness coupled with widespread profound poverty that requires self-reliance during a time of continual struggle for survival. Haitians are strongly oriented toward family and community (Dubois, 2012; Farmer, 2011; Miller, 2000; WHO, 2010). They are also a very religious people. Most Haitians follow either Catholicism or a Protestant faith, often in conjunction with Vodou (or Voodoo) beliefs and practices which are widespread and prevalent (Khoury, Kaiser, Keys, Brewster, & Kohrt, 2012; Miller, 2000; WHO, 2010). In her evaluation of ethnomedical beliefs of Haitians, Miller (2010) stated that "... concepts of reciprocity and continuity between living persons, between the living and the ancestors, and between the living and the supernatural are pervasive to Haitian life whether the person serves the Voodoo spirits or not" (p. 207). Khoury et al. (2012) identified Vodou as the predominant worldview of Haitians. "The majority of Haitians, including those who identify as Catholics

and to a lesser extent, Protestants, espouse the Vodou worldview" (p. 515).

The complex Haitian worldview has evolved from the influences of multiple competing factors shaped by adversity. Haitians exhibit tight kinship and family bonds and also perceive strong control from dead ancestors and spirits. They are surrounded by a multitude of international governmental and nongovernmental aid organizations yet possess a strong sense of self-reliance. Haitians are strongly influenced by traditional Catholic or Protestant religious traditions but have strong beliefs in the practices of Vodou traditions. The complex and multifaceted social structure dimensions of the Sunrise Enabler that influence Haitian cultural beliefs and practices are presented to assist healthcare clinicians to better understand their Haitian patients.

■ CULTURAL AND SOCIAL STRUCTURE DIMENSIONS

Ethnohistory

Because all people are shaped and influenced by their past experiences, having knowledge about the *ethnohistory* of a cultural group (or client) of interest is vital for understanding the culture. As conceptualized by Leininger, ethnohistory involves "... the past facts, events, instances, and experiences of human beings, groups, cultures, and institutions that occur over time in particular contexts that help explain past and current lifeways about culture care influencers of health and wellbeing or death of people" (McFarland & Wehbe-Alamah, 2015, p. 15). Most healthcare providers generally ask new patients detailed questions about their personal history, family medical history, previous diagnoses, illnesses and medications, religious preferences, and personal habits (good and bad) as part of developing a fundamental understanding of each person and to assist in the provision of quality care. The transcultural nurse or healthcare provider also gathers the cultural ethnohistory of the patient, their family, and cultural group.

Haiti is a country of approximately 10 million people located about 600 miles southeast of Miami, Florida (Embassy of the Republic of Haiti, 2015) and has a rich national ethnohistory. Over 900,000 Haitians who have either emigrated from Haiti or been born in the United States to Haitian parents currently live in the United States (Migration Policy Institute [MPI], 2014). In addition, an estimated 1.5 million Haitians have immigrated to various countries around the world (PAHO, 2012). These numbers are significant considering that the current population of Haiti is around 9.8 million people (PAHO, 2012). Haiti is recognized by the United Nations (UN), the World Health Organization (WHO), and the Pan American Health Organization (PAHO) as the most impoverished nation in the Western hemisphere (PAHO 2006, 2012; UN, 2012; WHO, 2012). As such, it has a higher degree of the most adverse health indicators (rates of HIV/AIDS; tuberculosis; infant and maternal mortality; malnutrition; and diarrheal diseases) than any other Western hemisphere nation (Archer & Le, 2013; Durham et al., 2015; PAHO, 2012). As a result of extreme poverty and absent social and health service infrastructures, most Haitians have never received ongoing primary health care nor evaluation and/or treatment for common chronic diseases such as hypertension, diabetes, or asthma (PAHO, 2012).

Historically, Haiti has had a weakly functioning government and no formal public education system (Farmer, 2011; Katz, 2013; WHO, 2010). With the resultant widespread functional illiteracy, lack of health promotion and teaching, and daily subsistence-level poverty, most Haitian people have very little knowledge or understanding about health promotion, disease prevention, or healthy lifestyle practices. Most Haitians must work six or seven days a week to earn enough money to survive, so obtaining routine health care or purchasing medications for unseen "silent" illnesses (such as hypertension or diabetes) has not been viewed as a priority (Farmer, 2011; Miller, 2000; PAHO, 2012).

The world has learned a great deal about Haiti since the devastating 7.0 magnitude earthquake struck the island in January 2010. Much of the capital city of Port-au-Prince was destroyed and nearly all of the government infrastructure was leveled. Over 200,000 people died (some estimates range up to 300,000 people) and 1.5 million people were left homeless. Much of the governmental, law enforcement, educational, health care, financial, utility, and transportation capabilities of Haiti were severely compromised or rendered inoperable (Archer & Le, 2013; Farmer, 2011; Katz, 2013; PAHO, 2012; UN, 2012; WHO, 2010; World Bank, 2015).

In October 2010, Haiti experienced the largest cholera epidemic of any country in modern history (Archer & Le, 2013; Barzilay et al., 2013; Farmer, 2011), the source of which was attributed to a United Nations peacekeeping unit that had recently arrived in Haiti from an Asian country (Farmer, 2011; Katz, 2013). Because Haiti had not previously experienced a cholera outbreak, the already overburdened healthcare system nationwide was severely strained. During the next two years, over 600,000 Haitians (representing more than 6% of the overall population) from all 10 compartments (Haitian states or provinces) became infected with cholera, 330,000 were hospitalized, and over 7,400 died (Barzilay et al., 2013). Nevertheless, the hardworking and industrious Haitian people remained resilient and perseverant in the midst of these concurrent natural disasters.

Self-reliance and long-standing community support have enabled Haitians to repeatedly rebuild after each onslaught as they continued their daily lives (Farmer, 2011; WHO, 2010). The presence of multiple international nongovernmental organizations (NGOs) including various healthcare service agencies has been a characteristic way of life in Haiti for decades. Because an extensive array of international healthcare and social service providers have continued to work with the Haitian people, ethnohistorical and cultural understandings of Haitian people are essential for the provision of culturally competent, safe, effective, and meaningful care.

Cultural Values, Beliefs, and Lifeways

Ferguson, Desir, and Bornstein (2014) conducted a literature analysis about cultural orientation in rural Haitian early adolescents. They found that despite serial macrotraumas (major earthquakes or hurricanes) and poverty-related microtraumas (unemployment; local corruption; lack of nutrition, education, and adequate housing), most Haitians were still optimistic about their futures. "Despite severe challenges, rural Haitian early adolescents demonstrate remarkable allegiance to their home country, culture, and traditional family values" (Ferguson et al., 2014, p. 621). Even after outside cultural exposures to international tourists, NGO teams, the Internet, and television that have provided a comparative awareness of their own economic poverty and governmental political strife, Haitians still maintain a strong sense of nationalistic pride and hopefulness for their futures (Ferguson et al., 2014). Family, community, and spirituality have been important factors in maintaining this pride and in supporting the Haitian cultural identity through many external and internal adversities (Nicholas, Jean-Jacques, & Wheatley, 2012).

Kinship and Social Factors

Haiti has a strong social class hierarchy that stratifies people based on their level of education (including language), family economic status, and skin color (Archer & Le, 2013; WHO, 2010). Haiti has two official languages, French and Creole (*Kreyol*) (Embassy, 2015). While everyone speaks Creole, only people from the educated and upper socioeconomic classes are typically fluent in French, which is the official governmental and medical language (Archer & Le, 2013; WHO, 2010; Winters & Derrell, 2010). Those who speak French typically have lighter skin color and are from historically wealthy families who make up the upper class elite in Haiti (WHO, 2010).

Family is very important in Haitian culture. Broad-based extended family and friendship networks are the foundation of Haitian culture (Allen, Marcelin, Schmitz, Hausmann, & Schultz, 2012; Farmer, 2011; Ferguson et al., 2014; WHO, 2010). Most Haitians live in small rural communities, which are traditionally clusters of houses organized around a central courtyard called a *lakou* (Miller, 2000). These small communities may be led by a Vodou priest who functions as the government, religious leader, and healthcare provider (Miller, 2000; WHO, 2010). Children are often raised by multigenerational families within these communal settings. Close community and kinship bonds result in members watching out for each other. This helps Haitians to develop the inner resilience needed to face difficulties such as illness, trauma, disaster, and death (Ferguson, Desir & Bornstein, 2014). Common-law unions are not unusual and polygamy is a known practice especially in rural communities. Religious marriage ceremonies are preferred by most Haitians as encouraged by the culturally predominant Catholic religion (Miller, 2000; WHO, 2010). Dubois (2012) summed up the importance of kinship factors to the Haitian people in the midst of chronic adversity by saying, "… to survive, they continue to depend, as they long have, on their informal rural and urban networks and on deeply rooted practices of self-reliance" (p. 366).

Throughout Haiti, elders are respected members of their families and communities where traditional gender responsibilities also predominate (WHO, 2010). Women are typically responsible for cooking, laundry, child rearing, and market purchases; men are commonly involved in agriculture, construction, or other physical labor and are responsible for the financial support of their wife (or wives) and children (Miller, 2000; WHO, 2010). In urban settings, it is very common to see women sitting along the main streets selling fruits and vegetables, operating small packaged-food stands, selling used clothing or shoes, or cooking rice and beans or fried food over a small charcoal fire. Children are typically well-disciplined and generally respectful of adults. Spanking and physical beatings are commonly used by adults for correcting children or providing discipline (WHO, 2010).

Kinship bonds are maintained even when family members emigrate to other countries such as the United States, Canada, or elsewhere in the Caribbean (Allen et al., 2012; MPI, 2014; WHO, 2010). Strong social interconnectedness with family and friends are maintained across geographic distances. This was especially evident during the earthquake and cholera disasters in 2010 when Haitians living abroad sent massive amounts of relief aid, thousands returned to help in rescue and rebuilding efforts, and many in the United States suffered psychological distress despite being elsewhere from these events (Allen et al., 2012). The Haitian diaspora living in the United States sent an estimated $1.1 billion to relatives in Haiti during 2012 (MPI, 2014). This family connectedness between those in Haiti and their global diaspora has been termed "transnationalism" (Allen et al., 2012). Haitians living outside their native country remain considerably influential to Haiti's national economic, social, and governmental processes (Allen et al., 2012; Dubois, 2012; MPI, 2014).

One of the negative aspects of Haitian culture is the widespread prevalence and seeming acceptance of childhood slavery (Balsari, Lemery, Williams, & Nelson, 2010; Gupta & Agrawal, 2010; WHO, 2010). Haiti has the distinction of being the first independent nation in the world created through rebellion by slaves to establish a free country for themselves. Nevertheless, an estimated 300,000 children (approximately 3% of the national population) are given or sold into slavery by their families, often to more economically affluent families or individuals as domestic help who are then frequently mistreated and abused (Balsari et al., 2010; Gupta & Agrawal, 2010; WHO, 2010). Haitian child slaves known as *Restaveks* (or *Restavecs*) cook, clean house, fetch drinking water from distant sources, do laundry, empty human excrement receptacles, clean outhouses, and generally do whatever else their owners require.

An estimated one-third of all Haitian households with children contain such "vulnerable children" and approximately one-half of these children do experience physical and/or sexual abuse (Gupta & Agrawal, 2010). The United Nations International Children's Emergency Fund (UNICEF, 2015) estimates that 24% of children in Haiti are involved in child labor and 86% receive violent discipline, although these terms are not defined. It is estimated that tens of thousands of Haitian children have experienced childhood abuse and neglect. Healthcare practitioners need to remain aware about abuse, that it is frequently perpetuated through ensuing generations. They need to be vigilant in evaluating their patients or clients with cultural or family histories or who show signs or symptoms of abuse. Although the Haitian government does acknowledge child slavery and related abuse, thus far there has been little official attempt or effort to eliminate the use of Restaveks or prosecute their abusive owners (Balsari et al., 2010; Gupta & Agrawal, 2010). Multiple international organizations with Internet websites (Restavek Freedom Foundation, Restavec Freedom Alliance, Jean R. Cadet Restavek Organization, End Slavery Now) document the plight of Restaveks and exert global pressure to end these practices.

The average fertility rate in Haiti in 2012 was 3.2 births per woman, which is significantly reduced from the estimated 5.2 rate in 1990 (UNICEF, 2015). However, birth rates are higher in the larger rural areas of the country where most births occur outside of a health facility; are not attended by a healthcare professional or midwife; and may not be documented with issued birth certificates (Chatterjee, 2008; PAHO, 2012; UNICEF, 2015). Lack of access to birth control can be attributed mainly to unaffordability, unavailability, and/or prohibitions from traditional Catholic religious teachings. As a result, only an approximate one-third of Haitian women use contraception (UNICEF, 2015). The lack of contraception and resulting high birth rate coupled with severe poverty and the inability to feed multiple children has resulted in abandoned children left to fend for themselves or to be sold or given away (Balsari et

al., 2010; Chatterjee, 2008; Gupta & Agrawal, 2010). Furthermore, the presence of hundreds of unregulated "orphanages" housing children who are not truly orphans (having been given or sent there for economic reasons by their families) has resulted in illegal adoptions and the trafficking of thousands of children worldwide (Balsari et al., 2010; Gupta & Agrawal, 2010). More recently, the Haitian government has started to close many of these orphanages and to more tightly regulate international adoptions.

Domestic abuse of women is common with 20% to 25% of women having reported themselves as victims of sexual or physical abuse (PAHO, 2012). Until 2005, rape was not considered a criminal offense in Haiti. In their economic analysis of gender inequality in Haiti, Padgett and Warnecke (2011) found that women were considered to be of lower status than men and with lower education and literacy rates. Whenever a family had insufficient food, the women and girls were typically fed less than their male counterparts or even allowed to go hungry (Padgett & Warnecke, 2011). In some businesses, female workers were paid less than male workers, sometimes earning only one-third as much for comparable work (Padgett & Warnecke, 2011).

Overall, Haitians maintain strong family and friendship ties both within the country and across international borders. Most Haitians exhibit traditional gender roles, live within multi-generational family units, and demonstrate respect for elders. Social structures and interconnectedness are important aspects of Haitian culture. From the perspective of Culture Care Theory, it is important for healthcare clinicians to understand the family and kinship dynamics of their clients or patients and who will be involved in decision making. It is essential for health care professionals to understand the social structure factors influencing their culture care situation, notably in Haitian culture a history of abuse or neglect. Despite being a former slave colony whose citizens fought for freedom, definite socioeconomic segregation and skin color stratification still exist nationally.

Spiritual, Religious, and Philosophical Factors

As a former French colony, Haiti's residents are predominantly Catholic with approximately 80% identifying themselves as Catholic and another 16% as

Protestant, the majority of the latter being Baptist (10%) or Pentecostal (4%) (Embassy, 2015). One unique characteristic of Haitian culture is the deeply ingrained religious belief in Vodou (or Voodoo), which is practiced by most Haitians and frequently integrated into both Catholic and (to a lesser extent) Protestant rituals and ceremonies (Archer & Le, 2013; Dubois, 2012; Kidder, 2003; Saussy, 2010; Vonarx, 2011; WHO, 2010). The Embassy of the Republic of Haiti website maintains that approximately one-half of Haitians practice Vodou (Embassy, 2015). One saying often heard is that "... Haiti is 80% Catholic but 100% Vodou" (Archer & Le, 2013, p. 188). In 2003, Vodou was recognized as one of the official religions of Haiti (Nicholas et al., 2012).

Vodou is especially predominant in rural areas and among the most impoverished people and those with the least education (Miller, 2000). "Vodou serves as the longstanding conceptual framework for understanding concepts of personhood and explanatory models of illness in rural Haiti. Furthermore, it establishes a systematic set of ethical guidelines" (Khoury et al., 2012, p. 516). Vodou is not just a religious practice "... but constitutes a healthcare system which includes healing practices, health promotion and prevention of illness, and promotion of personal wellbeing. Vodou provides information on how to promote, prevent, and treat health problems with theories of illness, treatment interventions, and prescriptions for behavior" (WHO, 2010, p. 6).

Vodou priests (*houngans or oungans*) and priestess' (*manbo or mambo*) are believed to cast spells or curses or heal with incantations or mystical powers; this belief among the Haitian people can greatly affect their willingness to accept Western pharmaceutically based health care (Khoury et al., 2012; Miller, 2000; Vonarx, 2011; WHO, 2010). In his literature review, Vonarx (2011) discussed how Vodou is a comprehensive healthcare system for many Haitians that combines religion, medicine, and mental health care. Spiritual beings (*loa or lwa*) include the spirits of deceased relatives or community members or leaders who are believed to exert control in positive or negative ways upon the living (Miller, 2000; WHO, 2010).

Most Haitians will attribute illness and disease to either natural or supernatural causes (Miller, 2000; Vonarx, 2011). Natural illnesses may be those with familiar symptoms and definite durations including commonly known conditions such as respiratory, vaginal, or urinary infections, skin diseases, and malaria (Miller, 2000; Vonarx, 2011). Supernaturally induced diseases are those which may suddenly occur, exhibit unfamiliar symptoms, and may be prolonged or not easily cured. Mental illnesses are poorly understood by most Haitians and usually ascribed supernatural causation (Khoury et al., 2012; Miller, 2000; Vonarx, 2011; WHO, 2010). Many Haitians will first seek out a Vodou houngan priest to heal their physical or mental illness and will only consult a Western-trained healthcare provider if this priest is unable to resolve the issue. The prevalence of Vodou practitioners throughout the rural communities of Haiti in addition to the lack of Western-trained healthcare providers and/or the affordability of treatment tends to reinforce the use of traditional Vodou health care for primary care (Miller, 2000; Vonarx, 2011; WHO, 2010).

As stated previously, Haitians are more likely to assume supernatural causation to account for any illness that is not readily explainable, such as the cholera epidemic (Grimaud & Legagneur, 2011; Vonarx, 2011). This disease exhibited rapid onset with seemingly strange and previously unencountered symptoms (profuse pale watery diarrhea) and significant mortality which were all interpreted as having a supernatural origin. In their analysis of community beliefs and fears during the 2010 cholera outbreak in Haiti, Grimaud and Legagneur (2011) discovered that many Haitians initially attributed this outbreak to Vodou and because of this misattribution and fear, dozens of Vodou practitioners were murdered in one community.

Rituals and funerals are especially important Haitian cultural beliefs (Grimaud & Legagneur, 2011; James, 2011). The mass burials necessitated by the 2010 earthquake and subsequent cholera epidemic caused significant emotional distress and trauma to uncounted numbers of families because of their inability to provide culturally congruent burial care (Grimaud & Legagneur, 2011). Haitians believe the dead have continued influence over their families and communities through Vodou rituals and communication, dreams, and the generational cycle of death and rebirth (Miller, 2000; Vonarx, 2011; WHO, 2010). Patron spirits are believed to pass down through generations. Hence, the importance of proper honor and respect through funeral ceremonies, gravesite worship, and continued prayer to the spirit of the deceased are regarded as vital by most Haitians (James, 2011; Miller, 2000; Vonarx, 2011; WHO, 2010).

Haitians are a very spiritual people, whether Catholic, Protestant and/or Vodou. "Religion in Haiti offers a sense of purpose, consolation, belonging, structure, and discipline. Religion can increase self-esteem, alleviate despair, and provide hope in very difficult and trying circumstances" (WHO, 2010, p. 8). Culturally competent healthcare clinicians need to learn about and integrate the religious and spiritual beliefs of the people (McFarland & Wehbe-Alamah, 2015). Western-educated healthcare clinicians with *etic* knowledge may dismiss Vodou practices as superstitious. However, it is vital to gain an *emic* understanding of the importance of Vodou within the cultural and religious beliefs of a Haitian patient and their family in order to provide safe, effective, meaningful, and culturally congruent care. Gaining *holding knowledge* about these important Vodou practices by Western-educated nurses and other healthcare professionals presents a significant culture care challenge in the provision of culturally congruent care for Haitians.

Economic Factors

Recognized by the UN, WHO, and PAHO as the most impoverished nation in the Western Hemisphere (PAHO, 2006, 2012; UN, 2012; WHO, 2012), Haiti had a gross domestic product (GDP) per capita of $820 in 2013, ranking it near the bottom at 165 of the 189 countries evaluated (World Bank, 2015). Over one-half of Haitians earn below the national poverty level of $2.44 per day with almost a quarter of all Haitians living in extreme poverty on less than $1.24 per day (World Bank, 2015). Based on data prior to the 2010 earthquake, the income disparity between the very rich and the very poor in Haiti was the second highest in the world (Padgett & Warnecke, 2011).

Unemployment in Haiti is a huge factor. In rural areas, more than one-third of Haitians are unemployed. In the capital city of Port-au-Prince, more than one-half of adults are unemployed (PAHO, 2012; UN, 2012). The lack of infrastructure (e.g., paved and maintained roadways; dependable electricity; reliable communication; mail service; clean water; and trash/sewage services) has resulted in difficulty attracting industry or business to the country (Padgett & Warnecke, 2011). Only about 34% of Haitians have access to electricity, which has frequent power outages; only

24% of the roads are paved, and many are in very poor repair (Padgett & Warnecke, 2011). The largest income component of the national GDP comes from funds sent by the Haitian diaspora. These external contributions amounts to an estimated 20% of the GDP (Archer & Le, 2013; MPI, 2014; Padgett & Warnecke, 2011). Haiti is noted as the most external remittance-dependent country in the world, with an approximately 44% of the homes in Port-au-Prince receiving financial support from relatives outside of Haiti (PAHO, 2012). The next largest GDP segment is agriculture related to subsistence farming and the countless street vendors (Refer to Figure 13.1).

The lack of government-provided social services and a complete absence of any governmental financial support (e.g., American style "welfare," food stamps, or social security income) has meant that virtually all Haitians must work to have income or provide support for costs of basic family living. The Biblical admonishment, "… If anyone will not work, neither shall he eat" (2 Thessalonians 3:10) is a fact of life in Haiti. It is readily apparent to visitors that Haitians are hardworking people. Those who own motorbikes or scooters will offer their services as a moto-taxi, and often transport one to three additional people and/or packages on the back of theirmotorcycle. People rapidly gather around a broken down vehicle to help repair it in hopes of earning a few Haitian *gourdes* (currency). Children walk between cars stopped at roadway intersections and wash dusty windshields with squirt bottles and dirty rags in hopes of being paid by a caring driver. Women line the city streets selling their produce from baskets. Some set up stands where they cook and sell rice and beans from their charcoal fire heated cooking pot. Used clothing and shoe merchants are everywhere (Refer to Figure 13.1). The lack of industrial equipment means that most jobs are accomplished by manual labor. A dozen men may load and unload a truck full of cinder blocks or bags of concrete. Similarly, construction sites will have dozens of men, most of whom mix concrete by hand and carry bricks up rickety ladders tied together from sticks. Although impoverished financially, Haitians are very hardworking in their attempts to stay alive and earn a living for themselves and their families.

The severe poverty experienced by most Haitians necessitates that almost all income goes to provide basic life necessities such as food, shelter, clothing, and

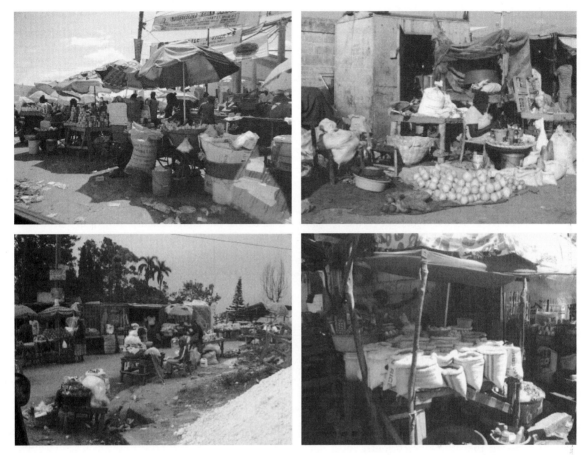

FIGURE 13.1 • Haitian street vendors selling fruits, vegetables, rice, clothing, etc. © Robert Kelch (2017).

charcoal (for cooking). Money is generally not available for health care or medicine, even if health care were available. Very few Haitians seek out medical care unless absolutely necessary. Healthcare providers need to remain aware about how the provision of care will be funded or paid for, such as whether services and/or pharmaceuticals will be given free of charge or at a nominal cost to patients.

Educational Factors

Approximately 47% of urban and 80% of rural populations of Haiti are unable to read (PAHO, 2012; WHO, 2010). The official government literacy rate for all Haitians over the age of 15 years is 52.9% (Embassy, 2015). About one-half of school-aged children do not attend school (PAHO, 2012; UNICEF, 2015; U.S. Agency for International Development [USAID], 2013; WHO,

2010). Very little education is provided by the government; more than 90% of academically enrolled children are at private schools operated by religious, humanitarian, or other nongovernment organizations (Brown, 2010; PAHO, 2012; USAID, 2013). Approximately 72% of the educated population have had only primary (elementary) level education, often atinadequately staffed and poorly equipped schools (PAHO, 2012; UNICEF, 2015; USAID, 2013; WHO, 2010). The Haitian government has been financially and organizationally unable to educate teachers; build or staff schools; develop educational standards; or promote education (PAHO, 2012; UNICEF, 2015; USAID, 2013). NGOs have helped fill this gap, but are only able to provide basic education to a portion of Haitian children.

Haitian children who are able to attend a school, with tuition frequently funded by various Western sponsors or organizations, are very appreciative. Each school requires specific uniforms, and it is common to see groups of children in different colored uniforms passing each other on their way to or from the various schools in a metropolitan or urban area such as Port-au-Prince, Cap-Haitien, or Les Cayes. Lack of books and supplies means that much of their education takes place through verbal recitation, memorization, and/or writing on an old chalk board. Most children desire to learn both French and English so as to have more opportunities for gainful future employment.

With the high illiteracy rate in Haiti, the design of any health promotion or disease management program must be individualized to the education level of the people who will be receiving these services (Owais, Hanif, Siddiqui, Agha, & Zaidi, 2011). Culturally congruent care must first be tailored to the culture. Accordingly, in Haiti, verbal or visual health education that incorporates simple diagrams, pictures, or graphics are needed to best depict key or important educational points.

Environmental Factors

Haiti and the Dominican Republic share the mountainous Caribbean island of Hispaniola with Haiti occupying the Western third of the land mass. Approximately 9.8 million people occupy 10,714 square miles, making it a very densely populated nation (Archer & Le, 2013; Embassy of the Republic of Haiti, 2015). Located near the Equator, the sun shines brightly most days and temperatures remain fairly constant year round, ranging from 85°F to 100°F (29°C-38°C) during the day and 65°F to 85°F (18°C-29°C) at night. The rainy season occurs from May through July followed by hurricane season from August to November (Archer & Le, 2013). Given the hot and humid climate, Haiti is plagued by mosquito-borne illnesses such as malaria, dengue, and parasitic-borne lymphatic filariasis (The Centers for Disease Control and Prevention [CDCP], 2015; PAHO, 2012). Many Haitians have been affected by these vector-borne diseases. As recently as 2002, approximately 30% of Haitians had been infected with filariasis although massive drug administration campaigns since the earthquake have been implemented to try to eradicate this disease (PAHO, 2012). Most Haitians have had malaria at least once during their lifetime with an estimated 3% prevalence rate (PAHO, 2012). Dengue fever and typhoid fever are also endemic throughout the country (PAHO, 2012). The mosquito-borne chikungunya virus—long endemic in

Africa, South Asia, and the Pacific—swept through the Caribbean basin including Haiti starting in December 2013 causing severe arthralgia and fever for those infected (CDCP, 2015). Notwithstanding, there are no governmental or nongovernmental programs or efforts attempting environmental control or chemical eradication of mosquitoes in Haiti (PAHO, 2012).

Haiti has often been assaulted by hurricanes and tropical storms (PAHO, 2012). In 2008, four separate hurricanes struck Haiti killing more than 800 people and destroying or damaging approximately 100,000 homes (PAHO, 2012). Tropical storms and hurricanes continue to plague the nation with death and destruction almost annually. Much of this destruction is due to the severe deforestation of Haiti's mountainous terrain resulting in frequent mudslides from heavy rainfall. These massive mudslides wash away the tightly packed, poorly constructed mountainside houses, kill dozens of people, and leave many homeless (Archer & Le, 2013; Brown, 2010; Winters & Derrell, 2010).

Diarrheal diseases caused by the lack of clean water and safe sanitation remain a major environmental and healthcare concern (PAHO, 2012). Only about 48% of rural residents and 78% of urban residents have access to clean drinking water. The cholera epidemic of 2010 caused widespread morbidity and mortality due to ingesting fecally contaminated water. Cholera is now endemic to Haiti due to the lack sanitary waste disposal that perpetuates the disease cycle. Improved sanitation facilities such as enclosed latrines and toilets are available to only 17% of rural and 34% of urban residents (Archer & Le, 2013; PAHO, 2012). Human and animal excreta are visible on the open ground in both rural and urban areas (PAHO, 2012).

These findings were confirmed by one author's (Kelch) personal observations during numerous trips to Haiti between the years 2009 to 2015 who noted household, personal trash, and biomedical waste littering the countryside and most waterways. In many areas, piles of accumulated garbage were eventually burned, releasing toxic smoke throughout densely populated areas. The rivers and stagnant bodies of water were used for bathing and laundry, and drinking and cooking water sources were significantly contaminated with trash and excreta.

Lack of utility infrastructures in Haiti means the majority of residents have no reliable source of electricity (Padgett & Warnecke, 2011). Propane tanks are available for cooking although most people cook over small charcoal fires especially in rural areas. This massive requirement for charcoal has resulted in the substantial deforestation of trees throughout the countryside (Archer & Le, 2013; Winters & Derrell, 2010). The prevalence of cooking fires, trash fires, and overall dusty-dirty conditions have caused significant adverse health effects, especially for children. Respiratory infections and diarrheal diseases account for over one-half of all childhood deaths before the age of five years (PAHO, 2012). Several major causes of childhood mortality (malnutrition, injuries, malaria, and tuberculosis) are thus environmentally linked (PAHO, 2012).

These environmental factors influence virtually all Haitians both physically and emotionally. Culturally congruent care decisions and actions must take into account the environment in which patients live, as depicted in the Sunrise Enabler (McFarland & Wehbe-Alamah, 2015). Acute treatment of a child or adult with diarrheal disease achieves very little if the person will continue to use the contaminated water sources that initially caused the illness because there is no access to safe sanitation. Similarly, acute treatment of a child with exacerbated asthma provides only temporary relief when living in a dusty, smoke-filled environment. Proper disposal of medical and human waste in sanitary landfills, hazardous waste disposal sites, or medical waste incinerators are also key to controlling many diseases (PAHO, 2012).

Political and Legal Factors

The political history of Haiti has been tumultuous and difficult. Its first recorded history dates from 1492 when the island of Hispaniola was discovered by Christopher Columbus in his search for the "New World." Columbus landed on the northern coast near the location of what later became Cap-Haitien, Haiti's second largest city (Archer & Le, 2013; Farmer, 2011). The island was initially inhabited by Taino Indians but during subsequent years slaves were brought from Africa to work on farms and plantations (Archer & Le, 2013; Brown, 2010; Farmer, 2011). Both the Spanish and French claimed parts of Hispaniola. The Western portion (Haiti) eventually came under the jurisdiction of France while the Eastern two-thirds of the island was controlled by the Spanish and subsequently became the Dominican Republic (Archer & Le, 2013; Brown, 2010; Farmer, 2011; Winters & Derrell, 2010). In 1791, a slave revolt began that lasted 13 years and

ended in 1804 with the creation of Haiti as the first independent nation in Latin America (Archer & Le, 2013; Brown, 2010; DuBois, 2012; Farmer, 2011).

Haiti is a former slave nation that has experienced continual upheavals. Violent changes in government leadership occurred more than times from 1804 until 1915 when U.S. President Woodrow Wilson sent American military troops to occupy Haiti and maintain peace (Archer & Le, 2013; DuBois, 2012; Farmer, 2011; Katz, 2013). American forces continued to occupy and control Haiti until 1934 while attempting to develop the country and structure its government based on American standards (Archer & Le, 2013; DuBois, 2012; Katz, 2013). Throughout the 20th century Haiti experienced governmental corruption, violent overthrows, and sociopolitical oppression that resulted in almost continual political, economic, and social instability (DuBois, 2012; Farmer, 2011; Katz, 2013). "Papa Doc" Duvalier and later his son "Baby Doc" Duvalier ruled from 1957 through 1986 through oppressive dictatorships and corruption, embezzling and diverting tens of millions of dollars for personal use or profit (DuBois, 2012; Farmer, 2011; Katz, 2013). During this regime, tens of thousands of Haitians were imprisoned or killed by police and military squads to suppress opposition to governmental control (DuBois, 2012; Farmer, 2011; Katz, 2013). In 1990, Catholic priest Jean-Bertrand Aristide was democratically elected to office as a hopeful reformer, but was forced from office and from Haiti during a coup d'état (DuBois, 2012; Farmer, 2011; Katz, 2013). He later returned to Haiti and was re-elected and in 2004 was again forced from office (DuBois, 2012; Farmer, 2011; Katz, 2013). Subsequent and more recent government leaderships have continued to be characterized by instability and ineffectiveness (DuBois, 2012; Farmer, 2011; Katz, 2013).

In addition, a huge restitution debt owed to France for losses suffered by the slave rebellion of 1791-1804 has plagued Haiti over the past two centuries (Archer & Le, 2013; Chatterjee, 2008, Dubois, 2012; Farmer, 2011). The 150 million francs that Haiti agreed to pay France in 1825 is estimated to be the modern equivalent to $21 billion (Chatterjee, 2008). Although this external debt was finally repaid with interest in the 1950s, the repayment diverted money away from the national budget that could have been used to build infrastructure and develop programs that could have enhanced living and health conditions for all Haitians.

In 1990, the United Nations sent a peacekeeping force to Haiti to help maintain control during the turbulent Duvalier coup period. Since that time, different peacekeeping forces have occupied the country, including the one designated in 2004 as the United Nations Stabilization Mission in Haiti (MINUSTAH) that has continued to patrol the countryside and assist the Haitian police force maintain civil order and control (Dubois, 2012; PAHO, 2012). Viewed by most Haitians as an uninvited occupying military force not generally welcome, the dislike of MINUSTAH intensified when the post-earthquake cholera epidemic in 2010 was found to have originated from a UN base located in the central highlands (Farmer, 2011; Katz, 2013).

Another unique characteristic of Haiti is the prevalence of numerous international organizations whose presence seemingly implies to Haitians that they are unable to run their own country. MINUSTAH, USAID, WHO, and PAHO, in addition to thousands of large and small NGOs from numerous countries and thousands of international missionaries from diverse religious backgrounds, are spread throughout this small country (Farmer, 2011; Katz, 2013). Dubois (2012) called Haiti a "... Republic of NGOs" (p. 351) and further stated that the nation is characterized by "... a bewildering patchwork of foreign aid organizations playing a central role in Haiti's economic and political life" (p. 351). Coordination of these efforts by the Haitian government is lacking and no reliable information exists about the number of organizations in residence or what these various missions or endeavors comprise. Furthermore, these uncounted entities receive very little oversight or control from the Haitian government while providing many basic civil services and having significant influence over much of Haitian life (Dubois, 2012).

The Haitian history of sociopolitical revolution and revolt; government upheavals, corruption, and embezzlement; and extreme poverty and disparities for the majority of the people (a small percentage of the elite live in luxury) has resulted in very little respect for or belief in their government for leadership or any reliance for the provision of essential civic services or human rights protections (Dubois, 2012; Farmer, 2011; Padgett & Warnecke, 2011; Winters & Derrell, 2010). They have thus developed self-reliance, community networking, and informal support systems that enable them to persevere through difficult times.

In their historical, political, and cultural analysis of the two different but adjacent countries of Hispaniola (Haiti and Dominican Republic), Winters and Derrell (2010) stated that Haiti is "... a hysteretic state, one in which the past does not simply shape the present, but where history itself has been an obstacle to change" (p. 598). Whereas Haiti has been characterized by more than 200 years of almost continual instability, corruption, poverty, and crisis upon crisis, the Dominican Republic has developed fairly well and is much more stable and prosperous. Winters and Derrell further contend that the cumulative effect of history, politics, ideology, religious values, and culture has resulted in Haiti's "... downward spiral of underdevelopment" (p. 599). James (2011) emphasized this historical effect on 21st century Haiti in her evaluation of the sense of insecurity felt by all or most Haitians, stating, "... Cycles of political, economic, and social ruptures have established insecurity as an ontological state of being in Haiti. Routines of rupture have created conditions in which trauma has become an ongoing, existential reality for many citizens." (p. 357). James detailed how government-sponsored or sanctioned arrests, assaults, imprisonments, rapes, and murders over prior decades, and particularly during the two Duvalier dictatorships, were attempts to destroy the tight social and kinship bonds that characterized the Haitian people. Nicholas et al. (2012) in their analysis of the mental health challenges faced by Haitians discussed the chronic history of political turmoil, government instability, social unrest, insecurity, and poverty that has adversely affected them. The researchers also pointed out the positive cultural aspects of family linkages, community networks, and strong spirituality as stabilizing factors that have strengthened the Haitian people throughout their history of adversity.

In providing culturally congruent care to Haitians, an understanding of their tumultuous political history is therefore quite important. A distrust of authority figures as well as health care or service providers may present challenges in gaining their acceptance of Western healthcare approaches (Miller, 2000). Leininger's Stranger-to-Trusted Friend Enabler, developed to help researchers and healthcare providers gain the trust and friendship of new people, would be beneficial to clinicians providing care for Haitians (Wehbe-Alamah & McFarland, 2015a). Culturally conditioned self-reliance, along with strong beliefs and frequent practices of Vodou, may result in patients seeking Western healthcare only as a last resort when their illness, disease, or injury has progressed to an advanced stage.

Each of the various social structure factors of the Sunrise Enabler are essential components in the discovery of the beliefs, practices, worldview, lifeways, and culture of most Haitians. Each factor influences each Haitian in unique and individual ways. Although the majority live in poverty, a small minority Haitians are affluent. Some Haitians strictly adhere to Catholic, Baptist, Pentecostal, or Vodou beliefs and practices while others blend elements together from two or more religious beliefs and traditions. Some children have been exposed to abuse or slavery, while fortunately many others have not. Those Haitians living in rural agricultural and seaside fishing areas, such as Les Cayes, have better nutrition than those residing in the slums of Port-au-Prince. Health care and social service professionals need to be aware of the various ethnohistorical and cultural factors that are major influencers upon the Haitian people. Such holding knowledge, awareness, and sensitivity are essential to assess or identify the value and meaning of these factors so as to provide culturally congruent care for the Haitian patient, family, community, or group.

Healthcare Considerations

Haiti's climate allows many fruits and vegetables to be grown year-round and are sold daily by street vendors. Outside of the city, most Haitians work at subsistence-level farming (Archer & Le, 2013). From 2009 through 2015, author Kelch noted that poverty and chronic hunger were dominant in many areas in Haiti, and that many people ate starchy, high-bulk, and filling foods such as rice, beans, and spaghetti as opposed to native fruits and vegetables (Kelch, Wehbe-Alamah, & McFarland, 2015). Starchy foods were typically seasoned with high sodium flavorings such as *Maggi* bouillon, readily found at street vendors and small shops throughout Haiti. Vegetables, when consumed, were usually eaten as part of a seasoned stew or added to a sauce served over rice. Many people were observed buying very inexpensive stalks of sugar cane and chewing the sweet pulp as a means of alleviating hunger. It was also common to see children and adults use their few coins to purchase a small package of crackers or cheese puffs to eat as a meal.

Very little obesity exists in Haiti, primarily due to the high prevalence of poverty and malnutrition, with less than 4% of Haitians considered to be overweight or obese (UNICEF, 2015). Very few Haitians own cars or motorbikes and thus rely on various forms of public transportation (mostly overcrowded "tap-tap" pickup trucks) that operate only on main roadways. Nearly every person walks extensively every day. Their thin stature and high-level of fitness developed from exertional activities of daily living helps counteract other adverse lifestyle health effects.

Even before the loss of many healthcare providers and facilities in the 2010 earthquake, Haitian medical care was considered inadequate by global health standards (Archer & Le, 2013; DeGennaro, DeGenarro, & Ginzburg, 2011; PAHO, 2012). Haitian physicians and nurses earned small salaries and frequently went unpaid for months (DeGenarro, 2011; DeGennaro et al., 2011; Garfield & Berryman, 2010). Prior to the earthquake, only 30% of healthcare facilities were public (or government managed), most located in the main cities (WHO, 2010). Approximately 50% of Haitian health services had been located in the capital city of Port-au-Prince although only about 20% of the country's population had resided there (PAHO, 2012). More than 70% of Haiti's healthcare services are provided by international volunteer organizations and NGOs. Even with this assistance, only about 40% of the population had access to healthcare services, primarily in urban areas (Brown, 2010; PAHO, 2012; WHO, 2010). Because cash payment for service was typically required prior to care at the public medical facilities, very few Haitians could actually afford to access basic or emergency medical care. As a result, reportedly 80% of Haitians seek "traditional medicine" (i.e., Vodou caregivers) first due to its low cost and accessibility (PAHO, 2012).

The 2010 earthquake destroyed the main government medical school and nursing school, both of which collapsed with many students and faculty inside (Archer & Le, 2013; DeGennaro et al., 2011; Farmer, 2011; Garfield & Berryman, 2012). Numerous hospitals and clinics were destroyed and more than 70% of the healthcare capability across the entire country was decimated (Archer & Le, 2013). Many of the Haitian nursing schools in operation prior to and after the earthquake were nonregulated schools without standardized nursing curricula or specific educational requirements. Since that time, several North American university medical and/or nursing schools have formed partnerships with Haitian medical and nursing schools to send clinical and academic instructors, medical residents, and nursing students to Haiti (Garfield & Berryman, 2012). They will help to redevelop the Haitian programs and provide training and mentorship to Haitian faculty during short-term trips to Haiti or through exchange programs with Haitian healthcare professionals to the U.S. (DeGenarro, 2011; DeGennaro et al., 2011; Garfield & Berrymam, 2010, 2012; Secor, 2011; USAID, 2013). Several large NGOs operating in Haiti (i.e., J/P HRO, Partners in Health, Project Medishare) have developed health professional mentorship programs. These international efforts to help rebuild the Haitian healthcare infrastructure will need to continue for many years (Archer & Le, 2013; Garfield & Berrymam, 2012). However, as with many other developing nations around the world, Haiti suffers from a "brain drain" as educated professionals (including physicians and nurses) emigrate to more affluent countries for more-lucrative employment opportunities, higher salaries, and significantly better living environments (Archer & Le, 2013; Chatterjee, 2008).

Haiti suffers from some of the worst health indicators in the world, with high levels of infant and maternal death, childhood malnutrition, diarrheal diseases, HIV/AIDS, TB, and sexually transmitted diseases (Chatterjee, 2008; PAHO, 2012; UNICEF, 2015). Adult chronic diseases such as hypertension, diabetes, and asthma are inadequately diagnosed or managed due to lack of available and affordable primary health care. The diagnosis and treatment of cancer, leukemia, and heart disease is essentially nonexistent for the vast majority of Haitians (PAHO, 2012). The prevalence of HIV is about 2.2% and isthe highest in the Western hemisphere (PAHO, 2012; UNICEF, 2015).

The lack of accessible healthcare facilities or trained birth attendants and midwives, especially in the rural majority of the country, results in only about 25% of pregnant women delivering their baby with the assistance of a medical attendant (PAHO, 2012). Many pregnant women with pregnancy or delivery complications are unable to reach a health facility or unable to pay for care and therefore die. As a consequence, Haiti has a maternal mortality rate of approximately 630 per 100,000 live births, also the highest in the Western hemisphere (Chatterjee, 2008; PAHO, 2012). When a mother dies, the newborn child will often not survive the first year of life even if delivered safely (Chatterjee, 2008). The infant mortality rate is 60 deaths per 1,000 live births (6%) and the mortality rate for children under five years of age is 76 deaths per 1,000 live births (7.6%) (PAHO, 2012; UNICEF, 2015). Both of these health indicators have been decreasing since 2005, but remain the highest across the Americas. Rates of chronic malnutrition are 18% to 32% throughout different regions of Haiti (UNICEF, 2015). Moderate to severe stunting of growth and development caused by malnutrition affects 22% of children resulting in lifelong short stature and probable cognitive disabilities (UNICEF, 2015). Anemia occurs in 61% of small children from six months to five years of age (PAHO, 2012). Because Haitians generally lack adequate routine health care and endure lifelong adverse living conditions, provider assessment of immunization status is an essential health need, especially for children as many Haitians have received very few of the recommended immunizations (PAHO, 2012; UNICEF, 2015).

Haitian mental health care is seriously deficient because of a lack of psychiatrists, psychologists, or trained mental health counselors throughout the nation (Khoury et al., 2012; Miller, 2000; Vonarx, 2011; WHO, 2010). Mental illness is often culturally ascribed to the supernatural or to evil spirits, necessitating emic or generic care by Vodou practitioners. Furthermore, Haiti has no formal licensing process for mental health providers (Nicolas, Jean-Jacques, & Wheatley, 2012). Mental health clinicians have indicated that Haitians are very reluctant to acknowledge mental illness, seek Western medical care (if it is even available), or take pharmaceutical medications for the treatment of mental health illnesses (Khoury et al., 2012; Miller, 2000; Nicolas et al., 2012; Vonarx, 2011; WHO, 2010). The high incidence of childhood sexual abuse, physical abuse, maltreatment, and neglect has a propensity for causing noncoping or maladaptive adverse behaviors as these children grow into adults and thereafter start their own families (Balsari et al., 2010; Gupto & Agrawal, 2010; Miller, 2000).

For healthcare providers who may wish to provide volunteer health care through any of the NGOs that operate in Haiti or help educate and mentor physicians, nurses, or other health care workers, they will encounter no real governmental regulations or licensing requirements. The *Ministère de la Santé Publique et de la Population* (MSPP; Haitian Ministry of Public Health and Population) provides essentially no oversight or regulation for NGOs that provide short or long term health care for the citizens of Haiti (Dubois, 2012; Garfield & Berryman, 2012; PAHO, 2012).

Nearly anyone can provide medical care or dispense pharmaceuticals in Haiti, regardless of education, experience, or licensure. Well-meaning Western volunteers provide health services that may be in excess of their formal education or licensure (PAHO, 2012; Durham et al., 2015). International short-term healthcare teams arrive in Haiti on an almost daily basis that may or may not be led by appropriately licensed providers. On multiple occasions, one author (Kelch) observed clinics in operation led by physical therapists, nurse aides, Licensed Practical Nurses (LPNs), or Emergency Medical Technicians (EMTs) who functioned as the healthcare provider, diagnosing illnesses and dispensing pharmaceuticals to Haitian patients. Pharmaceuticals accessible only by prescription in the United States and Canada are commercially available "over the counter" (PAHO, 2012) or openly dispensed by uneducated Haitian "drug vendors" who wander the streets carrying baskets of pre-packaged medications on their heads (Refer to Color Insert 4).

Vodou beliefs and practices are an integral part of Haitian cultural health beliefs and practices. Priests and priestesses are emic (generic) primary healthcare clinicians throughout much of Haiti, especially in rural communities. Herbal medicines and potions are routinely used, as are spells and incantations, to provide healing for both physical and mental illnesses (Miller, 2000; Nicolas et al., 2012; Vonarx, 2011; WHO, 2010). The Western healthcare practitioner must therefore carefully evaluate and consider Vodou beliefs and practices among their Haitian patients when coparticipatively developing care decisions and actions (Eipperle, 2015; McFarland & Wehbe-Alamah, 2015).

In their qualitative study about the unmet health needs of Haitian women, Urrutia et al. (2012) found similarity in the needs expressed by women living in both urban and rural settings. Both groups of women desired access to health care (including trained maternity care), clean water, proper sanitation, sufficient food to eliminate hunger and meet nutritional needs, and opportunities for education and employment.

Other issues important to the women included health education, affordable health care, improved proximity to health services, and better transportation options (Urrutia et al., 2012). The women studied expressed very little confidence in ability of the Haitian government to meet any of these needs but instead expected international NGOs to provide these services. The researchers noted the importance of NGOs working "from the bottom up" by asking community members what services they needed, seeking community input to prioritize projects, and getting their ideas about how to best implement project solutions (Urrutia et al., 2012).

Culturally congruent care integrates the complex cultural and social structure factors influencing Haitian patients. Most Haitians have minimal, if any, prior health care and probably no routine primary health care. Thus, chronic diseases such as diabetes, hypertension, asthma, or COPD may never have been diagnosed or treated. Sexually transmitted infections may not have been identified or treated and consequently could incur longer-term morbidity. Malnutrition may have caused permanent health disability or other health issues such as anemia. Inadequate or missed immunizations may have resulted in infections, disfigurement, and/or disability caused by various preventable and treatable communicable diseases. Vector-borne illness in any patient in the Caribbean basin is a likely occurrence. Mental illness, disaster related post-traumatic stress disorder (PTSD), or physical and emotional trauma from sexual or physical abuse can long affect individuals and carry over into extended family as well as future generations. Healthcare providers must evaluate and appropriately treat a multitude of issues when providing culturally appropriate care for Haitians. Etic perspectives about health, care, and treatment must not be allowed to supersede their emic values, beliefs, and experiences. This is the goal for providing culturally congruent, sensitive, meaningful, and beneficial care (McFarland & Wehbe-Alamah, 2015).

■ THE THREE MODES OF CULTURE CARE DECISIONS AND ACTIONS

Leininger developed three modes of culture care decisions and actions to enable transcultural healthcare professionals to *mutually discuss with the client* what cultural care practices can be preserved and/or maintained; accommodated and/or negotiated with minor changes; and repatterned and/or restructured (Eipperle, 2015). Using the modes, most culturally congruent care beliefs and practices can be maintained, some modified, and some eliminated (Eipperle, 2015; McFarland & Wehbe-Alamah, 2015). Based on an understanding of their ethnohistory and generic or folk care practices, the caregiver must assess, in collaboration with the client, which emic practices have no adverse effects on health, have cultural value or meaning, provide support or relief, and are thus safe to *preserve and/or maintain*. Some cultural practices may pose some unhealthy risk but can be *accommodated and/or negotiated* to protect the health and safety of the patient or family, and will need to be discussed with and agreed upon by those involved (Eipperle, 2015; McFarland & Wehbe-Alamah, 2015). Finally, some cultural practices or actions that are known to be dangerous or unhealthy, or cannot be implemented within health care constraints, should be changed (Eipperle, 2015). This *repatterning and/or restructuring* can be difficult and stressful for both practitioner and patient (and others involved), but is ultimately beneficial in the provision of optimum culturally congruent care. If done collaboratively and empathetically, healthcare providers can provide culturally congruent care -using the culture care modes of decisions and actions- that results in safe and beneficial outcomes while remaining acceptable and meaningful to the patient and/or family.

Culture Care Preservation and/or Maintenance

Culture care preservation and/or maintenance "… refers to those assistive, supportive, facilitative, or enabling professional acts or decisions that help cultures to retain, preserve, or maintain beneficial care beliefs and values or to face handicaps or death" (McFarland & Wehbe-Alamah, 2015, p. 16). It is vital for healthcare providers endeavoring to provide culturally congruent care to Haitian patients to acquire holding knowledge and a basic understanding of Haitian *emic* or folk beliefs, practices, and traditions. To preserve and/or maintain the culture care beliefs, traditions and practices of Haitians, a healthcare provider may strive to:

- Support Haitian family and community orientation, a caring attitude toward one another, and selfless giving toward others in need during times of personal stress as well as natural disaster. These

strong kinship bonds need to be maintained and supported. The healthcare provider can do so by involving family and friends in provision of care, as and when appropriate.

- Assess and support the strong spiritual beliefs and practices of most Haitians including beneficial Vodou beliefs and practices that give purpose and meaning to their lives, provide a strong sense of community, and promote expressions of sharing, caring, and helping.
- Empower and support the hardworking, industrious, and persevering work ethic exhibited by most Haitians.
- Provide mentoring and continuing education for local Haitian healthcare clinicians, who may lack the resources for continuing medical education or the capabilities for keeping abreast of the latest healthcare practices, procedures, or treatments.

Culture Care Accommodation and/or Negotiation

Culture care accommodation and/or negotiation "… refers to those assistive, accommodating, facilitative, or enabling creative provider care actions or decisions that help cultures adapt to or negotiate with others for culturally congruent, safe, and effective care for their health, wellbeing, or to deal with illness or dying" (McFarland & Wehbe-Alamah, 2015, p. 16). To accommodate and/or negotiate the needs of a Haitian patient and/or family, the healthcare provider may want to consider the following culture care actions:

- Negotiate increased consumption of fresh fruits and vegetables and decreased use of high sodium spices and flavorings, thereby promoting healthy nutrition.
- Accommodate multigenerational and/or extended family involvement in caretaking. This may require securing expanded space for multiple people or allowing family members or friends to rotate in to see a patient. Use of cellular phones may be accommodated to enable Haitian patients to communicate with significant friends or family living abroad and those unable to physically be present.
- Consider the language, education, and literacy level of Haitian patients when developing culturally appropriate health promotion and education resources. Educational and training posters with

culturally congruent pictures or graphics are an effective means of communicating health information to those who cannot or have difficulty reading.

- Integrate Western professional care (*etic*) such as pharmaceutical care with traditional cultural practices (*emic*) where appropriate, beneficial, and not harmful. This may involve integration of Vodou practices, symbols, amulets, or prayers. Traditional herbal potions or concoctions may need to be professionally evaluated and their use negotiated with the Haitian patient based on their overall safety or compatibility.

- Negotiate medical fees and pharmaceutical costs when providing care to Haitians in their native country in consideration for the extant Haitian poverty level. With many people earning only $1 to $2 per day and possibly supporting a family, healthcare providers need to identify how to provide services in a sustainable yet affordable way.

Culture Care Repatterning and/or Restructuring

Culture care repatterning and/or restructuring "… refers to assistive, supportive, facilitative, or enabling professional care actions and mutual decisions that would help people to reorder, change, modify, or restructure their lifeways and institutions for better (or beneficial) healthcare patterns, practices or outcomes" (McFarland & Wehbe-Alamah, 2015, p. 16). A key aspect of this mode is the mutual agreement or decision (between caregiver and patient or client, and/or their family) to make beneficial changes (Eipperle, 2015). A healthcare provider seeking to repattern and/or restructure the culture care beliefs or practices of a Haitian patient may:

- Evaluate whether relationships with immediate or extended family members are beneficial or adversely affecting care decisions. For example, older family members with strong Vodou beliefs may adversely influence a younger, more progressive family member regarding acceptance of Western medical treatments.

- Educate Haitian patients regarding disease processes, infectious pathways, and pharmacology. The Haitian people are a very spiritual people who ascribe much illness and disease to supernatural causes or to spells cast by Vodou priests or

priestesses. Lack of professional health care education coupled with commonality and accessibility of Vodou practitioners and traditional treatments may present challenges to patient acceptance of professional health care and treatment.

- Teach the value of consuming a nutritious, well-balanced diet. Poverty-induced malnutrition with insufficient caloric intake is a major issue in Haiti. It is a nation that grows a multitude of fruits and vegetables year-round, but one in which many people consume a predominantly rice and bean diet. This educational repatterning and/or restructuring while preserving cultural traditions is challenging and must be accomplished through shared trust and decision making.

- Evaluate the Vodou practitioners' homeopathic potions or medications and encourage discontinuing ones that are potentially toxic, harmful, or pose undesirable interactions with prescribed medications in use. Examples of potentially harmful traditional ritual practices include bloodletting (which pose a high-risk for blood-borne disease transmission), burning, tattooing, or cutting of flesh.

- Restructure attitudes of Haitian adults/society about misusing children as Restaveks or childhood slaves, and those who have already suffered physical and/or sexual abuse. This terrible treatment of children has been ongoing through multiple generations and will continue to perpetuate into future generations unless cultural acceptance of these practices is strongly and effectively *discouraged* through culture care repatterning and/or restructuring. In addition, efforts that promote care, caring, and respect to this vulnerable group (Haitian Restaveks children) who have already experienced these traumas need to be equally *encouraged* and promoted through similar culture care restructuring and repatterning.

- Develop and promote culturally acceptable means of water purification such as solar Pasteurization. Many Haitians are chronically dehydrated due to limited access to clean water which must be purchased and is limitedly affordable. Bleach sanitizing can be taught using accessible and affordable supplies along with individual and community-focused education about the importance of hydration.

- Teach Haitian patients basic hygiene practices during food preparation such as proper food handling and hand washing after toileting and prior to cooking and eating. Lack of formal health education has resulted in many Haitians not understanding the connection between hygiene and health, which has resulted in significant morbidity and mortality especially from preventable diseases (cholera).

- Educate Western healthcare practitioners visiting Haiti on a short-term basis about culturally specific and sensitive approaches to care. Appropriate pre-trip education, understanding, and adaptation of traditional Western professional practices are vital to the successful provision of health care in a developing nation such as Haiti.

- Use Leininger's Stranger-to-Trusted-Friend Enabler (Wehbe-Alamah & McFarland, 2015a) when providing care to Haitians to identify when trusted friend stage is reached. In a foreign culture, healthcare providers need to gain the trust and friendship of new people. As an "outsider" with *etic* knowledge, developing *emic* understandings come after the native people learn to trust and befriend the new person (visiting foreign professional healthcare provider).

- Restructure and/or repattern Haitian sanitation and economic infrastructure. This can be achieved by promoting and developing means for clean and safe sanitation and resources and by creating adequate employment opportunities. The lack of safe sanitation for waste and trash disposal are important environmental and healthcare concerns in Haiti.

- Advocate for adequate employment opportunities that allow Haitians to earn a living sufficient to buy food and other necessities of life which are vital to their long-term health promotion and disease prevention.

- Promote cooperation between NGOs. Many of the countless NGOs in Haiti are independent and autonomous with minimal, if any, interaction or cooperation with other organizations. Healthcare professionals need to develop collegial and inter-organizational relationships with other NGOs in order to provide synergistic and long-term care beneficial and sustainable for Haiti.

■ SUMMARY

The provision of culturally congruent, beneficial, and meaningful health care to people from diverse cultures, religions, or belief systems is an essential component of holistic nursing and professional care in an increasingly mobile and multicultural world. No longer can Western healthcare providers assume the ethnocentric view that "their way is the only way" when approaching patients. The Theory of Culture Care Diversity and Universality, developed by Madeleine Leininger to help transcultural nurses better understand people from diverse cultures, provides a framework for nurses and other healthcare professionals to guide them in providing safe, meaningful, and beneficial care to culturally diverse clients (McFarland & Wehbe-Alamah, 2015).

Many North American and other international healthcare clinicians from all professions are involved in the provision of short or long term care for native dwellers and the global Diaspora of Haiti. In this text, the influences on Haitian health and wellbeing were described through a review of the cultural and social structure dimensions of the Sunrise Enabler. It is essential that all healthcare clinicians develop holding knowledge about the major aspects of Haitian culture to provide its people with culturally congruent care. Their ethnohistory may be filled with adversity, but their culture has taught Haitians how to survive, endure hardships, and remain hopeful for a brighter future.

■ DEDICATION

This chapter is dedicated to the people of Haiti from whom much was learned about perseverance, commitment, community, and hospitality. It is also dedicated to the three nongovernmental organizations with whom author Robert Kelch has been affiliated and which have sought to educate, equip, employ, and empower Haitians. It is long-term partnerships of sustainable culturally appropriate caregiving that will eventually allow the Haitian people to develop, strengthen, and transform their nation into a more prosperous and healthier country.

■ DISCUSSION QUESTIONS

1. As a healthcare provider, how would you deal with a Haitian patient with a severe infection of an open foot wound who insists that his Vodou priest assured him it would be healed because of the ceremony performed and spiritual connections he made the night before?

2. During a week-long medical mission trip to Haiti to provide health care in a rural clinic, a group of obviously hungry and malnourished children linger near the door. Your team brought plenty of snack foods (granola bars, dried fruits, beef jerky, cracker packs, and candy) along for team use. Some members of the team want to give a few of the snacks to the children. Discuss your thoughts.

3. In a country with many nongovernmental organizations and volunteer aid organizations on site, discuss the potential advantages and disadvantages of a church or social service group sending a medical team of volunteers (miscellaneous healthcare professionals and nonmedical people) to Haiti to set up a temporary clinic in an impoverished area to assist the "poor people." You will have translators available and will be working through a local Haitian church.

4. You are a nurse in a large American East Coast metropolitan hospital responsible for admitting a new patient whom you are told is a recent immigrant from Haiti. Because the patient speaks minimal English, you request and receive a hospital staff member fluent in *Kreyol* who will act as your translator during the intake process. As you begin to fill in the sections of the patient record about medical history, family history, religious beliefs, etc., what will you ask based upon your general holding knowledge of Haitian culture?

■ REFERENCES

Allen, A., Marcelin, L., Schmitz, S., Hausmann, V., & Schultz, J. (2012). Earthquake impact on Miami Haitian Americans: The role of family/social connectedness. *Journal of Loss and Trauma, 17*(4), 337-349.

Archer, N., & Le, P. (2013). Haiti. In M. Krasnoff (Ed.), *Building partnerships in the Americas: A guide for global health workers* (pp. 186-205). Lebanon, NH: University Press of New England.

Balsari, S., Lemery, J., Williams, T., & Nelson, B. (2010). Protecting the children of Haiti. *New England Journal of Medicine, 362*(e25), 1-3. doi: 10.1056/nejmp1001820nejm.org

Barzilay, E., Schaad, N., Magliore, R., Mung, K., Boncy, J. …, & Tappero, J. (2013). Cholera surveillance during the Haiti epidemic – the first 2 years. *New England Journal of Medicine, 368*(7), 599-609.

Brown, G. (2010). The tragedy of Haiti: A reason for major cultural change. *The Association of Black Nursing Faculty (ABNF) Journal, 21*(4), 90-93.

Centers for Disease Control and Prevention. (2015). Health information for travelers to Haiti. Retrieved from http://wwwnc.cdc.gov/travel/destinations/clinician/none/haiti

Chatterjee, P. (2008). Haiti's forgotten emergency. *The Lancet, 372.9639*, 615-618.

DeGennaro Jr., V. (2011). Haiti needs continued support from foreign health professionals. *American Journal of Public Health, 101*(1), 4-5.

DeGennaro Jr., V., DeGennaro Sr., V., & Ginzburg, E. (2011). Haiti's dilemma: How to incorporate foreign health professionals to assist short-term recovery while capacity building for the future. *Journal of Public Health, 33*(3), 459-461.

Dubois, L. (2012). *Haiti: The aftershocks of history.* New York, NY: Metropolitan Books.

Durham, J., Marcos, M., Hill, P., & Paviignani, E. (2015). Haiti and the health marketplace: The role of the private, informal market in filling the gaps left by the state. *BMC Health Services Research, 15*(424), 1-10.

Eipperle, M. K. (2015). Application of the three modes of culture care decisions and actions in advanced practice primary care. In M. R. McFarland and H. B. Wehbe-Alamah (Eds.), *Leininger's culture care diversity and universality: A worldwide nursing theory* (3rd ed., pp. 317-344). Burlington, MA: Jones and Bartlett Learning.

Embassy of the Republic of Haiti. (2015). *About Haiti: Haiti at a glance.* Retrieved from http://www. http://haiti.org/index.php/economic-xm-affairs-xm/26-the-embassy/content/121-haiti-at-a-glance

Farmer, P. (2011). *Haiti after the earthquake.* New York, NY: Public Affairs.

Ferguson, G., Desir, C. & Bornstein, M. (2014). "Ayiti cheri:" Cultural orientation of early adolescents in rural Haiti. *Journal of Early Adolescence, 34*(5), 621-637.

Garfield, R., & Berryman, E. (2010). *After the earthquake: The recovery of nursing and nursing education in Haiti* [Paper from the Haiti Nursing Foundation]. Retrieved from http://www.haitinursing.org/Images/Garfield_Haiti%20Nursing%20Paper.pdf

Garfield, R., & Berryman, E. (2012). Nursing and nursing education in Haiti. *Nursing Outlook, 60*(1), 16-20.

Grimaud, J., & Legagneur, F. (2011). Community beliefs and fears during a cholera outbreak in Haiti. *Intervention, 9*(1), 26-34.

Gupta, J., & Agrawal, A. (2010). Chronic aftershocks of an earthquake on the wellbeing of children in Haiti: Violence, psychosocial health and slavery. *Canadian Medical Association Journal, 182*(18), 1997-1999.

James, E. (2011). Haiti, insecurity, and the politics of asylum. *Medical Anthropology Quarterly, 25*(3), 357-376.

Katz, J. (2013). *The big truck that went by: How the world came to save Haiti and left behind a disaster.* New York, NY: Palgrave Macmillan.

Kelch, R., Wehbe-Alamah, H., & McFarland, M. (2015). Implementation of hypertension and diabetes chronic disease management in an adult group in Les Bours, Haiti. *Online Journal of Cultural Competence in Nursing and Healthcare*, 5(1), 50-63. doi: 10.9730/ojccnh.org/v5n1a4

Khoury, N., Kaiser, B., Keys, H., Brewster, A., & Kohrt, B. (2012). Explanatory models and mental health treatment: Is Vodou an obstacle to psychiatric treatment in rural Haiti? *Culture, Medicine, and Psychiatry*, 36(3), 514-534.

McFarland, M. R., & Wehbe-Alamah, H. B. (2015). The theory of culture care diversity and universality. In M. R. McFarland and H. B. Wehbe-Alamah (Eds.), *Leininger's culture care diversity and universality: A worldwide nursing theory* (3rd ed., pp. 1-34). Burlington, MA: Jones and Bartlett Learning.

Miller, N. (2000). Haitian ethnomedical systems and biomedical practitioners: Directions for clinicians. *Journal of Transcultural Nursing*, 11(3), 204-211.

Migration Policy Institute. (2014). *The Haitian diaspora in the United States: July 2014*. Retrieved from http://www.migrationpolicy.org/research/select-diaspora-populations-united-states

Nicolas, G., Jean-Jacques, R., & Wheatley, A. (2012). Mental health counseling in Haiti: Historical overview, current status, and plans for the future. *Journal of Black Psychology*, 38(4), 509-519.

Owais, A., Hanif, B., Siddiqui, A., Agha, A., & Zaidi, A. (2011). Does improving maternal knowledge of vaccines impact infant immunization rates? A community-based randomized-controlled trial in Karachi, Pakistan. *BMC Public Health 2011*, 11(239), 1-8.

Padgett, A., & Warnecke, T. (2011). Diamonds in the rubble: The women of Haiti: Institutions, gender equity, and human development in Haiti. *Journal of Economic Issues*, 45(3), 527-557.

Pan American Health Organization. (2006). *The challenge of Haiti. Health: A right for all*. Retrieved from http://new.paho.org/hai/index.php?option=com_content&task=view&id=24&Itemid=122

Pan American Health Organization. (2012). *Health in the Americas, 2012 edition: Country volume-Haiti*. Retrieved from: http://www.paho.org/saludenlasamericas/index.php?option=com_docman&task=doc_view&gid=134&Itemid=

United Nations. (2012). *Haiti: Moving forward step by step 2012*. Retrieved from http://www.un.org/en/peacekeeping/missions/minustah/documents/UN-fact-sheets-2012-en.pdf

United Nations International Children's Emergency Fund. (2015). *At a glance: Haiti – Statistics*. Retrieved from http://www.unicef.org/infobycountry/haiti_statistics.html

U.S. Agency for International Development. (2013). *Haiti education*. Retrieved from http://haiti.usaid.gov/work/education.php

U.S. Agency for International Development. (2014). *Haiti: Nutrition profile*. Retrieved from http://www.usaid.gov/sites/default/files/documents/1864/USAID-Haiti_NCP.pdf

Urrutia, R., Merisier, D., Small, M., Urrutia, E., Tinfo, N., & Walmer, D. (2012). Unmet health needs identified by Haitian women as priorities for attention: A qualitative study. *Reproductive Health Matters*, 20(39) 93-103.

Vonarx, N. (2011). Haitian Vodou as a health care system: Between magic, religion, and medicine. *Alternative Therapies*, 17(5), 44-51.

Wehbe-Alamah, H. B., & McFarland, M. R. (2015a). Leininger's enablers for use with the ethnonursing research method. In M. R. McFarland and H. B. Wehbe-Alamah (Eds.), *Leininger's Culture Care Diversity and Universality: A worldwide nursing theory* (3rd ed., pp. 73-100). Burlington, MA: Jones and Bartlett Learning.

Wehbe-Alamah, H. B., & McFarland, M. R. (2015b). The ethnonursing research method. In M. R. McFarland and H. B. Wehbe-Alamah (Eds.), *Leininger's Culture Care Diversity and Universality: A worldwide nursing theory* (3rd ed., pp. 35-71). Burlington, MA: Jones and Bartlett Learning.

Winters, C., & Derrell, R. (2010). Divided neighbors on an indivisible island: Economic disparity and cumulative causation on Hispaniola. *Journal of Economic Issues*, 44(3), 597-613.

World Bank. (2015). *Haiti overview – context, strategy and results*. Retrieved from http://www.worldbank.org/en/country/haiti/overview#1

World Health Organization. (2010). *Culture and mental health in Haiti: A literature Review 2010*. Retrieved from http://www.who.int/mental_health/emergencies/culture_mental_health_haiti_eng.pdf

World Health Organization. (2012). *Haiti – health profile 2012*. Retrieved from http://www.who.int/gho/countries/hti.pdf

Ayurveda: Relevance in Culture Care

Joanna Maxwell (Basuray) and R. Amadea Morningstar

> *"Integrative care refers to safe, congruent, and creative ways of blending together holistic, generic, and professional care knowledge and practices so that the client experiences beneficial outcomes for wellbeing or to ameliorate a human condition or lifeway"* (Leininger, 2002, p. 148).

■ INTRODUCTION

The use of traditional or indigenous medicine is highly prevalent in Southeast Asia as a primary defense mechanism against illness and disease processes. Despite continual advancements in modern medicine, the health status of people worldwide is less than satisfactory. Millions of people living in Southeast Asia, Latin America, and African countries, as well as people living in rural or remote areas of other developing countries, do not have access to advanced Western health care. In countries such as India, Nepal, Sri Lanka, Thailand, and their neighboring countries, Ayurvedic medicine is the only available health care option (Wiwanitkit, 2010; World Health Organization [WHO], 2001). In addition, poor and low-income families in developed nations are not able to afford the cost of Western health care. More than 80% of people living in developing countries use generic/lay/folk healthcare methods or traditional medicine as their first-line defense against illness (Spudich & Menon, 2014; WHO, 2013). As Southeast Asian people migrate to Western countries, the use of Ayurveda is spreading and becoming regarded as a respected complementary healthcare approach among Asian and non-Asian residents in the Americas and in Europe (Spudich & Menon, 2014).

Prevalence of Ayurveda

Ayurvedic medicinal practices have been in use for more than 5,000 years in Southeast Asia and have spread far beyond this core region (Pole, 2006, pp. 5-6). Since ancient times, people have used indigenous knowledge of locally available medicinal plants to cure their diseases. This traditional natural healthcare approach in the region is important because it is closely connected to the people's culture. Indigenous Ayurvedic knowledge is handed down from one generation to the next. For this reason, people in these developing countries have a strong sense of connectedness with Ayurvedic medicine. The people associate their Ayurvedic knowledge with their grandmother, parents, uncle, or other close family members. The practical knowledge of Ayurveda is a part of family heritage (Manohar, 2014). Whenever a family or an individual immigrates to another area, they bring this special knowledge with them.

Ethnohistory of Ayurveda

Ayurveda is the oldest traditional healing system on the planet, rivaling the longevity of the Traditional Chinese Medicine system. Ayurveda originated during the ancient Vedic civilization of India (Hardiman, 2009). It arose from the four Vedas, the oldest Hindu religious books, and is closely associated with Vedic civilization in India. Sanskrit, one of the oldest language systems in Southeast Asia, is the language used for all Ayurvedic medical terms. *Ayurveda* translates from Sanskrit as "science of life" (Sharma, Chandola, Singh, & Basisht, 2007). The goal of this comprehensive approach is the integration of *mind, body, behavior*, and *environment*. Ayurvedic medicine uses medicinal plants, therapeutic foods, gems, breathing, and relaxation techniques as well as yoga, bodywork, and other therapies to promote optimal health (Morningstar, 2001, p. 7).

In the past, traditional Ayurvedic medical training was conducted on a *Gurukulam* educational basis wherein Ayurvedic practitioners focused on diagnosis, interventions, and the formulation of individualized medications for their patients based on the classical knowledge learned from their *Gurus* (teachers). In the present, however, Modern Ayurvedic physicians receive institutionalized education with a standardized course curriculum that covers the study of anatomy, physiology, and biochemistry, medicinal plants, and individualized medicinal preparations (Spudich & Menon, 2014). Ayurveda is also practiced at the community level by natural healers and Vaidyas (traditional practitioners of this healing system) who have family backgrounds in practicing Ayurveda rather than an institutionally-based education (Spudich & Menon, 2014).

■ INFLUENCE OF CULTURAL BELIEFS AND TRADITIONS ON HEALTHCARE PRACTICES

Cultural beliefs and traditions have a significant influence on people's health seeking behaviors, food choices, and perceptions toward health and wellness. The lack of understanding of culture, lifestyle factors, social roles, and foods in planning care will not help to achieve desired health outcomes. The beliefs and attitudes of Southeast Asians about health care are shaped by history and culture. For example, the religious view

of Hindus is that the causation of diseases and illness can relate in strong part to karma. Individuals consider prayers and rituals effective and important measures to change their perceived bad karma in having an illness (Pole, 2006, p. 7). Modern healthcare workers need to be aware of these health behaviors while providing care to patients from Southeast Asian cultures.

Because Ayurveda has been closely associated with Hinduism on the subcontinent of India and through its spread to the Western world (Pole, 2006, p. 8), some patients' health seeking behaviors and activities will have a close connection with their religious beliefs and practices, including their strong choice of vegetarian diet (Frawley, 1990, p. iv). Yet it is important to realize that not every Southeast Asian patient, or every patient using Ayurveda, will have these religious perspectives and preferences. The practice of Ayurveda among individuals and cultural groups in Southeast Asia and elsewhere reflects their uniquely diverse qualities. For example, Christian, Muslim, and Buddhist patients may practice Ayurveda differently (Pole, 2006, p. 8). Depending upon the intensity of symptoms and limitation of occupational and social roles, Southeast Asian individuals may choose to bring about changes in themselves by changing their lifestyle or by using folk remedies; by seeking advice from friends and family; by going to practitioners of complementary and alternative medicine; or by seeking professional help (Gupta, 2010). It is more likely for Southeast Asian patients to continue to use Ayurvedic medicine even though they have come to have treatment at a modern healthcare facility (Gupta, 2010). Healthcare providers should pay close attention to their detailed health history and carefully explain any possible side effects or interactions if biomedical pharmaceuticals are taken with any other medicines such as Ayurvedic herbs (Spudich & Menon, 2014).

India has a vast source of medicinal plants that are used in traditional medical treatments. Herbs, minerals, and organic matter are used in the preparation of herbal drugs. It has been an ancient practice and is an important component of the healthcare system in India. Pandey, Rastogi, and Rawat (2013) explained that 70% of the rural population depends on the traditional Ayurvedic system of medicine. Many healers and practitioners in India prepare formulations using their own recipes to distribute to patients (Spudich & Menon, 2014).

TABLE 14.1. The Elements, Perception, and the Senses in Ayurveda.

The Elements *Maha Bhutas*	Sense Faculties *Jnanendriya*	Sense Organs	Objects of The Senses *Tanmatras*
Ether (*akash*)	Hearing	Ears	Sound
Air (*vayu*)	Tactile perception	Skin	Touch
Fire (*tejas*)	Vision	Eyes	Form
Water (*ap*)	Taste	Tongue	Taste
Earth (*prithvi*)	Smell	Nose	Aroma

© R. A. Morningstar (2015).

■ AYURVEDIC MEDICINE PRACTICES

As a safe and effective alternative medicine practice, Ayurveda has been used for centuries. The indigenous knowledge of local people helps them to locate the local medicinal plants for use to achieve better health. Many Southeast Asian people are very dependent on nature, and close to nature (Patwardhan, 2014). That is why it has been easy for them to readily believe in the efficacy of Ayurveda and to use it for illness treatment (Cameron, 2011). Also, the easy accessibility, low cost, and minimal side effects are other reasons that rural people are drawn to use this traditional practice (Cameron, 2011; Patwardhan, 2014). The ties between Ayurveda and Hinduism also engender a strong feeling of connectedness in Southeast Asian people toward this effective and low-cost traditional medicinal practice (Patwardhan, 2014). While Ayurveda has also been influenced by Buddhism, Ayurveda and Hinduism have developed within the same cultural context for the past 2,500 years (Pole, 2006, p. 8). Many, but not all, Ayurvedic practitioners and patients are Hindu. This has influenced how Ayurveda is practiced, particularly in its valuation of vegetarian dietary choices (Frawley, 1990, iv).

There are about 15,000 medicinal plants that have been recorded in India and 7,000-7,500 plants are used in the community as treatments and cures (Parasuraman, Thing, & Dhanaraj, 2014). Some commonly used Ayurvedic medicines are: Ginger (*Zingiber officinale*), which is commonly prescribed for nausea, vomiting, motion sickness, and vertigo; garlic (*Allium sativum*), which is used as a natural antibiotic in Ayurveda and also lowers lipids and blood pressure; and turmeric (*Curcuma longa*), which is used as an antiseptic, antibacterial, anti-inflammatory, pain killer, and weight-reducing herb (Pradhan & Pradhan, 2011). Other interesting therapeutics include licorice root (*Glycyrrhiza glabra*), which is used as an anti-inflammatory for gastrointestinal disorders, as well as a mild laxative; it relieves muscle spasms, and acts as an adrenal tonic, but also is an antioxidant and may be cancer protective, i.e., prevents damage to genetic material that can eventually result in cancer. Yet licorice must be used with caution in patients with hypertension or those taking thiazide diuretics, laxatives, cardioactive glycosides, or corticosteroids (Pole, 2006, pp. 220-221). Gumar (*Gymnema sylvestre*) is another potent herb that has a glycolytic action and is used to regulate sugar metabolism, increase insulin production, and suppress the craving for sweets (Pandey et al., 2013). Due to its hypoglycemic action, if it is used by patients on diabetic medications, they need to be advised to monitor their blood sugar and medication dosage accordingly (Pole, 2006, p. 195).

Traditional Ayurvedic physicians trace the roots of this healing system to the Shad Darshan, the six primary East Indian philosophies of life, in particular, the East Indian philosophical system known as the Sankhya philosophy of creation. This school of thought describes the union of cosmic feminine and masculine forces to produce the consciousness of self-awareness, creative intelligence. Out of this intelligence comes our sense of individuality, the ego. From this individual consciousness springs subtle thought, the urge to action, habits, and the five senses (Lad, 2002, pp. 6-7). The objects of the five senses (*tanmatras*)—sound, touch, form, taste, and aroma—all arise as subtle attributes of the five elements, respectively, ether, air, fire, water, and earth (Refer to Table 14.1). Ayurveda thus bridges the most subtle consciousness to the most earthly manifestations of nature. It is a system of healing strongly rooted in nature, yet also in sophisticated meditative awareness. For these reasons, observational skills with patients are particularly

TABLE 14.2. The Doshas in Ayurveda.

DOSHA	VATA	PITTA	KAPHA
Attributes of the dosha	dry *(ruksha)* light *(laghu)* cold *(shita)* rough *(khara)* subtle *(sukshma)* mobile *(chala)* clear *(vishada)* dispersing	hot *(ushna)* sharp *(tikshna)* oily *(snigda)* penetrating *(sukshma)* light *(laghu)* mobile *(chala)* liquid *(drava)* sour, acid smell	heavy *(guru)* slow *(manda)* cold *(shita)* oily *(snigda)* slimy *(slakshna)* dense *(sandra)* soft *(mrudu)* static *(sthira)*
Elements related to the dosha	ether and air	fire and water	earth and water
Opposite attributes for healing and balance needed by the dosha	moist/liquid warm soft grounding slow oily slimy dense	cool grounding slow soothing fresh enough space	light dry warm sharp mobile subtle clear
Energetic qualities of the dosha	light, wiry	warm, pushy	slow, deep, solid
Mental qualities of the dosha	flexible, creative, generates lots of ideas	determined, assertive, fiery	steady, patient, "wait and see" attitude
Conditions needed by the dosha	safety, security	opportunities for creative expression	enlivening energy
What is offered by the dosha	new experiences	ability to transform; stick up for oneself	comfort zone
What a person needs to develop with primary constitution of the dosha	courage, perseverance	patience, willingness to wait, take a breath	openness to change
Key supports of the dosha	warm oil	cool influences	movement

© R. A. Morningstar (2015).
Note: the season, environment, climate, time of day, stage of life, digestive fire *(agni)*, and accumulated waste *(ama)* all can affect the balance of the doshas and their attributes.

valued in Ayurvedic practitioners (Morningstar & Desai, 1990, p. 7).

In Ayurveda, the treatment process is unique; its aim is more comprehensive than simply eliminating a symptom or a disease. An Ayurvedic treatment plan identifies the imbalance; seeks to eliminate the causes; addresses the illness; then seeks to rebuild and rejuvenate the body. The disease process *(samprapti)* is a six-step course of events. Three of these steps occur before a condition ever physically manifests with obvious symptoms (Lad, 2007). For this reason, an Ayurvedic approach can be particularly useful for preventive care, healing of chronic conditions, and treatment of idiosyncratic illness (Spudich & Menon, 2014).

Ayurvedic health and wellness

Health in Ayurveda is known as *Swastha* (*swa* meaning *self* and *astha* meaning *established*), which means that the *healthy person is one who is established in the self*. Ayurveda defines health as *a balance of three doshas* rather than the simple absence of disease. Ayurvedic science believes that the human body is made up of space, air, water, fire, and earth. Out of these five great elements, together called *Pancha Maha Bhuta*, arise the three biological energies known as the *doshas* that facilitate all bodily functions. The three doshas—known as *Vata* (Space and Air); *Pitta* (Fire and Water); and *Kapha* (Water and Earth)—function together to maintain health (Lad, 2002, pp. 30-31). When these doshas are in an appropriate proportion or balance within the body—along with a balanced digestive fire, balanced excretion of wastes, and healthy nourishment of the essential tissues—health (*Swastha*) is achieved. If the balance of any of these three doshas is disrupted by improper diet, lifestyle, or other day to day activities (such as excessive travel, overstimulation, or dehydration), this can lead to an imbalance or illness (Sharma et al., 2007).

An imbalance relates to specific disease processes for each of the three doshas. Vata governs the functions in the body that relate to *movement* (movement of food through the digestive system; oxygen transport by the blood; communication between nerves; and so forth; Lad, 2002, p. 39). Pitta relates to *transformation* (digestion of food; all enzymatic processes; and metabolic functions including the production and action of most hormones; Lad, 2002, pp. 39-40). Kapha supports the *structure and cohesion of the body* including muscular development and adipose retention (Lad, 2002, p. 40). Specific treatment modalities are chosen based on the imbalanced dosha and the disease process involved. For example, if Vata were out of balance, movement through the digestive tract in the process of elimination could be impeded, resulting in constipation. Ayurvedic methods to relieve this would focus on improving Vata's function and balance with warm moist foods, adequate fluids, lubricating oils, and regularity of routine (*dina charya*). Each of these methods would be used based on understanding the attributes of Vata and the anticipated bodily response to them (Morningstar & Desai, 1990, pp. 13-14).

Health is defined in Ayurveda as the balanced state of not only the three *doshas* (biological energies) but also the seven *dhatus* (essential tissues); the three *malas* (waste products: urine, feces, and perspiration); and *agni* (digestive fire). When all of these are in a simultaneously balanced state health (*Swastha*) exists (Sushruta Samhita, Chapter 15, verse 44, as cited in Lad, 2012, p. 1). In Ayurvedic medicine, the

practitioner assesses this balance through visual examination including inspection of the patient's tongue and fingernails; palpation including the radial pulses; and careful questioning. A patient's urine and feces may be examined and a food questionnaire may be completed (Lad, 2007, p. 95). In the East, the entire exam may take less than five minutes and rely primarily on the pulse assessment; in the West, Ayurvedic physicians often spend a half hour or more with each patient.

In Ayurveda, it is believed that each individual is born with a unique balance of the doshas (Refer to Figure 14.2 Constitutional Assessment form). This is their birth constitution or *prakruti* (Pole, 2006, p. 23). If there is more Vata (for example, 60%) than Pitta (30%) or Kapha (10%), in this balance the person would be considered to have a Vata constitution. Yet all three doshas would be present and interacting in the body, simply in different proportions. Each dosha has specific attributes that are easy to observe (Refer to Table 14.2). For example, Vata is dry, cool, light, and mobile. Someone with more Vata in their constitution might have a tendency toward dry skin, light bones, restlessness, and/or feeling chilled. A person of Pitta constitution would manifest more Pitta attributes, such as heat, oiliness, sharpness, or liquidity. These attributes could be seen in a tendency toward having red skin or inflammations, oily skin or hair, a direct manner of speaking, and/or a tendency to perspire easily. An individual with Kapha constitution would have more observable attributes, such as heaviness, slowness, coolness, and softness. Examples of these attributes could include heavy bones and/or weight, a tendency toward heavy sleep, taking longer to fill out a medical form, and skin cool and soft to the touch (Pole, 2006, p. 27).

In Ayurveda, the doshas are more than physical manifestations. They also describe psychobiological energies affecting not only physical signs and symptoms as described, but influences upon the mind and emotions. Someone with an excess of Vata would be likely to have a strong tendency toward worry, fear, and anxiety. A person with Pitta excess could have a hot temper. An individual with Kapha predominant in their constitution could be very loyal yet tend to withdraw in the face of stress. These would all be

TABLE 14.3. The Twenty Attributes of Ayurveda.

10 Opposite Pairs of Attributes *(Gunas)*

dry	oily
light	heavy
cold	hot
rough	smooth/slimy
subtle	gross
mobile	static
sharp	dull/slow
liquid	dense
soft	hard
clear	cloudy/sticky

© R. A. Morningstar (2015).

considered normal manifestations of doshic imbalance in Ayurveda (Morningstar & Desai, 1990, p. 13).

The three doshas and the five elements show up not only in individuals but also in environments, climate, seasons, and the weather. A cool damp area like Seattle in the winter or the foothills of the Himalayas in the fall would be considered to have more Kapha dosha at that time. Hot moist cities like New Orleans or Kolkata have more Pitta dosha. Areas that are dry, cool, and light like the arid mountains of New Mexico or the deserts of Rajasthan would be considered to have more Vata dosha (Lad, 2012, pp. 4-6).

In Ayurvedic theory, similar attributes aggravate while opposite attributes are used for healing. If someone is already hot and aggravated, putting them next to a hot fire will only make them more so. Inviting them out into a cool fresh shady area is more likely to help them calm down. This is the basic principle underlying Ayurvedic choices in healing modalities (Pole, 2006, pp. 19-20). The amount of each dosha in any individual can change over time (Lad, 2002, pp. 36-37). Their presenting state of balance or imbalance is known as the current condition or *vikruti* (Pole, 2006, p. 344). In the example cited, the person overheating by the fire would have an aggravated Pitta vikruti. Ayurvedic practitioners would assess both the constitution (*prakruti*) and current condition (*vikruti*) through taking of the pulse (Pole, 2006, pp. 28-29).

Ayurvedic treatment plans (*chikitsa*) take into account 20 key attributes, consisting of ten pairs of opposites (Pole, 2006, p. 20; Refer to Table 14.3).

These attributes can be applied in a variety of commonly used Ayurvedic healing modalities: Food, herbs, gems, colors, mantra/sound, yoga, breathing practices, steam, and rest. If we were to continue to work with the example of warm and cold, for someone who was chilled an Ayurvedic cook would offer a warming drink such as tea, which would include more warming (pungent) spices than cooling ones. Some examples of pungent spices include ginger, cinnamon, and cloves. If someone was too warm, cooling spices would be used like mint, coriander, or rose. Another pair of opposite attributes is heavy and light. If someone was heavy in weight, a light diet would be recommended including more vegetables and smaller portions (Pole, 2006, pp. 20-21). Some pranayama techniques and breathing practices could be used to strengthen digestive fire and shed weight (Lad, 2012, pp. 317-318).

For an individual with dry skin, *abhyanga* (oil massage) would likely be advised (Lad, 2012, pp. 171-172). In the case of constipation, high fiber foods, which are considered rough (like bran), might be recommended to some patients while slippery substances like aloe vera gel, which is smooth or slimy, would be suggested to others (Lad, 2012, pp. 366-367). Each remedy would be recommended for different cases. Each person is treated as an individual. For someone with an over-stressed nervous system, gross comfort might be recommended in the form of a feather bed (which is also soft) along with other subtle healing approaches such as suggesting a particular *yantra* (geometric healing painting) or *mantra* (chanted sacred syllables) (Lad, 2012, pp. 276-277). Gems and metals are also used therapeutically in Ayurveda through the wearing of prescribed pieces of jewelry such as a ring or necklace. Some items are considered warming such as gold and ruby; others have a more cooling influence, like silver, pearl, or sapphire (Lad, 2012, pp. 273-275).

In Ayurvedic therapeutic yoga, if a person had more Vata in their constitution, they would already be considered to have an abundance of mobile quality. They would instead be advised to slow down and hold stretching poses longer. Someone of Kapha constitution would receive the opposite recommendation; that is, to move more vigorously and more often (Lad, 2012, pp. 306-307).

TABLE 14.4. The Dhatus in Ayurveda.

Dhatu *	Essential Tissue	Primary dosha	Mala
Rasa	Plasma and Lymph	Kapha	Mucus
Rakta	Blood Cells	Pitta	Bile, Heat, Sweat
Mamsa	Muscles	Kapha	Ear Wax, Nasal Crusting, Tooth Tartar, Sebaceous Secretions
Meda	Adipose Tissue	Kapha	Sweat
Asthi	Bones and Cartilage	Vata	Hair and Nails
Majja	Bone Marrow, Nerves, Connective Tissue	Kapha	Tears
Shukra	Male Reproductive Tissue	Kapha	None or Secondary Sex Characteristics
Artava	Female Reproductive Tissue	Kapha	None or Secondary Sex Characteristics

© R. A. Morningstar (2015).

Dhatu: One of seven essential tissues in the body. They are nourished by the digestive tract and produce *ojas,* the body's vital energy cushion and immunity. They are cleansed as each tissue's wastes (*mala*) are carried away by the doshas.

TABLE 14.5. The Malas in Ayurveda.

The Three Primary Malas

Urine
Feces
Perspiration
Mala: Any waste product produced in the body

© R. A. Morningstar (2015).

The health status of each person along with their symptoms and ailments present a complex combination of conditions. A skilled Ayurvedic practitioner will take into account not only the doshas and their attributes but also the balance of the dhatus (Refer to Table 14.4) and the seven essential tissues as well as the three malas (Lad, 2012, p. 1). Someone with pernicious anemia would be considered to have a deficiency of *rakta dhatu* (Pole, 2006, p. 320). An individual with obesity has an excess of *meda dhatu* (Pole, 2006, p. 320). Particular healing recommendations would be made for each of these conditions. An in-depth discussion of the dhatus is beyond the scope of this chapter. Suffice it to say that the dhatus are treated both as channels (*srotamsi*; Lad, 2007, p. 297) and as solid tissue in Ayurveda (Lad, 2002, p. 103). Ayurvedic medicine focuses carefully on the details of the elimination of wastes as well (Pole, 2006, pp. 89-90) because an impediment in urination, perspiration, or elimination of feces can clog channels and obstruct healing

(Lad, 2007, p. 203; Refer to Table 14.5). Taste is very commonly used in Ayurveda for healing both for making dietary recommendations and in compounding herbal formulations. A skilled Ayurvedic practitioner will take into account the elemental make up and attributes of any experience including taste (Lad, 2012, pp. 277-279). Refer to Table 14.6 for more information about the Six Therapeutic Tastes in Ayurveda.

An Ayurvedic approach actively involves the patient. To apply this method of healing, an individual needs to be willing to eat specific foods and avoid others, take particular herbs, or follow prescribed basic lifestyle routines. Ayurveda asks more of the individual than the often more passive acceptance of treatment expected within Western biomedical settings or practices. It is better suited to some more than others, yet its benefits for health and longevity can be profound. While the application of Ayurveda initially may appear complex, once it is understood and practically applied, it can appeal to one's common sense and simplicity (Morningstar & Desai, 1990, p. 8).

Ayurveda and modern medicine

The various spices and herbs of Ayurveda have significant health benefits and are widely used in Southeast Asian countries. The common spices like coriander, cumin, ginger, garlic, and cinnamon have been researched and proven to have profound positive effects on heart

TABLE 14.6. An Ayurvedic Therapeutic Approach to The Six Tastes.

Rasa Taste	Maha Bhutas Elements	Guna Qualities	Virya Heating or cooling	Vipak Post-digestive effect
Sweet	Earth and Water	Heaviest; Most Moist; Cool	Cooling	Sweet
Sour	Earth and Fire	Light; Warm Liquid	Heating	Sour
Salty	Water and Fire	Heavy; Warm; Moist	Heating	Sweet
Pungent	Fire and Air	Hot; Dry; Light	Heating (hottest)	Pungent
Bitter	Air and Ether	Lightest; Dry; Cold	Cooling (coolest)	Pungent
Astringent	Air and Earth	Dry; Cool; Some Heaviness	Cooling	Pungent

Definitions
Rasa: Taste in the mouth
Virya: Energy, effect on stomach
Vipak: Long-term action, particularly on the wastes

Understanding Ayurvedic Herbal Formulations

Each formula includes	Example: A Curry or a Medicinal Tea
1. Leader or primary action (herb)	Turmeric
2. Assistant or complementary	Cayenne or ginger
3. Digestive or assimilative	Coriander, cumin, fennel
4. Cleansing or detoxifying	Fennel, black pepper or pippali, turmeric
5. Rejuvenative or tonic	Cardamom, coriander, or tulsi

(Lad, 2002, 2012; Morningstar, 2001; Pole, 2006; Shanbhag, 2007)

disease and the lowering of blood glucose (Sharma, et al., 2007). Asian cultures and food choices that place strong emphasis on using these spices are also helpful in achieving a health benefit. Ayurveda makes use of combination of different herbs to reduce side effects, cure disease, and reduce adaptive resistance. Most modern drugs are derived from Ayurvedic or other indigenous herbs; for example, the antihypertensive drug reserpine is derived from *Rauwolfia serpentine* (Fauzi, 2013). All drugs can have toxic effects if not used appropriately; the same is true for Ayurvedic drugs. One major constituent of Ayurvedic medications is *Aconitum heterophylum* whose roots are toxic. Metals like lead, mercury, and copper are also used in some Ayurvedic medications. Before these toxic plants and metals are used, they have to undergo extensive processes to remove the toxins and make them safe for human consumption. There are also instructions that, when followed, can counteract the side effects of Ayurvedic medications (Pole, 2006, p. 84). There have also been concerns within the Ayurvedic medical community about inadvertent heavy metal contamination in herbal preparations due to

pesticide contamination (Satake, 2011). The sustainable harvesting of wild plants is also of concern (Pole, 2006, pp. 77-78). Only an estimated 1% of Ayurvedic herbs and preparations not from the wild currently on the market have been organically certified (S. Pole, personal communication, April 17, 2013).

In the context of U. S. Food and Drug Administration regulations and other Western standards, a major disadvantage with Ayurvedic medicine is the lack of quality control methods to standardize the metal content of the drugs, including ways to determine whether the plants and metals have been appropriately processed so as to render them nontoxic (Thatte, Rege, Phatak, & Dahanukar, 1993). There are also no known means of monitoring whether proper instructions have been given about methods to counteract known side effects of the various drugs used with each person.

Ayurvedic medicine or practices are highly prevalent in Southeast Asia and increasingly common in Western countries. Ayurvedic medicinal plants are now easily accessible and are being used by the general population in Southeast Asian countries among those who have traditional knowledge; most Southeast Asian people have used them at least once in their lifetime. In addition, the authors have found that small numbers of people in Western countries are also using these plants to treat minor illnesses such as headache, stuffy nose, fever, dry mouth, and pain. Despite its widespread use and connection to people's lives, there has been little attention from most governments to promote Ayurveda, provider education, conservation of medicinal plants, and/or the inclusion of Ayurveda within modern healthcare systems. In 2014, the National Ayurvedic Medical Association (NAMA) called for new research and development efforts to advance Ayurvedic science. Optimally, the authors hope that traditional Ayurvedic practices could become scientifically standardized and integrated into modern healthcare practices to achieve better health outcomes for all people, especially those living in underdeveloped countries or rural/remote areas.

■ LEININGER'S CULTURE CARE THEORY FOR HEALTHCARE PROVIDERS

Leininger's Sunrise Enabler (McFarland & Wehbe-Alamah, 2015; refer to Color Insert 1) is a cognitive map depicting the social structure dimensions and the three care modes of decisions and actions that provide a means for providing culturally congruent care with beneficial outcomes when working with clients and patients from different cultures, health beliefs, and practice traditions. According to McFarland and Wehbe-Alamah (2015), every culture has generic (lay, folk, naturalistic) and usually some professional care to be discovered and used for culturally congruent care. Thus culturally congruent and acceptable generic and professional care practices can be integrated to achieve meaningful, beneficial, and optimal health outcomes.

Because planning and implementing health care for individuals and families is a daily activity for health professionals, the modes serve as an essential guide toward ensuring that care is culture specific, acceptable, and beneficial (Basuray, 2014; McFarland & Wehbe-Alamah, 2015). The three care modes of decisions and action plans are *culture care preservation and/or maintenance* to enable professional actions that facilitate people of the selected culture to

retain the values and ways used for healing and care; culture care accommodation and/or negotiation enable professional behaviors that help to modify cultural or professional health behaviors or lifestyle activities toward improving client health outcomes; and culture care *repatterning and/or restructuring* are provider behaviors that help people of the selected culture to change or modify their unsafe or harmful health behaviors within the context of their cultural values and beliefs (McFarland & Wehbe-Alamah, 2015, pp. 16-18). Further explanation and detail about the Sunrise Enabler and the care modes may be found throughout this text.

The Sunrise Enabler (Refer to Color Insert 1) can be used as a guide when gathering a detailed health, social, and/or family history to develop a clear picture of individual or family cultural values, beliefs, practices, or expressions; when learning about or assessing patients' healthcare needs and preferences; and when collaboratively or coparticipatively developing a mutually agreeable plan of care toward improved health outcomes (McFarland & Wehbe-Alamah, 2015, pp. 16-18). Table 14.7 shows suggested applications of the culture care modes for developing awareness about culturally competent care. The three case studies at the end of this chapter will help to exemplify application of Leininger's care modes of decisions and actions and the Sunrise Enabler (McFarland & Wehbe-Alamah, 2015) for clients who embrace Ayurvedic practices as well as Western medicine.

It can sometimes be challenging for healthcare providers to meet the needs of clients and patients who come from different cultures and concurrently practice alternative medicine (Basuray, 2014). Thus, healthcare workers should start by obtaining a detailed health history including any use of alternative medicine, diet and food patterns, and cultural beliefs and practices while planning a treatment and providing care. The treatment plan and care approaches include negotiating the action plan about how the client can change or modify their health behaviors. Within the framework of Leininger's modes of culture care decisions and actions, the healthcare-worker understands that cultural beliefs and practices for health promotion and health restoration after illness remain a *constant* focus throughout the duration of the provider-client relationship (McFarland & Wehbe-Alamah, 2015).

TABLE 14.7. Application of Culture Care Decision and Action Modes for Providers.

Sunrise Enabler Decision and Actions Modes	Ralph	Grace	Andrea
Culture Care Preservation and/or Maintenance	a. Ralph's cultural background (Pawleys Island), along with English language as his acquired second language, enables the provider to attend to Ralph's continued adjustments into the dominant American society during his lifetime. b. Ralph's travels during his tour of duty as well as having adopted the Buddhist faith, has resulted in his complex family, spiritual, and social history.	a. Grace is relatively healthy. A provider may be seeing her for routine primary care. b. Important to recognize Grace's introverted personality.	a. Andrea, born to Greek immigrant parents and raised in U. S., offers the provider the opportunity to recognize her as an individual with unique health-promoting behaviors, integrating Ayurveda and Western biomedicine. b. The provider addresses Andrea's age and her lifestyle adjustments within a culturally congruent framework.
Culture Care Accommodation and/or Negotiation	a. A provider could ask Ralph about his experience of the Ayurvedic cleansing therapy Pancha Karma and the benefits he has observed. b. A provider working with Ralph might want to get a clearer view of how he sees his health history and current needs. Open-ended questions, such as "Can you tell me more about that?" or "How was that experience for you?" could yield important information and build a mutually respectful relationship. Clarifying questions such as "I'm wondering what you mean by…" could enable the provider to be more certain that clear communication really is happening (Klienman, 1980).	a. A provider collaborates with Grace about her vegetarian diet when suggesting courses of action. b. Because she is introverted, a provider may have to put more focus on open-ended communication, to build rapport and a healthy relationship with her. It could be an opportunity for a provider to learn more about Ayurveda. c. A provider could ask Grace questions about her constitution *(prakruti)* and current condition *(vikruti)*, from her perspective. d. A provider could ask Grace: How has being back at home with her family and away from her college friends affected her health?	a. A mix of open-ended, close-ended, and clarifying questions could be useful to build rapport within the healthcare relationship, and keep the treatment on track. b. It is particularly important to take a careful medication history with Andrea, including any vitamin supplements or herbal medications as well as biomedical medications. Her providers would need to inform themselves about the needs of a patient with thalassemia, and monitor lab results closely, particularly in light of Andrea's relocation to an altitude of 7,000 feet.
Culture Care Repatterning and/or Restructuring	a. Through an established relationship with Ralph, the provider offers encouragement and feedback as well as acknowledges his success. b. Recommend that Ralph keep a diary or daily log for self-monitoring behaviors that could provide information to the practitioner.	a. The established trust in Grace's relationship with her provider is further enhanced through ongoing feedback and acknowledgement of her successes in establishing her healthful lifestyle.	a. Andrea's overall health condition should be reviewed by the provider on a regular schedule. b. Additionally, the provider's established relationship becomes critical when changes or adjustments are made in Andrea's life activities toward her goal of reaching optimal health.

Adaptation by R. A. Morningstar (R. Steele, personal communication with R. A. Morningstar, 12/29/14).

Principal Standard:
1. Provide effective, equitable, understandable, and respectful quality care and services that are responsive to diverse cultural health beliefs and practices, preferred languages, health literacy, and other communication needs.
Governance, Leadership and Workforce:
2. Advance and sustain organizational governance and leadership that promotes CLAS and health equity through policy, practices, and allocated resources.
3. Recruit, promote, and support a culturally and linguistically diverse governance, leadership, and workforce that are responsive to the population in the service area.
4. Educate and train governance, leadership, and workforce in culturally and linguistically appropriate policies and practices on an ongoing basis.
Communication and Language Assistance:
5. Offer language assistance to individuals who have limited English proficiency and/or other communication needs, at no cost to them, to facilitate timely access to all health care and services.
6. Inform all individuals of the availability of language assistance services clearly and in their preferred language, verbally and in writing.
7. Ensure the competence of individuals providing language assistance, recognizing that the use of untrained individuals and/or minors as interpreters should be avoided.
8. Provide easy-to-understand print and multimedia materials and signage in the languages commonly used by the populations in the service area.
Engagement, Continuous Improvement, and Accountability:
9. Establish culturally and linguistically appropriate goals, policies, and management accountability, and infuse them throughout the organization's planning and operations.
10. Conduct ongoing assessments of the organization's CLAS-related activities and integrate CLAS-related measures into measurement and continuous quality improvement activities.
11. Collect and maintain accurate and reliable demographic data to monitor and evaluate the impact of CLAS on health equity and outcomes and to inform service delivery.
12. Conduct regular assessments of community health assets and needs and use the results to plan and implement services that respond to the cultural and linguistic diversity of populations in the service area.
13. Partner with the community to design, implement, and evaluate policies, practices, and services to ensure cultural and linguistic appropriateness.
14. Create conflict and grievance resolution processes that are culturally and linguistically appropriate to identify, prevent, and resolve conflicts or complaints.
15. Communicate the organization's progress in implementing and sustaining CLAS to all stakeholders, constituents, and the general public.

The National Standards for Culturally and Linguistically Appropriate Services in Health and Health Care: A Blueprint for Advancing and Sustaining CLAS Policy and Practice (The Blueprint) is an implementation guide to help advance and sustain culturally and linguistically appropriate services within organizations. The Blueprint dedicates one chapter to each of the 15 Standards, with a review of the Standard's purpose, components, and strategies for implementation. In addition, each chapter provides a list of resources that offer additional information and guidance on that Standard.

FIGURE 14.1 • National Standards for Culturally and Linguistically Appropriate Services in Health and Health Care.
Source: U. S. Department of Health and Human Services Office of Minority Health (2013b).

AYURVEDA AND CROSS-CULTURAL COMMUNICATION

Healthcare workers need to also be aware of the U. S. national standards for Culturally and Linguistically Appropriate Services (CLAS). Fifteen standards were developed through the Office of Minority Health at the (U.S. Department of Health and Human Services [USDDHS], 2013b) regarding the provision of interpretation assistance for persons who speak a language other than English as well as "… provide effective, equitable, understandable, and respectful quality care and services that are responsive to diverse cultural health beliefs and practices, preferred languages, health literacy, and other communication needs" (USDDHS, 2013b; refer to Figure 14.1). Effective cross-cultural communication is essential for establishing therapeutic relationships. Culturally sensitive care facilitates communication and helps both clients and healthcare providers to make informed decisions about how to address identified care or health needs and to safely integrate alternative preparations with biomedical medications. As Ayurveda is a part of life for many Southeast Asian people and a growing number of Western individuals, culturally sensitive communication helps to identify and avoid possible adverse reactions and eventually increase patient satisfaction and beneficial outcomes (Basuray, 2014; Sharma et al., 2007)

Vignettes 1 and 2 that follow describe a daily account of how two individuals living in United States use Ayurvedic principles and activities in their lives. The accounts of Susan and Janice serve as examples for developing appropriate culture care awareness by healthcare providers.

VIGNETTE 1

Susan

A typical autumn day in the life of Susan, a young working urban dweller in the U. S. using Ayurvedic healing products and practices might look like this:

6:00 AM: Rise, shower, oil the body with warm sesame oil (*abhyanga*).

6:30 AM: Do breathing practices (*pranayama*), yoga and stretches, meditation.

7:30 AM: Consume a spoonful of *Chyvanaprash* (healing mix of herbs, ghee, and sugar or honey), hot decaffeinated herbal chai and a bowl of hot oatmeal with cardamom and cinnamon, followed by ¼ teaspoonful of a special blend of dry powdered herbs (to support digestion) mixed into a little hot water.

7:45 AM: Leave for work after feeding her dog.

8:30 – 11:30 AM: Teach yoga classes.

12 noon: Meet a friend at an Ayurvedic (vegetarian) restaurant for lunch. She chooses mung dal *kichadi* (a cooked stew of split mung dal, rice, vegetables, and spices), steamed vegetables, a chapatti, and hot ginger tea with honey. She says a prayer over the food and squeezes a little lemon on the kichadi and vegetables. The friends have an animated discussion. She forgot to bring her post-meal digestive herbs; instead she orders a small plain *lassi* (yogurt w/ hot water) spiced with cumin seeds, to finish the meal.

1:30 – 5:30 PM: Runs errands and works at her part-time job with a computer software firm. She tries to take a little break in the middle of the afternoon to rest and be quiet, but a friend is having a crisis so she spends the 15 minutes allotted on her cellular phone instead. She does eat a few soaked, peeled almonds and sips some hot tea as she listens to her friend.

6:00 PM: She puts a sweet potato and some fresh mung soup in the toaster oven to heat while she walks her dog at a local dog park.

6:45 PM: She enjoys the soup with chopped cilantro on top, and adds a dollop of ghee (clarified butter) to her steaming hot sweet potato. Her beverage is cumin-coriander-fennel seed tea, with each herb in equal proportions. She is still hungry, so she has some dates stuffed with walnuts.

7:20 PM: A friend calls and asks her out for coffee/chai. She goes back into the center of town.

9:00 PM: She gets home and takes some *triphala* (a traditional Ayurvedic combination of *amalaki, bibhitaki,* and *haritaki,* respectively in Latin as well as some *Emblica officinalis, Terminalia belerica,* and *Terminalia chebula*) to support elimination. She plays with her dog and listens to a TED talk on her computer.

10:00 PM: She starts to get ready for bed. She heats up some milk with a pinch each of ginger, cinnamon, and nutmeg. She oils the soles of her feet with sesame oil and a few drops of essential oil of lavender and brushes her teeth.

10:20 PM: Susan turns off any electronic equipment in her apartment and says a short prayer and meditates briefly. Once she has ensured her pet is settled, she retires.

VIGNETTE 2

Janice

A typical spring day in the life of a retired 65-year-old married woman living in the U. S. using Ayurvedic healing products and practices might look like this:

5:30 AM: Rise, shower, oil the body with warm sesame oil (*abhyanga*) and rinse nose with saline solution (*neti*).

6:30 AM: Do breathing practices (*pranayama*), yoga and stretches, meditation.

8:30 AM: In the kitchen, Janice takes a probiotic capsule, followed by an 8-ounce glass of fresh carrot, kale, ginger, and lemon juice. She follows this with ½ teaspoon of a rejuvenating blend of Ayurvedic herbs in hot water. Her husband Fred is having bacon and eggs with toast (he does not follow Ayurvedic health practices). They are tolerant of one another's choices although each sometimes jokes about the other's breakfast. She has been on a 40-day cleansing program since Easter.

10:00 AM: Janice goes into town on errands.

12:00 PM: Returns home, hungry.

12:30 PM: Serves her husband and herself each a large bowl of vegetable soup with hot corn tortillas and a large salad. He puts extra grated cheese in his soup; she adds sunflower seeds and a little avocado to her salad. She has cumin-coriander-fennel tea; he has iced club soda. She completes the meal with more of the rejuvenating herbs in hot water.

2:00 PM: Their son, Bob, drops by with their two grandchildren, aged 2- and 4-years, for her to watch. They play actively for an hour and then she puts them both down for a nap. She reads quietly for a while, then goes out to putter in the garden. When the children awaken at 4:00 PM, she has a snack of apples and juice waiting for them. She drinks some room temperature *tulsi* (basil, *Ocimum sanctum*) tea and eats some apple slices. They go outside to gather rocks for a painting project for their mom on Mother's Day.

5:30 PM: Bob returns to pick up the children.

5:45 PM: Janice warms up the soup from lunch adding extra spices and some cubed tofu to it and steams some root vegetables. Fred joins her; they both have tulsi-cinnamon-rose tea and squeeze some fresh lime over their vegetables. Fred has a couple of slices of smoked turkey; Janice does not. They both have a couple of oat-almond cookies. She completes the meal with more of the rejuvenating herbs as usual.

7:00 PM: Fred goes to play poker with his friends in town; Janice enjoys a quiet night at home. On a different evening, she might go in to town for yoga or chanting (*kirtan*).

9:30 PM: Fred returns. Janice has her evening Ayurvedic remedy of ½ teaspoon of bhumyamalaki (*Phyllanthus fraternus*) in hot water.

10:00 PM: Janice retires after a short meditation practice; Fred is watching the news on TV.

■ ROLE OF HEALTH CARE PROVIDER IN AN INTEGRATED FRAMEWORK

In the authors' view, one of the most significant advances within modern health care uses complementary and alternative methods as an integrated approach to planning and treatment practices. This could be particularly important in locales where Ayurveda is not a predominantly applied form of complementary practice and therefore has not been institutionalized such as in Western industrialized nations. The integration of Ayurveda, as well as other alternative forms of therapy, into Western medicine practices has the potential to have a profound impact upon improving people's lives by providing them effective healthcare options. The National Ayurvedic Medical Association in the United States has established standardized educational requirements, scopes and standards of practice, and educational course requirements for different levels of Ayurveda practitioners, from Ayurvedic health counselors to Ayurvedic doctors (NAMA, 2013). For example, the Ayurvedic doctor is required to be knowledgeable about the current pharmacotherapeutics of the Ayurvedic herbal medicines from a designated list (NAMA, 2013). The integration of Ayurveda into Western medical practices could provide opportunities for both types of practitioners to provide optimal generic and professional care to the client (Fauzi, 2013).

Although Ayurveda cannot be used to cure cancer or certain other disorders, it has been used to work together with Western medicine to produce therapeutic benefits and lower the risks from adverse effects of treatment such as providing benefits to the body in the management of cancer-related cachexia (Jain, Kosta, & Tiwari, 2010). In addition, it has been reported in the U. S. that Ayurveda helps manage the symptoms of a wide range of diseases including inflammatory conditions and immune dysfunctions (such as rheumatoid arthritis) and digestive disorders (Sharma, et al., 2007) when introduced early as a healthcare modality. The National Institutes of Health (NIH) reported on a clinical study that showed that in 79% of cases where Ayurveda was used, the health of patients in the U. S. with various chronic diseases showed measurable improvement after Ayurvedic treatment (USDDHS, 1994). Several modern clinical trials have been funded by the National Center for Complementary and Alternative Medicine (NCCAM) to determine the effectiveness of Ayurvedic treatment for specific disorders (USDDHS, 2013a). One recent positive finding has been reported that "…A 2011 preliminary clinical trial found that osteoarthritis patients receiving a compound derived from *B. serrata* gum resin (also known as frankincense) had greater decreases in pain compared to patients receiving a placebo" (USDDHS, 2013a). Researchers have also been trying to evaluate the effects of Ayurveda on patients with schizophrenia and diabetes; however these studies have shown inconclusive results thus far (USDDHS, 2013a).

Ayurveda and Western medical approaches could be used to deal with different aspects of the same illness. For example, the effects from modern chemotherapy and palliative therapy could be ameliorated through the use of supportive traditional Ayurvedic rejuvenation therapies (Spaudich & Menon, 2014). The Kottakkal Arya Vaidya Sala, Amala Cancer Research Center in India and the American University of Complementary Medicine in Los Angeles, California, USA are examples of institutions with programs that have integrated Western biomedical science and traditional Ayurvedic medicine into their patient care approaches (Spaudich & Menon, 2014). Although more research needs to be focused on such an integrated approach, it nevertheless affords an opportunity to expand care options while at the same time reducing health access disparities in the world.

For healthcare workers, one primary cultural competency goal would be to identify the common Ayurvedic medicines and practices prevalent in their geographical area. This goal could be achieved through clinical practice experiences, literature review, webinar participation, and personal interviews with Ayurvedic practitioners. The authors believe education about Ayurveda is key for healthcare clinicians as well as clients or patients. Healthcare workers could start by learning to understand the differences among various belief systems; what constitutes health seeking behavior; the factors involved in family influence; and the Ayurvedic medicines used. Furthermore, cultural competency skills acquired by healthcare workers who have provided care for Southeast Asian individuals with a strong cultural tradition of using Ayurvedic medicine can be assessed through self-report surveys; attending workshops; and by direct observational assessment. Most importantly, client education about Ayurvedic medicines needs to include information about the importance of making purchases from reliable, certified Ayurvedic practitioners with quality products who are known within the community (Pole, 2006, p. 77). The provider in a Western healthcare system needs to also encourage clients to share information about their use of Ayurvedic remedies and treatments currently being used so as to prevent drug interactions. Clients should ask about the side effects of Ayurvedic medicines (and other generic care or herbal remedies); inquire about any potential interactions with prescribed and over-the-counter pharmaceutical medications; and seek information regarding the specific instructions to follow for each Ayurvedic herb taken (Pole, 2006, pp. 83-84).

Finally, the authors emphasize that another important competency goal is to foster awareness about Ayurveda by healthcare workers so that they can be informed about their patients' potential use of Ayurvedic medicine. One approach for this goal would be to have the Ayurvedic *materia medica* available in all healthcare settings in regions where Ayurveda is practiced. Conducting surveys and/or interviews with hospital and clinic staff would help to determine the prevalence of Ayurvedic medication usage. The authors recommend that the survey include questions for healthcare providers about their perceived value for being able to access this Ayurvedic reference. The overall goal is to develop collaboration regarding Ayurvedic medicine as another cultural competency goal for healthcare professionals and educators. Healthcare practitioners need to *collaborate* with clients about integrating Ayurvedic modalities into their plans of care regarding their general health and wellness and/or in the management of disease symptoms or treatment side effects. This would not only increase client satisfaction as an active coparticipant with their healthcare provider being active in the patient's plan of care, but also promote the provision of culturally congruent and culture-specific care (Basuray, 2014). The developed integrated plan of care should be revaluated by either a questionnaire or an interview at a follow-up visit or after hospitalization or surgery to determine its effectiveness (Basuray, 2014).

As more people become interested in using alternative or complementary medicine, Western medicine practitioners have begun to value the integration of standardized Ayurvedic practices with biomedicine (Fauzi, et al., 2013). The combination of modern diagnostic tools, mass production of Ayurvedic medicines, and integrated therapeutic approaches with Western medicine could contribute to the further development and innovation of traditional Ayurveda (Fauzi, et al., 2013). In addition, the acceptance and use of these blended approaches represents an effective alternative for millions of people who either wish to try or use alternative medicine or do not have full access to modern health care—which would thereby significantly reduce health disparities. The title of the revered Ayurvedic medical text *Charak Samhita* translates as "They Who Walk Everywhere." The Ayurvedic physician Shalmali Joshi interpreted this to mean that Ayurvedic medicine has been uniquely able to adapt itself to a wide variety of cultural settings and practices (S. Joshi, personal communication, June 18, 1996).

Patients who practice Western forms of health care could benefit greatly from adapting Ayurveda traditions. Considering the recent push toward preventive medicine in the United States, Ayurveda could be integrated into this healthcare system. It is important to stress personal responsibility for health and the empowerment of people so that individuals take control of their health and work to identify root causes instead of relying on quick, convenient medications. Clients and patients who rely on Western treatments for their illnesses and health conditions could be encouraged to try simple and more familiar Ayurvedic methods such as pranayama and yoga. Educational materials such as brochures that promote the benefits of Ayurveda could present simple options for making lifestyle changes and educate people about taking responsibility for their health and wellness.

Traditional (generic/lay/folk) medicinal practices are widely used around the world (WHO, 2001). These practices are closely linked to the people's cultural beliefs, values, and expressions; their health behaviors; and the availability and accessibility of modern healthcare services (Basuray, 2014). In Southeast Asia, people have been using Ayurveda to treat illness and maintain optimal health for centuries (WHO, 2001). Traditionally, Ayurveda is culturally associated with ancient Hindu traditions and religious practices. This tested and trusted method of alternative treatments is used by many Southeast Asian people as their first-line method of defense against disease (Rastogi, 2010). Others who have used modern Western medicine and have been dissatisfied with these approaches or outcomes have come to Ayurveda to treat or to palliate their symptoms

(Spudich & Menon, 2014). The authors have found that people use their traditional knowledge of Ayurveda and medicinal plants and other therapies to treat problems like headache, gastrointestinal problems, sexual dysfunctions, cold and respiratory problems, infertility problems, and lagging energy among other ailments. With more research, training, and anecdotal documentation of indigenous knowledge, the greater likelihood that that this ancient Ayurvedic science with its roots in peoples' cultures can be preserved as a dynamic and evolving healthcare approach. This method of traditional healing might contribute to the development of new Western and Ayurvedic medicines and possibly increase access to care. With integration into Western medical care, Ayurveda could also help to reduce health disparities worldwide.

■ SUMMARY

Culture has a strong influence on people's perceptions of health, their health behaviors, and the means and rationales they use to seek health care (Basuray, 2014). Healthcare providers need to be culturally competent in order to provide care for clients who have different cultural values and beliefs (Basuray, 2014). Furthermore, it is *essential* to be aware of ones' own cultural values; we need to continually assess ourselves so as to avoid cultural imposition practices when providing care for culturally diverse persons (Hubbert, 2006, pp. 352-353). Healthcare workers can develop Ayurvedic cultural competency through exposure, experience, self-motivation, and dedication to learning about diverse cultures and their practices. Ayurveda is a preventive form of health care that emphasizes conservation of wellness. According to Lad (2002), Ayurveda "… understands the importance of individualized responses to the stresses and conditions of life" and treats the patient accordingly. As a result, Ayurvedic practitioners spend ample time recording the patient's medical history. These practitioners inquire about diet, lifestyle, personal habits, and physical environment to ensure a holistic understanding of the patient. For example, by focusing on arterial pulse mapping, Ayurvedic practitioners gain the ability to recognize disease processes through differences in a patient's map (Lad, 2002). Furthermore, family involvement is expected and honored in Ayurveda (Ramakrishna & Weiss, 1992). Relatives are expected to provide psychological support and help the patient to successfully implement their care

regimen. According to Ramakrishna and Weiss (1992), these methods have been recognized as effective in Eastern India for thousands of years.

Furthermore, supporters of Ayurveda have conducted studies to confirm that Ayurveda relieves stress and anxiety, reduces plaque and atherosclerosis, and alleviates pain and disability in people with chronic conditions (Ehrlich, 2011). There have been other advances in the field, including the development of the software AyuSoft (2015), which helps practitioners through the process of care decisions and actions; supports highly individualized therapy; and "… maximizes therapeutic efficacy and patient safety" (Patwardhan, 2014, para x). When providing care for clients who have been using alternative medicines, healthcare workers need to be open and accepting about their beliefs and alternative practices in order to develop positive and effective therapeutic relationships (Morningstar, 2001).

Western biomedical science and traditional healthcare practices such as Ayurveda can be integrated together to provide effective care for a larger share of the global population (WHO, 2001). One cultural competency goal for healthcare professionals and educators regarding Ayurvedic medicine would be to work together with the client to integrate the holistic approach of Ayurveda into plans of care for health and wellness as well as for the management of symptoms. It is possible that Western practitioners may also personally benefit from their contact with this ancient science with its strong emphasis on healthy self-care habits and respect for the natural world.

In the long-term, it would be ideal to have healthcare practitioners integrate aspects of Ayurveda healing into their own practices. These practitioners can meet cultural competency goals by attending a series of seminars and reading reliable textbooks and peer-reviewed journals about Ayurveda (e.g., textbooks by Vasant Lad or the *Ayurveda Journal of Health*). They could utilize evidence-based practice by researching particular healing methods in Ayurveda that concern their specialty. Within an *integration method,* the authors believe that Western healthcare providers could start by studying the specific Ayurvedic format used in taking a patient's history. Although it may appear similar to some Western formats regarding areas such as diet, lifestyle, and environment, Ayurvedic practitioners are distinctly referring to the *doshas*, and therefore, the nature of interview

Vata	Pitta	Kapha
Physical Assessment		
_____Light bone structure and/or prominent joints	_____Average bone structure	_____Heavy bone structure
_____Thin, also may be unusually tall or short	_____Medium, well proportioned frame	_____Ample build
_____Dry skin, rather cool*	_____Oily skin	_____Thick skin, cool, moist
_____Dry hair*	_____Oily hair, may be balding or prematurely gray	_____Thick hair
_____Cold hands and feet, little perspiration	_____Warm hands, perspire easily	_____Cool hands, moderate perspiration
_____Brittle nails	_____Flexible nails, yet fairly strong	_____Strong, thick nails
_____Narrow, somewhat pointed tongue	_____Medium width tongue, maybe unusually red	___ Wide slightly swollen tongue*
Client Report		
_____Has a hard time gaining weight	_____Can gain or lose weight relatively easily	_____Gains weight easily; has a hard time losing it
_____Prefers warm climate, sunshine, moisture	_____Prefers cool, well-ventilated climate and places	_____Any climate is fine as long as it is not too humid
_____Variable appetite	_____Good appetite, irritable if they miss a meal	_____Likes to eat; fine appetite, yet can skip meals without physical problems if necessary (even if not preferred)

FIGURE 14.2 •Constitutional Assessment. © R. A. Morningstar (2015).

questions differ from the nature and types of questions asked by Western practitioners (Refer to Figure 14.2).

Furthermore, encouraging patients to take responsibility for their own health and endorsing lifestyle management techniques before considering prescriptions would be a beneficial approach for all health practitioners to take. Adding simple and familiar Ayurvedic techniques such as pranayama, yoga, and diet modification to their treatment regimens would improve the health of their clients. Facilities or offices would provide

CONSTITUTIONAL ASSESSMENT

Place an "X" next to the choice that best describes the client.
Occasionally, more than one choice may need to be made.

Vata	Pitta	Kapha
____Bowel movement can be irregular, hard, dry or constipated	____Easy & regular bowel movement often, at least 1x to 2x/day, can be loose	____Regular daily bowel movements, steady, thick, heavy
____Digestion sometimes good, sometimes not	____Digestion usually good	____Digestion fine, sometimes a little slow
____Like to stay physically active	____Enjoy physical activities, especially competitive or intense ones	____Love leisurely activities most
____Client feels more mentally relaxed when moving	____Client finds exercise can help keep emotions from going out of control	____Exercise keeps client's weight down in a way diet alone does not; it may even ward off depression.
____Tends toward fear, anxiety or worry under stress	____Tends toward anger, frustration, irritability under stress	____Tends to avoid difficult situations or want to withdraw under stress
____Light sleeper	____Usually sleeps well	____Sound, heavy sleeper
____Variable thirst	____Usually thirsty	____Rarely thirsty
____Thin as a child	____Medium build as a child	____Plump or a little chunky as a child

• Note: these may also indicate a thyroid imbalance rather than a constitutional indicator.

The most accurate assessment of constitution is made by a skilled pulse assessment. However, this assessment form can give a rough estimate of constitution (*prakruti*). The column with the most checks generally indicates the primary constitution. If there are two columns marked nearly as often, the client could have a dual dosha constitution: Vata-Pitta, Pitta-Kapha, etc. Rarely, all three will be relatively equal, in which case a Tridosha or Vata-Pitta-Kapha type results.

If most of the answers are in one column, yet there are a few answers in another column, this may indicate a current imbalance (*vikruti*). For example, if primarily Pitta aspects have been checked for the client but "brittle nails" and "light sleeper" were also marked, and these changes have only been true for the client in the last few years, this could indicate that while they have a Pitta constitution, they are also working with a Vata imbalance (vikruti).

FIGURE 14.2· *(Continued)*

supplemental information (e.g., aforementioned brochures) for lifestyle improvement. The focus of the patient education materials does not necessarily need to be on Ayurveda, but rather the valuable techniques extracted from Ayurveda.

Three case studies below exemplify diverse applications of Leininger's Theory of Culture Care Diversity and Universality by using the social structure factors of the Sunrise Enabler to guide in the application of the three care modes of decisions and actions by healthcare practitioners for provision of health education and culturally congruent and culture specific care (McFarland & Wehbe-Alamah, 2015). Ayurvedic medicine exemplifies generic care practices that can readily be integrated with professional or Western health care or medicine practices in a complementary manner within the United States toward achieving optimal health outcomes.

■ CASE STUDIES FOR DISCUSSION

Case study one: Ralph

Ralph is from Pawleys Island off the coast of South Carolina. His native language is Gullah. As a child, hearing or speaking English frightened him. However, he is now fluent in English and has earned a graduate degree in psychotherapy. Although his early spiritual experiences were in the African Methodist Episcopal Church, he has become a well-known teacher in the Theravedan Buddhist tradition. In his professional practice, Ralph treats people with stress conditions using psychotherapy and mindfulness meditation training techniques. He also has friends in the Hindu community who are followers of Baba Neem Karoli, a Hindu sage who died in India in the 1970s. Ralph is married; his wife is also not a native English speaker. He has a grown son from a former relationship who lives in another city. Ralph served in the U. S. Army during the Vietnam War and has health issues related to his exposure to Agent Orange. He has been active in international Agent Orange conferences since they began in 2006. He has used Ayurvedic medicine as a primary health care modality for several decades. Its modalities of herbal medicine and prayer remind him of his grandmother's early health care for him. He has used its effective detoxification system of *Pancha Karma* many times and appreciates the vegetarian diet included in this tradition.

Reflections for discussion

- What are some of the issues present in Ralph's case that could impact the quality of care he receives?
- What do you need to be mindful about when working with clients/patients such as Ralph?

Factors to consider for Ralph

- English as a second language.
- A person with extensive and sophisticated training, dealing with potential underlying traumas of war.

Case study two: Grace

Grace is a 24-year-old woman who grew up in northern New Mexico in a tight-knit Anglo (Caucasian) family in the United States. She is a native English speaker and also speaks Spanish. She is a college graduate and plans to pursue additional graduate education in creative writing. Although she has an introverted personality, she had many friends in college. She is generally healthy with only occasional visits to healthcare providers as needed. Her family also tends to be introverted. They have strong interests in climate change, environmental health, and justice; Grace shares these concerns. She has chosen to follow a vegetarian diet since childhood; this has been her own personal choice. She has grown up receiving integrated care from a nutrition educator knowledgeable in both Ayurveda and Western nutrition. Now, as a young adult, she has chosen to pursue more Ayurvedic care and education. This has included *Pancha Karma* treatment from a clinic an hour away from her home. She has returned to live in her home town before pursuing a graduate degree in an unrelated field.

Reflections for discussion

- What cultural considerations might a provider take into account while treating Grace?

Factors to consider for Grace

- Dietary issues: She is a vegetarian following Ayurvedic perspectives.
- Adjustment issues: She is back home after years of living on her own.
- Stress: It is possible that she is experiencing stress due to the transitional nature of her current life.

Case study three: Andrea

Andrea was born in the U. S. of first generation Greek parents 60 years ago. Andrea is an only child; her mother is still living. She is a native English speaker. A college graduate, she has moved around the country with her husband, supporting him in his work. Recently they relocated to a rural, high-altitude area, taking a new job. Although they do not have any children, they have a strong nurturing relationship with their two dogs. Andrea has a number of health issues that necessitate frequent visits to healthcare providers, both Western and complementary/alternative.

She takes a number of prescribed pharmaceutical medications for physical and mental health; she also uses vitamin supplements and Ayurvedic and Western herbal preparations. She became interested in Ayurveda seven years ago and is knowledgeable about Ayurvedic principles of lifestyle and cooking. Although she has been interested at times in vegetarian diet, she has a genetic condition (thalassemia) that makes eating meat a necessity. She is willing to do this. Her recent move to a higher altitude has exacerbated her health issues, especially the fatigue.

Reflection for discussion

- What cultural considerations might a provider take into account while treating Andrea?

Factors to consider for Andrea

- Adjustment issues: Andrea and her husband have moved from an urban area to a rural area in a different state at a higher altitude, necessitating social and physical adjustments.
- Interactions between biomedical/pharmaceutical and alternative remedies are possible.
- Stress and aging: She is facing a variety of challenges related to life changes and aging.
- Family issues: As the only child in a tight-knit Greek family, demands and expectations from her mother could increase stress levels.

■ DEDICATIONS

To Madeleine Leininger, in deep gratitude for life-long learning on culture care. *Joanna*

To my teachers, students, and clients, with deep appreciation. *Amadea*

■ REFERENCES

Basuray, J. M. (2014). *Culture and health: Concept and practice* (2nd ed.). Ronkokoma, NY: Linus Publications.

Cameron, M. (2011). Why not Nepali Ayurveda? Conservation, development and cultural diversity. *Studies in Nepali History and Society*, 16(1), 63-82.

Ehrlich, S. D. (2011, October). *Ayurveda*. Baltimore, MD: University of Maryland Medical Center. Retrieved from http://umm.edu/health/medical/altmed/treatment/ayurveda

Fauzi, F. M., Koutsoukas, A., Lowe, R., Joshi, K., Fan, T-P., Glen, R. C., & Bender, A. (2013). Linking Ayurveda and Western medicine by integrative analysis. *Journal of Ayurveda & Integrative Medicine*, 4(2), 117-119. doi: 10.4103/0975-9476.113882. Retrieved from http://www.ncbi.nlm.nih.gov/pmc/articles/PMC3737444/

Frawley, D. (1990). *Introduction*. In R. A. Morningstar and U. Desai, *The Ayurvedic cookbook*. Twin Lakes, WI: The Lotus Press.

Gupta, V.B. (2010). Impact of culture on healthcare seeking behavior of Asian Indians. *Journal of Cultural Diversity*, 17(1), 13-18.

Hardiman, D. (2009). Indian medical indigeneity: From national assertion to global market. *Social History*, 34(3), 263-283.

Hubbert, A. O. (2006). Application of culture care theory for clinical nurse administrations and managers. In M.M. Leininger & M. R. McFarland (Eds.), Culture Care Diversity and Universality: A worldwide nursing theory (2nd ed., pp. 349-379). Sudbury, MA: Jones & Bartlett.

Jain, R., Kosta, S., & Tiwari, A. (2010, November-December). Ayurveda and cancer. *Pharmacology Research*, 2(6), 393-394. doi: 10.4103/0974-8490.75463. Retrieved from www.ncbi.nlm.nov/

Klienman, A. (1980). Patients and healers in the context of culture: An exploration of the borderland between anthropology, medicine, and psychiatry. *Comparative studies in health systems and medical care* (3rd ed.). Berkeley, CA: Quantum Books, University of California Press.

Lad, V. (2002). *Textbook of Ayurveda: Fundamental principles* (Volume 1). Albuquerque, NM: The Ayurvedic Press.

Lad, V. (2007). *Textbook of Ayurveda: A complete guide to clinical assessment* (Volume 2). Albuquerque, NM: The Ayurvedic Press.

Lad, V. (2012). *Textbook of Ayurveda: General principles of management and treatment* (Volume 3). Albuquerque, NM: The Ayurvedic Press.

Leininger, M. M. (2002). Part I. Toward integrative generic and professional health care. In M. M. Leininger & M. R. McFarland (Eds.), *Transcultural nursing: Concepts, theories, research, & practice* (3rd ed., p. 148). New York, NY: McGraw-Hill.

Manohar, P. R. (2014). Ayurvedic education: Where to go from here? *Ancient Science of Life*, 33(3), 143-145.

McFarland, M. R., & Wehbe-Alamah, H. B. (2015). The theory of culture care diversity and universality. In M. R. McFarland and H. B. Wehbe-Alamah (Eds.), *Leininger's culture care diversity and universality: A worldwide nursing theory* (3rd ed., pp. 1-34). Burlington, MA: Jones and Bartlett Learning.

Morningstar, R. A. (2001). *The Ayurvedic guide to polarity therapy*. Twin Lakes, WI: The Lotus Press.

Morningstar, R. A., & Desai, U. (1990). *The Ayurvedic cookbook*. Twin Lakes, WI: The Lotus Press.

National Ayurvedic Medical Association. (2014). *Professional scope of practice*. Retrieved from http://www.ayurvedanama.org/?page=ScopesOfPractice2

Pandey, M., Rastogi, S., & Rawat, A. (2013). Indian traditional Ayurvedic system of medicine and nutritional supplementation. *Evidence-Based Complementary and Alternative Medicine*, Volume 2013, Article ID 376327, e1-12.

Parasuraman, S., Thing, G., & Dhanaraj, S. (2014). Polyherbal formulation: Concept of Ayurveda. *Pharmacognosy Reviews*, *8*(16), 73-80 doi: 10.4103/0973-7847.134229. Retrieved from http://www.ncbi.nlm.nih.gov/pmc/articles/PMC4127824/

Patwardhan, B. (2014). Bridging Ayurveda with evidence-based scientific approaches in medicine. *The EPMA Journal*, *5*(19). Retrieved from http://www.epmajournal.com/content/5/1/19

Pole, S. (2006). *Ayurvedic medicine: The principles of traditional practice*. Philadelphia, PA: Churchill Livingstone Elsevier Limited.

Ramakrishna, J., & Weiss, M. G. (1992, September). Health, illness, and immigration: East Indians in the United States. *The Western Journal of Medicine*, *157*(3), 265-270.

Rastogi, S. (2010). Building bridges between Ayurveda and Modern Science. *International Journal of Ayurveda Research*, *1*(1), 41-46. doi: 10.4103/0974-7788.59943

Satake, A., & McDaniel, A. (2011). *India: Second opinion*. Retrieved from http://www.pbs.org/frontlineworld/stories/india701/interviews/ayurveda101.html

Sharma, H., Chandola, H. M., Singh, G., & Basisht, G. (2007). Utilization of Ayurveda in health care: An approach for prevention, health promotion, and treatment of disease. *The Journal of Alternative and Complementary Medicine*, *13*(9), 1011-1019.

Shanbhag, V. (2007). *Science of synergistic herb combining in traditional Ayurvedic formulas*. Retrieved from www.ayurvedanama.org/resource/resmgr/docs_conferencepro

Spudich, A., & Menon, I. (2014). On the integration of Ayurveda and biomedicine: Perspectives generated from interviews with Ashtavaidya Ayurveda physicians of Kerala. *Current Science*, *106*(11), 1500-1504.

Thatte, U. M., Rege, N. N., Phatak, S. D., & Dahanukar, S. A. (1993). The flip side of Ayurveda. *Journal of Postgraduate Medicine*, *39*(4), 179-182. Retrieved from http://www.jpgmonline.com/article.asp?issn=0022-3859;year=1993;volume=39;issue=4;spage=179;epage=82,182a;aulast=Thatte

U. S. Department of Health and Human Services, National Institutes of Health. (1994). *Alternative medicine: Expanding medical horizons. A report to the National Institutes of Health on Alternative Medical Systems and Practices in the United States* [Publication 94-066]. Washington, DC: U. S. Government Printing Office.

U. S. Department of Health and Human Services, National Institutes of Health, National Center for Complementary and Integrative Medicine. (2013a). *Ayurvedic medicine: An introduction* [Fact Sheet]. Rockville, MD: National Center for Complementary and Integrative Medicine. Retrieved from http://nccam.nih.gov/health/ayurveda/introduction.htm

U. S. Department of Health and Human Services, Office Public Health and Science, Office of Minority Health. (2013b). *National Standards for Culturally and Linguistically Appropriate Services in Health Care final report*. Rockville, MD: Author. Retrieved from http://www.hdassoc.org/wp-content/uploads/2013/03/CLAS_handout-pdf_april-24.pdf

Wiwanitkit, V. (2010). Use of Indian (Ayurveda) style alternative medicine in Thailand. *International Journal of Ayurveda Research*, *1*(4), 282. doi: 10.4103/0974-7788.76797

World Health Organization. (2001). Legal status of traditional medicine and complementary/alternative medicine: A worldwide review. Author. Retrieved from http://apps.who.int/medicinedocs/en/d/Jh2943e/8.7.html

World Health Organization. (2013). *WHO traditional medicine strategy: 2014-2023*. Geneva, Switzerland: Author. Retrieved from http://apps.who.int/iris/bitstream/10665/92455/1/9789241506090_eng.pdf

Transcultural Nursing and Health Care in Taiwan

Lenny Chiang-Hanisko

> *"Discovering diverse cultures and their care needs expands nurses knowledge and provides better ways to care for people" (Leininger, 1984).*

■ INTRODUCTION

Taiwanese Americans represent a culturally distinct group in the United States. Many Taiwanese and Taiwanese Americans were born in Taiwan and migrated to the United States to study, live, and work. Understanding their lifeways, values, and related culture care beliefs is necessary if nurses are to provide meaningful care and ensure beneficial outcomes. The culture care knowledge presented in this chapter is based upon the author's lifelong journey with the Taiwanese culture and her research studies using Leininger's (1991) Theory of Culture Care Diversity and Universality (also known as the Culture Care Theory or CCT).

Although Taiwanese share in the rich heritage of Chinese culture, Taiwan and China are distinctly different. Unlike China, Taiwan has been shaped through the centuries by Portuguese, Spanish, Dutch, and English powers as early as the 16th century and from later colonization by Japan. Due to its separate historical, sociopolitical, and economic development from China, current Taiwanese culture is fundamentally a mix of native Aboriginal, Japanese, Western (mainly American), and Chinese cultures. Although Taiwan and China share the same written script and official

language (Chinese Mandarin), Taiwan also has its own native languages, the most prominent being Hakka and Fujianese. Combining high educational standards with an advanced technological and industrial economy, Taiwanese support and practice an open and liberal democracy resulting in a high-level of political freedom. It is important for health care providers to recognize and understand the uniqueness and diversity of Taiwan in order to provide culturally-based care that is congruent with Taiwanese values, beliefs, and practices.

■ ASSUMPTIVE PREMISES

The following assumptions and premises are helpful to fully understand the Culture Care Theory (Leininger, 2002) and its relationship to transcultural nursing care and to guide culturally-based care and caring.

1. For people of Taiwanese decent or heritage, culture care expressions, patterns, and practices are influenced by their worldviews, social structures, and environmental contexts.
2. Culture care is holistic and is the most comprehensive means to discover the values, beliefs, and patterned lifeways that enable Taiwanese Americans to maintain their wellbeing and health, to improve

their human condition, and to deal with disabilities or death.

3. The Taiwanese culture has generic (lay, folk, and naturalistic) and professional care that needs to be discovered and used for culturally congruent care practices.

4. Culturally congruent care occurs when Taiwanese values, beliefs, expressions, and patterns are explicitly known and used appropriately, sensitively, and meaningfully with Taiwanese Americans.

5. Cultural conflicts, stresses, and pain indicate a lack of culture care knowledge and a failure to identify the needs of Taiwanese Americans receiving care.

■ ORIENTATIONAL DEFINITIONS

The following definitions by Leininger (1991) were adapted by the author (Chiang-Hanisko, 2002) and were used to guide the discovery and elaboration of Taiwanese values, beliefs, and lifeways.

- *Culture Care:* Refers to the subjectively and objectively learned and transmitted values, beliefs, and patterned lifeways that assist, support, facilitate, or enable Taiwanese Americans to maintain their well-being and health; to improve their human condition and lifeways; or to deal with wellness, handicaps, or death.

- *Worldview:* Refers to the way Taiwanese Americans look out on the world or their universe to form a picture of a value stance about their life or world around them.

- *Cultural and Social Structure Dimensions:* Refer to the dynamic patterns and features of interrelated structural and organizational factors of the Taiwanese culture (subculture or society). These include religions, kinship, political, economic, educational, technological and cultural values, and ethnohistorical factors as well as how these factors may be interrelated and function to influence human behavior in different environmental contexts.

- *Generic (Folk or Lay) Care:* Refers to culturally learned and transmitted indigenous folk (home-based) knowledge and skills used by Taiwanese Americans to provide assistive, supportive, enabling, or facilitative acts toward or for another individual, group, or institution with evident or anticipated needs to ameliorate or improve a human lifeway or health condition or to deal with disabilities or and death situations.

- *Culturally Congruent (Nursing) Care*: Refers to those cognitively based assistive, supportive, facilitative, or enabling decisions or actions that are tailor-made to fit with individual, group, or institutional Taiwanese cultural values, beliefs, and lifeways to provide or support meaningful, beneficial, and satisfying health care services.

- *Taiwanese Americans*: Refers to individuals who were born and raised in the country of Taiwan, or who identify themselves to be of Taiwanese decent or heritage, and have immigrated to the United States.

■ ETHNOHISTORY OF TAIWAN

Taiwan, also known as Formosa (a name given by Portuguese explorers meaning *beautiful*), is an island in the western Pacific Ocean between the East and South China Seas located midway between Japan and Korea to the north and Hong Kong and the Philippines to the south (Refer to Figure 15.1). Taiwan stretches approximately 245 miles from north to south and 90 miles from east to west. With a land area of 13,900 square miles, the island is about the size of Switzerland with approximately two-thirds covered by forested mountains. Taipei is both the largest city and the capital of Taiwan (Copper, 2012).

The fact that Taiwan is surrounded by the Pacific Ocean, thus being isolated both geographically and socially from its neighbors, may account for its "separatist tradition." The island was initially inhabited by nine different aboriginal cultural groups considered to be of Malay or Polynesian origin. Until the Ming dynasty (1368-1644), Taiwan was not yet clearly identified in Chinese court records. Around the year 1430, the admiral-explorer Cheng Ho determined its exact location after which its present name was used in official sources (Copper, 2012).

During the 16th century, the Portuguese sighted but bypassed Taiwan. Afterward, the Dutch and Spanish began setting up trading stations, missions, and forts on the island. In 1661, the Dutch were driven out by the pirate Koxianga who later made the island a refuge for supporters of China's deposed Ming dynasty (Rubenstein, 2007).

In 1895, Taiwan was ceded to Japan as recompense in the wake of the Sino-Japanese War and entered yet another colonial period lasting 50 years. Japan's colonization of the island took place in the face of strong

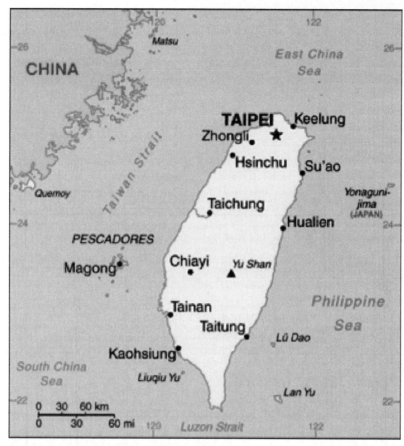

FIGURE 15.1 · Map of Taiwan, U. S. Department of State (2014).
Retrieved from https://travel.state.gov/content/passports/en/country/taiwan.html

hostility from both the Taiwanese and aboriginal peoples. Japan began to culturally convert the island by making Japanese the official language of government and education (Republic of China [Taiwan], 2014b, p. 305). Many older Taiwanese people are still able to speak Japanese (Copper, 2012). After World War II, Taiwan was restored to National Chinese control (Rubenstein, 2007).

In 1949, as a result of the civil war on Mainland China, the Chinese communists defeated Chiang Kai-shek's National Forces and took control of China (Republic of China [Taiwan], 2014b, p. 302). Chiang moved his government to Taiwan and under the Kuomintang Party, kept the idea of reuniting Taiwan with China as an important goal of their group (Wu & Dai, 2014). After Chiang Kai-shek and his eldest son died numerous social, political, and economic reforms were developed, strengthening the pro-independence party and resulting in a higher degree of self-sovereignty and autonomy from mainland China (Corcuff, 2002).

At present, Taiwan has a population of more than 23 million people (Republic of China [Taiwan], 2014a) that is divided into four main ethnic groups (Copper, 2012). The first group, the aborigines, were originally identified to be of Malay or Polynesian origin. The next two groups are the *Hakka* who came from southern China near Hong Kong and the *Fujianese* who came from China's Fujian Province directly across the Taiwan Straits (Copper). By the year 1000 A.D., there were a large number of Hakka settled in western Taiwan (Copper). The Fujianese began migrating across the Taiwan Strait nearly a thousand years ago with many making the journey between the 14th and 17th centuries (Copper). Being separated from China for so many years has made the Hakkas and Fujians culturally distinct from other Chinese. The fourth ethnic group is composed of Chinese who came to Taiwan from various parts of China after World War II. They are often referred to as Mainlanders (Copper).

In more recent times, the challenges and needs of Taiwanese Americans and Chinese Americans have received increasing attention among social scientists. As the Taiwanese population continues to increase in the United States, the distinction between Taiwanese Americans and Chinese Americans needs to be understood. The history of Chinese-descended immigrants and their characteristics have changed drastically since the first migrations. Not only has the total number of Chinese-descended immigrants increased, but also the composition of recent immigrants is strikingly different from previous groups (Zhou, 2009). Early Chinese immigrants were often laborers with low levels of education (Zhou, 2009). In contrast, recent Taiwanese and Chinese immigrants are often highly educated and skilled professionals (Zhou, 2009, p. 80).

Although growing Western influences have inundated the country, the Taiwanese have preserved their identity and a considerable part of their traditional premodern culture (Storm & Harrison, 2007). As more Taiwanese migrate to the United States, it is important for nurses to understand the cultural history and healthcare needs and practices that are culturally specific to Taiwanese immigrants.

■ CULTURAL AND SOCIAL STRUCTURE DIMENSIONS

Leininger (1995) stated that one of the greatest challenges in nursing is to know and understand people in their familiar or naturalistic living contexts in different places in the world. Each year, thousands of immigrants from all over the world arrive in the United States bringing their homeland values, beliefs, and lifeways including health and illness practices. One of the largest Asian groups to immigrate to the United States are people of Chinese ancestry, numbering over 2.2 million (Pew Research Center, 2014a). Included in this group are Taiwanese immigrants who, despite residing in the United States for long periods of time, continue to practice their traditional cultural lifeways.

Such transcultural practices need to be studied and understood by transcultural nurses. The author's professional observations and research findings are interspersed throughout the culture-specific information that follows, with the goal to present her personal, professional, and research experiences about the Taiwanese culture.

Worldview

Taiwan's worldview can be best described as a continual struggle for independence, often viewed as a source of strength and inspiration. The issue of independence dominates political, social, and economic debate among Taiwanese people and can stir strong emotions. Since the 17th century, Taiwanese independence has been an ongoing struggle against occupying groups that included the Dutch, Spanish, Japanese, and Chinese Nationalists led by the Kuomintang. The quest for sovereignty has been complex with some pro-independence groups advocating for Taiwan to become a distinct entity from China, promoting its own Taiwanese language, and reducing political and economic links with the mainland. In contrast, other Taiwanese support the status quo or existing state of affairs and already view Taiwan as an independent nation with a high degree of autonomy and self-rule. Although many Taiwanese do not deny that they are ethnic Chinese or of Chinese descent, they seek legal and political separation from the Chinese national identity rather than one based upon the use of racial, ethnic, or ancestral designations. On the whole, people from Taiwan will usually refer to themselves as Taiwanese instead of Chinese. For those living abroad, although they may be referred to as Chinese American, they will think of themselves as Taiwanese. They are quick to distinguish that while China is mainly Chinese in culture, Taiwan is a rich blend of culture and history due to multiple outside or foreign influences.

Cultural Values, Beliefs, and Lifeways

Cultural values of Taiwanese people are rooted in the search for harmony and balance as a caring modality (Chiang-Hanisko, 2002). Taiwanese believe that keeping unity between humans and heaven is an essential part of existence and is integral to how the world is viewed. Harmony, balance, and unity emanate from the individual but are expressed in a familial and collective expression at a societal level (Chiang-Hanisko,

2002). An appreciation of nature is important to achieve harmony as a caring modality in one's life.

Taiwanese believe the search for harmony and balance is often divided into matters that are either internal or external in nature and are often referenced in Taiwanese diet and medicine (Chiang-Hanisko, 2002). The forces of *Yin* and *Yang* (e.g., the dual principles of male and female, or positive and negative) are reinforced through the importance of hot and cold concepts in Taiwanese food and medicine. These principles are part of a philosophy that fosters a balance between humans and nature, which are reflected in the Taiwanese worldview (Chiang-Hanisko, 2002; Republic of China (Taiwan), 2014e). Illness is regarded as an imbalance of *Yin* and *Yang*; this theory suggests that to maintain caring for good health, one needs to have good eating habits as well as proper goals in life. Body equilibrium is maintained on a hot day by eating cool foods like fruits and vegetables and avoiding meats, oil, fatty dishes, and alcohol. On cool days, plenty of stimulating foods should be eaten like meats and high-protein meals. Herbs and home remedies are widely used to restore balance.

Religion and Philosophy

Taiwan is a highly tolerant society. Freedom of religion is considered by the people of Taiwan to be a fundamental human right and is written in the Constitution of the Republic of China (Republic of China [Taiwan], 2000). Religion in Taiwan embodies a diversity of religious beliefs and practices due to its long multicultural history. According to a recent report published by the Religion and Public Life Project of the Pew Research Center (a nonpartisan think-tank based in Washington, DC), Taiwan has the second-highest religious diversity in the world (Pew Research Center, 2014b). Buddhism, Taoism, and folk religions are its traditional religions. The Dutch introduced Protestant Christianity to Taiwan, the Spanish brought Catholicism, and the Japanese spread Shintoism. While a majority of the population consider themselves Buddhist or Taoist, many Taiwanese follow some form of traditional folk religion deeply rooted in Chinese culture (Republic of China (Taiwan), 2014b). Modern Taiwanese may adapt new beliefs with old practices such as worshiping popular deities or ancestor worship (National Museum of Taiwan History, 2010).

Confucianism is also important to understanding the Taiwanese (Chiang-Hanisko, 2002). A Taiwanese person may call themselves a Buddhist, a Taoist, or even a Christian, but they never cease to be Confucian. The Confucian philosophy contains elements of moral, social, and political thought that gives meaning to living, dying, family life, childbearing, maintenance of health, and cause of illness. The principles of Confucianism represent both a guide for serving society and respecting family as well as a mindset of values that deeply permeates Taiwanese life.

Kinship and Social Structure Factors

Although many Taiwanese feel pressured to change their traditional values as Taiwan continues its economic prosperity as one of the wealthier countries in Asia, traditional values based upon the philosophy and teachings of Confucius still help to define how Taiwanese view the family (Chiang-Hanisko, 2002). Traditional Confucian values make family needs a priority over the needs of an individual family member, and children are expected to make sacrifices to meet the needs of their parents (Chiang-Hansiko, Adamle, & Chiang, 2009). Paternalism and filial piety imply that older family members should be respected while younger family members should abide by elders' decisions (Chiang-Hansiko et al., 2009). Confucian teachings stress the importance of maintaining harmony in family relationships and keeping the family name honorable (Chiang-Hanisko, 2002).

Family-centered relationships based upon a kinship system, inherent in Confucian ideology, form the nucleus of care patterns in contemporary Taiwanese society (Chiang-Hansiko et al., 2009). Confucian scholars wrote about the responsibility of a patient's family in times of illness during the Sung Dynasty (960-1279), "Only those who understand the art of medicine can be called children who fulfill their duties toward their parents" (as cited by Unschuld, 1979, p. 57). Other scholars added, "Whoever leaves the cure of diseases to common physicians neither possesses compassion, nor does he fulfill his duties toward his parents. The knowledge of medicine is indispensable in the assistance of one's relative" (as cited by Unschuld, 1979, p. 57).

The tradition of family members taking responsibility for care decisions on behalf of an ailing relative is still practiced in Taiwanese society (Chiang-Hansiko, et al., 2009). Family members are called upon to be gatekeepers in filtering information between health-care professionals and their sick relative. They are involved in the continuum of care including assessment, diagnosis, treatment decisions, and ongoing evaluations. Patient and family are viewed as one entity (Chiang-Hansiko, et al., 2009). Equally important, however, is the recognition of acculturation as an ongoing process resulting in intergenerational family differences. Taiwanese Americans may share in all, some, or none of the beliefs and practices of traditional Confucian values.

Economy and Technology Factors

Over the past 60 years, Taiwan has transformed itself from an agricultural island to a high-technology industrial economy (Yeh & Chi, 2014, p. 263). The country has progressed through various states, including the use of agriculture to support industry during the 1950s when import restrictions were imposed; the export years of the 1960s; the building of infrastructure through the Ten Major Construction Projects during the 1970s; the liberalization of government and private businesses leading to internationalization of the 1980s; and finally the explosive growth of information technology in the 1990s (Republic of China [Taiwan], 2014d). Taiwan has become an indispensable member in the modern global chain of high-technology industries with sizable investments in semiconductor research and development, image display, biotechnology, communications, and information services (Republic of China [Taiwan], 2014c). As a developed capitalist economy, Taiwan ranks as the 21st largest in the world by purchasing power parity (United States Central Intelligence Agency, 2013) making its economy the 17th freest nation in the 2014 index of economic freedom (The Heritage Foundation, 2014). Recent arrangements have relaxed cross-strait barriers between Taiwan and China to promote economic revitalization and a more open economic relationship. Despite these trade arrangements, opposition to engaging with China is cause for concern by some because of fears that sovereignty will be lost.

Educational Factors

Taiwanese continue to greatly value education that imbues Confucian traditions valuing disciplined study and academic achievement. An ancient Chinese saying, "… all pursuits except studying are of little value"

epitomizes the deep respect held by Taiwanese families toward education. Traditionally, Taiwan has had an extremely competitive educational climate where a high school graduate would have about a 20% chance to enter a university (Republic of China [Taiwan], 2013). The educational climate could be further characterized as having a high-stakes testing structure that acts as an access gatekeeper to higher education. Taiwanese parents have been known to make lifestyle sacrifices, even to the point of compromising their standard of living, in the pursuit of education for their children (Republic of China [Taiwan], 2013). Perhaps a cultural response to this hyper-competitive educational environment has been the development and proliferation of buxibans (補習班) or supplementary education schools in Taiwan (Republic of China [Taiwan], 2013). Parental investment in buxiban activities as an enhancement to formal classwork is seen as a necessary step to gain access to higher education and, ultimately, a means to enable economic and social mobility (Republic of China [Taiwan], 2013). Each year, a large number of Taiwanese students choose to study abroad. While many do return to Taiwan after graduation, others pursue overseas career opportunities, often deciding to permanently emigrate to the country where they had chosen to study. Buxibans have even been transplanted to Taiwanese immigrant communities in the United States (Zhou & Kim, 2006).

Nonetheless, the current state of education in Taiwan is changing. After unprecedented expansion of higher education in the 1990s in response to global competition, Taiwanese society is faced with a low birthrate and an aging population (Republic of China [Taiwan], 2013). It is expected that a number of universities will need to merge or close after 2016 when the cohort of 18-year olds is anticipated to decline for the first time (Tsai, 2010; Chang, 2014). The Ministry of Education is working to reorient the Taiwanese educational system so as to remain globally competitive because the country is dependent on exporting such products as semiconductor chips; electronic equipment; communication technology; industrial machinery; and optical, technical, and medical equipment (Republic of China [Taiwan], 2010). These new educational goals for the years between 2014 and 2023 are intended to support creativity, interdisciplinary ability, information competence, global mobility, employability, and citizenship (Republic of China [Taiwan], 2013).

Currently, the Taiwanese have achieved a literacy rate of approximately 98%, an indicator of national competitiveness (Chou, 2014).

■ CULTURAL THEMES

Culture Reflected in National and Cultural Identity

These culture themes are based upon findings from the author's research conducted over many years and her experiences as an invited and visiting scholar to Taiwan as well as her own life experiences as a native Taiwanese. The characterization of Taiwanese identity has been a central issue of discussion in Taiwan society for several decades with many citizens envisioning themselves as part of a nation separate from mainland China. Two factors that influence how Taiwanese define their national and cultural identity are *the cultural commonality between Taiwan and China* and *the uncertainty of political separation from mainland China* (Huang, Liu, & Chang, 2004). These authors contend that the Taiwanese identity dilemma is rooted in the dynamic interplay between these two elements—cultural commonality and political division. While Taiwanese may recognize and accept themselves as ethnic Chinese, increasingly they contend that Chinese culture is only one part of Taiwanese culture. The struggle to seek political and legal separation from China has become a source of cultural regeneration wherein the Taiwanese people assert themselves to safeguard their ethnic and national identity. The fact that Taiwan is already autonomous from China fuels their desire to defend and preserve their fundamental human rights such as freedom of expression, religious tolerance, and political debate. Protection of freedom, democracy, and human rights are core values of Taiwan's people.

The issue of reunification can be a sensitive and complex matter with many Taiwanese people—especially with those who have family residing in mainland China. While some Taiwanese may be cautious about discussing preferences toward reunification, they will certainly express a desire for democracy and an open political system. The continuing cycle of conflict and struggle, followed by negotiation and accommodation, and the changing political landscape in the region and broader global community, will no doubt recreate Taiwanese views of nation, culture, and society but within a traditional Taiwanese context.

Culture Care Means Preserving Traditional Folk Health Care Beliefs

Taiwanese Americans are willing to spend a great deal of time, effort, and money to obtain Chinese medicine for their promotion of health and prevention of illness. They believe it is important to prevent illness and will go through much effort to do so. Most believe that chemical substances in the body could endanger health. Many maintain that Western medicine is chemically based while Chinese medicine is more natural. A common belief is that *Western medicine* could actually *inhibit health* but taking *Chinese medicine* helps to *promote health*. Chinese medicine is viewed as more holistic while Western medicine is seen as primarily addressing localized symptoms (Sun et al., 2013).

In Taiwanese culture, traditional healing practices often exist side-by-side with modern medicine. Taiwanese Americans use various Taiwanese home remedies such as acupuncture, cupping, and plant and animal treatments like deer horn and ginseng. When available, Chinese and Western medicine may be used together. For those Taiwanese living in the United States, many may have limited access to Chinese medicine and resort to the use of Western medicine.

Caring Expressed as Unconditional Emotional and Physical Support of Taiwanese Loved Ones

The expression of emotions is a universal phenomenon and can show considerable variation worldwide. Emotions play an essential role in how people relate to each other and can result in social harmony or discord. Ethnographic studies suggest that emotions in Chinese culture are to be tempered and emotional control is respected (Soto, Levenson, & Ebling, 2005). For those who practice traditional Chinese medicine, manifestation of extreme emotions can even result in illness and disease (Soto et al., 2005). Taiwanese expression, perception, and self-regulation of emotions are undoubtedly influenced by cultural tradition, social ideals, and Confucianism. The display of negative, excessive, or unrestrained emotions may disturb and disrupt social and familial harmony; therefore such expressions are devalued and have little social significance. In this context, emotions are acceptable as long as they do not have a negative effect on social or family relations. Caring is often viewed as loving someone by providing an action but not necessarily by emotional and verbal responses. Caring is characterized as a process of continuous overt activities and deeds that reflect the inner expression of love. Among ancient Chinese thinkers, as reflected in the Analects of Confucius and Mencius, emotions are viewed within a moral context and are reflective of a person's character (Munro, 2002; Virag, 2014). Taiwanese may use this historical framework to associate emotions with good ethical judgments expressed through actions, work, and deeds to help others, but not necessarily with verbal communication.

■ LEININGER'S CULTURE CARE MODES OF DECISIONS AND ACTIONS

In accordance with Leininger's theory (1991, 2006), three culture care modes derived from knowledge of culture as well as care meanings and values are used to guide nursing decisions and actions. They are cultural care preservation and/or maintenance; cultural care accommodation and/or negotiation; and cultural care repatterning and/or restructuring. The author has also drawn upon the rich text of her own observations and experiences which are interspersed among the research findings that follow.

Cultural Care Preservation and/or Maintenance

Culture care preservation as filial love reflects the importance of family relationships for Taiwanese Americans (Chiang-Hanisko, 2010). Culture care means family closeness, and care is family-centered. Nursing decisions and actions need to be planned with this context in mind. Family decisions about treatment may be more important than the individual's decision (Chiang-Hansiko et al., 2009). It is necessary to include family members in every aspect of care, from preventing illness to maintaining health. Culture care preservation and/or maintenance of family love (filial love) by including significant family members in caring and treatment activities is essential.

Cultural Care Accommodation and/or Negotiation

Harmony and balance as culture care must be accommodated or negotiated for Taiwanese Americans. For example, illness is viewed as an imbalance between

Yin (cold) and Yang (hot), so nurses need to provide this balance of cold and hot to be culturally sensitive caregivers. Nurses need to accommodate this value by facilitating the Taiwanese to keep their traditional diets and medicine for internal and external equilibrium.

Holism and spiritual life values demonstrated as caring ways need to be accommodated or negotiated for Taiwanese Americans. Older generation Taiwanese Americans do not separate illness of the body from illness of the mind, so it is important for nurses to view the whole person within this cultural context. This mode of accommodation includes nursing care that recognizes and promotes the connection between cultural, psychological, and spiritual care as well as physical care actions. For those Taiwanese Americans who believe that promoting a peaceful mind state represents caring and brings health, nurses need to accommodate and facilitate the use of spiritual care with professional nursing care practices for healthy recoveries.

Cultural Care Repatterning and/or Restructuring

Culture care repatterning and/or restructuring may be difficult for nurses who do not understand Taiwanese Americans. Taiwanese Americans may utilize a variety of treatment approaches combining Chinese with Western medicine (Chiang-Hanisko, Tan, & Chiang, 2014). Some treatments are accomplished through self-care while others are provided by professional caregivers. Most Taiwanese Americans expect quick results from Western medicine, so it is necessary for nurses to emphasize the importance of taking medicine when there may be no immediate visible effects. Taiwanese Americans often have beliefs about causes of illness and what treatments should be used, which may not be consistent with those of Western health care. This implies that nurses need to develop an understanding of Taiwanese cultural beliefs about care and health so they can effectively work with the patient to accept, alter, or decline Western care practices. With older generation Taiwanese Americans, it may be culturally unacceptable to violate their traditional beliefs about health and care practices. Restructuring nursing decisions and actions would be needed where traditional Taiwanese folk health care and professional nursing practices are in conflict or if changes are necessary when transitioning from traditional to professional care.

Furthermore, repatterning or restructuring nursing decisions and actions needs to be conducted by helping clients understand the possible consequences and side effects of combining Western medicine prescribed by their provider with Chinese herbal remedies. Careful and sensitive repatterning or restructuring care practices also provides a sense of trust between patient and healthcare provider that then develops from an understanding and acceptance of the client's cultural beliefs.

■ SUMMARY

This chapter examined the unique lifeways and worldviews of Taiwanese and Taiwanese Americans rather than merging all Chinese (Taiwan, mainland China, Hong Kong, Singapore, etc.) into one cultural group. An island state such as Taiwan has absorbed and assimilated many foreign influences due to colonization and therefore is distinctly different from other countries of Chinese heritage economically, socially, and politically. Taiwan's advanced industrialized and technologically progressive economy supported by a democratic political system is vastly different from China where market reforms are incomplete as it attempts to shift from a centrally-planned economy to a market-based economy. Therefore, wide variations in the culture care meanings and beliefs between Taiwanese Americans and Chinese Americans are to be expected.

The Theory of Culture Care Diversity and Universality enhances the understanding of culture as an important dimension of care, especially as nurses work to understand how Taiwanese people conceptualize illness, health, and wellbeing. The framework of Leininger's theoretical tenets of cultural diversities and universalities about human caring is key for guiding nurses to adapt care toward being culturally congruent with Taiwanese clients. As change takes place in Taiwan, nurses need to have competency in identifying and supporting customs, traditions, and beliefs, and the continual evolution and adaptation of care, toward greater universality for the Taiwanese people.

■ DEDICATION

This chapter is dedicated to my mentor, Dr. Madeleine Leininger, who visited Taiwan in 1998 to plant the seeds for transcultural nursing.

■ DISCUSSION QUESTIONS

1. What are the commonalities and differences of culture care expressions, beliefs, and practices between the Taiwanese and the Chinese cultures?
2. Discuss how healthcare professionals could use the discovered themes discussed in this chapter to assist with the development of culturally congruent care in clinical practice.
3. In what ways can Leininger's three culture care modes of decisions and actions facilitate the provision of culturally congruent care for Taiwanese Americans?
4. Discuss some challenges that may be encountered when providing (or planning to integrate into practice) culturally congruent care with Taiwanese clients.
5. In what ways does the Taiwanese worldview, social structure factors, and environmental context influence their cultural care expressions, beliefs, and practices?

■ REFERENCES

Chang, J. (2014). Number of universities should be reduced: Education minister. *The China Post*. Available at http://www.chinapost.com.tw/taiwan/national/national-news/2014/09/25/417973/Number-of.htm

Chiang-Hanisko, L. (2002). Taiwanese Americans cultural care meanings and expressions. In M. M. Leininger & M. R. McFarland (Eds.), *Transcultural nursing: Concepts, theories, research and practices* (3rd ed., pp. 415-428). New York, NY: McGraw-Hill, Inc.

Chiang-Hanisko, L. (2010). Paradise lost: How older adult Taiwanese immigrants make decisions about their living arrangements. *Journal of Cultural Diversity, 17*(3), 99-104.

Chiang-Hansiko, L., Adamle, K., & Chiang, L. (2009). Cultural differences in therapeutic humor in nursing education. *Journal of Nursing Research, 17*(1), 52-61.

Chiang-Hanisko, L., Tan, J., & Chiang, L. (2014). Polypharmacy issues in older adults. *The Journal of Nursing, 61*(3), 97-104.

Chou, C. P. (2014, November 12). Education in Taiwan: Taiwan's colleges and universities. *Taiwan-U.S. Quarterly Analysis, 16*. Retrieved from http://www.brookings.edu/research/opinions/2014/11/taiwan-colleges-universities-chou

Copper, J. F. (2012). *Taiwan: Nation, state, or province?* (6th ed.). San Francisco, CA: Westview Press.

Corcuff, S. (2002). *Memories of the future: National identify issues and the search for a new Taiwan*. Armonk, NY: M. E. Sharpe.

The Heritage Foundation. (2014). 2014 Index of Economic Freedom. Retrieved from http://www.heritage.org/index/country/taiwan

Huang, L., Liu, J. H., & Chang, M. (2004). 'The double identity' of Taiwanese Chinese: A dilemma of politics and culture rooted in history. *Asian Journal of Social Psychology*, 7(2), 149-168.

Leininger, M. M. (1984). *Care: The essence of nursing and health*. Detroit, MI: Wayne State University Press.

Leininger, M. M. (1991). *Cultural care diversity and universality: Theory of nursing*. New York, NY: National League of Nursing.

Leininger, M. M. (1995). *Transcultural nursing: Concepts, theories, research, and practice*. Blacklick, OH: McGraw-Hill, Inc.

Leininger, M. M. (2002). Part I: The theory of culture care and the ethnonursing research method. In M. M. Leininger & M. R. McFarland (Eds.), *Transcultural nursing: Concepts, theories, research and practices* (3rd ed., pp. 71-98). New York: McGraw-Hill, Inc.

Leininger, M. M. (2006). Cultural care diversity and universality theory and evolution of the ethnonursing method. In M. M. Leininger & M. R. McFarland (Eds.), *Cultural care diversity and universality: A worldwide nursing theory* (2nd ed., pp. 1-41). Sudbury, MA: Jones and Bartlett.

Munro, D. J. (2002). Mencius and an ethic of the new century. In A. K. Chan (Ed.), *Mencius, context, and interpretations*. Hawaii, HI: University of Hawaii Press.

National Museum of Taiwan History. (2010, July 1). *Watch Taiwan: No. 6*. Retrieved from http://www.nmth.gov.tw/Portals/0/epaper/en/06/coverstory05.html

Pew Research Center. (2014a). *7 facts about world migration*. Retrieved from http://www.pewresearch.org/fact-tank/2014/09/02/7-facts-about-world-migration/

Pew Research Center. (2014b). Pew research religion & public life project: Global religious diversity. Retrieved from http://www.pewforum.org/2014/04/04/global-religious-diversity/

Republic of China (Taiwan). (2000). *Constitution of the Republic of China*. Retrieved from http://www.taiwan-documents.org/constitution01.htm

Republic of China (Taiwan), Ministry of Economic Affairs, Bureau of Foreign Trade. (2010). *The Bureau of Foreign Trade news release*. Retrieved from https://www.moea.gov.tw/Mns/.../wHandNews_File.ashx?news

Republic of China (Taiwan), Ministry of Education. (2013). *Human resource development* [White paper]. Retrieved from http://epaper.edu.tw/news.aspx?news_sn=21968

Republic of China (Taiwan), Directorate General of Budget, Accounting, and Statistics, Executive Yuan. (2014a). *National statistics: Republic of China (Taiwan)*. Taipei, Taiwan: Author. Retrieved from http://eng.stat.gov.tw/mp.asp?mp=5

Republic of China (Taiwan), Executive Yuan. (2014b). *The Republic of China Yearbook 2014*. Taipei, Taiwan: Author.

Republic of China (Taiwan), Ministry of Economic Affairs, Industrial Development Bureau. (2014c). *Industrial development in Taiwan, R. O. C.* Retrieved from http://www.moeaidb.gov.tw/external/ctlr?PRO=english.About01&lang=1

Republic of China (Taiwan), Ministry of Economic Affairs, Small and Medium Enterprise Administration. (2014d). *Taiwan's economic development*. Retrieved from http://www.moeasmea.gov.tw/ct.asp?xItem=72&CtNode=263&mp=2

Republic of China (Taiwan), Ministry of Foreign Affairs. (2014e). *Chinese medicine in Taiwan*. Retrieved from http://www.mofa.gov.tw/en/News_Content.aspx?n=D63485FC2A6F4D3C&sms=CE9D6F5CD437EB7A&s=71383ADCFFA42811

Rubenstein, M. A. (2007). *Taiwan: A new history*. New York, NY: M. E. Sharpe.

Soto, J. A., Levenson, W., & Ebling, R. (2005). Cultures of moderation and expression: Emotional experience, behavior, and physiology in Chinese Americans and Mexican Americans. *Emotion*, 5(2), 154-165.

Storm, C., & Harrison, M. (2007). Methodologies, epistemologies and a Taiwan studies. In C. Storm & M. Harrison (Eds.), *The margins of becoming: Identity and culture in Taiwan*. Wiesbaden, Germany: Harrassowitz Verlag.

Sun, D. Z., Li, S. D., Liu, Y., Zhang, Y., Mei, R., & Yang, M. H. (2013). Differences in the origin of philosophy between Chinese medicine and Western medicine: Exploration of the holistic advantages of Chinese medicine. *Chinese Journal of Integrative Medicine*, 19(9), 706-711.

Tsai, H. C. (2010). The policy implication of the over-supply and demand in Taiwan's higher education. *Bulletin of Humanities and Social Science*, 11(3), 36-41.

United States Central Intelligence Agency. (2013). Gross Domestic Products (GDP; Purchasing power parity). *CIA World Factbook*. Retrieved from http://www.cia.gov/library/publications/the-world-factbook/fields/2001.html

Unschuld, P. (1979). *Medical ethics in imperial China: A study in historical anthropology*. Los Angeles, CA: University of California Press.

Virag, C. (2014). Early Confucian perspectives on emotions. In V. Shen (Ed.), *Dao companion to classical Confucian philosophy*. Toronto, Canada: Springer.

Wu, C-L., & Dai, S-C. (2014). From regime transition to liberal democracy: The case of Taiwan. In E. S. K. Fung & S. Drakeley (Eds.), *Democracy in Eastern Asia: Issues, problems and challenges in a region of diversity*. New York, NY: Routledge.

Yeh, C. E., & Chi, G-C. (2014). The development of Taiwan's high-technology industries. In S. T. Lee & J. F. Williams (Eds.), *Taiwan's struggle: Voices of Taiwanese*. Plymouth, UK: Rowman & Littlefield.

Zhou, M., & Kim, S. S. (2006). Community forces, social capital, and educational achievement: The case of supplementary education in the Chinese and Korean immigrant communities. *Harvard Educational Review, 76*(1), 1-29.

Zhou, M. (2009). *Contemporary Chinese America: Immigration, ethnicity, and community transformation*. Philadelphia, PA: Temple University Press.

16

The Sunrise Enabler's Application in Conflict Resolution for Nurse Administrators and Managers

Ann O. Hubbert

> *"Transcultural nursing administration knowledge is imperative in order to develop creative transcultural administrative goals and practices" (Leininger, 1996).*

■ INTRODUCTION

Nursing administrators and managers are leaders who directly affect all aspects of health care and education throughout the United States. Nurses in these leadership roles face difficult challenges throughout both the health care and educational systems because they are called upon to address diverse issues such as rising health care costs, quality of care, and equity of access to care. The American Nurses' Association (ANA) (2014) continues to strongly advocate to federal policymakers and regulators that nurses are crucial for effective transformational changes to occur within the health care and educational systems.

The ANA's commitment to ensuring contributions from within and by the profession is anchored in the knowledge that nurses who are educated and practice within a holistic framework are imperative for effective implementation of the reforms necessary for improved access and optimal delivery of all health care. These challenges also present nursing leaders with new opportunities to facilitate interprofessional and multidisciplinary cooperation based on application of Leininger's Theory of Culture Care Diversity and Universality (Culture Care Theory) (Leininger, 1991, 1995, & 2006) in their participative/collaborative decision and action processes with multicultural individuals and groups.

An effective leader recognizes that his/her organization is represented by diverse as well as similar cultural groups including but not limited to professional disciplines, health care providers, clients, families, students, faculty, insurers, donors, network/systems, and volunteers amongst an overall organizational culture. Often, leaders must respond and intervene to address anxieties faced by employees in the midst of organizational changes, which may start as minor disagreements but lead to dysfunctional processes and negative outcomes within the organization. These anxieties may manifest as conflicts among and/or between individuals or groups within the same organization or partner organizations that join together in new business models.

All organizations have a variety of cultures that influence the decisions and actions made within the organization; the philosophy, values, and mission of the organization; and the formation of any collaborative partnerships. Transcultural nursing administration provides the direction for successful communication, collaboration, assessment, and action amidst the complexities of such relationships among and between organizational cultures. A transculturally focused nursing administrator recognizes the negative impact on the delivery of services when conflicts are addressed solely as being "problematic acting out behaviors" without recognizing relevant cultural contexts.

This chapter discusses transcultural nursing administration as a specific foundation for nursing administration decisions and actions using the constructs of Leininger's Culture Care Theory (CCT) to successfully resolve conflicts among or between organizations and employees (Leininger, 1991). Toward this end, specific constructs—culture care universal values; assumptive premises; the Sunrise Enabler; and the three modes of culture care decisions and actions—are discussed to provide the reader with a working knowledge on how to explicate the CCT into an applicable approach for conflict resolution at any organizational level.

■ LITERATURE REVIEW

Leininger (1996) held that transcultural nursing administration was an imperative for working successfully as an administrator within a multicultural world in the areas of management, education, and service. She maintained that administrative practices can influence quality outcomes and prevent unfavorable conflicts. This focus remains a foundation for contemporary nursing administrators as they search for ways to resolve conflicts that arise among and between the vast numbers of cultures represented within the organizational structure. Too often, administrators may disregard the value of acknowledging that transcultural issues exist within all organizations. Some organizations may focus on ethnic cultural differences, while maintaining a uniculturally oriented (one culture) view of the administrative role.

These phenomena are significant considering that contemporary nursing leaders function within many cultures that transcend organizations (Schein, 2010). Diverse cultures (organizational cultures, professional cultures such as nursing and medicine, donors, community representatives, fiscal officers, and state and federal regulatory bodies) influence the operation of organizations and guide the development of standards of practice for professional subcultures.

Leininger's (1995) description of a dominant culture versus a subculture within nursing is useful when considering the variety of cultures and subcultures within organizations that administrators may work with on a continual basis. Increasingly, small interprofessional groups or teams are coming together to work toward developing innovative new policies and actions; these teams can evolve as yet another subculture within the main organization. Cultural biases may exist between interprofessional cultures or even subcultures within organizations and lead to unproductive cultural clashes and conflicts. Ludwig-Beymer (2008) described the need to create culturally competent organizations, or face the challenges presented by cultural conflicts including clients' reluctance to access health care services, which may ultimately lead to health care inequities.

Slavkin (2010) defined leadership in the 21st century health care environment as "the act that signifies making a difference." He discussed leadership skills as sustaining, improving, or changing directions as required within simple or complex organizations with the recognition that there is not one organizational culture, but varying numbers of cultures and subcultures with which the employees and clients identify. Slavkin's definition supports the earlier works and vision of Leininger (1996) who sought to stimulate a worldwide imperative for transcultural nurse administrators to provide leadership in nursing administration and health care to create a "… different and rewarding world for academic nursing education and clinical practice" (Slavkin, 2010, p. 33).

Nurse administrators are expected to be proactive in role modeling leadership skills that can "make a positive difference" (Slavkin, 2010, p.35) to avoid conflicts when organizational changes may impact the norms, values, and practices of professional and client cultures within organizations. Change, innovation, and transformation are dynamic processes that require the blending or assimilation of subgroups by nurse leaders who represent diverse professional, political, and organizational cultures (distinct nursing interests, clients, faculty, students, interprofessional partners, collaborating institutions, and donors). The realities of such diverse expectations include phenomenal levels of accountability in the midst of fewer resources, higher levels of regulation, and frustrations among professionals and consumers that too often lead to conflicts among and between groups.

Administrative leadership is immersed in sustaining, improving, or changing strategic directions in small cultures or large multicultural groups that function within simple or complex organizational cultures (Slavkin, 2010). Scott (2010) recognized that tensions between groups in health care organizations exist despite growing calls for groups to join together in new alliances to evaluate and implement best-evidences for practice, safety, financial stability, and sustainability. Administrators are expected to demonstrate leadership skills with a wide array of cultures within their organization; if dysfunctional elements surface during a change implementation, the administrator is expected to facilitate the change evolution processes through successful negotiation with the involved subcultures to achieve a positive outcome (Schein, 2010).

Among the vast array of leadership development approaches available, two national experts (Wakeman [2010] and Johansen [2012]) with strong, in-depth contemporary programs focused on teaching leadership tenets, compliment and support the work conducted by Leininger since the 1950s. In 2013, the American Association of Colleges of Nursing (AACN) selected Wakeman (2013a, 2013b), as the professional highlighted speaker for the annual academic deans' and business officers' leadership development conference to share her expertise with nurse administrators in higher education. Wakeman's (2010, 2013a, & 2013b) is well known for her work in reality-based leadership that has positive, complementary, and supportive guidelines for transcultural administrators.

The desire to "solve the conflict quickly" can lead to leadership decisions or actions that imply a "right versus wrong" assessment of the conflict without allowing the resolution process to evolve new positive outcomes. Through her extensive work with organizational groups, Wakeman (2010) identified ambiguity as the most frequent cause of conflict occurring between individuals or groups (p. 127). She discovered three prominent aspects of ambiguity of group processes that can easily lead to conflict among group members: goals for the group, roles within the group, and procedures the group is to follow. Administrators are encouraged to provide clarity in these three areas to avoid ambiguity that can result in false assumptions and personality differences that lead to conflict and decreased possibilities for the group to achieve success.

The second nationally recognized individual is futurist Bob Johansen (2012). His book titled, *Leaders*

Make the Future, offers guidelines for leaders to be successful in what he terms a "tough decade." His work is nationally highlighted for nursing administrators' professional development in the AACN's member-community's leadership book club (AACN, 2014). Johansen's work (2012) encourages leaders to "... flip problems into opportunities" (p. 189) and to rebalance their skills for the challenges faced by being able to see beyond the polarities of present situations to create harmonious alignment among and between groups. He also recommends that leaders acquire a background in cultural anthropology and skills similar to ethnography, the knowledge base from which the Culture Care Theory and the Ethnonursing Research Method were developed by Leininger (1991).

Johansen (2012) referred to "polarized conflicts," and encouraged leaders to avoid the temptation of "picking sides" and/or delivering quick judgments (p. 113). In addition, both Johansen (2012) and Wakeman (2013b) emphasized the importance of administrative self-assessment skills, corresponding directly to the Culture Care Theory, which offers a guide for administrators to discover their own cultural beliefs, biases, and practices (Andrews & Boyle, 2012, pp. 20 - 23). Accordingly, an administrator's self-assessment is essential to identify and address any self-biases when considering or preparing for conflict resolution.

Ludwig-Beymer (2008) offered an in-depth review of culturally competent health care organizations; her work emphasizes the urgency for administrators to acquire cultural competency with multiple cultures within health care organizations. She also highlights the significance of having administrators conduct organizational cultural assessments to identify any barriers to care that may exist. Conflicts within any organization impede the effectiveness of the mission and outcomes. Andrews and Boyle (2012) stressed the importance for nurses to first engage in their own cultural self-assessment before providing culturally congruent care to patients; this precept holds true for transcultural administrators as well (p. 20).

The administrators' ability to have insight into personal biases, values, and beliefs allows them the opportunity to overcome their own ethnocentric tendencies and to gain an open perspective of the views presented by diverse groups or individuals experiencing conflicts. Because it is impossible for one administrator to hold expert knowledge about all the diverse cultures within his/her organization and existing partnerships, the Culture Care Theory provides a sound theoretical foundation in the quest toward achieving competence with conflict resolution as a transcultural administrator.

THEORETICAL FRAMEWORK

Leininger's Culture Care Theory was developed in the 1950s and has a scientifically sound and humanistic knowledge base that has evolved over six decades (Leininger, 1991, 2002a; McFarland and Wehbe-Alamah, 2015). The theory is foundational for working among and between diverse cultures and subcultures. It has been used as a guide for nurse administrators and managers (Hubbert, 2006; Ludwig-Beymer, 2008) working within health care systems, the nursing discipline, and diverse interprofessional teams. The Culture Care Theory provides administrators with clear guidelines that enable them to recognize and work with differences and similarities among groups susceptible to or experiencing cultural clashes.

Leininger's Sunrise Enabler (See Color Insert 1) guides ethnonursing researchers as they study cultures in relation to a selected domain of inquiry (Leininger, 2002b) and has been widely used by practicing nurses to expand views of care and conduct cultural assessments (McFarland & Wehbe-Alamah, 2015). The Sunrise Enabler is a key cognitive map of the theory that enables the transcultural administrator to study a conflict situation from the perspectives of several represented cultures simultaneously and offers a simple approach to "bring the theory into action" in conflict resolution.

The three modes of culture care decisions and actions depicted in the Sunrise Enabler provide ways that can be used on a daily basis by administrators to address any cultural clash or conflict. The culture care modes can be used to assist an administrator to discover and understand the cultural views represented in a conflict using a professional and nonjudgmental approach to achieve resolution based on a theoretical foundation. Used as a guide in this manner, the Sunrise Enabler enhances an administrator's creative and sound decision-making approaches in conflict resolution (Hubbert, 2006). As organizations evolve, conflicts are likely continue to emerge. Transcultural administrators may utilize their knowledge and

application of the Culture Care Theory to grow, creatively reimagine, and contribute to the redefinition of their organizations time and time again.

ORIENTATIONAL DEFINITIONS

The following are orientational definitions of key terms used in this chapter:

- *Transcultural nursing administration:* defined by Leininger (1996, p. 30) as "a creative and knowledgeable process of assessing, planning, and making decisions and policies that will facilitate the provision of educational and clinical services that take into account the cultural caring values, beliefs, symbols, references, and lifeways of people of diverse and similar cultures for beneficial or satisfying outcomes."
- *Culture of nursing:* defined by Leininger (1995, p. 208) as "the learned and transmitted lifeways, values, symbols, patterns, and normative practices of members of the nursing profession."
- *Subculture of nursing:* defined by Leininger (1995, p. 208) as "a group of nurses who show distinctive values and lifeways that differ from the dominant or mainstream culture of nursing."
- *Cultural bias:* defined by Leininger (2002, p. 51) as "a firm position that one's own values and beliefs must govern the situation or decisions."
- *Culture clash:* defined by Leininger (2002, p. 58) as "conflict among or between groups with different values, beliefs, or lifeways that are tense and cause overt problems."
- *Polarized conflicts:* defined by Johansen (2012, p. 113) as "conflicts between groups with opposing views, and often are dilemmas rather than problems that can be solved."
- *Cross cultural grace:* defined by Johansen (2012, p. 113) as "means of being nimble, poised, and engaging which leaders need; an ability to listen and learn from people who are very different from them and perhaps different in a disturbing way."
- *Cultural pride:* defined by Johansen (2012, p. 113) as "a person's pride of their culture, but not necessarily cultural knowledge."
- *Worldview:* defined by Leininger (2002, p. 83) as "the way an individual or group looks out on and understands their world about them as a value,

stance, picture, or perspective about life or the world."

- *Ethnocentrism:* defined by Leininger (2002, p. 50) as "the belief that one's own ways are the best, most superior, or preferred ways to act, believe, or behave."

■ ASSUMPTIVE PREMISES

Leininger presented 11 major theoretical tenets and predictions of the Culture Care Theory, (McFarland & Wehbe-Alamah, 2015, p. 8); three are presented here as significant for the discussion of transcultural nursing administrators' decisions and actions in conflict resolution. Administrators who have the skills to assess organizational groups as cultures will find these assumptions provide key ways of understanding diverse levels of organizational conflict and dissatisfaction.

The first theoretical assumptive premise, "… culture care expressions, meanings, patterns, processes, and structural forms are diverse but some commonalities exist among and between cultures" (McFarland & Wehbe-Alamah, 2015, p. 8) offers support for diverse professional cultures within any organization as unique cultures themselves. Nurses who practice in a distinctive or specialty area (i.e., pediatrics, critical care, or long-term care) identify with that specific nursing culture and thus as a subculture and exhibit all levels of cultural pride (wearing identifying professional symbols as part of their dress or uniforms; displaying certification identification; or choosing a group color or style of uniform). Similarly, among nursing educators, many provide their educational expertise by working with or teaching specific populations of students (undergraduate versus graduate; freshmen versus senior; a medical-surgical class versus one on ethics) or through their preference to teach classes rather than conduct research. A transcultural administrator who possesses cross cultural grace (Johansen, 2012, p. 113), realizes that cultural pride has many levels, that worldviews vary, and that there are times within an organization when all members will need to unify in accepting a worldview that benefits or sets the direction for their organizational culture.

Conflicts arise among diverse subcultures of nurses within any organization for a myriad of reasons. Yet,

they all share commonalities by being members of the larger culture of nurses as an entity within their workplace, state, or national professional organization as well as nationally through their licensures and/or certifications. Organizationally, the diverse cultures or subcultures that exist within nursing represent the larger culture of the profession of nursing, which is itself diverse from the cultures of other professions (such as medicine, pharmacy, social work, financial officers, and many types of volunteer workers) that often coexist within health care organizations. Similarly, departments, schools, or colleges of nursing are culturally diverse from other schools or colleges that comprise complex educational institutions. In the context of the main or dominant organizational culture, all of these cultures come together as the culture of "Organization X." This organization may have many diverse cultures that share commonalities as employees and interested parties of Organization X. Often, organizations combine into new systems; as Organization X joins Organization Y, a new system emerges as Organization Z.

Challenges escalate when structural missions, visions, philosophies, and policies affect employees with the evolving organization's cultural perspectives. Nursing's cultures and subcultures, for example, are directed to merge multiple levels of policy toward creating consistency and commonality throughout a new system. For example, nurses from blended pediatric care units with diverse care philosophies from within one or more organizations may be tasked to create a "new culture" of care/caring with common values, beliefs, and practices of pediatric nursing. The array of cultures represented becomes massive and cultural conflicts may result. The challenge for the transcultural administrator is to bring these diverse cultures together while acknowledging their differences and promoting their commonalities to allow for productive and efficient work. Transcultural administrators need to recognize their organizations' diverse cultures and their corresponding values, beliefs, and behaviors and provide a knowledge foundation for the organization to embrace diversities and identify shared commonalities.

A second theoretical assumption that is pertinent and important for each culture is that "…culture care values, beliefs, and practices are influenced by and embedded in the worldview, social structure factors, and the ethnohistorical and environmental contexts" (McFarland & Wehbe-Alamah, 2015, p. 8). For example, a clinical health simulation educational center within a school of nursing may be led by a worldview that is different from that of all other cultures within the school. The center's national accreditation standards and guidelines for practice that are quite specific for the nursing culture may not generally be known or understood by other faculty and staff even though the clinical simulation center and its culture are part of the school's overall culture and worldview.

The third theoretical assumption "…culturally congruent and therapeutic care occurs when culture care values and beliefs are known and used sensitively with people of diverse or similar cultures" (Leininger, 2002c, p. 19) has direct implications for administrative conflict resolution. An administrator who can calmly and confidently assess and understand the diverse and similar cultures represented is more likely to reach a unifying outcome. For example, nurses from different client centered areas (emergency services and inpatient units) may experience cultural conflict when implementing a new process where they feel their area is misrepresented (culture of the emergency services versus the culture of the inpatient units). Both of these "diverse cultures" hold views they believe are at risk in this "cultural clash." Both groups also represent the overarching dominant nursing culture of the organization, which has its own views and beliefs on how employee/staff behaviors can best serve clients. Most conflicts are not "black and white, or right or wrong" so it is crucial for the effective transcultural administrator to gain a solid understanding of these diverse and common cultural values and beliefs.

■ CULTURE CARE VALUES IN NURSING ADMINISTRATION

Leininger's Culture Care Theory and the Ethnonursing Research Method, have resulted in the discovery to date of approximately 178 care/caring constructs (McFarland & Wehbe-Alamah, 2015, pp. 11-13) that help nurses understand the meanings of care held by cultures who have their own definitions. These identified care/caring constructs are similarly valued by diverse cultures and can be used by administrators working with various organizational cultures to achieve a common clarity of purpose. The relevance of three caring/care constructs—respect, listening, and being present—are discussed in relation to transcultural administrators' approaches to conflict resolution.

The first care/caring construct for transcultural administrators to embrace in their decisions and actions for conflict resolution is respect (Horn, 2002; Leininger, 1998). Transcultural administrators need to role model respect for individuals and their views, expertise, and contributions to the organization even if these are not in alignment with the administrator's own views. Leadership behavior that models respect for all participants involved in a conflict provides a positive direction in the midst of confusion. Wakeman (2010) identified five steps for leaders to redirect negativity in times of conflict; one step is to "see others through a lens of respect" (p. 140). Wakeman's specification of respect as crucial for leaders dealing with conflict supports the Culture Care Theory's care/caring construct of "respect as vital for leaders as they work with individuals or groups that are expressing stress-induced inappropriate behaviors" (Mixer, 2015, p. 377).

Respect is represented by a leader's willingness to interact with conflict by looking beyond the negativity toward respecting the individuals and their goals and not jumping to conclusions reached through the lens of an ethnocentric viewpoint related to deciding what is "right." An ethnocentric view can negatively influence the opportunity to learn and/or create new levels of understanding. Johansen (2012) referred to a view of knowing there is only one right way as a "threshold of righteousness" (p. 112) meaning every other view is wrong. Transcultural administrators often deal with these extreme views among individuals or groups. Having the knowledge and skills to assess the origin of these views is highly beneficial. Another level of respect for a transcultural administrator is respect for one's self and one's leadership. This continual process of self-assessment needs to become a routine aspect of administrative responsibility. Respect for what is known and unknown as a leader can be empowering and add clarity to carrying the leadership role (Johansen, 2012).

A second care/caring construct for transcultural administrators is listening (Horn, 2002; Leininger, 1998). A transcultural leader strives to exhibit behaviors of active listening in times of conflict. Active listening by a leader can be a powerful approach that gives groups immersed in conflict an opportunity to tell their story about what is important to them in the identified strife. A leader's ability to listen and learn from the views of people who are different from one another offers all participants equal consideration and a way to move toward a process of conflict resolution (Johansen, 2012, p. 113). An administrator who can emphasize the importance of listening and provides the structure for listening during conflict takes great strides toward achieving clarity amidst confusion and possibly even chaos. Times of stress, confusion, ambiguity, uncertainty, and complexity create anxieties that dominate over clarity (Johansen, 2012, p. 43). The structure provided by a transcultural administrator who actively listens is a step of progress toward calming anxieties.

The third relevant care/caring construct is being present (Horn, 2002; Leininger, 1998), which is further defined in this context for transcultural administrators as "helping, facilitating, providing assistive acts, being connected, and providing attention to the groups or individuals involved in the conflict situation" (Hubbert, 2006). Being present can be embodied by various behaviors and activities such as walking to someone's office or work area to speak with them instead of relying on a written or oral message, finding ways to be visible on a routine basis away from an administrative suite, being accessible through scheduled "open door" appointments, facilitating times for interested parties to gather with the administrator for discussions and casual conversations, and even taking (or scheduling) a quick response time to communicate with employees expressing frustrations.

In times of conflict, transcultural administrators can exhibit behaviors of being present through actions of respect and listening. Administrative presence can lead to confidence among those embroiled in a conflict, conveying the message that they have not been abandoned or ignored by administration to work the situation out themselves. Wakeman (2013a) advocated the idea of administrators "being present" by recognizing their role is truly to support the mission and goals of the organization in every way possible (p. 131), including how they respond to the frequent employee question, "Do you have a minute?" The response made at that moment will clearly convey an administrator's ability to be present and can be as simple as saying, "Let me see who I can find to help you" in a way that acknowledges the employee's concern.

■ THE THREE MODES OF CULTURE CARE DECISIONS AND ACTIONS

The Culture Care Theory's three modes of culture care decisions and actions (McFarland & Wehbe-Alamah, 2015, p. 16) are a valuable guide for administrators to follow as a foundation for administrative decisions and actions in their provision of direction, insights, and clarity in conflict resolution. They are discussed individually to explain how an administrator can apply each mode effectively while respecting the cultures represented within the conflict, listening to and acknowledging their views and/or beliefs, and actively facilitating a resolution.

Culture care preservation and/or maintenance refers to assistive, supportive, facilitative, or enabling professional acts or decisions that helps cultures retain, preserve, or maintain beneficial care beliefs or values (McFarland & Wehbe-Alamah, 2015, p. 16). An administrator who begins by addressing a conflict with this mode will consider what assistance is desired by each culture represented. For example, with representatives of two disciplines coming together to implement a new corporate policy, or two faculty members who disagree over a new curricular direction, an administrator can initiate the discussion by asking, "Tell me what is important for you to preserve in the midst of this change, confusion, or ambiguity?" Both cultures represented can then respond with what the essence of the matter may be regarding their concerns. The administrator's professional application of culture care preservation and/or maintenance through active listening can be invaluable toward achieving consensus as both cultures share their views, values, and beliefs about the conflict.

Culture care accommodation and/or negotiation refers to those assistive, accommodating, facilitative, or enabling creative provider care actions or decisions that help cultures adapt to or negotiate with others for culturally congruent, effective care (McFarland & Wehbe-Alamah, 2015, p. 16). Administrators addressing conflicts among cultures within organizations will need to be flexible by using accommodation and/or negotiation of policies, processes, or practices depending on the situation. There may be some directives impacting the cultures within organizations that administrators simply will not be able to change with negotiation, such as a corporate merger, which will need to be explained.

This culture care mode provides the means for the administrator and the participant cultures to mutually decide through accommodation and/or negotiation what is needed for them to work together within the reality of the situation [merger] causing the conflict. This mode helps the administrator identify where the ambiguity and lack of alignment between the cultures exist by addressing issues or questions such as: Is there a goal that is unclear that both cultures need to participate in? Is either culture confused about its role in the situation causing conflict? Do both cultures understand the processes or procedures? What can be negotiated or accommodated to reach a resolution agreeable to both cultures? Gaining clarity about what is known, unknown, or assumed by each culture is crucial. Administrative presence using this mode is essential as it conveys the message to all cultures involved that their distress has been acknowledged and that a resolution will be forthcoming as opposed to remaining in a state of ongoing confusion, ambiguity, and conflict.

Culture care restructuring and/or repatterning refers to those assistive, supportive, facilitative, or enabling professional actions and mutual decisions that would help people to reorder, change, modify, or restructure within their organization for better outcomes (McFarland & Wehbe-Alamah, 2015, p. 16). An administrator can guide the participant cultures to consider what practices or processes are negative, detrimental, obstructive, or harmful and therefore need to be repatterned or restructured to achieve conflict resolution. Administrators can facilitate these changes through respectful assessment of the cultures' views, beliefs, and values, and acknowledgement of the time and effort they devoted to the resolution process.

■ CASE SCENARIO

The presented scenario addresses many aspects of the Sunrise Enabler and brings the culture care modes into the conflict resolution process as a means for the readers to enhance their own understanding of the use and application of the culture care modes in transcultural nursing administration. Each mode is discussed in the context of applicable cultural and social structure dimensions from the Sunrise Enabler (McFarland & Wehbe-Alamah, 2015, pp. 17-18) which influence cultural worldview, values, and beliefs during conflict situations.

The scenario occurs at a university with a recent mandate directing that a new course in the health sciences college be offered and taught as an interprofessional class with joint participation by students and faculty from the disciplines of nursing, social work, respiratory therapy, radiological sciences, community environmental sciences, and kinesiology. There were faculty disagreements between these professional schools, as diverse worldviews existed among the faculty about the university, the college, and even faculty roles within their own school. The varied faculty worldviews guided decisions and actions, as faculty identified with one professional discipline's culture to a greater extent than with the worldview of the larger university organization.

The development of this new course, a common curricular faculty role responsibility, required faculty from multiple cultures to come together to work toward a common goal. The faculty tasked with this course development project also represented distinct professional cultures and worldviews that led to clashes in views and beliefs about the value of the task and resulted in conflicts and emotional angst. The "new course directive" affected curricula in all of the disciplines (cultures), which required many levels of change processes including intense work effort by the faculty task force; potential accreditation updates; and faculty consensus and a series of votes about the new course.

The project faculty belonged to the larger culture of the university and their professional disciplines who ultimately report to the same administrative team at the university (beyond their own professional schools). It appeared logical from a university and college administrative perspective that a task force of diverse faculty, representing all the schools, was formed to accomplish the goal of developing the new course. However, conflicts quickly arose when the task force members began to identify that "my discipline's way of doing this is the right way versus your discipline's approach." When conflicts develop, the main goal becomes lost because emotions heighten along with the ensuing disagreements and confusion.

An astute transcultural administrator can use the application of the three modes of culture care decisions and actions to address the conflict in this scenario. First, clarification of the goal for the task force by the administrator would provide a foundational basis for the group. For example: "We have a mandate by the university to create a one credit interprofessional course in ethics that will be taken together by all students from our college in combined sections. These sections will be taught by faculty representing all schools in the college following the same agreed upon course objectives and outcomes. Our deadline is to submit our college course to the university curriculum team in six months. Our goal is to create this course with approval by all members of this task force; it is then to be shared with all of our schools for final approval. We can all realize our task force has different views as to how we can best accomplish this goal and that there is no one absolute direction we must follow. Each member represents a unique professional culture (nursing, social work, respiratory therapy, radiological sciences, and community environmental sciences) and that each is very successful in our college. To accomplish our goal, we will use the three modes of culture care decisions and actions to assure that each profession's views are acknowledged and understood."

After establishing a clear goal, a transcultural administrator can initiate a process of cultural self-assessment among the professional educational cultures represented in the task force. Each professional culture represented is asked to reflect on the following self-assessment questions and then discuss their culture's views and beliefs:

- What are recognized key ethical values and beliefs within our professional culture that influence our current choice of curriculum?
- Do we have any strong values, beliefs, or biases about the other professions in our college? Can any values, beliefs, or biases be considered ethnocentric? Could any of these cause cultural imposition on other cultures in our college or in this assigned task force?
- What might the consequences be for our larger college culture if this process is unsuccessful? Who could be affected?

After a discussion of responses to these cultural self-assessment questions, the three modes of culture care decisions and actions can be applied in the task force conflict resolution process.

Culture care preservation and/or maintenance begins with introductions by the task force members; the transcultural administrator asks: "As you introduce yourself, please share with us what is important for your school/discipline to preserve as we approach this curricular change." One professional school may want to preserve their already complex course schedule as they perceive that it has no room for any additions or alterations. Another school may express that the topic of ethics is already well addressed in their curriculum and believe they do it well [enough]. Yet, another school may share that their national organization has required curricular standards about the teaching of ethics and they want to be assured the interprofessional course will meet these criteria. Multiple schools may express the need to preserve their faculty assignments without variation or alteration due to budgetary (school) or financial (personal) issues. Some faculty may want to preserve their status of having all of their classes offered on campus rather than in an online format. As the introductions progress, diverse and sometimes similar cultural views and beliefs are expressed and thus also become part of the transcultural and conflict resolution learning experience for all involved.

Cultural and social dimensions that may be identified in this scenario through application of this mode include educational factors, economic factors, and kinship and social factors. Educational factors important to the various team members include their curricula already in place. Revisions entail multiple levels of processes, accreditation criteria, and the effect on other courses in curricula–all of which must be considered. In addition, the task force must also determine which faculty members are qualified and desire to teach this new course. Economic factors of concern may elicit a series of questions: Budgets are tight… how do we teach a new class? My work assignment is full, will I be paid to develop this course? We have double the number of students than other schools; are we going to be compensated for that? Kinship and social factors also come into play as this may be one of the few times this diverse team is asked to work together as a college of which they are all members; in the past they may have only emphasized their representation of school and discipline.

Culture care accommodation and/or negotiation, identifies what can be negotiated between the cultures represented, including some levels of accommodating specific criteria. To accomplish this, acknowledging the team members' discussions of what they desire to preserve as a representative of their culture is a crucial step that facilitates learning about the other cultures within their college and moving beyond any preconceived assumptions and ethnocentric views. This mode offers the direction for discussions among the cultures as they learn about each other and move beyond their own worldview.

Cultural and social dimensions applicable in this case scenario for the represented faculty cultures include technology and kinship/social factors, which also influence the environmental context. Several of the schools have active online courses with faculty who are strong advocates for these integrated course methodologies. The faculty relate that their students (kinship) are very positive about taking online courses (technology). Course evaluations provide evidence of student satisfaction and success of online education in their schools. However, another faculty member represents a school that has limited online offerings because their faculty place a high value on campus experiences. Their student evaluations reflect a higher value for those courses than for online courses. Negotiations commence between the cultures represented in the curriculum team as they acknowledge what similar views they share: Desire to have a successful outcome as representatives of the college, a positive course experience for all students, faculty opportunities to share their expertise in a new manner, and meeting the goals of the team in a timely manner.

Faculty may agree to have multiple sections with options for students to take the course online, on campus, in a block weekend schedule, or a hybrid combination of several delivery methods. They could decide to recruit faculty based on their interests in the topic, create faculty teaching teams, or acquire a curriculum coordinator who has an assignment to work with this course specifically with all the represented schools. Student outcomes can be established with a plan for how to assess both the process and the identified outcomes. Revisions can be made thereafter in the future. The creative opportunities are endless and offer new avenues for faculty and students in interprofessional education.

Cultural care repatterning and/or restructuring is the plan for what needs to be repatterned or restructured in order to avert a negative outcome. Decisions are made using this mode for specific actions that will eliminate harmful tendencies and result in positive outcomes for the cultures represented, leading to successful accomplishment of the goal of the task force. The worldview of the college and individual professional cultures is relevant to recognize again at this point of assessing and planning for a successful development of the new course offering to meet the goal of establishing an interprofessional ethics class for all students in the college. Ethnocentric views are restructured in consideration of the common good. Each professional school has national accreditation standards (worldview) that need to be taken into consideration. In addition, the college as a larger culture embraces the worldview of the mission of the university; curricular processes for course revisions; and the commitment that faculty members are in charge of the curriculum. The college's worldview also is repatterned to include a vision for evolution with future plans for increased interprofessional courses, student activities, and community service.

The opportunities for success are influenced by and related to the creativity of the task force members as they progress through the culture care modes. As these various college subcultures of the professional schools work together using the three modes of culture care decisions and actions, they also evolve in their identification of a new subculture: The interprofessional subculture of the college.

■ SUMMARY

The application of Culture Care Theory is a strong beneficial framework for nurse administrators and managers within any facet of the health care system including professional preparatory education. The Culture Care Theory is a broad, holistic theory that uses the Sunrise Enabler as a cognitive map to guide nurse administrators as they explore and individualize culturally sensitive options for conflict resolution. A nursing administrator or manager dealing with daily conflict can apply the three modes of culture care decisions and actions. Administrators can create a handout, a pocket card, or a bookmark with the culture care modes written out in simple format and present it to the individuals involved in a cultural clash as a written guideline to direct their participation toward a positive and creative conflict resolution. As an administrator facilitates the use of the culture care modes with the parties involved, the written document will provide clarity and help to keep them focused on their purpose—conflict resolution.

Contemporary nursing administrators work in multicultural, interprofessional institutions as leaders with strong influences on care practices, policies, educational directions, and business models within health care systems. As nurses, they have opportunities to guide the processes for care and conflict resolution decisions and actions using the Culture Care Theory with a clear, holistic, and distinct approach. There are many leadership development program options for nursing leaders from a wide array of disciplines. The Theory of Culture Care Diversity and Universality, as a foundation of transcultural nursing administration, is a highly relevant, simple, and sustainable theoretical direction that will continue to advance administrative nursing as a discipline and profession.

■ DEDICATION

My work is dedicated in respect, honor, and loving memory to Dr. Madeline Leininger, a teacher, mentor, and friend.

■ ACKNOWLEDGEMENT

I would like to acknowledge my administrative team colleagues from Boise State University College of Health Sciences for their interprofessional collaborations within our curricula: Tim Dunnagan, EdD, Dean; Vivian Schrader, EdD, RN, Chair, Nursing; Denise Seigart, PhD, RN, Chair, Nursing; Dale Stephenson, PhD, CIH, Director, School of Allied Health Sciences; Karla West, PhD, Director, Counseling Services University Health Services; Lester, Jody, MA, RRT, Chair, Respiratory Care; and Leslie Kendrik, MS, RT, Chair, Radiologic Sciences.

■ DISCUSSION SCENARIOS

Scenario 1. You are a nurse manager in an outpatient family practice clinic for maternal child care. It has come to your attention that a nursing staff member is concerned about the behaviors of a client, Maria Lopez, a young mother who brings her two children (ages three years and six years) in for care frequently due to their asthma and severe allergies. Maria has stated in her family history that she and her family moved to this community three years ago after immigrating to the U.S. from Mexico and living with extended family in another state for two years. Her husband works in a factory in your community. Maria works in a Hispanically oriented food market. Her mother and aunt also live with them. Her aunt is employed in a restaurant, and her mother helps care for the children. Maria speaks minimal English, but her six-year-old daughter speaks English fairly well for a young child.

During a team staffing meeting, one of the senior nurses emotionally discussed with staff that Maria was "noncompliant" with the team's instructions, indicating that otherwise "…there would be better control with the children's symptoms" and that "…We just need to let her know there are consequences to this type of behavior." The nurse's remarks evoked some head nods, but another new nurse added, "…I disagree. Just because we are busy and do not feel we have enough time to spend with Maria does not mean we should label her as noncompliant with the implication that she does not listen to us or care about her children." As the manager, you can see that both nurses are now quite emotional about this situation.

As the preceptor to a nursing student who is taking a leadership course, you have decided to have the student join you as an observer in a meeting with Maria. The purpose of the meeting is to perform a cultural assessment of Maria and her family as a first step to addressing the conflict situation that exists between the senior nurse and Maria's family. When you tell the staff of your decision, the senior nurse responds, "Well, plan for extra time as she will probably not come alone and always has someone else with her who does not speak any English."

As a transcultural administrator/manager, apply the three modes of culture care decisions and actions for the questions that follow.

1. Select dimensions of the Sunrise Enabler's cultural and social structure dimensions relevant for the cultures represented by the nurses and Maria's family. Discuss why they are important for nurses to understand when working with Mexican American clients and families when they seek health care. Which dimensions apply to the subcultures of the nurses (i.e., the senior nurse versus new nurse; manager versus staff)?

2. Using culture care preservation and/or maintenance, consider both the nursing culture and Maria's culture. Clearly identify what needs to be preserved and/or maintained for both cultures as the process moves forward. Why?

3. Using culture care accommodation and/or negotiation, identify for the cultures in the conflict/s what needs to be accommodated and what can be negotiated.
4. Using culture care repatterning and/or restructuring, discuss how successful repatterning can occur between the nursing culture and Maria's culture to optimize her positive healing process. Identify what you would strive to repattern in this scenario.

Scenario 2. The Chair of the undergraduate baccalaureate nursing program has been approached by two classmates of a student during the second semester of the program. The students are concerned that although the school policies for receiving a grade have technically been followed, they feel their peer has unfairly received a C grade. Their friend, Tommy, is a member of the Navajo nation and is attending college away from his home state. They share with you that after the exam review session, Tommy realized that the faculty member had incorrectly marked several of his correct responses as wrong and deducted those points. Correcting the difference in the points would be enough to change his grade from a C to a B, but he says nothing and accepts the exam grade as is. His classmates are quite distraught and want to start a petition against the faculty member who they describe as "incompetent and careless." The students fear the C grade will negatively affect Tommy and his future success in the nursing program.

As a transcultural administrator/manager, discuss application of the three modes of culture care decisions and actions for the questions that follow.

1. Select dimensions of the Sunrise Enabler's cultural and social structure dimensions relevant for the cultures represented by the students and the faculty. Discuss why they are important to understand in this scenario. How are the identified dimensions influenced by the worldviews of the cultures represented?
2. Using culture care preservation and/or maintenance, consider both the student culture and the faculty culture. Clearly identify what needs to be preserved and/or maintained for both cultures as the process moves forward. Why?
3. Using culture care accommodation and/or negotiation, identify for the cultures in the conflict/s what needs to be accommodated and what can be negotiated.

4. Using culture care repatterning and/or restructuring, discuss how successful repatterning can occur between the identified cultures. Identify what you would repattern in this scenario.

Scenario 3. Two faith-based hospitals located in the same town have announced that they are merging into one corporation. As a result, both of the nursing departments are being reorganized into one corporate nursing division, with the goal of having all policies come into alignment within one year. Imagine that you are a nurse manager who is asked to facilitate the policy development process for the home health and hospice services emerging from departments within these two institutions. You have recently attended an international Transcultural Nursing Society conference where you participated in sessions focused on transcultural nursing administration and are eager to put your new knowledge into positive action. However, you know there is strong resistance within your own hospital organization to the upcoming mandated changes based on prevalent comments from the nursing staff such as "Our identity will be gone!".... "Why was this decision made so quickly?" .... "How many of us will lose our positions?".... "We have always been the *best* hospital!".... "Our standards will only be lowered." Anxieties have begun to increase as the merger date approaches. Because you have attended multiple management sessions about the merger, you do not share these views and do not want these conflicting thoughts to lead to dissatisfaction and confusion.

As a transcultural administrator/manager, you begin with an organizational cultural assessment conducted within the units of the two institutions. How would you first organize this process using the three modes of culture care decisions and actions for the questions that follow?

1. Select dimensions of the Sunrise Enabler's cultural and social structure dimensions relevant for the cultures represented by the nurses of the two institutions. Discuss why they are important to understand in this scenario. How are the identified dimensions influenced by the worldviews of the cultures being discussed?
2. Using culture care preservation and/or maintenance, clearly identify what to be preserved and/or maintained for both cultures as the process moves forward. Why?

3. Using culture care accommodation and/or negotiation, identify for the cultures in the conflict/s what needs to be accommodated and what can be negotiated.

4. Using culture care repatterning and/or restructuring, there is a successful repatterning that can occur between the identified cultures. Identify what you would strive to repattern in this scenario.

■ REFERENCES

American Association of Colleges of Nursing. (2014, October 8). *AACN's virtual book club* [Leadership Discussion Board]. Retrieved from https://mail.google.com/mail/u/0/?ui=2&ik=a082e45f87&view=pt&search=trash&th=148f01f803917d24&siml=148f01f803917d24

American Nurses' Association. (2014, June 18). *Health care reform: Health care transformation: The affordable care act and more.* Retrieved from http://nursingworld.org/MainMenuCategories/PolicyAdvocacy/HealthSystemReform/AffordableCareAct.pdf

Andrews, M. M., & Boyle, J. S. (2012). Culturally competent nursing care. In M. M. Andrews and J. S. Boyle, J. S. (Eds.), *Transcultural concepts in nursing care* (6th ed., pp. 17-37). Philadelphia, PA: Lippincott Williams & Wilkins.

Horn, B. (2002). Urban USA transcultural care challenges with multiple cultures and culturally diverse providers. In M. M. Leininger and M. R. McFarland (Eds.), *Transcultural nursing concepts, theories, research & practice* (3rd ed., pp. 263-270). New York, NY: McGraw-Hill.

Hubbert, A. O. (2006). Application of culture care theory for clinical nurse administrators and managers. In M. M. Leininger and M. R. McFarland (Eds.), *Culture care diversity and universality; A worldwide nursing theory* (2nd ed., pp. 349-364). Sudbury, MA: Jones and Bartlett.

Johansen, B. (2012). *Leaders make the future ten new leadership skills for an uncertain world* (2nd ed.). San Francisco, CA: Berrett-Koehler Publishers.

Leininger, M. M. (1991). The theory of culture care diversity and universality. In M. M. Leininger (Ed.), *Culture care diversity & universality: A theory of nursing* (pp. 5-68). New York, NY: National League for Nursing Press.

Leininger, M. M. (1995). Overview of Leininger's theory of culture care. In M. M. Leininger (Ed.), Transcultural nursing: *Transcultural nursing concepts, theories, research & practice* (pp. 93-112). New York, NY: McGraw-Hill.

Leininger, M. M. (1996). Founder's Focus: Transcultural nursing administration: An imperative worldwide. *Journal of Transcultural Nursing, 8*(1), 28-33.

Leininger, M. M. (1998). Dominant culture care (emic) meanings and practice findings from Leininger's theory. *Journal of Transcultural Nursing, 9*(2), 45-48.

Leininger, M. M. (2002a). Essential transcultural nursing care, concepts, principles, examples, and policy statements. In M. M. Leininger and M. R. McFarland (Eds.), *Transcultural nursing concepts, theories, research & practice* (3rd ed., pp. 45-69). New York, NY: McGraw-Hill.

Leininger, M. M. (2002b). The theory of culture care and the ethnonursing research method. In M. M. Leininger and M. R. McFarland (Eds.), *Transcultural nursing concepts, theories, research & practice* (3rd ed., pp. 71-98). New York, NY: McGraw-Hill.

Leininger, M. M. (2006). Culture care theory and uses in nursing administration. In M. M. Leininger and M. R. McFarland (Eds.), *Culture care diversity and universality: A worldwide nursing theory* (2nd ed., pp. 365-379). Sudbury, MA: Jones and Bartlett.

Ludwig-Beymer, P. (2008). Creating culturally competent organizations. In M. M. Andrews and J. S. Boyle (Eds.). *Transcultural concepts in nursing care* (5th ed., pp. 197-225).

McFarland, M. R., & Wehbe-Alamah, H. B. (2015). The theory of culture care diversity and universality. In M. R. McFarland and H. B. Wehbe-Alamah (Eds.), *Leininger's culture care diversity and universality: A worldwide nursing theory* (3rd ed., pp. 2-34). Burlington, MA: Jones and Bartlett Learning.

Mixer, S. J. (2015). Application of culture care theory in teaching cultural competence and culturally congruent care. In M. R. McFarland and H. B. Wehbe-Alamah (Eds.), *Leininger's culture care diversity and universality: A worldwide nursing theory* (3rd ed., pp. 369-387). Burlington, MA: Jones and Bartlett Learning.

Schein, E. H. (2010). *Organization culture and leadership.* San Francisco, CA: Jossey-Bass.

Scott, E. S. (2010). Perspectives on healthcare leader and leadership development. *Journal of Healthcare Leadership, 2,* 83-90. Retrieved from http://www.dovepress.com/perspectives-on-health care-leader-and-leadership-development-peer-reviewed-article-JHL#

Slavkin, H.C. (2010). Leadership for health care in the 21st Century: A personal perspective. *Journal of Healthcare Leadership, 2,* 35-41. Retrieved from http://www.dovepress.com/leadership-for-health-care-in-the-21st-century-a-personal-perspective-peer-reviewed-article-JHL#

Wakeman, C. (2010). *Reality-based leadership.* San Francisco, CA: Jossey-Bass.

Wakeman, C. (2013a). *The reality-based rules of the workplace.* San Francisco, CA: Jossey-Bass.

Wakeman, C. (2013b). *Reality-based rules of the workplace – know what boosts your value, kills your chances, and will make you happier at work* [Workshop]. American Association of Colleges of Nursing Summer Seminar, July 21-24, 2013, Vail, CO.

Enhancing the Role of the Transcultural Nurse in the Global Environment

Mary Brigid Martin and Marilyn A. Ray

▪ *"No culture can live, if it attempts to be exclusive"* (*Mahatma Gandhi*)

▪ INTRODUCTION

Leininger (2002) predicted that by the year 2015 health care systems must be transculturally based (p. 577) to care for diverse cultures of the world. The "mother" of transcultural nursing was ever so intuitive: This reality is already upon nurses and the call to be culturally astute as a caregiver amid turbulent global dynamics has never been more necessary. Local, national, and world events indicate transcultural understanding and development are evolving, sustainability at all levels is of great concern, and social conflicts persist, causing human rights violations, social injustice, and other detriments to humanity.

The time is now for nurses to practice to the full extent of their education and enact their capacity as cultural experts within nursing and the interdisciplinary domain. Nurses, especially nurses educated as transcultural nurses, have the knowledge and skills to interpret issues and make decisions through a transcultural lens. McFarland and Leininger (2011) attested that collaborative caring is needed to achieve global cooperation. Many opportunities exist for nurses to support policy and enact practice that upholds equity, as issues that seem international in nature, such as human rights and social justice values (Ray & Turkel, 2014), are of concern locally, particularly when caring for the vulnerable.

Within nursing, there is a philosophy and "...ethic of social caring—a practice of how we think after identifying through critical reflection, dialogue, reasoned argumentation, beliefs, values of human dignity, human rights [respect for human dignity] and social justice (or fairness) that must be woven into the cultural fabric of daily life" (Ray & Turkel, 2014, p. 132). Nurses must know the international organizational initiatives that aim to improve the quality of life worldwide. Local is global and global is local. Consider the issues related to poverty, food insecurity, challenges encountered by immigrants, drug abuse, human rights violations, and violence all over the world. The roles of advocate for human rights and social justice and as interdisciplinary collaborators will serve to define nurses' place in the global arena.

These phenomena pose opportunities for the 13 million nurses worldwide (International Council of Nurses [ICN], 2014) to re-examine the use of Leininger's *Theory of Culture Care Diversity and Universality*. In this chapter, the theory (with Sunrise Enabler) serves as a guiding framework to discover evidence-based knowledge that influences the understanding of sociocultural factors that define health, and the adaptation of nursing practice in our increasingly culturally diverse world. Global nursing begins at home, wherever that may be. This chapter addresses how cultural values related to social structural dimensions, including kinship and social factors, religious and/or philosophical factors, economic factors, educational factors, environmental, technological, and political/legal factors, critically influence the health and well-being of our increasingly interconnected global humanity.

■ THE ROLE OF THE TRANSCULTURAL NURSE IN THE GLOBAL ENVIRONMENT

The role of the nurse in the global environment requires attention to the increasing migration of populations and health disparity/minority health worldwide, and the need for the provision of culturally congruent care in health care practices. These issues deserve the attention of the millions of nurses globally because they also have meaning locally. Culturally astute nurses will keep abreast of international news and events and have knowledge of key organizations that unite nursing and health care interests, such as the ICN (2014) and the World Health Organization (WHO, 2014).

Migration, Health Disparities, Minority Health, and Culturally Congruent Care

Migration is a dynamic and diversifying force in global development. Migrating people seeking opportunities for improved living and working conditions is an international phenomenon. Many nations are attempting to deal with and understand issues of political power and control, conflicts, sectarianism, terrorism, poverty, famine, and disease, while at the same time addressing humanitarian needs by facilitating transcultural understanding and peaceful solutions (Ray, 2010a, 2010b). In 2013, 232 million people worldwide were immigrants (3.2% of the global population) compared with 175 million in 2000 and 154 million in 1990 (United Nations Department of Economic and Social Affairs [UNDESA], 2013). That same year, nearly half of all immigrants lived in only 10 countries worldwide, with the U.S. having the largest number (45.8 million), followed by Russia (11 million); Germany (9.8 million); Saudi Arabia (9.1 million); United Arab Emirates (7.8 million); United Kingdom (7.8 million); France (7.4 million);

Canada (7.3 million); Australia (6.5 million); and Spain (6.5 million) (UNDESA, 2013). Some nations are making attempts to deal with immigration concerns. For example in the United States, President Barack Obama took executive action to influence immigration law that would help five million undocumented immigrants remain in this country (American Immigration Council, 2014).

While nurses worldwide may encounter immigrants in their practices, Western countries lead the way as host countries—the United States with 13% of the population, Australia with 19.6%, and Canada (18.9%; UNDESA, 2013). Populations that migrate often face discrimination and isolation and may compete with other groups for access to resources including health care (Pacquiao, 2008). Historic and present social contexts, prejudice, and bias also impact differences in care by influencing discriminatory behaviors among providers (Ray, 2010a, 2010b, 2016; Smedley, Stith, & Nelson, 2002). While progress has been made in reducing disparities, the Institute of Medicine (2012) has attested that further data collection is needed to improve the multifaceted environmental and mental health issues that influence disparities, minority health, and cultural competence. Health disparities are not only moral and professional imperatives, they are civil rights injustices that must be eliminated (American College of Physicians, 2010). Nurses are well positioned to advocate for equity in the provision of health care and in support for patient rights, whether institutionally (as in a hospital patient bill of rights), nationally (as in civil rights), or globally (as in human rights, as cited in the Universal Declaration of Human Rights (U. N., 2014a).

The Transcultural Nursing Society, the International Association for Human Caring, and the International Council of Nurses are nursing organizations that are advancing and enhancing knowledge of culturally congruent care. Culturally congruent care practices will be expected from nurses worldwide who care for diverse populations (Leininger, 2002). Within this perspective, it is important to recognize that nearly half of the world's migrants are women (UNDESA, 2013) who will require care from nurses with knowledge of transcultural maternal-child health and elder care.

While the title transcultural nurse is limitedly recognized worldwide, most nurses in the world will not carry a certification credential as a transcultural nurse. Nonetheless, it is imperative that basic, advanced, and continuing nursing education worldwide be designed to include content about cultural diversity and culturally congruent care, particularly about the populations for whom these nurses provide direct care. In the United States for example, the American Association of Colleges of Nursing (AACN, 2008, 2011) has included culture, caring, and complexity as central constructs for both undergraduate and graduate curricula (France & Ray, 2013). Complexity sciences illuminate the notion of the interconnectedness of all things (human-environment integrality), choice-making within networks of relationships, and transcultural caring dynamics (Ray, 2010a, 2010b, 2016). These phenomena are articulated within the concept of culture itself and identified differently in culture theories and international organizations; thus, highlighting what is necessary for student learning now and in the future (Ray, 2010a, 2010b, 2016).

Key International Organizations

Learning about the initiatives of international organizations such as the U.N., WHO, and ICN may reveal the universal nature of nurses' roles and human needs and in turn support global awareness of key needs and developments that influence health, caring, and healing.

The United Nations

The initiatives of the United Nations (U.N.) (2014b) include sustainable development; environmental and refugee protection; disaster relief; counter-terrorism; disarmament and nonproliferation; human rights; gender equality and the advancement of women; promotion of democratic, economic, and social development; international health; and food production. Smith (2006) explained that the U.N. is the only universal membership and general-purpose international organization in the world, and as such, is the main venue to pursue these efforts. An important initiative of the U.N. is the 2015 Millennium Development Goals (MDG) (United Nations Development Program [UNDP], 2014) developed more than a decade ago that created a framework for international development. The MDGs encompass multiple dimensions of ongoing efforts spearheaded by the U.N. and its affiliated governmental agencies and nongovernmental

organizations (NGOs). Interdisciplinary collaboration builds bridges for problem solving, therefore, it is important for nursing organizations to know which avenues exist to connect with the work of the U.N. These include the primary options for organizations and institutions to either apply for designation as an U. N.-affiliated NGO or apply for designation as a WHO-affiliated collaborating center. Further information is available online at the respective organizational websites for specific application requirements.

The Universal Declaration of Human Rights was agreed upon by the U.N. General Assembly on December 10, 1948 after the Second World War in an effort to proclaim that the violence that had occurred therein would never recur (U.N., 2014a). This is the legal document that outlines the basic rights and freedoms of mankind and addresses such issues as discrimination, torture, disabilities, and the rights of women, children, migrants, minorities, and indigenous peoples (U.N., 2014a). The Declaration was intended to provide minimum human rights standards for all nations; the challenge has been compliance with this international law in the face of inherent sociocultural differences between countries. The U.N. supports this international law across all nations in the interest of ensuring a world that is free from discrimination, slavery, genocide, and murder (U.N., 2014a). Nurses must know that all persons have a right to culture but that cultural rights are not unlimited, nor shall they be used at the expense of another (Ayton-Shenker, 1995).

The World Health Organization

The WHO is the health authority within the United Nations that provides direction on global health issues; formulates the international health research agenda, standards, and policies; and tracks and evaluates global health trends (WHO, 2014). The WHO is divided into six regions across the globe: Region of the Americas (Pan American Health Organization); Eastern Mediterranean Region; African Region; European Region; Southeast Asia Region; and Western Pacific Region (WHO, 2014). Within each region there are institutions designated by the WHO that coordinate and facilitate its programs to advance health locally, nationally, and internationally (WHO, 2014). Nurses may become involved in conferences and other activities by networking with collaborating centers located in their area and may even seek the distinguished status as of becoming a collaborating center through formal processes with the WHO.

The International Council of Nurses

Founded in 1899, the ICN is a partnership of more than 130 national nurses associations that represents nurses worldwide and promotes quality nursing care, global health policy, the progression of nursing knowledge and the profession itself, and the competency of and satisfaction within the global nursing workforce (ICN, 2014). Nurses may obtain free membership in the ICN as part of their national nurses' association membership, such as the American Nurses' Association. An extensive website presents activities and initiatives of the ICN at http://www.icn.ch/membership.

■ THE ROLE OF THE NURSE IN THE UNITED STATES ENVIRONMENT

The Patient Protection and Affordable Care Act (PPAFA) was signed into law by President Barack Obama on March 23, 2010, with a final decision to uphold the law issued on June 28, 2012 by the U. S. Supreme Court (The White House, 2012). This legislation underscores the provision of quality, affordable health care for all Americans; public programs toward improving quality and efficiency of health care, prevention of chronic disease, development of the health care workforce, transparency and integrity of health care programs, improving access to innovative medical therapies, community living assistance and services, revenue provisions, and reauthorization of the Indian Health Care Improvement Act (Indian Health Service, n. d.). While The PPAFA law was proposed so as to put consumers in charge of their own health care, the new law also gives Americans the stability and flexibility to make informed choices about their health (The White House, 2012). Because this law has provisions for improving the health care workforce, it will behoove transcultural nurses to raise their voices to facilitate culturally relevant care for all citizens through practice, administration, policy development, research (including leading interdisciplinary research teams), and the advancement of cultural competence (Cultural Competence Project, 2014). Culturally competent nurses are well positioned to assist health care consumers to understand insurance options in considering their resources and unique family needs (Ludwig-Beymer, 2014).

The aforementioned organizations are integrating local, national, and global health concerns in their goals and directives related to practice, policy, education, and development. Contemporary nurses must be aware of the work of these organizations and integrate their principles into their own practices in the interest of culturally congruent, equitable, optimal patient care for all populations.

■ TRANSCULTURAL NURSING INHERENT IN GLOBAL NURSING PRACTICE

Nurses who demonstrate transcultural nursing competence aim to maintain and preserve human rights, a global concern for the wellbeing of humanity. Transcultural nursing care "…upholds the universal human right to cultural justice" (Miller et al., 2008, p. 6). In the United States and abroad, nurses may role model human rights advocacy in their communities and practice arenas and inform about policy related to civil and human rights issues. Nurses possess skills that empower their role as advocates for human rights regardless of their country of origin and practice. It is essential that the nurses know policy about patient and civil rights pertinent to their institutional affiliations and country of practice respectively, as well as internationally recognized human rights, such as the Universal Declaration of Human Rights (U. N., 2014a).

■ LEININGER'S THEORY OF CULTURE CARE DIVERSITY AND UNIVERSALITY

Leininger (1977) was the first nurse-anthropologist in the world. In her studies and research, Leininger discovered that understanding the relationship between culture and care was the most crucial challenge of nursing, stating that anthropology is "…the study of culture, the blueprint for man's [humans'] way of living, and only by understanding culture can we hope to gain the fullest understanding of man [human] as a social and cultural being" (Leininger, 1970, p. vii). "…Care [and caring] is a universal phenomenon that has endured beyond specific cultures, and has brought forth important humanistic attributes of care-givers and care-recipients (Leininger, 1977, p. 2). Leininger stated that there was a need to blend the two worlds of nursing and anthropology/caring and culture for understanding the practice of nursing and to form new conduits for thought and research (Leininger, 1970; Ray, 2010a, 2010b; Ray, Morris, & McFarland, 2013).

■ SOCIAL STRUCTURAL DIMENSIONS OF THE SUNRISE ENABLER

The idea of human rights or the evolution of understanding the values of human dignity of people from all cultures were always a central part of Leininger's Theory of Culture Care Diversity and Universality (Leininger, 1985, 2002; McFarland & Leininger, 2006; McFarland & Wehbe-Alamah, 2015). Her focus as a transcultural nurse was on caring as the essence of nursing and the call for caring as a foundation to transcultural nursing practice (Leininger, 1977). Within this framework, as a nurse and as an anthropologist, Leininger claimed that "…caring is one of the oldest and most universal expectations for human development and survival through our long history and in different places in the world" (1977, p. 2). The following paragraphs describe the holistic nature of transcultural nursing within the context of understanding the dynamic social structural phenomena of Leininger's Sunrise Enabler (cultural values, beliefs and lifeways, kinship and social factors, religious and philosophical factors, economic, educational, environmental, technological, political, and legal factors) (Leininger, 1977, 2002; Leininger & McFarland, 2006; McFarland & Wehbe-Alamah, 2015). Throughout history, mankind has cocreated governing societies, for social survival in the world, that ultimately influence health, healing, and wellbeing locally and globally. Please refer to **Sunrise Enabler (Color Insert 1)** to appreciate how Leininger's theory relates to the MDGs and the manner in which the interrelationship between local and global health (and vice versa) exists within the discipline and practice of transcultural nursing.

The overarching factors of the Sunrise Enabler (as previously stated) identify specific social structure domains and are dynamic. Social structural phenomena are, in essence, the social determinants of health and wellbeing in diverse cultures. They "hold within them" values, beliefs, and attitudes and determine meaning and action in nation states. Subsequently, they facilitate the direction or holistic ways in which

problems can be solved. For example, political, economic, legal, kinship, religious structures, and social-cultural determinants must be understood so that political leaders, clerics, and health care professionals can facilitate understanding of how social-cultural factors influence caring, health, healing, dying, and death (McFarland & Leininger, 2006; Ray, 2010a, 2010b). Nurses sensitive to the cultural needs of patients, families, and communities must consider these social-culture factors across the care continuum: admission, history taking, patient assessment, provision of care, and discharge planning (McFarland & Leininger, 2006; Ray, 2010a, 2010b). Socio-cultural factors, illuminated in the Millennium Development Goals (MDGs), are identified as follows:

1. Eradication of extreme poverty and hunger
2. Achievement of universal primary education
3. Promotion of gender equality and empowerment of women
4. Reduction of child mortality
5. Improvement of maternal health
6. Combating of HIV/AIDS, malaria, and other diseases
7. Ensuring of environmental sustainability
8. Development of a global partnership for development (UNDP, 2014)

The MDGs are global health care priorities that relate directly to the social structure factors of the Sunrise Enabler. All Sunrise Enabler factors and all MDGs impact the health and quality of life of people around the world. The following explication of the social structure factors provide context for these relationships between the factors of the Sunrise Enabler and the MDGs.

Cultural Values, Beliefs, and Lifeways

Cultural values, beliefs, and lifeways facilitate increasing migration from area to another because of war and ideological conflict, poverty, food insecurity, crime, and unsafe social environments that negatively affect health and wellbeing. For example, MDG 6, which addresses HIV/AIDS, also entails the spread of life threatening communicable diseases (such as Ebola from West Africa) related in part to increased international travel. MDG 6 and MDG 2 (universal primary education) raise concerns for the spread of disease and child exploitation within violent crime, gangs, drug use, organized crime, human/sex trafficking, and child abuse/abandonment.

Kinship and Social Factors

There is a changing definition of family in many parts of the world; for example, the Lesbian, Gay, Bisexual, and Transgender population, and the interest of their civil/human rights and unique health needs. Consider the work at hand to accomplish MDG 3 that addresses gender equality and empowering women, MDG 4 that addresses child mortality rates, and MDG 5 that addresses maternal health issues. These MDGs help us to see the needs of women and the fact that, as stated earlier, within migratory patterning, more than 50% of the people migrating are women (UNDESA, 2013).

Religious and/or Philosophical Factors

Diverse groups and regions in conflict have created increased migrations by groups from diverse backgrounds who have culture specific care needs across the care continuum—birth, illness, health maintenance, and end of life. Philosophically, consider the ambitions of MDGs 2, 3, 4, and 5 that speak to the imperative for universal education, care for the needs of women and children (maternal-child health), and gender equality and the empowerment of women.

Philosophically, consider the ambitions of MDGs 2, 3, 4, and 5 that speak to the imperative for universal education, care for the needs of women and children (maternal-child health), and gender equality and the empowerment of women.

Economic Factors

Most countries around the developing world are influenced by the lack of resources for combating poverty; feeding populations; building housing and infrastructures such as roads, sanitation devices, and clean water supplies; and overall maintaining a safe way of life. MDG 1 addresses the eradication of extreme poverty and hunger that, in part, is influenced by economics (UNDP, 2014). MDG 6 addresses HIV/AIDS and other diseases as previously described that have not only negative health outcomes but also a negative economic impact. MDGs 7 and 8 address environmental sustainability and global partnerships for development. These MDGs address the fact that all nations must work toward global sustainability as

they claimed they would be when they signed the U.N. Millennium Declaration in 2000 (UNDP, 2014). The global economy and the international corporate economy are interconnected; hence when there are ebbs and flows, these dynamics have worldwide impact affecting financial resources, employment, banking, housing markets, and personal disposable income (UNDP, 2014).

Educational Factors

Education is the key to health and wellbeing and supports knowledge of cultures, transcultural interaction, health and health care. Within nations, migration takes place to gain access to education; here is a need for parity in education for all, especially for women and children (UNDP, 2014). Consider MDG 2, which addresses the achievement of universal primary education; educational disparity, and the persistence of child labor worldwide that leads to compromised quality of life for the youth of the world (UNDP, 2014).

Environmental Factors

Protection of the environment for the sake of health and wellbeing has always been a challenge to the world community, whether nations are developed or developing. Consider MDG 7 that addresses environmental sustainability; many nations are in the business of economic wellbeing as opposed to environmental wellbeing even though health means wealth. On November 11, 2014 in China, the Chinese Prime Minister Xi Jinping and U.S. President Barack Obama (the two biggest economies and greenhouse gas emitters) formed an agreement that they will partner closely on a broad-ranging package of plans to improve the climate, reduce carbon pollution in preparation for negotiations toward a new climate treaty in Paris in 2015 (McDonnell & West, 2014).

Technological Factors

Technology has changed the world. Computer technology, Internet access, and social media over the last few decades have influenced most cultures to the extent that they refer to the notion of the *cybersphere* reshaping human reality (Floridi, 2014). Computers and social media have connected people from all parts of the world with both good and bad consequences. Technology aids to facilitate education in new ways. At the same time, technology has facilitated more time spent on computers, which can be either healthy or unhealthy in terms of forming relationships with technology that influence our lifestyles (such as Internet and gaming addictions); sedentary lifestyles; isolation/decreased social contact; cyber-bullying; privacy issues; personal safety/security with Internet/social media use (Floridi, 2014).

Political Factors

Ongoing wars, ethnic cleansing, and genocide in Syria and other countries in the Middle East, Africa, and the Ukraine/Russia, to name but a few, have resulted in millions of people being displaced. Countries who bear the influx of refugees and who compete for already limited resources experience backlashes of violent crime, drug use, organized crime, human trafficking, and child abuse/abandonment/exploitation—the unsavory outcomes of war (Ray, 2010a, 2010b; Wolfe, 2011). Power, control, and other factors of political systems have influenced the decline of health in many nations causing increased suffering, hunger, lack of adequate housing or shelter, illness, and human misery. We must look at MDGs 1, 7, and 8 to engage and be committed to forming global partnerships that will sustain humanity and the environment, and facilitate the development of a peaceful world for the growth and development of humanity and the human spirit.

Legal Factors

Legal agreements are what bind nations together. The MDG agreement established in 2000 for international cooperation and development (for initiation by 2015) was signed by all 189 U.N. member states (UNDP, 2014). They embraced these goals in good faith. Regulations and/or binding agreements affect the lives of all people; the hope is the MDGs will similarly/positively affect the lives of people around the world who live in signatory nations. It is the nurse's responsibility to meet standards, uphold legislation in practice, and at the same time engage in policy development that will encourage commitment to the MDGs as well as the goals of the WHO, ICN, and other organizations such as the Transcultural Nursing Society that are committed to addressing the culture care needs of people around the world.

MDG Post 2015 Agenda

While there have been advances in the achievement of the MDGs by the 2015 deadline, this has not been consistent among all countries. Further progress is imperative. The U. N. Secretary-General in 2012 formed a U. N. System Task Team on the Post-2015 U. N. Development Agenda that addresses a broader focus including Sustainable Development Goals (SDGs) such as sustainability of cities, climate change, protection of forests and oceans, as well as continued focus on poverty, food insecurity, health, and education (U. N., 2015).

■ THREE MODES OF CULTURE CARE DECISIONS AND ACTIONS

Leininger was the first nursing theorist who accomplished what is now known as translational science or translational research and practice (Ray et al., 2013). Leininger's Theory of Culture Care Diversity and Universality and the Sunrise Enabler provide a framework for learning what is needed to become aware, understand, facilitate, and direct patient care in terms of the three modes of culture care decisions and actions. By outlining the social structural dimensions (factors), such as the Kinship and Social Factors; Religious and Philosophical Factors; Cultural Values, Beliefs, and Lifeways; Political and Legal Factors; Economic Factors; Technological and Educational Factors, Leininger showed the influencers on care expressions, patterns, and practices. She identified the fact that for individuals, families, groups, communities, or institutions in diverse health contexts, there was an interplay between generic (folk) care, professional care-cure practices, and nursing care practices that guided transcultural care decisions and actions for *culture care preservation and/or maintenance*; *culture care accommodation and/or negotiation*; and *culture care repatterning and/or restructuring* (Leininger, 1985, 1991; McFarland & Wehbe-Alamah, 2015; Ray et al., 2013). Leininger's modes of culture care decisions and actions for culturally congruent nursing care in the global environment call for attention to the needs of an increasingly diverse patient population (Ray et al., 2013). The three culture care modes directly relate to decision making that supports choice, patient safety, and optimal health outcomes.

Culture Care Preservation and/or Maintenance

This culture care mode identifies the fact that when we engage with people of another culture, we must be cognizant and sensitive to what should be understood, preserved, and maintained in a cultural practice (Leininger, 1985, 1991). For example, it is unethical for a nurse to try to change a familial care pattern on his or her own without consultation with the patient or family member. Although everything in culture is dynamic and constantly changing, especially when people interact with each other, it is the nurse's responsibility to be sensitive about how he or she communicates so that caring patterns are respected and honored for maintenance of wellbeing within a culture.

Culture Care Accommodation and/or Negotiation

This culture care mode provides a means for the transcultural nurse to address how to accommodate culture care or negotiate change based on evidence-based science and care practices for patient safety (Ray et al., 2013). For example, with a person not familiar with taking an antibiotic for a bacterial infection, for culturally congruent care for health and wellbeing, one must examine the culture care practices that the patient and family use and also negotiate with them regarding the taking of a medication that will facilitate a possible biological cure of the disease.

Culture Care Repatterning and/or Restructuring

This culture care mode provides for cultural repatterning. For example, in sub-Saharan Africa the Ebola crisis persists having killed more than 4,000 people (Matua, 2015). Seeking understanding of the cultures of sub-Saharan nations in general in terms of Ebola, for example, calls for repatterning of local cultures (Matua & Locsin, 2016). This repatterning involves modifying the African people's relationship with food sources, discovering how to improve the safety of their interactions with people infected with the disease, and developing and promoting better understandings of the human side of Ebola outbreaks (Matua, 2015). But how can this issue be approached culturally, emotionally, economically, morally, and politically? What does repatterning and/or restructuring of deep seated cultural practices mean?

Leininger stated that for potential emotional, moral, and political changes to occur in nations (such as those suffering with Ebola), the social structural factors of Leininger's Sunrise Enable and three modes of culture care decisions and actions can be used to guide the change process (2002). Transcultural communication with key leaders in health care, nursing, medicine, politics, and the survivors themselves is necessary to first determine what cultural patterns can be preserved and/or maintained, and how culturally congruent care needs can be accommodated and if needed negotiated to improve care, health, healing, wellbeing, and policies. Culture care repatterning and/or restructuring is used to address policies and practices that are unsafe or lead or harmful outcomes for health and wellbeing. Policies are complex adaptive systems generated from knowledge of ethnohistory, but are only as strong as the commitment to understanding the culture of the people or citizens at large in diverse nation-states.

Culturally congruent care requires that the nurse holds a great deal of knowledge about a frequently encountered culture including its ethnohistory, caring and curing practices, levels of education, and preferred means of communication. With transcultural understanding, caring, and loving kindness, a nurse is able to communicate kindly and sincerely with members of a nation for the purposes of changing a culture for their safety, wellbeing, and health. Often culturally congruent care requires "living with people of a culture" to gain understanding. Sometimes, this understanding does not happen. Health, wellbeing, dying, or death are complex phenomena and require of us and others hope for a future that will be better than the past or the present. "Respect for persons, cultivating humanity through a commitment to peace, power, justice, and caring are uncompromising" (Ray & Turkel, 2014, p. 144).

◼ SUMMARY

Leininger's contribution to theory development and her understanding of transcultural nursing knowledge has changed the world of nursing. As a human scientist, she had the intuition, knowledge, assertiveness, and sheer will to take risks. She stated that caring was the essence of nursing and, as an anthropologist and transcultural nurse, caring for self and others was the oldest form of human expression (Leininger, 1981). She did this at a time when others were advancing a more positivist notion of the discipline; she highlighted the fact that the culture care needs of people of the world would be fulfilled by nurses educated in transcultural nursing and caring (Leininger, 1981). She was creative, an innovator, a scientist, theorist, mentor, teacher, and a friend. She developed the view in ethnonursing research (her innovation) "from stranger to friend," and indeed, she was.

The background of nursing knowledge has transitioned from a receptive phase wherein nursing knowledge was attained from other disciplines, to a self-generative phase wherein knowledge focused on nursing itself, and then on to a transformative phase wherein nursing knowledge has the capacity to influence nursing practice and disciplines other than nursing (Newman, Smith, Dexheimer, Pharris, & Jones, 2008). The time is now for nurses with transcultural expertise to inform other disciplines, as we possess a definitive body of knowledge derived from both nursing and the social sciences including anthropology, psychology, and political science. Nurses hold a crucial place in understanding cultures through interdisciplinary collaboration at all levels of education, practice, and research and can provide a health perspective that may otherwise be overlooked by non-health professionals.

The role of the nurse in the global environment commands attention to ongoing migration patterns, especially in the context of local practices. In our proximity to patients, nurses are posited to research causes of health disparities and provide leadership for culturally congruent care practices that promote optimal patient outcomes. Leininger's (2002) prediction that health care systems must be transculturally based (p. 577) conveys not only the timeliness of the matter, but distinguishes the leader of transcultural nursing as indeed forward thinking and undoubtedly caring about the world's people.

■ DEDICATION

The authors dedicate this work to caring nurses worldwide and all humanitarian aid workers who so selflessly give of themselves to others—often at the risk of their own lives.

■ DISCUSSION QUESTIONS

1. Discuss each of the factors of the Sunrise Enabler in relation to a patient in a recent nursing situation. How do each of these factors influence the wellbeing and quality of life of this patient?
2. Reflect upon each of the factors in the Sunrise Enabler in relation to yourself. How does this self-reflection affect your perspective about how these factors influence your own wellbeing and quality of life?
3. Describe two ways transcultural nursing knowledge may benefit policy development in your health care workplace.
4. Describe two organizations nurses may access for information on international health issues.
5. Research one nongovernmental organization (NGO) in the region where you live. Discuss how the expertise of a transcultural nurse/nurse (either volunteer or paid) may benefit the organization.
6. Research a job opening at a nongovernmental organization (NGO) that may be suitable for a nurse, locally or beyond. What are the application process and job requirements? Do you meet them? Would you consider such work?
7. Research a health care organization that engages in international work, such as Doctors Without Borders. Can you see where there is a fit for the services of transcultural nurse/nurse? How? Where? When and for how long? What is the role description and compensation, if any?
8. Identify an international news event that has occurred or is currently occurring outside of your country. How has it affected your personal perspective, professional practice, or a patient(s) or policy/procedure in your practice setting?

■ REFERENCES

American Association of Colleges of Nursing. (2008). *Tool kit of resources for cultural competent education for Baccalaureate nurses*. Retrieved from http://www.aacn.nche.edu/education-resources/toolkit.pdf

American Association of Colleges of Nursing. (2011). *The essentials of master's education in nursing*. Washington, DC: Author.

American College of Physicians. (2010). *Racial and ethnic disparities in health care*. Philadelphia, PA: Author.

American Immigration Council. (2014). *Executive action on immigration: A resource page.* Retrieved from http://www.americanimmigrationcouncil.org/executive-action-immigration-resource-page

American Nurses' Association. (2015). *Members and affiliates.* Retrieved from http://nursingworld.org/FunctionalMenuCategories/AboutANA/WhoWeAre

Ayton-Shenker, D. (1995). *The challenge of human rights and cultural diversity.* United Nations Department of Public Information. Retrieved from http://www.un.org/rights/dpi1627e.htm

Cultural Competence Project. (2014). *Transcultural nursing theories and models.* Retrieved from http://www.ojccnh.org/project/theories-models.shtml

Floridi, L. (2014). *The fourth revolution: How the infosphere is reshaping human reality.* Oxford, UK: Oxford University Press.

France, N., & Ray, M. (2013). Studying caring sciences in nursing: The foundation of the discipline and profession of nursing at Florida Atlantic University, USA. In K. Vaidya (Ed.), *Nursing for the curious: Why study nursing?* Canberra, AU: Curious Academic Publishers [Kindle version].

Indian Health Service. (n.d.). Affordable Care Act. Retrieved from http://www.ihs.gov/aca/

Institute of Medicine. (2012). *How far have we come in reducing health disparities? Progress since 2000: Workshop summary.* Washington, DC: The National Academies Press.

International Council of Nurses. (2014). *About ICN.* Retrieved from http://www.icn.ch/about-icn/about-icn/

International Association for Human Caring. (2015). *Vision and goals* [Statements]. Retrieved from www.humancaring.org

Leininger, M. M. (1970). *Nursing and anthropology: Two worlds to blend.* New York: John Wiley.

Leininger, M. M. (1977). The phenomenon of caring: Caring: The essence and central focus of nursing. *American Nurses' Foundation (Nursing Research Report), 77*(1), 2; 14.

Leininger, M. M. (Ed.). (1981). *Caring: An essential human need.* Thorofare, NJ: Slack.

Leininger, M. M. (1985). Ethnography and ethnonursing: Models and modes of qualitative data analysis. In M. M. Leininger (Ed.), *Qualitative research methods in nursing.* New York, NY: Grune & Stratton.

Leininger, M. M. (1991). *Culture care diversity and universality: A theory of nursing.* New York, NY: National League for Nursing Press.

Leininger, M. M. (2002). Transcultural nursing and globalization of healthcare: Importance, focus and historical aspects. In M. M. Leininger and M. R. McFarland (Eds.), *Transcultural nursing: Concepts, theories, research & practice* (3rd ed., pp. 3-44). New York, NY: McGraw Hill.

Leininger, M. M., & M. R. McFarland. (Eds.). (2006). *Culture care diversity and universality: A worldwide nursing theory* (2nd ed.). Sudbury, MA: Jones & Bartlett.

Ludwig-Beymer, P. (2014). Health care reform and the transcultural nurse. *Journal of Transcultural Nursing, 25*(4) 323-324.

Matua, G. (2015, March 6). *Ebola: The untold stories of survivors (Volume 1).* Create Space Independent Publishing Platform (https://www.createspace.com/).

Matua, G., & Locsin, R. (2016). "Like a moth to a flame." Ebola and the culture of caregiving in Sub-Saharan Africa. In M. Ray (Ed.). *Transcultural caring dynamics in nursing and health care* (2nd ed.). Philadelphia, PA: FA Davis.

McDonnell, T., & West, J. (2014, November 11). BREAKING: The U. S. and China just announced a huge deal on climate—and it's a game changer. Retrieved from www.motherjones.com/environment/2014/11/obama-just-announced-historic-climate-deal-china

McFarland, M. R., & Leininger, M. M. (2011, October 21). *The culture care theory and a look to the future for transcultural nursing* [Keynote Address]. Presented at the 37th Annual Conference of the International Society of Transcultural Nursing, Las Vegas, NV.

McFarland, M. R., & Wehbe-Alamah, H. B. (Eds.). (2015). *Leininger's culture care diversity and universality: A worldwide nursing theory* (3rd ed.). Burlington, MA: Jones & Bartlett Learning.

Miller, J., Leininger, M., Leuning, C., Pacquiao, D., Andrews, M., Ludwig-Beymer, P., & Papadopoulos, I. (2008). Transcultural Nursing Society position statement on human rights. *Journal of Transcultural Nursing, 19*(1), 5-7. doi: 10.1177/1043659607309147

Newman, M., Smith, M., Dexheimer Pharris, M., & Jones, D. (2008). The focus of the discipline revisited. *Advances in Nursing Science, 31*(1), E16-E27. doi: 10.1097/01.ANS.0000311533.65941.f1

Pacquiao, D. (2008). Nursing care of vulnerable populations using a framework of cultural competence, social justice, and human rights. *Contemporary Nurse, 28*(1-2), 189-197. Retrieved from www.ncbi.nlm.nih.gov/pubmed/18844572

Ray, M. (2010a). Creating caring organizations and cultures through communitarian ethics. *Journal of the World Universities Forum, 3*(5), 41-52.

Ray, M. (2010b). *Transcultural caring dynamics in nursing and health care.* Philadelphia, PA: FA Davis.

Ray, M. (2016). *Transcultural caring dynamics in nursing and health care* (2nd ed.). Philadelphia, PA: FA Davis.

Ray, M. A., Morris, E. M., & McFarland, M. R. (2013). Qualitative nursing methods: Ethnonursing. In D. E. Polit and C. T Beck (Eds.), *Nursing research: Generating and assessing evidence for nursing practice* (8th ed.). Philadelphia, PA: Wolters Kluwer|Lippincott, Williams, & Wilkins.

Ray, M., & Turkel, M. (2014). Caring as emancipatory nursing praxis: The theory of relational caring complexity. *Advances in Nursing Science, 37*(2), 132-146.

Smedley, B., Stith, A., & Nelson, A. (2002). *Unequal treatment: Confronting racial and ethnic disparities in health care.* Washington, DC: National Academy Press. Retrieved from http://www.iom.edu/~/media/Files/Report

Smith, C. (2006). *Politics and processes at the United Nations: The global dance.* Boulder, CO: Lynne Rienner Publishers.

The United Nations. (2014a). *The universal declaration of human rights.* Retrieved from http://www.un.org/en/documents/udhr/

The United Nations (2014b). *U. N. at a glance.* Retrieved from http://www.un.org/en/index.shtml

The United Nations. (2015). *Millennium Development Goals and beyond 2015 – action 2015.* Retrieved from http://www.un.org/millenniumgoals/beyond2015-overview.shtml

The United Nations Department of Economic and Social Affairs. (2013). *Population Division International Migration.* Retrieved from http://esa.un.org/unmigration/wallchart2013.htm

The United Nations Development Program. (2014). *The Millennium Development Goals.* Retrieved from http://www.undp.org/content/undp/en/home/mdgoverview.html

The White House. (2013). *A more secure future. What the new health law means for you and your family.* Retrieved from http://www.whitehouse.gov/healthreform

The World Health Organization. (2014). *About WHO.* Retrieved from http://www.who.int/about/en/

The Transcultural Nursing Society. (2015). *Mission, vision, philosophy, values, and goals* [Statements]. Retrieved from http://www.tcns.org/

United States Department of Health and Human Services. (2013). *The patient protection and affordable care act.* Retrieved from http://www.hhs.gov/healthcare/rights/law/

Wolfe, A. (2011). *Political evil: What it is and how to combat it.* New York, NY: Vintage Books.

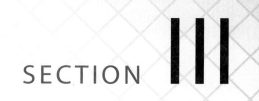

SECTION III

Culture Care Theory, Research, and Practice in Diverse Cultures and Settings

Culture Care Theory and Translational Science: A Focus for Doctor of Nursing Practice Scholarship

Marilyn R. McFarland

> *"Transcultural nursing is changing the ways nurses are discovering and learning about people of diverse and similar cultures with their caring, health, and wellbeing needs. Learning, teaching, and applying transcultural nursing theoretical and research-based knowledge is one of the most significant developments of this century and will be even greater in the 21st century"* (McFarland & Leininger, 2002, p. 527).

■ INTRODUCTION

In 2006, American Association of Colleges of Nursing (AACN) member institutions voted to support a clinical doctorate in nursing (AACN, 2006a), and published the *Essentials of Doctoral Education for Advanced Nursing Practice*, which detailed the curricular elements and competencies required by all doctor in nursing practice (DNP) programs (AACN, 2006a). These *DNP Essentials* outline eight foundational competencies required of all DNP graduates regardless of specialty (AACN, 2006a). Essentials II and VII respectively address scientific underpinnings for practice, organizational and systems leadership for quality improvement, and collaboration for improving patient and population health. Doctor of nursing practice graduates are to be prepared to uniquely contribute to nursing science by evaluating, translating, and disseminating research into practice. Essential II emphasizes the DNP graduate's role in assimilating nursing science and practice with the complex needs of humankind (AACN, 2006a). Related key DNP skills include the development of clinical practice guidelines, designing evidence-based interventions, and

evaluating practice outcomes. Essential VII is focused on preparing DNP graduates to lead interprofessional teams in the analysis of multifaceted practice and systems issues through effective communication and collaborative skills; this Essential also emphasizes the skills needed to synthesize the psychosocial dimensions and cultural influences related to population health (AACN, 2006a). Doctors of nursing practice take a leadership role in the development and implementation of practice models, standards of care, and other scholarly projects to improve patient and population health based on experiential knowledge and evidence-based research (AACN, 2006b).

In 2010, a university in the Midwestern United States (U. S.) admitted the first class of bachelor of science in nursing graduates as BSN-to-DNP students. The graduate faculty recognized that the Doctor of Nursing Practice curriculum should focus on demonstration of the scholarship of integration and application, as described by Boyer in 1990, by preparing nurses to evaluate and implement evidence-based best practices for the improvement of patient care and health outcomes. In addition, the philosophy of the School of Nursing (SON) faculty at the university is rooted in leadership education, scholarship, cultural competence, and nursing service (University of Michigan-Flint [UMF], p. 2). Cultural competence is a process taught by nurse educators to prepare students to co-participate as registered nurses with clients in planning and accessing care in a manner that is culturally congruent with their unique health and healthcare practices as diverse individuals, families, cultural groups, institutions, or organizations (UMF, p. 2). There is a required transcultural healthcare course taught by transcultural nurses holding advanced certifications (CTN-A; Transcultural Nursing Society, n. d.) for all DNP students during their first semester, which in part, provides students with foundational information about major transcultural theories and models and their application to healthcare practice, education, and research as well as opportunities to explore cultural diversities and similarities of diverse populations locally, nationally, and globally.

In 2009, Edwardson compared the scholarly DNP program project with the PhD/DNSc dissertation requirements by describing similarities and differences of the final product requirements for the two types of nursing doctoral degrees (Edwardson, 2009, as cited by Zaccagnini & White, 2015, p. 421). It was explained that both approaches to problem-solving needed to be systematic and rigorous, and the literature reviews should be in-depth and rigorous. The PhD/DNSc dissertation topic is narrow and the investigation is tightly controlled to prevent extraneous influences, whereas the DNP project is a project adapted to real-world situations and the extraneous influences cannot be controlled. Both types of research projects are based on theoretical concepts and literature (Edwardson, 2009, as cited by Zaccagnini & White, 2015, p. 421). The final product for both research approaches should meet the institution's academic requirements for scholarly work (AACN, 2006a).

■ DNP EVIDENCE-BASED POPULATION HEALTH PROJECTS

The Doctor of Nursing Practice Population Health Evidence-Based Project creates opportunities for the advanced nursing practice community to collectively meet the challenges for improving the population's health. This DNP scholarly project is designed to facilitate the development of qualified, knowledgeable, and experienced advanced practice nurses prepared to focus on the integration of population health into their practices to improve health outcomes (AACN, 2015). In 2010, the Director of the National Institute of Nursing Research, Dr. Patricia Grady, stated:

The findings from basic studies in healthcare science drive progress toward deeper discoveries about the mechanisms of both health and disease, but their usefulness and impact may not be readily apparent. Improving how we apply these findings in real world settings promises to advance the capacity of science to address the increasingly complex health care challenges in our world today. The application of scientific findings to clinical practice is the function of a rapidly expanding field of science known as *translational research*. (Grady, 2010, p. 164)

Grady (2010) described the stages of translational research work in two directions—to continually develop and re-evaluate an intervention across diverse settings and populations, and to proactively integrate data from real-world settings into the inception, design, and development of new basic and applied research studies. Wendler, Kirkbride, Wade, and Ferrell (2013), after completing a concept analysis, defined *translational research* (TR) as:

…. A feasible scientific inquiry that tests the implementation of evidence based interventions at the organizational and/or individual level, measuring implementation uptake….TR requires communication and collaboration between and among researchers and clinicians …is framed theoretically and is process and outcomes driven. Antecedents to translational research include having scientifically strong evidence available and an organizational infrastructure that supports engaged leaders and clinicians…Consequences of translational research include improved organizational and patient outcomes…new knowledge development and organizational and individual learning. The result of successful translational research is sustained practice change that benefits patients and closes the research practice gap. (Wendler, Kirkbride, Wade, & Ferrell, 2013, pp. 223-224)

Titler (2014) also stated that, "…an emerging body of knowledge in translation science provides an empirical base on effective implementation strategies to promote adoption of evidence-based practices in real world settings" (p. 269). In 2015, the AACN issued a white paper clarifying the research requirements for the DNP degree as focused on the generation of knowledge through the innovation of practice change, translation of evidence, and implementation of quality improvement processes in practice settings to improve health outcomes for patients (p. 2). DNP practice-scholarship is demonstrated when the principles of nursing scholarship are combined with the eight *DNP Essentials* to produce a graduate prepared to improve health and care outcomes. The integration of these new or refined skills improves outcomes through organizational or systems leadership, quality improvement processes, and translation of evidence into practice, among other ways (AACN, 2015, p. 2). Graduates of both research- and practice-focused doctoral programs are prepared to generate new knowledge. However, *research-focused* graduates are prepared to generate knowledge through rigorous research and statistical methodologies that may be broadly applicable or generalizable. *Practice-focused* graduates are prepared to generate new knowledge through innovation of practice change; the translation of evidence; and the implementation of quality improvement processes in specific practice settings, systems, or with specific populations to improve health or health outcomes. New knowledge generated through practice innovation, for example, could be of value in other practice settings. Such new knowledge is considered *transferrable* but is not considered *generalizable*. DNP graduates *generate evidence* through their practice to guide improvements in practice and outcomes of care (AACN, 2015, pp. 2-3).

In 2015, the AACN clarified the translation of evidence into practice in DNP scholarship as "…the mechanism that provides knowledge development within a discipline" (p. 2). To clarify the difference between *the development* and the *application* of research-focused scholarship and practice-focused scholarship, the *DNP Essentials* state, "…Rather than a knowledge-generating research effort, the student in a practice-focused program generally carries out a practice application-oriented final DNP project" (AACN, 2006a, p. 3). As DNP programs have evolved, questions have emerged regarding the *development of new knowledge,* which have been—in some instances—sources of debate within and among nursing education and practice communities. It has become increasingly understood that DNP knowledge-production is measured on the basis of its contribution to improved outcomes rather than its contribution to generalizable knowledge (AACN, 2015). Therefore, DNP programs focus on the translation of new science and its application and evaluation.

■ TRANSCULTURAL NURSING AND TRANSLATIONAL RESEARCH

Leininger (2002) emphasized both research and practice when she wrote about the future of transcultural nursing and the importance of "…the active advancement and use of transcultural nursing based knowledge and practices to serve a growing multicultural world" in 2002 (p. 577). Marion et al. (2016) in their American Nurses' Association Standard 8 implementation article offered discussion about integrating culturally congruent practices throughout the nursing process, and the important need for cultural competence in advanced practice nursing. Historically, transcultural nurse researchers have primarily used either qualitative and/or quantitative knowledge discovery methods to do original research to improve the cultural competence of nurses and to improve health outcomes for patients (Marion et al., 2016). More recent transcultural translational research projects, such as the one by Courtney and Wolgamott (2015), have been conducted with evidence-based practice and translational study designs by advanced practice DNP students with a focus on clinical practice and are discussed in the section that follows (Bhat, Wehbe-Alamah, McFarland, Filter, & Keiser, 2015; Coleman, Garretson, Wehbe-Alamah, McFarland, & Wood, 2016; Kelch, Wehbe-Alamah, & McFarland, 2014).

■ EXEMPLARS OF DNP TRANSLATIONAL PROJECTS GUIDED BY THE CULTURE CARE THEORY

Culturally Competent Hypertension and Diabetes Care

Leininger's Culture Care Theory (McFarland & Wehbe-Alamah, 2015) was used as a guide by a DNP student to design, implement, and evaluate an evidence-based hypertension (HTN) and Type 2 diabetes (T2DM) management program for rural primary clinic staff members at a nongovernmental organization (NGO) in Haiti (Kelch, Wehbe-Alamah, & McFarland, 2015).

The purpose of his project was to determine whether a sustainable HTN and T2DM identification and treatment program could maintain blood pressure (BP) below 140/90 and T2DM hemoglobin A_{1c} levels below 7.5% among Haitian NGO employees during a five-month period (Kelch, Wehbe-Alamah, & McFarland, 2015). The organization's employees included Haitian teachers, childcare and laundry workers, cooks, groundskeepers, nurses, and security staff. During the five-month research period, new employees hired by the organization were also enrolled into the program. Although the schoolteachers and two clinic nurses had some formal training, many of the staff had minimal formal education, and several were functionally illiterate. The clinic staff had provider access for their *acute* healthcare needs from visiting American healthcare teams sponsored by another NGO that cared for the rural population, but they had never had access to professional evaluation and management for their *chronic* health conditions. This NGO desired assistance to develop a culturally congruent and sustainable evidence-based primary healthcare program for adult staff to evaluate and treat their chronic health conditions. This management program was based on health promotion concepts and medical guidelines for the treatment of diabetes and hypertension from the American Diabetes Association (2014) and the World Health Organization (2011, 2012), both organizations offering guidelines for diabetes care, that latter for use in low-resource settings.

During his three separate trips to Haiti over a five-month period, the DNP student (Kelch) evaluated 48 participant staff members and when indicated treated them for hypertension and type 2 diabetes and provided culturally congruent health education to enhance their health knowledge and promote sustainability of the treatment regimen (Kelch, Wehbe-Alamah, & McFarland, 2014). The project produced recommendations for establishing a primary care and disease management program in Haiti and a model for possible transferability to other low-resource countries worldwide. In addition, the project demonstrated how to secure and involve local clinical staff; secure local project funding; work with local suppliers of medications and equipment; form intra-organization partnerships; and design culturally congruent clinical and educational interventions for staff (Kelch, Wehbe-Alamah, & McFarland, 2015).

Culturally Competent Palliative and End-of-Life Care

As DNP students and faculty, Bhat, Wehbe-Alamah, McFarland, Filter, and Keiser (2015) recognized that despite efforts to promote patient-centered care and respect for client choices across the healthcare continuum, cultural considerations about palliative care, including end-of-life (EOL) care, remained poorly understood. A translational research study was designed and implemented on a palliative care and hospice unit in a 1,070-bed Midwestern teaching hospital. Leininger's Culture Care Theory (2006) provided the framework to study and structure the development of an educational program to introduce plans of care influenced by cultural values, beliefs, expressions, and practices during the patient assessment process (Bhat, Wehbe-Alamah, McFarland, Filter, & Keiser 2015). The purpose of this translational research project was to determine whether registered nurses (RNs) working in a combined palliative care and hospice (PCH) unit acquired increased cultural awareness, sensitivity, and culturally competent behaviors after completing a cultural education program consisting of three web-based modules and to also ascertain whether the nurses' cultural assessments of patients improved afterward.

The study used a quasi-experimental design; fifteen registered nurses participated in the cultural competence education modules. A pre-intervention and post-intervention electronic chart audit identified patients' documented cultural assessment data that had been completed by nurses upon patient admission. The nurses also completed the Cultural Competence Assessment tool preintervention and postintervention. Analysis of the postintervention data showed the nurses had increased their cultural awareness, sensitivity, and improved their cultural assessment and documentation skills. These findings support the use of web-based education and show how this format can translate cultural competency knowledge into nursing practice. Providing this education to nurses was an important component in creating an environment that provided culturally congruent palliative care. This study served as a beginning step for implementing cultural competency training for nurses and for determining the transferability potential of the educational program to other palliative and hospice care units in similar healthcare institutions (Bhat, Wehbe-Alamah, McFarland, Filter, & Keiser 2015).

Reducing Avoidable Readmissions Effectively (RARE)

This translational project was also conceptualized within Leininger's Culture Care Theory (McFarland & Wehbe-Alamah, 2015) and used the principles from the Reducing Avoidable Readmissions Effectively (RARE) campaign (Minnesota Hospital Association and Stratus Health, 2014) to determine whether educational strategies about a culturally congruent nursing discharge process would improve nurses' cultural competence (Coleman, Garretson, Wehbe-Alamah, McFarland, & Wood, 2016). The outcomes these researchers evaluated were whether the instructional intervention changed the nurses' practice behaviors; reduced 30-day emergency department (ED) visits; or reduced readmissions for bariatric surgery patients at a U. S. Midwestern teaching hospital (Coleman, Garretson, Wehbe-Alamah, McFarland, & Wood, 2016). This project incorporated pre- and post-testing of staff nurses who had completed an online cultural competency course entitled, "Delivering Culturally and Linguistically Competent Nursing Care." A two-month pre- and post-intervention chart review of nursing documentation was conducted regarding culturally competent discharge planning that also compared patient emergency department visits and hospital re-admission rates when bariatric surgery had been performed (Coleman, Garretson, Wehbe-Alamah, McFarland, & Wood, 2016). Content analysis of nursing comments and responses to open-ended questions about their views of the educational program and subsequent patient outcomes provided important project sustainability information.

This project successfully educated the nurse participants and enhanced the cultural congruence of the discharge process. It also resulted in a statistically significant improvement in the nurses' knowledge of culturally and linguistically competent nursing care as evidenced by their enhanced and increased documentation using the new culturally congruent discharge plan process after completing the educational program. Thus, not only did the nurses gain knowledge about the importance of delivering culturally congruent and specific care, but they also applied what they had learned by integrating culturally congruent care into the patient discharge process.

Pre- and post-implementation chart reviews did not demonstrate any *statistically significant* results for decreased patient emergency department visits or hospital readmissions within 30 days of discharge. However, the *number* of emergency department visits within 30 days were reduced during the two-month time period of the intervention demonstrating *clinical significance*, which is important in translational research (Coleman, Garretson, Wehbe-Alamah, McFarland, & Wood, 2016). The researchers also stated there was potential transferability of this project for other patient populations at risk for post-procedure complications.

These three transcultural research projects, focused on improving the cultural competence of nurses and the provision of culturally congruent care for patients, are exemplars of transcultural translational studies conducted by advanced practice DNP nursing students. These projects were focused on the implementation of evidence-based educational programs and practices toward improving care and health outcomes for patients from diverse backgrounds in underserved clinical settings. They have potential transferability within other culturally competent educational programs as well as for culturally congruent care practices in diverse clinical settings. It is the recommendation of this author that DNP students be encouraged to work with interdisciplinary colleagues using transcultural theories and models such as the Culture Care Theory (McFarland & Wehbe-Alamah, 2015) to implement translational research projects as their practice-focused scholarship to generate new transcultural nursing knowledge. Through these innovations of practice change; translations of evidence; and implementations of quality improvement processes in specific clinical settings, systems, or with specific populations from diverse and similar cultures, they will meaningfully improve the health and health outcomes of the people served (AACN, 2015, p. 2).

■ SUMMARY

The importance of transcultural scholarly research projects within a translational research design conducted by DNP advanced practice nursing students was the focused discussion for this chapter, as well as the importance of using evidence-based transcultural knowledge to improve the cultural competence of nurses and the provision of culturally congruent care for patients. These projects increasingly need to be conducted within intradisciplinary and interdisciplinary partnerships using multi-site venues to make the best use of student and faculty time, followed by published dissemination through mainstream nursing journals (Broome, Riner, & Allam, 2013). The scholarship of the student earning a DNP has been compared with Boyer's model of the scholarship of application. Boyer (1990) stated that a *scholar* asks, "…How can knowledge be responsibly applied to consequential problems…and to individuals as well as institutions" (p. 21). The core transcultural concepts of *cultural competence* and *culturally congruent care* (McFarland & Wehbe-Alamah, 2015) have been described within the context of the Culture Care Theory and transcultural nursing. Continued emphasis is required on the convergence of translational research methods and these core transcultural constructs. The scholarship of application by advanced practice nurses was demonstrated through descriptions of their exemplar DNP transcultural translational research projects.

ACKNOWLEDGEMENTS

I gratefully acknowledge the diligent work and dedication of all transcultural nurse researchers, educators, clinicians, and scholars who design and conduct original research studies and scholarly translational projects that contribute new knowledge to the discipline and practice of nursing.

DEDICATION

This chapter is dedicated to the DNP students who have chosen to conduct translational research projects within a transcultural nursing focus.

DISCUSSION QUESTIONS

1. Discuss the evolution of the translational DNP project.
2. Discuss the value of conducting transcultural nursing studies with a translational methods design.
3. Brainstorm ideas for DNP translational research projects guided by a transcultural nursing theory.

REFERENCES

American Association of Colleges of Nursing. (2006a, October). *The essentials of doctoral education for advanced nursing practice.* Silver Spring, MD: Author.

American Association of Colleges of Nursing. (2006b). DNP nursing curriculum planning solutions: A guide to accredited curriculum design and proper book selection. Silver Spring, MD: Author. Accessible at http://www.dnpnursingsolutions.com/about-dnp-program-guide

American Association of Colleges of Nursing. (2015, August). *The doctor of nursing practice: Current issues and clarifying recommendations: Report from the task force on the implementation of the DNP.* Silver Spring, MD: Author.

American Association of Colleges of Nursing. (2017). *Fact sheet: The doctor of nursing practice (DNP).* Silver Spring, MD: Author.

American Diabetes Association. (2014). *Diabetes treatment guidelines, education, and health promotion strategies.* Retrieved from http://www.diabetes.org/

Bhat, A., Wehbe-Alamah, H. B., McFarland, M. R., Filter, M. S., & Keiser, M. (2015). Advancing cultural assessments in palliative care using web-based education. *Journal of Hospice and Palliative Nursing, 17*(4), 348-355.

Boyer, E. L. (1990). *Scholarship reconsidered: Priorities of the professoriate* (p. 21). Princeton, NJ: Carnegie Foundation for the Advancement of Teaching.

Broome, M. E., Riner, M. E., & Allam, E. S. (2013, August). Scholarly publication practices of doctor of nursing practice-prepared nurses. *Journal of Nursing Education, 52*(8), 429-434. doi: 10.3928/01484834-20130718-02

Coleman, S. K., Garretson, B. C., Wehbe-Alamah, H. B., McFarland, M. R., & Wood, M. (2016). RESPECT: Reducing 30-day emergency department visits and readmissions of bariatric surgical patients effectively through cultural competency training of nurses. *Online Journal of Cultural Competence in Nursing and Healthcare, 6*(1), 31-51. doi: 10.9730/ojccnh.org/v6n1a3

Courtney, R., & Wolgamott, S. (2015). Using Leininger's theory as the building block for cultural competence and cultural assessment for a collaborative care team in a primary care setting. In M. R. McFarland and H. B. Wehbe-Alamah (Eds.), *Leininger's culture care diversity and universality: A worldwide nursing theory* (3rd ed., pp. 345-368). Burlington, MA: Jones & Bartlett Learning.

Grady, P. A. (2010). News from NINR: Translational research and nursing science. *Nursing Outlook, 58*(3), 164-166.

Kelch, R. H., Wehbe-Alamah, H. B., & McFarland, M. R. (2015). Implementation of hypertension and diabetes chronic disease management in an adult group in Les Bours, Haiti. *Online Journal of Cultural Competence in Nursing and Healthcare, 5*(1), 50-63. doi: 10.9730/ojccnh.org/v5n1a4

Leininger, M. M. (2006). Culture care diversity and universality theory and evolution of the ethnonursing method. In M. M. Leininger and M. R. McFarland (Eds.), *Culture care diversity and universality: A worldwide nursing theory* (2nd ed., pp. 1-41). Sudbury, MA: Jones and Bartlett.

Marion, L., Douglas, M., Lavin, M. A., Barr, N., Gazaway, S., Thomas, E., & Bickford, C. (2016, November 18). Implementing the new ANA standard 8: Culturally congruent practice. *OJIN: The Online Journal of Issues in Nursing, 22*(1). doi: 10.3912/OJIN.Vol22No01PPT20

McFarland, M. R., & Leininger, M. M. (2002). Transcultural nursing: Curricular concepts, principles, and teaching and learning activities for the 21st century. In M. M. Leininger and M. R. McFarland (Eds.), *Transcultural nursing: Concepts, theories, research, and practices* (3rd. ed., p. 527). New York, NY: McGraw-Hill.

McFarland, M. R., & Wehbe-Alamah, H. B. (2015). The theory of culture care diversity and universality. In M. R. McFarland and H. B. Wehbe-Alamah (Eds.), *Leininger's culture care diversity and universality: A worldwide nursing theory* (3rd ed., pp. 1-34). Burlington, MA: Jones & Bartlett Learning.

Minnesota Hospital Association, & Stratus Health, Institute for Clinical Systems Improvement. (2014). *Reducing avoidable readmissions effectively*. Retrieved from http://www.rarereadmissions.org/about/index.html

Titler, M. G. (2014). Overview of evidence-based practice and translation science. *Nursing Clinics of North America, 49*(3), 269-274.

Transcultural Nursing Society. (n. d.). *Advanced certification requirements (CTN-A)*. Accessible at http://www.tcns.org/Certificationctnarequire.html

University of Michigan-Flint, School of Nursing. (2017, April 12). *Graduate nursing student handbook*. Flint, MI: Author. Accessible at https://www.umflint.edu/sites/default/files/users/chelswin/graduate_nursing_student_handbook_-_2017-2018_4-12-17_revisions.pdf

U. S. Preventative Services Task Force. (2008). *Screening for type 2 diabetes mellitus in adults*. Retrieved from http://www.uspreventiveservicestaskforce.org/uspstf/uspsdiab.htm

Wendler, M. C., Kirkbride, G., Wade, K., & Ferrell, L. (2013). Translational research: A concept analysis. *Research and Theory for Nursing Practice, 27*(3), 214-232. doi: 10.1891/1541-6577.27.3.214.

World Health Organization. (2011). *Use of glycated haemoglobin (HbA1c) in the diagnosis of diabetes mellitus*. Retrieved from http://www.who.int/diabetes/publications/report-hba1c_2011.pdf

World Health Organization. (2012). *Guidelines for primary health care in low-resource settings*. Retrieved from http://www.who.int/entity/nmh/publications/phc2012/en/index.html

Zaccagnini, M. E., & White, K. W. (2015). *The doctor of nursing practice essentials: A new model for advanced practice nursing* (2nd ed.). Burlington, MA: Jones & Bartlett Learning.

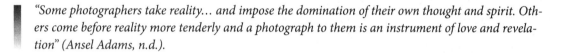

CHAPTER

19

Engaging in the Sacred Song of Diversity: The Art of Cultural Immersion

Edith J. Morris

> *"Some photographers take reality… and impose the domination of their own thought and spirit. Others come before reality more tenderly and a photograph to them is an instrument of love and revelation" (Ansel Adams, n.d.).*

■ INTRODUCTION

The quote by Ansel Adams captures the essence of cultural immersion. Immersion into a culture different from one's own needs to be approached with compassion and a joy for learning to see the world in a new way. It must not be one of *cultural imposition** where the dominant cultural ways are viewed as superior (*ethnocentrism*) and are imposed on the lifeways of another. Immersion is a learning experience that not only changes the way one thinks about and views the world, but an approach that promotes peace and healing in communities and in the world. It is important that we make efforts to understand one another and to respect our *differences* (diversities), but even more importantly, that we mutually enjoy our shared *similarities* (universalities). The search for *truth in meaning* about people's beliefs and values about health, wellbeing, illness, and death is an imperative for ethnonursing researchers and transcultural healthcare providers (HCPs) and requires proficiency in both the *art* and *science* of nursing. Equally vital is the cultural immersion process which is necessary in order to provide culturally congruent care based on truthful and credible data from the people.

The purpose of this chapter is to explore the art of cultural immersion by discovering its *ontological** (ways of being) and *epistemological** (ways of knowing) components. The ontology of nursing is about how we are present within the discipline and relates to the art of nursing while the epistemology is the empirical or science part of nursing. Immersing in a culture requires both empirical knowledge (science) and metaphysical knowledge (art) flowing in a simultaneous, intertwined, and endless harmony so that one [form of knowledge] becomes indistinguishable from the other. The art of nursing has been described as a "…complicated undertaking that involves the temporal acquisition and synchronous use of empirical and metaphysical knowledge and values; it is not static, but dynamic to each nursing situation" (Finfgeld-Connett, 2008, pp. 384-385). Carper (1978) described four ways of knowing in nursing: The <u>art of nursing</u> which includes *personal knowledge* gained through experience accompanied by *esthetic knowledge* which is expressive, creative, and subjective; *ethical knowledge* or the moral component of nursing; and finally the <u>science of nursing</u> which is the *empirical knowledge* essential within the discipline. Carper has described three ways of knowing from within the art

* Term definition located in chapter Glossary.

of nursing and one from within the science of nursing. Yet, so much more weight has historically been given to the science of nursing as the profession strives to gain its rightful place alongside medicine and other professional and scientific healthcare disciplines. Through narratives about personal experiences of immersion into different cultures, I will share how the art of nursing encompassed the science to enable successful cultural immersions.

The influences of social cultural values, beliefs, and meanings about life, death, wellbeing, and safety need to be primary considerations in order to enable healthcare professionals to provide culturally congruent care whether conducting research or engaging in direct/hands-on clinical care. Entering into another's culture can be challenging as one is entering their sacred beliefs, values, and life meanings, which define the responses and actions of the other. Being accepted into another's culture is an honor bestowed on the entrant by the local people of that culture—one which must be treated with the greatest respect (Leininger, 1991).

As a transcultural nursing researcher, the question that I am most often asked is how was I able to gain acceptance and trust in a culture and a subculture that was so different from my own. This question seems to have arisen because I am a White, late middle-aged, middle-class woman from a small White/European American community who chose to base her doctoral dissertation on a qualitative ethnonursing field study conducted with African American adolescent gang members (Morris, 2004).

Because stories are an effective way to express and teach complex concepts, I have chosen to tell the story of my cultural immersion journeys wherein I was able to achieve cultural acceptance and trust in communities very different from my own. It is also the story of the many adolescents and adults that travelled with me and openly shared their stories. Because of their willingness to be openly sharing, I was able to acquire knowledge that would not have been possible to learn in school or from a textbook by dwelling with the people themselves. It is my hope that this chapter will assist and encourage the readers as they enter and immerse with diverse cultures to learn about their cultural beliefs, values, practices, and lifeways.

More than 20 years ago as a doctoral student, I began my journey in transcultural nursing with my mentor Dr. Madeleine Leininger, a nurse anthropologist who developed the Theory of Culture Care Diversity and Universality along with the Ethnonursing Research Method. Prior to meeting her, I had not given much thought to culture and health care or even that culture had any major influence on health. My first transcultural class at Wayne State University in Detroit, Michigan, USA, inspired me to begin a continuing and ever-evolving journey that has forever changed my worldview as well as the way that I conduct research and provide health care to patients. It was not so much learning and understanding new cultures that enraptured me, but it was being able to see the world through the lens of a diverse culture and to integrate this new transcultural paradigm into my own thought processes. Gaining an understanding of the actions and reactions of others by experiencing their cultural lifeways changed the way I thought about *culture* and *health* and how I viewed my patients who were from diverse backgrounds. In my clinical practice, I began to ask questions about cultural values and practices that related to health care. I found people were anxious to share this information with me and that it did make a difference as to how we choose to address health and wellbeing or problems and concerns related to their care.

■ ENABLERS THAT ASSIST WITH THE CULTURAL IMMERSION PROCESS

Leininger (1991) created enablers to assist the researcher or HCP in conducting healthcare research among diverse cultures. Two of the six enablers, the Observation-Participation-Reflection Enabler (OPR) and the Stranger-to-Trusted Friend Enabler, were designed to guide the researcher during their cultural immersion (Leininger, 1991). The OPR Enabler and the Stranger-to-Trusted Friend Enabler are most often used concurrently to assist the researcher or HCP to initiate the research study or clinical data collection processes.

The OPR facilitates the researcher or HCP entering and remaining with the people to observe and study their cultural lifeways in relation to nursing and other healthcare phenomena in a systematic and reflective way (Leininger, 1991). The OPR has four phases that begin with a strictly *observation phase* as the researcher enters the culture; it then moves to an *observation phase with limited participation*; and ultimately to *active participation* with the culture, which includes intimate conversations where cultural rituals and truths are shared—this is when the full immersion occurs (Leininger, 1991). The final phase of the OPR is the *reflection phase* where findings from the cultural immersion are confirmed with the key and general informants (Leininger, 1991, 2002c; Ray, Morris, & McFarland, 2013; Wehbe-Alamah & McFarland, 2015b). These phases do not progress in a strictly linear fashion, but rather go back and forth until the immersion is completed.

The Stranger-to-Trusted Friend Enabler "…enables the researcher or HCP to move from the status of stranger to trusted friend in order to ensure that authentic, credible and dependable data are obtained" (Leininger, 1991, p. 82). This enabler requires that the researcher or HCP first start by examining their personal beliefs, values, and lifeways so as to more fully understand themselves before entering into the world of the culture they are about to study (Leininger, 1991). The researcher enters the culture as a stranger who may not be fully trusted and is therefore tested by the insiders who observe and judge reactions and behaviors of the outsider/researcher as information is conveyed or shared. Genuine sharing of local secrets, stories, and cultural information will not take place until the outsider (researcher) becomes as trusted as one would trust a close friend. Once the researcher has gained this level of trust, the rich *emic** cultural data will be shared by the cultural informants/participants [*insiders*] (Leininger, 1991). The Stranger-to-Trusted Friend Enabler is used throughout the cultural immersion experience and during the data collection and analysis processes as the researcher evolves in building a strong and trusting relationship with each participant or cultural group (Leininger, 1991, 2002c, 2006b; Ray et al., 2013; Wehbe-Alamah & McFarland, 2015b).

■ LITERATURE REVIEW

Cultural immersion as described in the healthcare literature means that *time* and *presence* within a culture are necessary components toward acquiring *cultural competence** with any given cultural group (Campinha-Bacote, 2002). The literature discusses cultural immersion experiences almost exclusively in relation

to short-term graduate and undergraduate service-learning experiences focused on gaining clinical knowledge with another culture and for longer-term graduate student cultural research. The longer immersion experiences enable the researcher to earn the people's trust so that informants/participants become more likely to share truthful and authentic data. Cultural immersion experiences have been reported as lasting from two days to four months and are generally located geographically onsite within the cultural context of the people or group of interest (Amerson, 2012; Anderson, Friedemann, Buscher, Sansoni, Hodnicki, 2012; Harrowing, Gregory, O'Sullivan, Lee, & Doolittle, 2012)—although one study did report immersion by email (Guo, Wang, Corbin, Wynn, & Statz, 2014).

The major purpose of the undergraduate cultural immersion experience is to promote *cultural awareness** (Camphina-Bacote, 2002) yet prevent cultural *imposition* (Leininger, 2002b). Cultural awareness has been defined by Camphina-Bacote (2002) as the self-examination and in-depth exploration of one's own cultural and professional background; it involves recognizing one's biases, prejudices, and assumptions about individuals who have different values, beliefs, and lifeways. The process of cultural immersion leads to a new cultural awareness without threat of imposition, which thus allows the individual to achieve a level of *cultural competence**.

Cultural immersion experiences for undergraduate students tend not only to be shorter but also less intense and focused on addressing healthcare concerns (Heppner & Wang, 2014; Isaacson, 2014; Thrackrah, Thompson, & Durey, 2014). The value of cultural immersion for undergraduate service learning experiences has been *qualitatively* documented in the literature through the use of journaling and interviews and *quantitatively* through the use of several transcultural assessment scales. These scales have included the Multicultural Counseling Inventory (MCI; Sodowsky, Taffe, Gutkin, & Wise, 1994); Cushner's Inventory of Cross Cultural Sensitivity (ICCS; Loo & Shiomi, 1999); the Inventory for Assessing the Process of Cultural Competence Among Health Care Professionals-Student Version (IAPCC-SV; Campinha-Bacote, 2007); and the Transcultural Self Efficacy Tool (TSET; Jeffreys, 2000; Jeffreys & Dogan, 2010).

Quantitative study results about the value of culture immersion have been mixed. Guo et al. (2014)

conducted a pilot study using a quantitative design and the Multicultural Counseling Inventory (MCI) supplemented by the use of structured descriptive questions to gain further insights. The qualitative questions were emailed to a cross-sampling of the participants taken from the quantitative portion of the study in lieu of going into the field and conducting face-to-face interviews. These researchers reported statistical significance on the knowledge subscale and in the overall MCI total scores from pre- to post-test administration. However, they found no statistically significant differences in the cultural awareness and relationship subscales. This study also included a qualitative analysis, which found that through the email immersion experiences, the participants were able to recognize their own stereotypes and racism more clearly.

Jones, Neubrander, and Huff (2012) were unable to achieve statistically significant differences in cultural attitudes on Cushner's Inventory of Cross-Cultural Sensitivity (ICCS), which can be attributed to the small sample size in this study. However, their later study included a qualitative component that identified changes in personal and professional growth and also in values and attitudes about the culture studied when compared to their own culture through self-examination of the researchers' personal cultural beliefs. In another mixed-methods study, Isaacson (2014) investigated the levels of effectiveness of the immersion experience in relation to length of time for the field experience using Campinha-Bacote's (2007) IAPCC-SV. One group spent four days immersed with an indigenous group on the Northern Plains Reservation while a second group resided for two weeks with a faculty mentor on the reservation. The researcher found that although the first group did acquire *cultural awareness*, the levels of *cultural competence* significantly increased in the second group, which was attributed to their length of immersion experience. The qualitative data was collected through written *critical reflective journaling** and the narrative interpretation was guided by *hermeneutic phenomenological methodology**. Themes generated from this study revealed that these students moved from an initial preconceived negative perception of this indigenous population to having transformed thinking, which enabled them to better understand the daily struggles of this cultural group.

One large quantitative study yielded statistically significant results using pre- and post-test measures in overall self-efficacy with the TSET (Halter et al., 2014). Larsen and Reif (2011) led another smaller quasi-experimental study using the TSET to determine the effect of cultural immersion and cultural education classes upon undergraduate students' transcultural competence. In this study, a group of students who had taken part in a cultural immersion was compared to a group who had not had any immersion experience but who had taken cultural education classes. The cultural immersion group scored significantly higher on the TSET than the cultural education group. These findings lend support to the value of cultural immersion experiences toward the development of cultural competence among undergraduate students.

The qualitative studies reviewed varied in their methodology but generally used exploratory, descriptive, or narrative approaches (Heppner & Wang, 2014; Ingulli, Doutrich, Allen, & Dekker, 2014; Thackrah, Thompson, & Durey, 2014). As may be expected with qualitative studies, thematic findings were varied depending upon the research question or the domain of inquiry under study. However, one consistent theme was identified that centered on the value of the cultural immersion as an eye-opening experience. These qualitative study researchers concluded that undergraduate students gained valuable cultural knowledge (Heppner & Wang, 2014; Ingulli et al., 2014; Thackrah et al., 2014) and made important connections within the cultural community (Thackrah, et al., 2014). Through their immersion experiences with a diverse people, the students did gain knowledge from their experiences; however, there was no change in the level or depth of their understanding of the social constructs of the observed culture (Harrowing et al., 2012).

■ CULTURAL IMMERSION PROCESS

There are some important baseline rules to keep in mind as one begins the immersion process into a culture that is not one's own. The healthcare professional (HCP) or researcher is entering into another's sacred space, and therefore, must bring a spirit of humbleness by not only being aware of one's personal biases but also by putting them aside and entering with a sense of authenticity. In all instances, the researcher is the *learner* and the participants are the *knowers* (Leininger, 1991, 2002c, 2006a; Wehbe-Alamah & McFarland, 2015b).

The benefits to the researcher or HCP who enters with an open mind are countless and include gaining a new paradigm of thought–one that will offer new insights into the world of the local people. It is important to understand that the HCP or researcher, being of a particular culture, may not fully know his/her own culture because of intrinsic *acculturation* and *ethnocentrism* (Leininger, 2000). Ethnocentrism is the "…belief that one's own culture is superior in every way to all others" (Haviland, Prins, McBride, & Walrath, 2013, p. 401). Ethnocentrism often presents itself when well-meaning students participate in service-learning assignments, believing that their own healthcare practices are superior and attempt to impose their practices on the people of the culture in which they are a *guest*. It is important that all health care and related teaching be done within the [*emic**] context of the culture of the local people and not from the [*etic**] perspective of outsiders.

Undergraduate Student Cultural Immersion Experiences

Cultural immersion experiences are best initiated by first assessing one's own culture and one's understanding of the roots of your own beliefs, values, and lifeway practices. Although immersing into another culture will enrich understanding your own culture, it is nevertheless important to begin by first thoroughly examining your own cultural origins. In doing so, personal biases may be recognized, acknowledged, and set aside so as to be able to enter into a diverse culture without cultural bias or stereotyping. The length of time necessary for an outsider to gain the trust of the local people depends upon the cultural group being studied; age, gender, and other demographics of the informants; the purpose of the study; the amount of time the researcher has had previous contact with the particular group under study; and the level of trust a particular group has developed with the researchers, healthcare providers, and other study professionals.

Cultural immersions for undergraduate students seeking to gain experience in another culture does not require the same amount of time needed to develop the desired level of trust as does the researcher seeking a deeper level of immersion. Healthcare student or undergraduate researchers collecting data from adults usually can accomplish immersion in a shorter time, especially if the HCP is already known to the individual(s). The researcher will typically need a longer period of immersion with children and adolescents in order to obtain accurate healthcare data (Morris, 2004). Further, if the researcher is from a dominant or different culture than the study participants, the researcher will need a substantively longer period of immersion to reach a trust level with them. (Morris, 2004, 2012, 2015). People involved in the justice system are often more reluctant to share information because their level of trust in other people is generally low (Morris, 2004). These paths to successful cultural immersion have become known to me over time given my immersions with different cultural groups and having guided many doctoral students through the cultural immersion process. The quality of an educational service-learning experience or the ability to obtain credible and truthful research data about another culture first and foremost requires a successful cultural immersion.

Graduate Student or Researcher Cultural Immersion Experiences

At the graduate level, most immersion experiences are related to experiencing a culture for research purposes. This immersion is longer and lasts until the student researcher has gained the trust of members of the culture under study. The period of time involved varies according to the culture and the subculture that one is entering, but it has generally been found that immersion to gain trust for research purposes takes a minimum of three months (McFarland, 2002). For cultures or subcultures where there is reason to distrust outsiders, the process can take much longer. As previously noted, Leininger's (1991) OPR and Stranger-to-Trusted Friend Enablers serve as guides for the researcher in knowing when an adequate level of trust has been achieved with the local people. When trust is achieved, in-depth data collection can begin.

■ PERSONAL CULTURAL EXPERIENCES

Cultural Background

Born and raised in a relatively high-context culture myself—a small tightly-knit Welsh American community—I quickly grasped the influence of cultural beliefs, values, and practices along with the pivotal role they played in daily life. At that time, I did not fully understand how much my own cultural background influenced every decision I made and every behavior that I expressed. I also came to realize that one cannot categorize and stereotype cultural values and beliefs due to the influential processes of *acculturation*, *cultural assimilation*, and *cultural accommodation*. *Acculturation* refers to a "…massive cultural change that occurs in a society when it experiences intensive first-hand contact with a more powerful society" (Haviland, et al., 2013, p. 400) or a "…process by which an individual or group from Culture A learns how to take on many, but not all, values, behaviors, norms, and lifeways of Culture B" (Leininger, 2002a, p. 56). An example of this would be the arrival of the Europeans in the Americas and their powerful domination over the indigenous cultures. *Cultural assimilation* is the "…absorption of an ethnic minority by a dominant society" (Haviland et al., 2013, p. 400) or the "…ways an individual or group from one culture very selectively and usually intentionally selects certain features of another culture without necessarily taking on many or all attributes of lifeways that would declare one to be acculturated" (Leininger, p. 56). The African American culture in the United States may be an example of this process.

Cultural accommodation is a "…process by which people resist assimilation by modifying its traditional culture in response to pressures by a dominant society in order to preserve its distinct ethnic identity" (Haviland et al., 2013, p. 400). The Amish culture may be one example of cultural accommodation as evidenced by their avoiding the use of electricity, electrical appliances, or motorized transportation such as cars or farm implements, but integrating solar energy or propane fuel from an on-site tank (but not natural gas that connects to a central piping system) for conveniences such as hot water. As I reflect on my small Welsh American community, I recall examples of all three of these processes occurring simultaneously. In more recent times, that community has assimilated yet has also culturally accommodated in ways that have allowed retention of some elements of its original cultural identity.

One cannot assume that a culture can be known through textbooks or one's preconceived ideas about a particular social or cultural group. Immersion within the specific culture to be studied is necessary in order

to gain insights and experience nuances from within a particular group of people. It is good to begin by reading and studying the known generalities of a culture; but in order to gain in-depth understanding and knowledge, immersion with the local people is of critical importance. Hall (1959, 1969, 1976, 1983), an American anthropologist who studied indigenous cultural groups in North America, developed a theory of high- and low-context cultures. He described *high-context* cultures as valuing interpersonal relationships that are strong and lasting; through these relationships decisions are made that affect the wellbeing of the culture and the community. Communication is largely nonverbal and contextual and overshadows the verbal message. Rules are known to the [*emic**] insiders of the *culture* but are not explicitly expressed. *Relationships* are valued over timeliness, change occurs slowly, and knowledge is embedded in the social structure of a high-context culture (Hall, 1959, 1969, 1976, 1983). Becoming accepted into a high-context culture requires a longer immersion period on the part of an [*etic**] *outsider* interested in studying the culture from within. In contrast to high-context cultures, *low-context* cultures share fewer life activities; relationships are short term with few acquaintances; there is less sharing of intergenerational knowledge; social-cultural boundaries become more blurred; and sociocultural change tends to be more rapid (Hall, 1976, 1983).

Personal Cultural Immersion Experience

To further explain the concept of cultural differences and the influences related to acculturation, I will use my personal cultural experiences as examples. As mentioned, I was born and raised in a relatively high-context Welsh American culture. Most of the people in the community were second-generation immigrants from Wales who held firmly to their Celtic values from the "old country." The process of acculturation began as outside influences entered the community through the formation 'outside' marriages, friendships, and employments. It was common for some of these outsiders to think of the Welsh as part of English culture — after all was not Wales part of Great Britain or the United Kingdom (U. K.)? However, because the Welsh culture is very different from English culture in its values and lifeway practices, cultural pain and cultural imposition often resulted. Leininger (2002c), Hubbert, (2006), and Knecht and

Sabatine (2015) defined *cultural imposition* as the act or process of forcing one's values, beliefs, or lifeways onto people from another culture. To further complicate the cultural issues of this small community, there were some minor nuances of cultural difference and dialect depending on what part of Wales from which one had immigrated. North and South Wales were culturally different then, and remain so, just as different as Northern Ireland and Protestant Ireland are from one another. The U. K. is a relatively small geographic area connected by a common government; yet, England, Scotland, Northern Ireland, and Wales are each very distinct in their cultural values, beliefs, practices, and lifeways. It is, therefore, incorrect to assume that by knowing one culture from within the U. K. assures that all cultures within the U. K. are known.

It is a disservice to any culture or subculture to assume that one can know a particular culture by reading about it in a textbook. Cultural immersion is necessary in order to fully understand and learn the truths from within a particular culture. Based on the above discussion, it would seem that *full* cultural competence of someone from outside the culture is not possible. It may even be difficult for those from within the culture to achieve given that one may only become fully aware and knowledgeable of one's own culture largely through the study of another's culture (Leininger, 1991, 2002a, 2002b; 2006b; Wehbe-Alamah & McFarland, 2015a, 2015b).

A number of years ago, I was able to experience my own cultural immersion in Wales. My ability to immerse into the Welsh culture was nearly immediate. Values, beliefs, practices, and lifeway experiences were the same as those I had grown up with, but even more so. Many sociocultural dimensions such as language, philosophical factors, and cultural events were the same. Remarkably, the physical characteristics of the Welsh resembled those of family and friends from the small community where I had lived during my early years. Immersing in the culture of Wales was enlightening and comfortable, as I was in an environment that was familiar to me. When one is from a high-context culture, and returns to the geographical origin of that particular culture, then immersion generally occurs rapidly, if not immediately. It is a valuable experience to return to the origins of one's culture in that it solidifies and offers insights into one's own personal cultural values, beliefs, practices, and lifeways, and thus opens a door to appreciating and fully understanding the diversity that also exists in other cultures.

■ SELECTED CULTURAL IMMERSION EXPERIENCES

First immersion experience in a diverse culture

Transitioning into the Research Domain

After admission into my doctoral program and with my first transcultural nursing course behind me, I was committed to studying the health of adolescents based on their culture. As a nurse practitioner in an adolescent clinic located in a juvenile detention center and juvenile prison, I became intensely interested in the subculture of youth gangs. Wanting to make my dissertation study as succinct as possible, and upon Dr. Leininger's advice, I realized the importance of also choosing an ethnic culture because the identification of a gang subculture, if there was one, could be supported through the findings of the study. I had contact through the juvenile justice system with three different cultures having adolescents who claimed gang membership: African American, European American, and Latino. Any one of these cultural groups had an adequate number of potential participants to support a qualitative ethnonursing study.

After careful consideration, I chose to study African American adolescent gang members because I believed they were quite open and honest about their lifeways, because I also believed they would accept me into their culture and subculture if I could gain their trust, and in addition because they were not of my own cultural background. Furthermore, I had had several in-depth conversations with African American adolescent gang members in my role as nurse practitioner that led me to believe that I was perceived by them as having the ability to move from a stranger to a trusted friend with this group.

I remember one such conversation with a young African American man who talked openly about race and racism and how his feelings toward White people had developed during his life. He continued to talk about his fears of prejudice, racial wars, and violence. He stated that he was not so afraid of dying on the street as he was afraid of where he would go after his death. He went on to say that his fear was that he would go to Heaven, which he believed was for White people. This was a long and in-depth discourse on race relations that I believed reflected that a mutual trust had developed between us, particularly *because* of our ethnic differences. I remember this conversation vividly and it was this interaction that gave me confidence in my ability to earn trust from people of a culture different from my own. At this point I was excited about the idea of immersing into another culture, to begin to view the world through fresh eyes and make new discoveries. With this new level of confidence, I was ready to move forward.

Many peers and colleagues questioned my decision to study African American adolescent gang members because this was a group that was known to have difficulty trusting others. Because I was not of their culture, it was believed that I would not be able to gain their trust and hence would not learn truths from them. Some of these detractors suggested that I should at least study my own culture, but Dr. Leininger's question (personal communication, April 1995) was an affirmation to me: "…How can you ever bring about peace and healing unless you understand the world from another's [point of or world] view?" Her words provided me with ongoing encouragement throughout my journey whenever I was being doubted or questioned by others.

Obtaining Institution Review Board Approval

The Institution Review Board (IRB) and the Vice President for Research further questioned my ability to conduct the study. The IRB invoked restrictions as to how and where I could collect the data, citing concerns about my safety. My arguments were that I could not adequately collect data and learn truth from the study participants if I could not be with them in their daily lives. The IRB finally relented, yielding to my desire to conduct a field study. I assured the IRB members that I would not be with the adolescent gang members during any criminal activities nor when the participants needed to be "about their business." Indeed, the adolescents were very careful that I was not exposed to any danger when I was with them. I have never before or since felt safer in a high-crime inner city area than when I was doing fieldwork with the gangs. The key to learning truths about the culture and subculture and for being safe was an adequate and thorough cultural immersion. A thorough immersion reveals the authenticity of the

researcher, which is vitally important to the members of the culture that one has entered.

One area where the IRB would not concede was that I could not collect data in the jail nor would they allow me to be out on the street randomly selecting gang members to join the study. I needed to have a community center or school as my main contextual setting. As it turned out, doing so was helpful for finding participants and for collecting data. Because I was familiar with some of the gang members in the detention center, but not with those in school or at the community centers, I needed to immerse more intensely than I would have otherwise, had the study taken place in the setting where I was better-known. The immersion experience was crucial toward my becoming part of the environment of African American adolescent gang members and gaining their trust, although it did require time and patience as a good cultural immersion always does. Final IRB approval was contingent upon securing a Certificate of Confidentiality from the National Institutes of Mental Health, which I applied for and received. The Certificate of Confidentiality meant that past and current crimes (except for abuse) discussed within the context of the research were exempt from being subpoenaed into a court of law. After 18 months of being under IRB review, and with the Certificate of Confidentiality in hand, my study was approved and I was able to begin data collection.

Gaining Participant Trust

During immersion and the development of close relationships with study participants or patients, boundaries between the researcher or HCP and participant/patient may and often do become blurred. This blurring is necessary in order for the researcher to understand cultural lifeways from the perspective of the participant while at the same time not completely crossing the lines of professional objectivity or violating the participants' personal space (Finfgeld-Connett, 2008). For example, during my data collection for this particular study, I participated in both school and some non-school activities with the gang members. However, at no time did I have prior knowledge of nor did I participate in any of their criminal actions. At times, some criminal actions were reported to me after-the-fact and we would discuss them, but at that point they were within the bounds of the Certificate of Confidentiality and not reportable as long as they did not involve abuse. Reporting versus maintaining the confidentiality of the research participant can become an ethical dilemma for the researcher. This quandary is what led to many of the discussions I had with gang members. We eventually resolved it by establishing a shared mutual understanding that if I broke trust with the adolescent gang members, then I would no longer receive truthful and credible data. Assuring truth was essential because many future social actions and interventions could be based on findings from the research. HCPs are not protected by the Certificate of Confidentiality and are bound by law to report any criminal actions. The participants in my study were well aware of these distinctions.

For this study, I chose a small charter school as the central context of my immersion experience. My first day happened to coincide with the day of the terrorist attack on the World Trade Center and the Pentagon. While we watched these events unfold on television, we were informed that the third plane was flying just above the school at the very same time. The events of that day seemed to heighten the immersion process as I was in the same room with the person who would become the gatekeeper to my study participants. The gatekeeper allows the researcher entrance into the culture and promotes acceptance by letting the potential participants and their parents/guardians know that the researcher is *safe territory* (Leininger, 1991, 1995, 2002c). The gatekeeper is one of the most important people for having a successful immersion and for conducting a cultural field study, and in performing the data analysis. I quickly learned that this gatekeeper, a volunteer at the school, held the confidence of all of my potential participants when I heard them calling her "mom." She was vitally important in helping me to in obtaining signatures for the informed consent and assent documents.

I spent time with the gatekeeper (immersed) for several weeks learning about the culture, the school, and the students and faculty. She invited me to attend Parent-Teacher Association (PTA) meetings, faculty and staff meetings, and school-sponsored dances and activities throughout the early part of my immersion. I evolved into a *presence* at the school before any information about the study became known or data collection took place. Early on, I was introduced during a school assembly by the school principal; students were told that I would be spending time at the school conducting research for my dissertation. The research was not mentioned again for another three months.

As time progressed, the immersion experience moved into the classrooms where I spent time with the students, still primarily as an observer but interacting more each day by helping them with homework and just talking to them. I ate lunch with them in the cafeteria where I was able to have more casual conversations and get to know them better. The students began to initiate conversations with me and we entered the initial friend status described by Leininger (1991) in her Stranger-to-Trusted Friend Enabler. At this point, I was known but still not fully trusted; gaining trusted status was crucial to learning truths about the culture. My observation status gradually evolved into having some participation and then into active involvement as described in the Observation-Participation-Reflection Enabler (OPR; Leininger, 1991). I had begun the immersion process in late August and by late November, I felt ready to begin the process of describing my research to the potential participants and evaluating whether I had achieved a trusted level with them. By that time, I had consents signed by most of the parents/guardians, but had not yet gotten the assents signed by the adolescents. With the assistance of the gatekeeper, the parents were willing and even anxious to have me talk to their children about gangs. The adolescents were initially slower to consider participating. I started out with 13 key participants (11 boys and 2 girls) who were willing to take part in the study. As time went on the sampling actually snowballed; the adolescent participants were recruiting more potential participants than I could handle for this in-depth qualitative study.

Even after the consents were signed, it was clear that the trust level had not been fully developed. The adolescents were still testing the waters; they told me that they had stolen telephones or participated in some other questionable action that I knew not to be true. I did not question them but rather let them tell me these things. Later, I realized that they were testing me to see if I was going to tell anyone. When they realized/discovered that I did not reveal any of this information, I was then able to move to a deeper level of trust with the adolescents.

Although I had discussed the Certificate of Confidentiality with the adolescents and what it meant, they continued to test me to see if I would actually follow through and keep their confidences. I further told the adolescents that if they expressed plans to hurt themselves or someone else, such information would not be kept confidential—although the latter was not required by the Certificate of Confidentiality, which specifically addressed elder abuse and child abuse to others, but did not include acts of self-harm or abuse to nonvulnerable people. I repeated these rules each time I met with them so they were clear on what I would keep confidential and what I would report. Early data that was collected when I was unsure of truth was not included in the final data analysis. The adolescents' trust and confidence in me strengthened as the data collection process proceeded and was evidenced by their behavior in my presence, the depth of their stories, and confirmation of their stories (when able).

Evolution of the Immersion Experience

Immersion continued throughout the field study, continually evolving into deeper and deeper levels of engagement and truth-sharing. As the layers of mistrust and distrust were peeled back, I got closer to the core, basic truths of the culture. As deepening feelings of connectedness with the students developed, I experienced a new level of understanding about urban African American adolescents in gangs. This connection and level of communication was not language-dependent, but rather a kind of tacit *knowing* that a level of trust had emerged—one that would yield truth in the data. This is part of the *art of nursing*; it is not cognitive, not empirically verifiable, but remains in the metaphysical realm as described by Finfgeld-Connett (2008). It was as if a *gestalt** had occurred; actions and behaviors made sense to me where before I may have dismissed these behaviors as meaningless or silly. Every word, every behavior had a deep, rich meaning for me. There were also instances where I could forsee certain reactions or behaviors from the adolescents whereas before they would have taken me by surprise. It was at this point that I realized communication was occurring without the use of language. Language was no longer necessary for *understanding* and there was no known language to describe the experiential knowledge gained through this form of enlightenment. It was at this point that I knew I had reached full immersion into the African American subculture of adolescent gangs.

It was also evident that I had to continue to work with them by intensive listening, reflecting my understanding

of what they said, and—most importantly—maintaining their trust in order to remain immersed with them at this level. This is a special moment recognized by every researcher who has ever achieved complete immersion. At this point, I felt all of my biases and prejudices had been lifted away. It was one of the most intense feelings of freedom I had ever experienced because I was able to understand their cultural lifeways in a way that I previously had not. I felt truly nonjudgmental because I *understood*. This is a difficult moment to express in words. The inability to fully describe how I knew I had achieved a successful immersion is part of the art of nursing where knowledge has been gained at a metaphysical (spiritual) level that is beyond the science of nursing.

There were several ways I maintained the in-depth level of immersion with the African American culture and the subculture of adolescent gangs. I had been giving the adolescent participants candy for their willingness to talk with me. One morning one of the participants came to me and handed me a crumpled dollar bill and two quarters. When I asked what this was for, he said that he had sold the candy that I had given him and that he thought this was really my money and not his. I assured him that the candy had been a gift to him and therefore this was his money. Hence, the idea was born to start a candy business. With approval from the principal and school board, the adolescents and I started a candy business. I bought bulk candy for them, and after expenses were paid, the sales provided a small amount of money for those who worked the business. The students were planning a trip to Washington, D. C. at the end of the school year and everyone who travelled to D. C. was to be given $25 for the trip from money that came from lunch-hour candy sales at the school. The gatekeeper kept the financial records; because of her trustworthy reputation with the adolescents, this also arrangement also helped them to maintain their trust in me. The adolescents looked forward to working in the candy store and would give me specific orders for what I should purchase. Their trust in me was maintained along with my level of immersion as we partnered in the noon-time candy business.

A Sad Occurrence

It was after the completion of my data collection but when I was still going to the school on a regular basis that one of the adolescent participants died as a result of suicide. I recall visiting him in the intensive care unit during my lunch hour, holding his hand and talking to him. I felt sad not only because I knew he had so much to offer the world, but also because he was the first one with whom I had felt truly immersed during that early period of my time at the school. He was one who came to me with the crumpled money because he had sold the candy I had given him. He was one of those adolescents who had recently turned 13 years old—things seemed to change for all of them when they hit their 13th year (Morris, 2012). He died after a week in the hospital, never having regained consciousness.

The young man's homegoing (funeral) service was beautiful cultural experience in African American spirituality for me. I attended the homegoing service with the adolescents from the school, many of whom had been participants in my research. The service lasted about two hours; the first hour being very quiet and solemn. The pastors spoke and friends and family gave testimonials and told stories. The first hour ended in a prayer and then the coffin was closed. Immediately upon its closure, the clergy leading the service broke into joyous singing and dancing. Soon the people were also standing, singing, and dancing. The mood was upbeat, lively, and joyous as if welcoming the deceased into his eternal heavenly home. They were celebrating because he had *gone home*. While it was an emotionally draining experience, it left me with a sense of peace, calm, and happiness. For me, this was not an immersion experience, but rather a post-immersion experience. It left me with a reinforced feeling of connectedness to the adolescents, the school staff, my gatekeeper, and the larger surrounding community.

Leaving the Research Domain

Once my data collection was over, I did not leave the adolescent participants from the school. Leaving the field in an appropriate and respectful way is as important as entering and immersing. I would emphasize the importance of remaining with the community after the completion of the data collection and analysis. This helps to prevent participant feelings of abandonment or of having been "used" for research purposes. It was also helpful to me to remain with this community with which I had built close relationships and friendships, offsetting my own feelings of loss and emptiness because the field work had concluded and the nature of

our relationships had changed. Spending time *leaving* the culture is equally as important as the time spent *immersing* into the culture, and generally requires a longer period of time—if, in fact, one ever does truly leave a place where strong relationships have been built. I continued to volunteer at the school for one to two days a week, and continued to talk to the participants. They seemed to know when I was coming, because they would always want to talk. I had to remind them that I no longer had the Certificate of Confidentiality and so what they said now could be subpoenaed into court. They were careful in refraining from talking about any criminal actions, and although our conversations remained in-depth, they did take on a different tone without that protection. I was appointed to the Board of Education for the school and served for approximately one year after the data collection period had ended. This allowed me to maintain a presence in the school until I moved out of the city about the same time that many of the student participants were moving on to other schools, so our separation thus occurred more naturally. However, I have maintained my relationship with the gatekeeper, so I am still able to keep abreast about all of the research participants.

Immersing in Other Similar and Diverse Cultures

Each cultural immersion is as different as the individual culture itself. I have more recently immersed with another culture of African American adolescents in a Midwestern city different from where my dissertation research took place. They are not gang members, but rather are part of a youth council that is actively involved in their community in a variety of ways. They are highly respected members of the community and the city in which they reside. After two years of immersion with this group, I arrived at a level of trust where research could begin. This immersion took much longer as I was not with them every day in school, but instead met with them once a week for a couple of hours at one of their regular youth council meetings. A gatekeeper who was an adult leader of the group and well respected by both the adolescents and the overall community invited me into the group. Getting to know the gatekeeper and the other adults who worked with the adolescents was a crucial first step.

I attended the weekly meetings as an observer for nearly two years before I moved into the active participation phase (Leininger, 1991). Serving as a group facilitator was the first activity where I assumed an active role with this group. During that particular meeting, I was surprised at their openness, not only in talking casually, but also with the questions that they asked me. For example, they wanted to know how I felt when they discussed racial issues or made some comments about White people. For me, this was evidence that we were able to cross racial lines and establish talking points where conversations about our differences as well as our similarities were informative, nonjudgmental, healing, and growth-producing.

Since facilitating that initial session, I have continued to lead sessions as well as participate in a number of field trips to cultural celebrations such as the Juneteenth Celebration, the Martin Luther King March, rap concerts, and movies related to African American history including "42" and "Selma." Having the adolescents in the car or riding a bus with them during these trips accelerates the immersion experience because we can converse on a more personal level, as well as allowing me to listen to their peer conversations with one another. When they are in my car, they select the radio stations that we listen to—their music, both words and rhythm, provides me with further cultural awareness and insight into their values and lifeway practices. There is also an unwritten rule about 'what is said in my car stays in my car'—within the parameters of what I can ethically keep secret. Walking alongside them in the Martin Luther King Day March was a powerful experience for me as we sang "We Shall Overcome." Again, this was one of those experiences where there are not words to adequately describe the feeling, but it is a metaphysical experience that runs deeper than conversation and language. These metaphysical feelings fall within the parameters of the *art of nursing*, which are indescribable in language, but are a *knowing* and a *feeling* of being in concert with those around you.

On occasion, the adolescents have asked me to help them organize parties and other events. For example, they wanted to have a surprise celebratory event for the adult leaders of their group to show their appreciation and they asked me to help them with food, cards, and planning. On another occasion they asked me to participate in the Kwanzaa celebrations *and* if I would be willing to bring the macaroni and cheese.

The adolescents have also invited me into their Youth Council leadership meetings and other formal activities of the Council. The more frequently I see them, the deeper the immersion becomes. Others have invited me to become Facebook "friends" with them, which has also been an immersion promoter in that I can be in contact with them more frequently than just at the weekly meetings. Being invited to participate in their insider activities has validated my acceptance into the group.

Many of the adolescents' parents/guardians or caregivers also participate in the weekly meetings, which has enabled me to immerse with other family members as well. At present, I am working with adolescents and adults in this community on an ethnohistory project. When I first entered into this community, I looked for historical documents as a means to gain a better understanding about them but found little information. Given that one of the goals of the Youth Council meetings has been to teach African American history and because they wanted older people and adolescents in the community to forge stronger connections, it seemed as though developing an ethnohistory of the community would be an ideal project toward meeting those goals. The adolescents were trained how to interview adults to elicit ethnohistorical stories about their community. A video-ethnohistory along with a written history is a future project that adolescents and adults in the community plan to work on together. The adolescents have voiced enthusiasm and are anxious to get started. I thought it laudable that they suggested also conducting a Jewish ethnohistory of the community, recognizing that it had been primarily Jewish before it was African American.

Attending the Youth Council Meetings with the adolescents in addition to the cultural community events taught me many things that I had not known about African American history. All of my time spent over the years as a student in the classroom and the time I spent reading about the culture did not inform me as fully as these classes taught by African Americans about African Americans and African history—in addition to attending numerous and varied community cultural events. It has become clear to me that all of the formal classes in which I have been the learner have been taught from an ethnocentric dominant cultural perspective! I would venture to suggest that elementary, secondary, and higher education history classes continue to be taught from this same ethnocentric perspective. Knowing cultural and ethnohistorical truths about ethnic and cultural groups of people is essential for the provision of quality health care and to promote community healing and peace. The lack of healthcare provider knowledge about people from cultures other than their own is no longer acceptable or excusable. Immersing with people of other cultures and ethnicities is a *must* in order to learn, understand, and be responsive to the healthcare needs of diverse populations.

I recently received funding notification that will allow me to begin an ethnonursing community-based participatory action study to learn about ways to make the community safer by designing interventions to prevent violence and promote safety and wellbeing within the community. These interventions will be developed by the adolescents and then tested at a later date in an intervention study. Funding will be sought from the National Institutes of Health (NIH) to further develop and test the health promotion strategies developed by members of the community.

Cultural Immersion in a non-English Speaking Country

A few years ago, I had the opportunity to travel to the University of Panama in a visiting faculty role to teach Leininger's Theory of Culture Care Diversity and Universality to doctoral students. All classes at the University were taught in Spanish and the country was largely Spanish-speaking. I was not fluent in Spanish. Most of the students at that time were non-English speaking and we were dependent upon the coordinator of the doctoral program for communication with one another. The coordinator of the program, Dr. Lydia de Isaacs, had organized my coming to Panama to teach so we both knew well in advance that language was going to be a barrier to my communication with the students. I soon learned that not only was she fluent in Spanish and English, but she was an excellent translator and trustworthy for interpreting my English into Spanish. Having a trustworthy translator is crucial for a successful cultural immersion when there are language differences. Although language is a barrier to communication, it is not a barrier to developing meaningful and lasting relationships that reflect a successful cultural immersion.

My first visit to Panama lasted a full seven days. In addition to teaching, I was offered the opportunity to partake in several cultural events. Independence Day (Panama's independence from Columbia) was one of the major holidays celebrated while I was there. The School of Nursing had festivities where I was able to experience traditional foods, dance, and clothing. There are so many things to be learned about a culture through its music, dance, and food. Stories about the culture and its ethnohistory are shared through the interpretations of the creative and performing arts. Experiencing the arts of this culture made it evident that language is only one piece toward knowing its lifeways, values, beliefs, and practices. My birthday also was celebrated during the Independence Day events, and the faculty and students sang "Happy Birthday" in Spanish along with a birthday cake that was inscribed with "Felicidades Edith." I felt a deep sense of gratitude and connection with these people which, for me, verified that this cultural immersion was going well. This immersion, although somewhat difficult because of the language barrier, was actually easier and quicker than my previous immersions. There were several reasons for this, including the ease of immersing with adults rather than adolescents, and that my role with them was as a teacher rather than as a researcher. They had anticipated my coming and were anxious to learn about Leininger's theory, making my acceptance into the culture much easier.

I spent most of each day in the classroom with Dr. de Isaacs and the students during my first visit. Toward the end of the week, there were a few brief periods where it was just the students and me in the classroom without the benefit of a translator, and yet we found ways to communicate. One of the primary tools we used, although not necessarily a reliable one, was Google© Translate. There was also gesturing and discovering that there were words that had basic similarities between the languages. Our communication had reached a much deeper level than mere language; I became aware of this toward the end of the week. As we got to know each other better, a soul-to-soul communication emerged that allowed us to know one another in a way that went beyond language or science and delved into art of nursing. I was also picking up a few Spanish words by this time, so that was helpful for filling in the gaps. During the late afternoons and evenings, I was able to experience other events in Panama City including the Market Place where I was able to meet many indigenous people who were selling their art works. Being immersed in the aesthetics of a culture, including music as well as art, is another way to learn about cultural and ethnic history, traditions, beliefs, values, and lifeway practices.

The following year, I was able to reconnect with the students and Dr. de Isaacs when we attended the Annual International Conference of the Transcultural Nursing Society. During the conference we spent much of the time together. Friendships between Dr. de Isaacs, the students, and myself became further solidified during this time and have remained strong since then. We continue to communicate both professionally and personally. Nine months later, I returned to Panama for ten days when I was a speaker at the Transcultural Nursing Conference in Santiago de Veraguas. I spent the remainder of my time there with the doctoral students assisting them with their research. I was also given the opportunity to accompany Dr. de Isaacs and her research team to the site of their field study in Koskuna where the Guna (an indigenous people) lived.

Being included in Dr. de Isaacs' field study with the Guna was a highlight of my second trip to Panama. This indigenous population was located just outside Panama City, Panama. With Dr. de Isaacs as the gatekeeper, I was able to participate in some of the research team's activities for the few hours that I was with them in the field. The team included nursing, sociology, education, psychology, and pharmacology researchers; the goal of the project was to improve the quality of life for the Guna people. Because I was in the company of Dr. de Issacs, the Guna were friendly and communicated openly with me in their native language or in English. I was able to walk the streets of the village, observe the children in the school, and browse about in a store that carried only the most essential items for meeting the needs of the village residents.

During this second visit to Panama, I stayed with Dr. de Isaacs rather than in a hotel. Being at her home allowed me to immerse deeper into the culture and learn more of the lifeways of the Panamanian people. By this time, the students were beginning to speak and understand English, and I was also a little better with my bit of Spanish. Communication through language was not the barrier that it had been during my first visit. I was also able to recognize some written words from the PowerPoint presentation at the conference. I even learned enough Spanish to say a sentence or two during my lecture! I have found that people whose first language is not English are very appreciative of efforts to speak or write to them their native language. I try to offer a few words, written or spoken, in the language of those with whom I am communicating whenever I am with different cultural groups. Attempting to speak the language of a culture is well worth the effort. It is meaningful to the people whose culture is being entered. These efforts do not have to be fluent or perfect; it is sufficient that the effort has been made. This is one concrete way of gaining respect from the people during the immersion process.

Three months afterward, I was able to again rejoin Dr. de Isaacs and three of the doctoral students at another transcultural nursing conference in the United States. Most of our time was spent reconnecting as friends and thus the cultural connection was maintained. Since that time, I have continued to communicate regularly with all of them through various electronic means; I write in Spanish and they write in English. In the near future, three of the doctoral students will be coming to the U. S. for their own international cultural experience wherein they will have the opportunity to immerse in a diverse culture outside of their country. I am honored and humbled that they chose to engage in that experience near where I now live.

■ SUMMARY

Cultural immersion is necessary to understand truths about a particular culture for researchers, healthcare providers, and students who want to learn how to conduct research or practice within a particular culture. The length of time needed to gain truths about a particular culture varies based on the context (high versus low) of the culture under study as well as the familiarity of the researcher/practitioner with the culture being studied. It is essential that the researcher or practitioner listen carefully and with a sincere interest in learning about the people's culture. Interest may be exhibited by the researcher/practitioner spending time within the culture by genuinely offering friendship to the people, along with an authentic interest in and enthusiasm about learning about their lifeways. It is important to have a guide such as Leininger's Stranger-to-Trusted Friend Enabler to confirm that an in-depth level of friendship and trust has been achieved in order to be assured that the shared information is credible and trustworthy. Once credible data has been acquired, it becomes useful and important for providing culturally congruent health care. It is vital to continually review and return to the people for substantiation of the data so as to ensure accurate truths about the culture are reported in the disseminated findings.

■ DEDICATION

It is indeed an honor to dedicate this chapter to the memory of Dr. Madeleine Leininger, my professor, mentor, constant supporter, and friend. Without her important insights, nurturing, patience, and caring, I would not have been able to achieve my goal of becoming a transcultural nurse.

It is also with gratitude and thankfulness that I dedicate this chapter to the everlasting memory of my dad and mom, John and Mildred Morris. Although my dad died when I was a freshman in college, he had always encouraged me to become a nurse. Mom was a constant source of encouragement throughout my many years in school and throughout my career as a nurse. Most of all, I am grateful that they instilled in me a deep sense and appreciation for humanitarianism, as well as providing the foundation that nourished my sense of social justice, equality, and fairness.

■ ACKNOWLEDGEMENTS

I wish to gratefully acknowledge three colleagues and friends without whose constant encouragement and guidance this chapter might never have come to fruition. Dr. Jean Anthony suggested the idea of writing a chapter where I could talk about my immersion experiences with adolescents from a culture vastly different from my own. Dr. Karen Burkett listened to my ideas about how to write this chapter and was always able to come up with just the right source to support my ideas and move me forward in the writing of the chapter. Rev. Peter Matthews was an avid listener, a valued supporter, and a constant source of encouragement for me. He stimulated my writing creativity by encouraging me to write in such a manner that thrust me completely out of my comfort zone and into a new and artful style of writing. Additionally, he made me aware of the hidden meaning of the word "privilege"--a word that I frequently used in relation to being allowed to enter another's culture. He suggested that I instead use the words "humbled" or "honored" as less offensive words. I can never again use the word

privilege without being reminded that this may not be a respectful word among many cultures, particularly when used by someone with Euro-American cultural origins.

Finally, I want to acknowledge my family: My husband Dave Morris and my daughters Sarah Morris, and Megan Morris, who have always been supportive of my efforts in many different ways—from listening to me go on for hours about my passions and ideas to proofreading multiple drafts of my manuscripts and lectures.

■ DISCUSSION QUESTIONS

1. You are travelling to a foreign country where you only know a few words of the language. As you leave the airport and head to the site of your fieldwork, how would you greet the people? What would you want to say first? (Assume that you have a trustworthy professional interpreter.)
2. You are entering a culture in your country that is different from your own. The culture that you are entering is suspicious of people from outside the culture, particularly professionals and researchers. What would you do to gain trust?
3. As a new researcher, you have become interested in studying the roots of your own culture in your indigenous country/native homeland. How would your cultural immersion be different from your immersion into a culture *different* from your own?
4. Discuss whether it is possible to fully immerse into a culture other than your own. Can you fully be accepted as a "new" member of that culture? Can you ever be trusted fully enough to gain truthful and credible data from the culture that you are studying?
5. How would you ensure ethical and legal parameters are met when you are reporting about a culture other than your own?

■ GLOSSARY

Cultural imposition: "…refers to the tendency of an individual or group to impose their beliefs, values, and patterns of behavior or another culture for varied reasons" (Leininger, 2002a, p. 52).

Ethnocentrism: "…refers to the belief that one's own ways are the best, most superior, or preferred ways to act, believe, or behave" (Leininger, 2002, p. 50).

Ontological: "...refers to the branch of metaphysics that studies the nature of existence or being" (Retrieved from http://www.dictionary.com/browse/ontological?s=t).

Epistemological: "...is the branch of philosophy that investigates the origin, nature, methods, and limits of human knowledge" (Retrieved from http://www.dictionary.com/browse/epistemological?s=t)

Emic: "...refers to local, indigenous, or insider's views and values about a phenomenon or experience (adapted from Leininger, 2002, p.84); influences care decisions and actions in primary care (Eipperle, 2015, p. 322).

Etic: "...refers to outsider's or more universal views and values about a phenomenon or experience (adapted from Leininger, 2002, p.84); influences care decisions and actions in primary care (Eipperle, 2015, p. 322).

Cultural Awareness: "...is the self-examination and in-depth exploration of one's own cultural and professional background" (Campinha-Bacote, 2002, p. 182).

Cultural Competence: "...is the ongoing process in which the health care provider continuously strives to achieve the ability to effectively work within the cultural context of the client (individual, family, community" (Campinha-Bacote, 2002, p. 181). This ongoing process involves the integration of cultural awareness, cultural knowledge, cultural skill, cultural encounters, and cultural desire.

Critical Reflective Journaling: "...assists students in the practice of interpretive thinking; helping them to (Isaacson, 2014, p. 251) 'unlearn past understandings and become a nurse who is adept at thinking from multiple perspectives and at challenging her own current assumptions and understandings'" (Issacson, 2014, as cited by Ironside, 2006, p. 484).

Hermeneutic Phenomenological Methodology: Involves reading and re-reading the text, and committing time for reflection and pondering. While dwelling with the text, "...the researcher periodically returns to the literature and the participants; journals, thoughtfully considering each participant's use of particular words (Ironside, 2008), respecting the 'languages own essence'" (Issacson, 2014, as cited by Heidegger, 1977/1993, p. 348).

Gestalt: "...a configuration or pattern of elements so unified as a whole that it cannot be described merely as a sum of its parts" (Retrieved from http://www.vocabulary.com/dictionary/gestalt); a simultaneous converging of ideas/concepts....a higher level synthesis / realization of thought and awareness.

■ REFERENCES

Adams, A. (n.d.). Quotation. Retrieved from http://thinkexist.com/quotation/some_photographers_take_reality-and_impose_the/223023.html

Amerson, R. (2012). The influence of international service-learning on transcultural self-efficacy in baccalaureate nursing graduates and their subsequent practice. *International Journal of Teaching and Learning in Higher Education*, 24(1), 6-15.

Anderson, K., Friedemann, M-L., Buscher, A., Sansoni, J., & Hodnicki, D. (2012). Immersion research education: Students as catalysts in international collaboration research. *International Nursing Review*, 54(9), 502-510. doi:10.1111/j.1466-7657.2012.01014.x.

Campinha-Bacote, J. (2002). The process of cultural competence in the delivery of healthcare services: A model of care. *Journal of Transcultural Nursing*, 13(3), 181-184.

Camphina-Bacote, J. (2007). *The process of cultural competence in the delivery of healthcare services: The journey continues* (5th ed.). Cincinnati, OH: Transcultural C.A.R.E. Associates.

Carper, B. A. (1978). Fundamental patterns of knowing in nursing. *Advances in Nursing Science*, 1(1), 13-24.

Eipperle, M. K. (2015). Application of the three modes of culture care decisions and actions in advanced primary care. In M. R. McFarland & H. B. Wehbe-Alamah (Eds.), *Leininger's culture care diversity and universality: A worldwide nursing theory* (3rd ed., p. 322). Burlington, MA: Jones and Bartlett Learning.

Epistemological. (n. d.). *Dictionary.com*. Retrieved from http://www.dictionary.com/browse/epistemological?s=t

Finfgeld-Connett, D. (2008). Concept synthesis of the art of nursing. *Journal of Advanced Nursing*, 62(3), 381-388. doi: 10.1111/j.1365-2648.2008.04601.x

Gestalt. (n. d.). *Vocabulary.com*. Retrieved from http://www.vocabulary.com/dictionary/gestalt

Guo, Y., Wang, S, Corbin, M., Wynne, C., & Statz, S. (2014). Cross-national emailing as cultural immersion in multicultural counselor training: A pilot study. *Journal of International Counselor Education*, 1(6), 28-45.

Hall, E. T. (1959). *The silent language*. New York: Double Day.

Hall, E.T. (1969). *The hidden dimension*. New York: Double Day.

Hall, E.T. (1976). *Beyond culture*. New York: Double Day.

Hall, E.T. (1983). *The dance of life*. New York: Double Day.

Haviland, W. A., Prins, H. E. L., McBride, B., & Walrath, D. (2013). *Cultural anthropology: The human challenge*. Belmont, CA: Wadsworth Publishers.

Heidegger, M. (1977/1993). *Basic writings*. New York, NY: Harper-Collings.

Heppner, P., & Wang, K. (2014). A cross-cultural immersion program: Promoting students' cultural journeys. *The Counseling Psychologist*, *42*(8), 1159-1187.

Harrowing, J. N., Gregory, D. M., O'Sullivan, P. S., Lee, B., & Doolittle, L. (2012). A critical analysis of undergraduate students' cultural immersion experiences. *International Nursing Review*, *59*(4), 494-501. doi: 10.1111/j.1466-7657.2012.01012.x

Hubbert, A. O. (2006). Application of culture care theory for clinical nurse administrators and managers. In M. M. Leininger & M. R. McFarland (Eds.), *Culture care diversity and universality: A worldwide nursing theory* (2nd ed., pp. 349-364). Sudbury, MA: Jones and Bartlett.

Ingulli, C., Doutrich, D., Allen, C., & Dekker, L. (2014). Opened my eyes: The meaning of an immersion experience for currently practicing nurses. *Online Journal of Cultural Competence in Nursing and Healthcare*, *4*(1), 6-16. doi: 10.9730/ojccnh.org/v4n1a1

Ironside, P. M. (2006). Using narrative pedagogy: Learning and practicing interpretive thinking. *Journal of Advanced Nursing*, *55*(4), 478-486. Retrieved from doi: 10.1111/j.1365-2648.2006.03938.x

Ironside, P. M. (2008). *Heideggerian hermeneutics*. Presentation given at the Institute for Heideggerian Hermeneutical Methodologies, Indianapolis, IN.

Isaacson, M. (2014). Clarifying concepts: Cultural humility or competency. *Journal of Professional Nursing*, *30*(3), 251-258. Retrieved from http://dx.doi.org/10.1016/j.profnurs

Jeffreys, M. R. (2000). Development and psychometric evaluation of the trans-cultural self-efficacy tool: Synthesis of findings. *Journal of Transcultural Nursing*, *11*(2), 127-136.

Jeffreys, M. R., & Dogan, E. (2010). Factor analysis of the transcultural self-efficacy tool (TSET). *Journal of Nursing Measurement*, *18*(2), 120-139.

Jones, A. M., Neubrander, J., & Huff, M. (2012). A cultural immersion experience for nursing students. *Global Partners in Education Journal*, *2*(1), 1-11.

Knecht, L. A., & Sabatine, C. K. (2015). Application of culture care theory to international service learning experiences in Kenya. In M. R. McFarland & H. B. Wehbe-Alamah (Eds.), *Leininger's culture care diversity and universality: A worldwide nursing theory* (3rd ed., p. 482). Burlington, MA: Jones and Bartlett Learning.

Larsen, R., & Reif, L. (2011). Effectiveness of cultural immersion and culture classes for enhancing nursing students' transcultural self-efficacy. *Journal of Nursing Education*, *50*(6), 350-354.

Leininger, M. M. (1991). Ethnonursing: A research method with enablers to study the theory of culture care. In M. M. Leininger (Ed.), *Culture care diversity and universality: A theory of nursing* (pp. 73-117). New York, NY: National leagues for Nursing Press.

Leininger, M. M. (1995). Transcultural nursing: Development, focus, importance and historical development. In M. M. Leininger (Ed.), *Transcultural nursing: Concepts, theories, research, & practice* (2nd ed., pp. 3-54). New York: McGraw-Hill Publishers.

Leininger, M. M. (2000). Founder's focus: Transcultural nursing is discovery of self and the world of others. *Journal of Transcultural Nursing*, *11*(4), 312-313. doi: 10.1177/104365960001100412

Leininger, M. M. (2002a). Essential transcultural nursing care concepts, principles, examples, and policy statements. In M. M. Leininger & M. R. McFarland (Eds.), *Transcultural nursing: Concepts, theories, research, & practice* (3rd ed., pp. 45-69). New York, NY: McGraw-Hill.

Leininger, M. M. (2002b). Ethical, moral, and legal aspects of transcultural nursing. In M. M. Leininger & M. R. McFarland (Eds.), *Transcultural nursing: Concepts, theories, research, & practice* (3rd ed., 271-299). New York, NY: McGraw-Hill.

Leininger, M. M. (2002c). Part I. The theory of culture care and the ethnonursing research method. In M. M. Leininger & M. R. McFarland (Eds.), *Transcultural nursing: Concepts, theories, research, & practice* (3rd ed., pp. 71-98). New York, NY: McGraw-Hill.

Leininger, M. M. (2006a). Culture care diversity and universality theory and evolution of the ethnonursing method. In M. M. Leininger & M. R. McFarland (Eds.), *Culture care diversity and universality: A worldwide nursing theory* (2nd ed., pp. 1-41). Sudbury, MA: Jones and Bartlett.

Leininger, M. M. (2006b). Ethnonursing and research enablers. In M. M. Leininger & M. R. McFarland (Eds.), *Culture care diversity and universality: A worldwide nursing theory* (2nd ed., pp. 43-81). Sudbury, MA: Jones and Bartlett.

Loo, R., & Shiomi, K. (1999). A structural and cross-cultural evaluation of the inventory of cross-cultural sensitivity. *Journal of Social Behavior and Personality*, *14*(2), 267-278.

Morris, E. (2004). *An ethnonursing culture care study of the meanings, expressions, and lifeway experiences of selected urban African American adolescent gang members* [Doctoral dissertation]. Available from ProQuest Dissertations and Theses database (UMI No. 3130357).

Morris, E. (2012). Respect, protection, faith and love: Major care constructs identified within the subculture of selected urban African American adolescent gangs. *Journal of Transcultural Nursing*, *23*(3), 262-269.

Morris, E. (2015). An examination of subculture as a theoretical social construct through an ethnonursing study of urban African American adolescent gang members. In M. R. McFarland & H. B. Wehbe-Alamah (Eds.), *Leininger's culture care diversity and universality: A worldwide nursing theory* (3rd ed., pp. 255-285). Burlington MA: Jones and Bartlett Learning.

Ontological. (n. d.). In *Dictionary.com*. Retrieved from http://www.dictionary.com/browse/ontological?s=t

Ray, M., Morris, E., & McFarland, M. R. (2013). Ethnonursing method of Dr. Madeleine Leininger. In C. T. Beck (Ed.), *Routledge international handbook of qualitative nursing research* (pp. 213-229). New York, NY: Routledge.

Thackrah, R., Thompson, S., & Durey, A. (2014). Listening to the silence quietly: Investigating the value of cultural immersion and remote experiential learning in preparing midwifery students for clinical practice. *BMC Research Notes*, *7*(685), 1-2. Retrieved from http://www.biomedcentral.com/1756-0500/7/685.

Sodowsky, G.R., Taffe, R.C., Gutkin, T.B., & Wise, S.L. (1994). Development of the multicultural counseling inventory: A self-report measure of multicultural competencies. *Journal of Counseling Psychology*, *41*(2), 137-148.

Wehbe-Alamah, H. B., & McFarland, M. R. (2015a). Leininger's enablers for use with the ethnonursing research method. In M. R. McFarland & H. B. Wehbe-Alamah (Eds.). *Leininger's culture care diversity and universality: A worldwide nursing theory* (3rd ed., pp. 73-100). Burlington, MA: Jones and Bartlett Learning.

Wehbe-Alamah, H. B., & McFarland, M. R. (2015b). The ethnonursing research method. In M. R. McFarland & H. B. Wehbe-Alamah (Eds.). *Leininger's culture care diversity and universality: A worldwide nursing theory* (3rd ed., pp. 35-71). Burlington, MA: Jones and Bartlett Learning.

CHAPTER 20

Culturally Competent Research Using the Culture Care Theory: Malaria Care in Maasailand

Cecily W. Strang and Sandra J. Mixer

> *"People of different cultures can inform and are capable of guiding professionals to receive the kind of care they desire or need"* (McFarland, 2010, p. 459).

■ INTRODUCTION

Across the globe, people remain at risk for diseases that are both preventable and curable. The environmental contexts, ethnohistories, and cultural lifeways of many indigenous populations influence barriers to professional care/cure practices that could improve their health. It is essential to discover culture-specific care desires and needs among diverse peoples and cultures in order to deliver safe and beneficial professional health care. The Theory of Culture Care Diversity and Universality (also known as the Culture Care Theory or CCT) and the Ethnonursing Research Method are relevant and useful to discover the care needs of human beings. Knowledge of these needs is necessary to provide culturally congruent health care that respects the values, beliefs, and practices of people of diverse or similar cultures.

The discovery and delivery of culturally congruent care requires culturally competent research. Nurse researchers are accountable to conduct rigorous studies in their pursuit to discover practices that will guide care decisions and actions. The research process, focused on the domain of inquiry (DOI; a health care phenomenon within a specific culture), includes respect for and discovery of the people's worldview,

social structure, environmental context, care expressions and patterns, as well as their cultural values, beliefs, and lifeways (McFarland & Wehbe-Alamah, 2015). Research findings can be synthesized to recommend safe and beneficial care practices that promote the wellbeing of people.

The purpose of this chapter is to provide an exemplar of culturally competent research using the culture care theory (CCT) and Ethnonursing Research Method. The theory and method served as the framework that enabled a Western researcher to conduct a study within a developing world context. The research was an ethnonursing study focused on the domain of inquiry of culturally congruent malaria care among the Maasai in the Kimana region of Kenya, East Africa (C. W. Strang, 2014). Overall research findings have been previously published (Strang & Mixer, 2015). This chapter presents a synthesis of literature and previously unpublished data from this study and the process of culturally competent research that led to the discovery of themes, care constructs, and care decisions and actions. The authors focus on understanding the unique culture of the Maasai, the importance of emic discovery, the invaluable use of CCT enablers, and the intricate and challenging process of language translation.

The primary researcher made numerous visits to Maasailand for over 26 years and immersed herself within their culture as a community health worker. Visits ranged from two to four weeks with one experience lasting two years. Respected by many in the community, she was honored with the gift of the Maasai name *Naserian*. During these visits, she heard little discussion of malaria care and no mention of malaria prevention during daily conversations. Maasai did not appear to feel fear or have a sense of defeat from the disease, possibly because they have always lived with it. However, when someone had malaria, the primary researcher noted that great concern was voiced and discussion centered on the severity of the illness and whether the person would live or die. In response to witnessing the burden of malaria among the Maasai people, the researcher sought to discover nursing care decisions and actions that would benefit their overall health, be receptively received, and remain culturally congruent within their traditional lifeways. Using the Maasai malaria care study as an exemplar, the authors encourage other ethnonursing researchers to explore their phenomenon of interest and discover care meanings, expressions, and practices of the cultural group being studied, whether individuals, families, community members, nursing students and faculty, or organizations.

MALARIA: GLOBALLY AND IN MAASAILAND

Malaria is preventable and treatable, yet this infectious disease continues to globally affect the health of millions as one of the top ten causes of sickness and death in developing, low-income countries (World Health Organization [WHO], 2015). Among the half of the world's population who live at risk, 300 million become infected and one million die; 90% of these deaths are among children under age five in Sub-Saharan Africa (WHO). The morbidity and mortality of malaria affect the overall health disparity and economic and political status of an individual, a community, and even an endemic nation (Kenya National Bureau of Statistics, 2011). Global interest in malaria care is consistent and focuses on three main aspects: *prevention* (U. S. President's Malaria Initiative, United States Department of Health and Human Services [USDHHS], 2012);

treatment (Centers for Disease Control, USDHHS, 2015); and *eradication* (National Institutes of Health, USDHHS, 2008). International and Kenyan national investments of time, funding, and human resources span a wide range of needs from quantitative and qualitative research to practical intervention strategies.

Although efforts by government and nongovernmental organizations (NGOs) have successfully decreased or eliminated malaria in various locations, the Maasai people of Kenya, East Africa continue to live at daily risk of infectivity. Only 14% of surveillance systems track the actual number of malaria occurrences worldwide and, because there are no surveillance strategies extant in Maasailand, the morbidity and mortality statistics for malaria among the Maasai in the Kimana region of Kenya are not fully known (WHO, 2013, 2015). Some statistics place this area as one of low transmission (WHO, 2013). However, the environment is conducive to endemic malaria. The area sits 1,200 meters above sea level (within the expected elevation for malaria of less than 2,500 meters) and is home to the female Anopheles mosquito (vector for malaria; USDHHS, 2015). In the Kimana region, there are areas with springs resulting in standing water and the nearby Amboseli National Park has year-round swampland. Further, the bi-modal rain pattern brings water and green grass to the dry expanse of the Rift Valley, which creates two high-transmission seasons. These are all factors conducive for mosquito propagation (USDHHS, 2015).

In addition, data gathered from the study informants supported the finding that malaria was a continued and primary health concern. Key informants who provided in-depth data about the DOI were traditional Maasai living in remote villages. General informants who provided additional reflective data about the DOI were Maasai and non-Maasai malaria care partners, pastors, and community members (McFarland & Wehbe-Alamah, 2015). Many informants participated in multiple interviews and provided confirmation of research findings. For example, two years prior to the study, the researcher traveled to the Kimana region to confirm that malaria was a primary concern of the Maasai and a significant need for malaria care research within their communities. The following question was posed to Maasai men and women, students, tribal elders, nurses in the local clinic, store owners, pastors, and government officials: "What is the number one health problem for Maasai in this area?" All but one responded, "Malaria!" (C. W. Strang, 2014).

Malaria care in any culture is multifaceted. Anyone who lives at high-risk can contract the disease, even those who use the best preventive measures. According to global experts (U. S. Centers for Disease Control and Prevention, the Kaiser Family Foundation, and the World Health Organization) *access to care*; *knowledge of preventive measures*; and *appropriate care to minimize consequences of active disease* are important best care practices for people at risk (USDHHS, 2012). The immediate concern is that this disease and its consequences are preventable (USDHHS, 2012). Barriers to effective malaria care frequently cited in the literature include insufficient infrastructure to enable prompt delivery of preventive measures (USDHHS, 2012); severity of illness secondary to poor baseline health in those infected (USDHHS, 2012); gaining a correct diagnosis prior to initiation of treatment (USDHHS, 2012); increased incidences of counterfeit drugs (USDHHS, 2012); factors related to climate change (WHO, 2015); lack of education and poor living conditions in homesteads (KFF, 2013); and lack of culturally appropriate communication strategies to initiate and sustain behavior change (WHO, 2015). The existence of these barriers was confirmed by the researcher during the ethnonursing study described. One healthcare informant stated that "...many Maasai present to the clinic with malaria symptoms, but we do not have the tests to accurately diagnose." Maasai informants acknowledged that professional care may be needed, but that they "...cannot walk to the hospital [with a sick child]. It is dangerous from wild animals and is too far.... We cannot hire transport because, during the rains when there is malaria, the roads are impassible." Another frequent comment was that "...the medicines at the government hospitals are not as strong as those from the private clinics" (C. W. Strang, 2014). It is important to partner with the host country and address their complex malaria care needs by focusing on strengthening infrastructure, improving the availability of supplies, and monitoring and evaluating malaria care measures (USDHHS, 2012).

In Maasailand, malaria is endemic–meaning it is in constant transmission with measurable new cases and has existed in this region for thousands of years (KFF, 2013). With a comprehensive literature review, only four studies were found that addressed malaria specifically within the context of the Maasai people. Two were ethnobotanical studies focused on herbs found within the Maasai geographic environment and traditionally used for malaria care (Bussmann et al., 2006; Koch, Tamez, Pezzuto, & Soejarto, 2005). One additional study examined Maasai perspectives toward health care that included malaria care in their review (Wanzala, Hassanali, Kibet, & Dossajee, 2005). Another qualitative study explored malaria beliefs and practices of pastoralists that also included Tanzanian Maasai (Malisa & Ndukai, 2009). No studies were found that explored the use of known professional care prevention and treatment modalities or the specific generic care uses of herbs for malaria care among the Kenyan Maasai. There were no studies found that addressed why morbidity and mortality statistics show low occurrence in the region, although local Maasai community members reported high occurrence.

■ THEORETICAL FRAMEWORK TO GUIDE CULTURALLY COMPETENT RESEARCH

The CCT with the ethnonursing method are appropriate to guide culturally competent qualitative research. Together, they provide an organizing framework for each step in the research process, beginning with the literature review to the development of the research questions and inquiry guide as well as during the analysis process and explication of the three care modes of decisions and actions. In addition, both the theory and the method guide researcher reflections and evaluations of comprehensive discoveries. Transcultural nurses serve diverse patient populations by addressing the culture care needs of individuals, families, groups, and/or communities. In addition, the CCT states that multiple influencers of care exist within every culture and that the ethnonursing method can be used to sensitively and competently discover largely unknown truths (McFarland, Mixer, Wehbe-Alamah, & Burk, 2012). An ethnonursing researcher needs to focus on showing respect for the people's cultural worldview, ethnohistory, cultural and social dimensions, and generic and professional care practices while discovering applications for culturally congruent care. Culturally congruent care is defined as "...culturally based care knowledge, acts, and decisions used in sensitive and knowledgeable ways to appropriately

TABLE 20.1. Themes and Patterns Synthesized from Discovered Meanings, Expressions, and Practices of Malaria Care Among the Maasai.

Theme One: Malaria Care is a Response by the Entire Maasai Community to Promote Community Wellbeing
   Pattern 1: Recognizing environment as cause and cure
   Pattern 2: Understanding of and familiarity with malaria
   Pattern 3: Responding as community in malaria care

Theme Two: *Enkai*, as Creator, is in Ultimate Control and is Resourced in Malaria Care
   Pattern 1: *Enkai* is Enkai
   Pattern 2: *Enkai* is creator and in control of the world
   Pattern 3: *Enkai* is resourced as a malaria care act

Theme Three: Malaria Care is a Planned Sequence of Traditional, Spiritual, and Professional Care/Cure Practices
   Pattern 1: Traditional care/cure practices are the first care act
   Pattern 2: Spiritual care/cure practices are a co-care act
   Pattern 3: Professional care/cure practices are an emerging care act
   Pattern 4: The Maasai environmental context influences facilitators and barriers to malaria care/cure practices

Theme Four: The Maasai Community is Resolute in Responding to the Malaria Illness
   Pattern 1: Maasai do not live in fear of the malaria illness
   Pattern 2: Maasai are curious to learn more about malaria care
   Pattern 3: Maasai do not depend upon political or nongovernment organizational support for malaria care

Reproduced, with permission from Strang, C. W., & Mixer, S. J. (2015, February 26). Discovery of the meanings, expressions, and practices related to malaria care among the Maasai. *Journal of Transcultural Nursing, 1-9.*

and meaningfully fit the cultural values, beliefs, and lifeways of clients for their health and wellbeing" (McFarland & Wehbe-Alamah, 2015, p. 14).

In the unique and beautiful sub-Saharan grasslands, the Maasai inhabitants continue their traditional lifeways and healthcare traditions. Malaria care has been minimally researched among the Maasai culture. The Ethnonursing Research Method was an appropriate qualitative approach to conduct a culturally sensitive research study to respectfully discover the rich knowledge of malaria care held by the Maasai people. The theoretical constructs of *care* and *culture* were discovered as influencers of malaria care within the Maasai emic perspective as described by four main themes and their supportive care patterns (Refer to Table 20.1; Strang & Mixer, 2015).

■ MAASAI CULTURAL AND SOCIAL STRUCTURE DIMENSIONS

The Sunrise Enabler is as a cognitive map that was used to visualize the domains of the CCT and guide comprehensive discovery based on the theory components throughout the entirety of the study (Refer to Color Insert 1). The review of literature and study findings

illustrating the rich Maasai cultural and social structure dimensions related to malaria care are synthesized as follows. Informant quotes organized within the CCT framework are summarized in Table 20.2.

Worldview

The worldview of the Maasai is a holistic perspective that interconnects the physical, mental, and spiritual realms. They exude pride as a people who are created by *Enkai* [God]. They continue to speak their oral language of *Maa*, uphold indigenous lifeways, and thrive among the provisions and challenges of the harsh environmental context in which they live. Their worldview was clearly reflected in the ethnonursing discoveries of their malaria care practices (C. W. Strang, 2014).

Environmental Context, Language Influences, and Ethnohistory

Maasailand, which straddles the Kenya/Tanzania border near Mount Kilimanjaro, comprises 150,000 square kilometers of the Great Rift Valley. The area has both wet and dry seasons, swamps, and a dry desert landscape. Implications of colonialism, which began in the early 1900s and escalated after WWII, have been far reaching (Homewood, Kristjanson, & Trench, 2009).

TABLE 20.2. Cultural and Social Dimensions of the Maasai and Malaria Care.

Factors	Maasai Informant Quotes
Environmental Context	"Malaria is especially a problem if it rains, … caused by long grass and stagnant water." "The mosquito bites before we light the fire at night, not during the day." "When you live near the water, you are more likely to get malaria." "It is important to know the specific part of each herb to use in malaria care… maybe the bark or leaf."
Language	*"Enk-agang'ani* is the same word used for malaria and for mosquito." *"Oltikana* means malaria and is also translated as fever." *"Enkeeya* translates to the following words: sickness, disease, and death."
Ethnohistory	"Herbs hold multiple purposes. They cause purging of the sickness," "aid in recovery when eat soup with herbs," and "prevent occurrence if you drink herbs all the time." * "Men collect herbs because they are strong. The roots are hard to dig out and herbs are located too far for women to travel safely." "I do not worry about my child getting malaria. My child *will* get malaria." *
Cultural Values, Beliefs, & Lifeways	"Malaria is in the blood, but affects the whole person." "In the morning you are ok, but by night you feel, you start shaking, headache, whole body feels very hot. So you say you are very sick: I have malaria!" "We believe the mosquito puts poison in the stomach, so we vomit and diarrhea to get rid of malaria." "You cannot get well unless you take the herbs with the tablets."
Kinship and Social	"My family nearby cares for me when I am sick." "The women wash the patient," "observe the sick person for signs of worsening illness or recovery," and "make recovery soup." "I take my child to the clinic for assessment and correct diagnosis."
Religious & Philosophical	*"Enkai* [God] is creator of the environment … the rain, the mosquitoes, and the herbs." "God is good, so we don't blame God for malaria." * "Every morning and evening hours I am telling God for malaria to disappear." "When my child gets sick, I start with prayer." *
Technological	"We mix the herbs with an *olkipire* [handmade stirring stick]." "We do not have a net. I put the child that sleeps with me under a blanket, so the mosquito does not bite her." "My neighbor has the radio for our village. You could advertise a malaria care seminar on the Maasai station." "I can get messages and call for help on my mobile [telephone]."
Political	"NGOs and elected officials do not care about health care." "The government has brought no nets this way." "The *liabon* [traditional healer] cannot help with malaria. The chief cannot help. Can you help?" "The current health system of Kenya does not understand the Maa culture or the inaccessibility of their community to health care facilities. They are pastoralists and the women and children suffer the most."

(Continued)

TABLE 20.2. Cultural and Social Dimensions of the Maasai and Malaria Care. *(Continued)*

Factors	Maasai Informant Quotes
Economic	"I [the herbalist] serve all the people around. I do not charge." "We have to sell livestock to [afford to] go to hospital. I ask permission from my husband to sell a goat or cattle, so I can take my child. If I cannot contact him, my neighbors will help me and I will somehow repay them." "We have not money to buy a net, but would use it if available and affordable."
Educational	"My parents taught me how to feed my children these herbs, so this disease can disappear." "People do not know the cause of malaria; they need education." "Is there a way to stop the sequence of events, from environmental cause, to illness, to the need for care and cure? Come back and teach us." "We are interested to learn more, because nobody loves to be sick." *

Reproduced, with permission from Strang, C. W. (2014). Discovery *of the meanings, expressions, and practices related to malaria care among the Maasai* [Doctoral dissertation]. Retrieved from http://trace.tennessee.edu/utk_graddiss/2734/
Note: Quotes noted with an * were published by Strang and Mixer (2015).

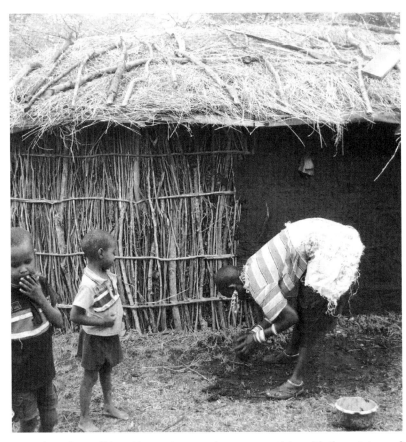

PHOTO 20.1 Construction of a traditional home by covering woven sticks with the mixture of cow dung, soil, and water. © C. W. Strang (2013).

The Maasai hold a unique sense of space and place in the environment that is deeply intertwined with their ethnohistory and worldview (Saitoti & Beckwith, 1980). Residents of the study area held the universal view that their environment, and thus most aspects of their life, was ultimately controlled by *Enkai* and not by themselves (Strang & Mixer, 2015). In their oral traditions in the Maa language, Maasai stories reflected that they are the chosen people of *Enkai* [God] and the receivers of land and all the world's cattle (Saitoti & Beckwith, 1980; F. F. Strang, 2004). Cattle have historically been at the center of the Maasai life and a measure of wealth for the family, village, and tribe (Thomson, 1885) — and remain so. The informants in this study were more traditionally oriented and their lifeways in the 21st century remained interwoven inseparably with the environment (Strang & Mixer, 2015). Sticks tied with grasses were covered with a mixture of mud from the earth and dung and urine from the livestock to form the walls of their homes. Hard-packed dirt constituted the floor and wood was the fuel used for cooking and heat. The forest served as the toilet. Most of their daily tasks involved resourcing provisions from their surroundings such as collecting firewood and water for village life, searching for grass and water for livestock, and collecting plants for medicinal care. Water sources varied from three to 20 km walking distance from a village circle or *enkang* (Wanzala et al., 2005). Because they lived predominately outdoors, the Maasai reported the "...mosquito bites were frequent and caused fevers and illness."

Healthcare and other decisions among the people are community and village-based rather than individually decided and determined by male elders in a traditionally patriarchal societal structure (Saitoti & Beckwith, 1980). As modernization encroaches into Maasailand, changes are occurring and traditional lifeways are challenged, including the availability and patterns of use for their pastoral rangelands; their traditional oral versus formal patterns of education; and their generic care versus professional healthcare practices (Hodgson, 2011). Maasai are beginning to reclaim their indigenous lifeways as a proactive adaptation to change (Hodgson). This activism reflects self-determination, engenders international support for indigenous peoples, and provides focus on the right of the indigenous Maasai to protect their land, resources, cultural identity, knowledge, and language (Hodgson).

However, none of the literature reviewed reported any current activism about health care in the rural Maasai villages. This dichotomy between traditional and contemporary Maasai culture highlights the challenges for professional caregivers who, although often not familiar with the unique Maasai culture, aim to offer beneficial, safe, and culturally congruent care that fits within the Maasai lifeway.

Cultural Values, Beliefs, and Lifeways

Each member of the Maasai community had a responsibility for the daily wellbeing of self and family as well as the village and community as a whole. Even a four-year-old child was responsible for daily tasks such as washing clothes or dishes, watching over a sibling, or collecting firewood near the village. When someone became sick with malaria, their chores had to be completed by others (Strang & Mixer, 2015).

Primary health care was provided at the local level by family or village members first, usually through use of herbs and traditional first aid measures. If this proved unsuccessful, the *laibon* [traditional spiritual leader/healer] or a Maasai herbalist was often consulted. Herbs held great value and were the common care act for treating malaria as well as other illnesses such as intestinal worms, stomach problems, and skin rashes. The roots, bark, and leaves from trees, shrubs, and other plants were resourced in medicinal care; there were specific plants used for malaria. Informants were confident in their knowledge and ability to recognize malaria symptoms and offer care using the appropriate herbs and correct dosages. A dramatic change has occurred in Maasailand regarding options for health care. Clinics now dot the landscape; some offer professional disease assessments and malaria care treatment (C. W. Strang, 2014; Strang & Mixer, 2015).

Beadwork is a traditional lifeway still practiced in all villages, mostly by women, and is one of the few possessions of the Maasai (Refer to Photo 20.2). Beadwork is a symbol of beauty, tradition, wealth, and gender, and symbolizes special life-event passages. Each Maasai informant wore traditional beadwork: Simple and intricate necklaces, earrings, and bracelets; bands worn around the head and waist; and/or beads sewn in decorative patterns onto fabrics, leather, or dried gourds. Informants mentioned that selling beadwork was one means to earn funds for professional malaria care (C. W. Strang, 2014).

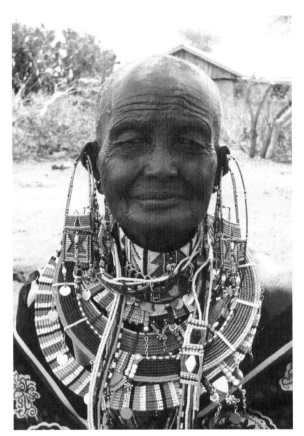

PHOTO 20.2 Maasai woman adorned with hand-crafted beaded jewelry. © C. W. Strang (2013).

Ceremonies

Within male or female age groups, transitions to new roles occur across their life span (Saitoti & Beckwith, 1980). Age-related rites of passage for males occur at approximately 10 to 15 year intervals, each celebrated with great ceremony. First, boys are initiated to warriorhood through circumcision and attain the status of *moran*. The next rites of passage are promotion to junior elder status, then to full elder. The moran live for a period of time in a separate warrior village, or *manyatta*, and are instructed by the elders on the lifeways of the Maasai (Saitoti & Beckwith, 1980). These traditions are in flux, as government pressure for Maasai to shorten the moran period has resulted in loss of instruction time on Maasai traditions and elevated younger men, less knowledgeable in the indigenous lifeways, to junior and full elder status (F. F. Strang, 2004). Age-related rites of passage for females are fewer and of shorter duration compared to the male ceremonies. For women, and traditionally after clitoridectomy, there are two other ceremonies: Marriage (often arranged by the father) and fertility (a ceremony to bestow a blessing for the bearing of many children; Mol, 1996). Most of the Maasai rites of passage ceremonies include expressive group singing and dancing (F. F. Strang, 2004).

Kinship Factors

In any social gathering traditional greetings using the correct etiquette are offered as an initial act to show respect toward community members. The physical and verbal acts of greeting depend upon the age of the greeting person and the greeted person. In the region of the study, Maasai persons of the same age use only words. Adults and children bow to be touched on the head when greeting an older person — an act showing respect and, in turn, to receive a blessing. Seniority based on the status of age remains a cultural value. In this patriarchal society, the oldest male elder in a village is held as their wisest decision maker; together, the most respected of these elders are the overall decision makers for the region (C. W. Strang, 2014).

Dwellings are arranged in a circular pattern surrounded by acacia thorn fencing to help protect women and children during the day and to keep domestic herd animals in and wild animals out at night. This circle of homes, or *enkang*, represents a unique kinship circle, the residence for up to 100 persons. This group may be composed of one male husband, his mother, one to four wives, and many children who are deeply loved within this tight polygamous or monogamous family structure (F. F. Strang, 2004; Wanzala et al., 2005).

Maasai men traditionally have cared for the animals and made family and community decisions (Mol, 1996). Maasai women traditionally have done most of the daily living chores such as build the home; search and collect firewood and water; cook; milk the animals; care for children; and pay for school and health care fees (Mol). Most of these traditional roles remain intact. The current Maasai diet includes milk, chai (mixture of tea, milk, and sugar), curd (soured milk), beans, meat, rice, and maize (C. W. Strang, 2014).

It was noted in several reviewed studies that it was difficult to gain access to female participants within the Maasai patriarchal society. However, mothers and grandmothers have been found to be the best sources of information regarding recent illnesses in the home

(Haasnoot, Boeting, Kuney, & van Roosmalen, 2010). Family structure was found to be very diverse — sometimes related by blood, sometimes by marriage — but representative of offering shelter to anyone in need. Usually, many family members lived together in a village setting. It is expected that all persons will be cared for (including orphans) and provided with the basics of life such as clothing, food, and an inside place to sleep. Daily chore responsibilities were assigned and the responsibility for children's fees to attend a nearby school was often provided (C. W. Strang, 2014; Strang & Mixer, 2015).

Religious and Philosophical Factors

Maasai are monotheistic, believing in one God, and that this one God is giver of life and wrath, rain, and mosquitoes; they generally discount witchcraft and superstition (Mol, 1996). Numerous buildings with crosses on the roofs were seen throughout the study area. Informants and guides confirmed that these structures were churches attended by Maasai (C. W. Strang, 2014).

Technological Factors

Examples of technologies used by the Maasai included wristwatches; flashlights (called *torches*); radios; and mobile telephones (Strang & Mixer, 2015). Mobile telephones are available, affordable, and commonly used among Maasai (Zurovac, Talisuna, & Snow, 2012). To use a mobile telephone in a low network area within Maasailand, one simply needs to climb the nearest hill to access a satellite link. The Maasai people also use mobile telephones to access the Internet, pay for goods, and transfer money: No bank, post office, or computer required (C. W. Strang, 2014).

Researchers have suggested use of such telecommunication technologies in developing countries also has the potential to improve malaria care by decreasing the communication gap between healthcare providers and malaria patients (Zurovac et al., 2012). In Kenya, mobile telephones have been used to conduct disease surveillance, perform medication treatment reviews with patients, and to provide education to healthcare workers via text messaging (Zurovac et al., 2012). Many Maasai had mobile telephones. Women often wore a pouch around their neck to hold their telephone and men slipped their telephones inside their belts (Strang & Mixer, 2015). Approximately half of the villages in the study also had a single radio which was shared among residents (C. W. Strang, 2014; Strang & Mixer, 2015).

Political and Legal Factors

For thousands of years, the Maasai roamed freely. However, in more contemporary times, wealthy Africans and non-Africans have moved into or are bordering Maasailand and government demarcation rules have reduced land resources available for use by the Maasai (Homewood et al., 2009). Such rapid change upon those who have long-occupied this land has affected their heritage. One change, among many, is the appearance of a few rural clinics offering some professional care and challenging traditional, generic care practices. Within the Maasai community, changes in traditional healthcare decisions and actions were made at several levels. Elders of the villages met together to discuss opportunities for change and decide what was best for the community as a whole. Young parent informants, who reported they had been to school and had had a science course, chose to use professional rather than generic care practices for their children. Informants, who were either government- or nongovernment-appointed leaders in Maasailand, all voiced a desire for opportunities to offer professional health care to Maasai in rural areas (C. W. Strang, 2014; Strang & Mixer, 2015).

Economic Factors

The Maasai informants reported the economic burden of malaria often relates to the cost of professional care and preventive measures. The benefit of using insecticide treated nets (referred to as ITNs) to prevent mosquito bites was often known; however, the nets were not affordable or accessible. Extra funds for malaria care are scarce in the Maasai community where most income is from subsistence livestock-keeping (Malisa & Ndukai, 2009). Beadwork or livestock had to be sold to raise money to take an ill person to a clinic when they were not cured by using traditional herbs. Private care centers offered higher-quality medicines but were more costly. Government facilities were usually attended because of their lower cost (C. W. Strang, 2014; Strang & Mixer, 2015).

Educational Factors

Oral stories and proverbs conveyed in Maa teachings by elders to the youth have been the main way of sharing traditional knowledge and lifeways (Saitoti & Beckwith, 1980). One large change in Maasailand is the opportunity for formal education. Sparsely located government or parochial schools were seen throughout Maasailand (C. W. Strang, 2014). Schools, conducted in English, teach the basics of science and often reclassify oral histories as myths. Some Maasai children attend school; however, they are still expected to remember their traditional roots. For example, one Maasai elder shared that, after he picked up his 12-year-old son from boarding school and prior to seeing his mother and siblings, the son was left in a remote location to herd the livestock for two weeks. Although it was important to receive an excellent school education, his son "...needed not to forget the traditional ways and who he was as a Maasai." In school, traditional malaria care practices are challenged and new understandings about diseases and the benefits of professional care are introduced (C. W. Strang).

■ CONDUCTING CULTURALLY COMPETENT RESEARCH

The primary researcher conducted a culturally competent research study with the use of the Culture Care Theory framework and the Ethnonursing Method. Cultural competence includes *cultural awareness* (affective dimension); *cultural sensitivity* (attitudinal dimension); *cultural knowledge* (cognitive dimension); and *cultural skills* (behavioral dimension; Rew, Becker, Cookston, Khosropour, & Martinez, 2003). Culturally competent researchers gather and use culture-specific knowledge in sensitive, creative, and meaningful ways (Papadopoulos, 2006). This is a continual process throughout the span of a study. This malaria care study provides an exemplar of the process of conducting culturally competent research in a developing world context.

The major constructs of the CCT were addressed in this study, beginning with the initial review of the literature to the identified culture care modes to maintain, negotiate, and/or repattern malaria care in a way that would benefit the health of the Maasai (McFarland & Wehbe-Alamah, 2015). As previously stated, the literature search was guided by the theoretical framework and included the topics of Maasai worldview, ethnohistory, and general literature on malaria and malaria care specific to the Maasai. Information from this literature was then compared to and

broadened with the discovered research findings. For example, the literature reviewed stated that the Maasai as a people were focused on community rather than individuals. The depth of this concept was confirmed by Maasai informant mothers who shared the following proverb: "Do not discriminate between all the children you are caring for, because maybe you will die [of malaria] and leave it to the other women in the village to care for your children."

The overwhelming response from informants and the community-at-large to the research study led to the discovery of a massive amount of rich data. The primary researcher attributes the depth of discovery about malaria care in Maasailand to her focus on using a caring approach throughout the study. It was a privilege to enter into the culture of those who suffer daily from a high occurrence of malaria and to seek traditionally-known emic knowledge that could then guide nursing decisions and actions toward offering best-practice malaria care among the Maasai people. The CCT and the Ethnonursing Method guided the discovery of this knowledge. The goal was to represent the Maasai culture and malaria care spirit of dignity and pride in a manner they would approve, bathed in respect and methodological sensitivity for their unique context. The respect shown the researcher by the Maasai community added credibility to the quality of the data collected and exemplified the researcher's ability to move from stranger to trusted friend. The nurse researcher obtained full support and permission from the Maasai senior chief and the elders to conduct this research. In addition, university Institutional Review Board (IRB) approval was obtained.

Focus on an Emic Perspective

In using the Ethnonursing Method, the researcher suspends *a priori* judgment, enters a new context as an etic (outside) observer, and undertakes fieldwork to understand the culture from the emic (inside) perspective (Polit & Beck, 2012; Wehbe-Alamah & McFarland, 2015a). In conducting culturally competent research, the researcher showed respect for the culture and care practices, affirmed the informants' stories as worthy of sharing, and made every effort to hear their emic perspective (C. W. Strang, 2014). The researcher must be cognizant of any biases, opinions, or preprofessional perspectives. To accomplish this task, the researcher becomes an active observer and listener; records observations, reflections, and internal conflicts in a reflective journal daily; and self-reflects orally or through email with a research mentor prepared in the ethnonursing method (Wehbe-Alamah & McFarland, 2015a).

The Maasai speak *Maa* which is primarily an oral language. Therefore qualitative ethnonursing and its use of in-depth interviews was congruent with the Maasai people who use storytelling as part of their oral traditions (C. W. Strang, 2014). The goal of the study was to discover the emic (generic/folk) and etic (professional nursing) care practices that would promote culturally congruent, safe, and beneficial malaria care that fit with the Maasai people's daily lives (McFarland & Wehbe-Alamah, 2015). From an etic perspective, the non-Kenyan, non-Maasai researcher was interested in discovering generic and professional malaria care practices among the Maasai. The researcher also made conscious efforts to move from stranger to trusted friend within the Maasai community and to immerse in the unique culture to uncover the Maasai emic perspective about malaria care. When the Maasai are approached in a culturally competent manner, community members are more likely to respond in open dialogue, thus strengthening study credibility and confirmability (Mixer, McFarland, Wehbe-Alamah, & Burk, 2012).

Use of Ethnonursing Research Enablers

An ethnonursing study seeks to discover emic knowledge because it is the most credible (McFarland, 2010). Discovery of such authentic data is facilitated through the use of ethnonursing research enablers (Wehbe-Alamah & McFarland, 2015). These enablers are used throughout the research process for the in-depth review of literature, data collection and analysis, and discovery of previously unknown cultural truths. These discoveries lead to culturally congruent nursing care decisions and actions. Four ethnonursing enablers (Sunrise Enabler, Observation-Participation-Reflection Enabler, Stranger-to-Trusted Friend Enabler, and Ethnodemographic Enabler) were used to conduct culturally competent research to discover the meanings, expressions, and practices of malaria care among the Maasai. The enablers are not intended to be used separately, rather are used in conjunction with one another to fully guide the researcher in rigorous, culturally competent inquiry (McFarland & Wehbe-Alamah, 2015).

Sunrise Enabler

The Sunrise Enabler is a conceptual map (Refer to Color Insert 1) of the social structure dimensions and major constructs of the CCT that guided the researcher to collect comprehensive emic malaria care data (McFarland & Wehbe-Alamah, 2015). The enabler is horizontally divided into upper and lower halves. The upper half, an image of a sunrise, depicts rays with each representing cultural factors that may influence the domain of inquiry (DOI). The dividing line, where the sun rays form, directs the conceptual focus toward the individual in the nurse-client relationship, and/or beyond to include families and communities. This flexibility was imperative for culturally competent research in Maasailand, a community-focused rather than individually-focused society. The upper half of the enabler, above the horizon, represents and reminds the researcher to seek the world, cultural, and holistic views of care, and environmental, contextual, and historical influencers of care. The lower half of the enabler represents and directs discovery toward generic and professional influences of care and options for transcultural nursing malaria care decisions and actions to improve health and wellbeing of Maasai people (C. W. Strang, 2014).

The Sunrise Enabler can be entered from any point as the researcher moves among potential care domains and influencers. Focused on the concepts of malaria care, the primary researcher accessed the Sunrise Enabler in several ways. As a visual aid, it was frequently reviewed as a reminder of the multiple factors that influence malaria care among the Maasai. The Sunrise Enabler also served to guide the comprehensive literature review, development of the ethnodemographic data and inquiry questions prior to entry into the field, and review of collected data to evaluate recurrent patterning and saturation.

Observation-Participation-Reflection Enabler

An important aspect of culturally competent research is for the researcher to set aside time to observe, participate, and reflect while in the study context. The Observation-Participation-Reflection (OPR) Enabler is a four-step process that guides the researcher's entry into and maintains focus on the natural environment of the informants (McFarland et al., 2012). The researcher progressed sequentially through the phases of this enabler, from being a general observer of the

Maasai people and their cultural lifeways to becoming an observer with some limited participation in daily living activities. Some longer-term nurse researchers may become trusted to participate fully in the people's daily lives while making detailed observations and reflections on culture care practices.

In Maasailand, the study experience began with a drive from the international airport to the study region located at the foot of Mount Kilimanjaro. Prior to scheduling any interviews, the first days were spent observing daily events of the local Maasai village residents; driving and hiking in the Kimana area; walking and shopping in a local market; visiting a church service and local clinic; and making copious field journal notes. Progression through all OPR phases was important to maintain perspective within the environmental context of the study and conduct culturally competent research.

A concerted effort was made by the nurse researcher to suspend prior knowledge of the culture and enter with an open perspective to enable discovery of emic knowledge. Prior to each interview and during the data analysis period, the researcher was cognizant to remain open-minded and suspend personal opinions from past experiences within the Maasai culture. To facilitate this effort, the researcher decided to conduct her study in an area of Maasailand where she had had minimal contact and was less well-known. Value and respect for the informants' emic ideas and interpretations of malaria care enhanced accurate data collection. The researcher desired to enable informants to share their story of malaria care in a way that made sense to them and was of value to them.

The researcher intentionally planned varied observation and participatory research experiences to gain cultural insights. With each outing, conversation, or drive through the region the researcher listened, watched, smelled, tasted, or touched the surrounding environment. The researcher lived in a camp environment in the research region located next to traditional Maasai villages. Each day the researcher could hear the laughter and cries of the children; greet the women on their daily trek to the nearby spring balancing laundry on their heads; smell the open fires needed to heat the water and cook meals; and drink chai with a neighbor who invited her to sit nearby on the cowskin hide and learn the art of beadwork. While shopping in the local market, the researcher would look for items relevant to malaria care such as herbs or insecticide treated nets. Other observation and participation events included attending a wedding and worship services, eating at a local restaurant, and visiting an orphanage and a local clinic. Usually a translator would assist with helping to understand and/or communicate during these experiences. The researcher continually made notations about each experience and the data analysis process in a field note journal (Refer to Photo 20.3).

Stranger-to-Trusted Friend Enabler

To help the nurse researcher move from a stranger to a trusted friend within the Maasai culture, the Stranger-to-Trusted Friend Enabler was used (Wehbe-Alamah & McFarland, 2015a). The Maasai people in the Kimana region needed to get to know the researcher and develop a trusting relationship so that study informants would be willing to share truthful, credible information. Although the researcher and her family had served intermittently over the past 26 years in Maasailand, this was only the researcher's second visit to the Kimana region.

A trusting relationship is essential for culturally competent research (Papadopoulos, 2006). Within the Maasai culture, the elders were the gatekeepers and they conveyed the trustworthiness of the researcher to community members, mostly through word of mouth. As a result, informants felt comfortable participating in the study and revealed insider, covert data about their culture and malaria care. In this study, these relationships supported the credibility of data and promoted safety for the researcher; as she traveled around the area her presence was not interpreted as a threat.

As early as the initial planning phase of the study, the researcher's purpose was to discover the Maasai emic perspective about malaria care. The researcher's demonstrated interest in their care needs during her trip prior to conducting the study helped to promote her position from a stranger toward a trusted friend within the Maasai community in the Kimana region (McFarland & Wehbe-Alamah, 2015a). The researcher believed that this led to a high rate of informant response during the study. Many mornings the researcher found Maasai men and women waiting outside her tent to share their stories about malaria care.

Ethnodemographic Enabler

This enabler was used to develop the ethnodemographic section of the interview guide. Ethnodemographic

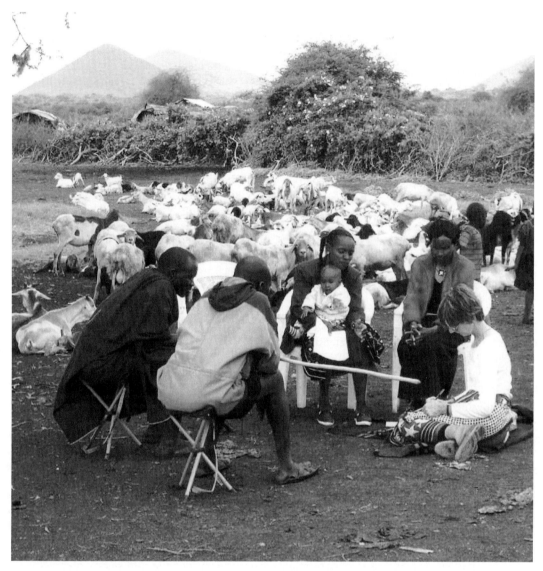

PHOTO 20.3 Interview setting most congruent with the lifeways of the Maasai. © F. F. Strang (2013).

data described the environment, history, social, cultural, ethnic, and geographic context and helped the researcher understand the context of malaria care and malaria care practices (Wehbe-Alamah & McFarland, 2015b). Examples of general ethnodemographic data sought in the Maasai context included the gender of informant and family members; sources of water and cooking fuel; home structure and type of toilet facility; and use of insecticide treated nets during sleep. Prior to the first interview, the researcher reviewed the Ethnodemographic Enabler with a traditional Maasai elder who resided in the area to ensure that a respectful, culturally competent research inquiry was conducted. It was advised that the researcher make one change and not ask how many children a person had. This question could be interpreted as similar to those asked by government census takers and might cause mistrust because the Maasai prefer not to be counted. Therefore, this question was removed from the inquiry guide.

Translation

The cultural congruency of all oral and written material is essential to conduct culturally competent research. The translation process is time-intensive and its importance cannot be over emphasized (Maneesriwongul & Dixon, 2004). A competent researcher makes every effort to protect all participants. In the Kimana region, many Maasai did not speak English and the researcher did not speak fluent Maa. Therefore, translation of the written and spoken word, informed consents, inquiry guide, and informant interviews needed to be undertaken in order to bridge the language barrier and conduct a respectful, culturally competent study.

Translation of Informed Consent and Inquiry Guide

The pre-study translation planning facilitated accurate comprehension of data among the researcher, interpreters, and informants. Detailed translation processes using the source language of English and the target language of *Maa* were conducted for the informed consent and inquiry guide (Maneesriwongul & Dixon, 2004; Polit & Beck, 2012). It was necessary for the informed consent form to be available in English and *Maa* for full study disclosure to all potential informants regarding its purpose, risks, and benefits. The inquiry guide was used during interviews. Cultural sensitivity was enhanced by use of appropriate vocabulary and careful phrasing of questions. Maasai and community gatekeepers from the Kimana district were asked by the researcher to participate in the translation process. Traditional Maasai and Maasai who had completed secondary school, signifying fluency in English, participated. The intricate translation process and inclusion of local villagers was interpreted by the Maasai as an expression of respectful inquiry and as a result unintentionally increased community trust in the researcher.

Initially, forward translation was conducted by English speaking Maasai who translated the English documents into *Maa*. Then, back-translation was performed by another group of Maasai who had access only to the *Maa* version of documents and translated them back into English. Monolingual testing was accomplished by Maasai community members reviewing documents in the *Maa* language for accuracy, comprehension, and culturally respectful language. Discrepancies were resolved. Finally, the primary researcher compared the initial and back translated English versions for accuracy of *Maa* translation and ensured IRB requirements were retained (Maneesriwongul & Dixon, 2004).

Translation During an Informant Interview

When the researcher is not fluent in the language of study informants, the use of translators within the study context will likely increase collaboration and trust between the researcher and the informants. Experienced researchers who have used the Ethnonursing Method have acknowledged that some meaning may be lost during the translation and interpretation processes (Purnell, 2013). It has also been discovered that using a trusted translator from the culture being studied is often perceived as a caring act, thus eliciting a higher level of credible information. On this basis, the researcher used only two translators during key informant interviews, which provided consistency throughout the study.

Purnell (2013) encouraged the nurse to develop important skills when using an interpreter such as looking at the informant and not the interpreter when asking or answering interview questions. This was found to be wise counsel. The nurse researcher noted in her field notes that:

> …As the interview process progresses, I realize that my skills in using an interpreter had become much smoother and more relaxed. I am interacting, for the most part, with the informant and not the interpreter. However, it took three to four interviews to become comfortable to allow the interpreter to be my voice and focus more fully on the informant. (C. W. Strang, 2014)

Another suggestion by culture care researchers has been to consider the informant's preference regarding translator gender (Purnell, 2013; Wehbe-Alamah, 2011). The researcher checked the cultural appropriateness of consistently using a female translator and was informed by Maasai elder gatekeepers that an interpreter of the same gender was not necessary with Maasai informants. Female interpreters were used during most of the study and no hesitation by men was noted in their willingness to participate or speak freely in the presence of a female interpreter.

The researcher made every effort to obtain accurate and truthful data. The interpreters selected were fluent speakers of both Maa and English and understood the concepts of translation and interpretation

(Maneesriwongul & Dixon, 2004). Two interpreters were present at all interviews where the informants spoke Maa. The researcher knew both interpreters, but they did not previously know one another. One interpreter was a trusted friend of the researcher for more than 25 years, a health care provider in Maasailand who was familiar with malaria illness, fluent in Maa and English, and from a region outside the research study area. The other interpreter was a resident of the research region, fluent in Maa and English, educated post-high school, but had remained a full participant in the Maasai culture. She was knowledgeable of Maasai traditions as she lived in a traditional Maasai village as the third wife of a Maasai elder. In addition, this local interpreter also knew the area. She was a great asset in suggesting informants that best fit with the DOI of the study. Also, having a Maa speaker from the region was beneficial when translating some colloquial language nuances.

The researcher had initially planned to use only one interpreter. However, upon her arrival in Kenya, the elder requested that his wife accompany the researcher as a guide and gatekeeper into area villages. This was an excellent accommodation in the plan as most interviews involved hours of walking through the bush. Without a guide, it would have been very difficult to find most of the villages. On the initial trek through the bush toward the village of the first scheduled interview, the two interpreters informed the researcher that they thought the three should now be known as "The Malaria Ladies." This dubbing of a group title was an affirmation to the researcher that all three of them had moved from strangers to trusted friends, which also added to the trustworthiness of the data translation and affirmed the usefulness of the enablers to the researcher. Both women expressed an eagerness to help their people, had personally suffered from and cared for their children with malaria, desired to learn more about malaria, and participate in the research process.

The process of working with the interpreters was key to this study. Both interpreters were Maasai and, as the study was reviewed with them prior to the first interview, both had expressed preconceived ideas of how the informants might respond. The nurse researcher realized that it was important for the interpreters to also bracket [set aside] their *a priori* knowledge. Therefore, before each interview and as

recorded in the field notes, the researcher reminded herself and the interpreters to "…pretend we have not heard any answers to these questions before and that we do not anticipate a specific answer. Also, we should expect and welcome diversity in the responses. To the interpreters' surprise, although many responses were similar, diversity was realized as well" (C. W. Strang, 2014).

Once the study began, the researcher needed to adjust her approach in order to demonstrate respect for the Maasai culture. First was the adjustment from translation to interpretation. The researcher would have preferred to have had the interviews directly *translated* (with frequent word-for-word accounts). However, it was culturally more appropriate to use an *interpretation* format that allowed each informant to first share longer, uninterrupted accounts of knowledge followed by the interpreter detailing the overall concepts conveyed (Polit & Beck, 2012).

Another needed adjustment was in how to categorize informants. The originally-proposed format was for all key informant interviews to be within individual contexts. Before one of the earliest key informant interviews, the researcher and interpreters had walked 45 minutes through the bush to reach the area where the informant lived. Upon arrival, the original informant was not available. However, an elderly, almost blind lady offered herself as a guide to a nearby village where others could probably assist us. This *kokoo* [grandmother/matriarch] led us on a 15-minute trek and presented us to the village. After describing the reason for our visit, we were all welcomed; five chairs were brought from homes and placed in a circle to accommodate the researcher, the two interpreters, the key informant, and the *kokoo*. Because the *kokoo* had invested herself into the venture, the informant expected her to be included in the interview experience. The researcher decided that, to provide a culturally congruent research experience, the interview should be adjusted to include both informants. The next decision was how to categorize informants. It regularly occurred that one answered the questions more freely and fully, while the other offered intermittent, brief comments and clarifications. Upon reflection of this interview and others with similar scenarios in the days ahead, the researcher developed a method to categorize the informants: One as the key informant and the other(s) as general informants. (Refer to Figure 20.1).

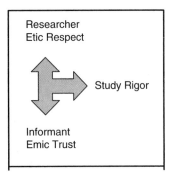

FIGURE 20.1 • Respect and trust promote rigor.
Reproduced, with permission from Strang, C. W. (2014). *Discovery of the meanings, expressions, and practices related to malaria care among the Maasai* [Doctoral dissertation]. Retrieved from http://trace.tennessee.edu/utk_graddiss/2734/

Results from Conducting Culturally Competent Research

Conducting culturally competent research contributes to the discipline and practice of nursing. The nurse researcher reflects on the study themes and patterns, explicates care constructs, and identifies professional care decisions and actions that will benefit the people by improving their health and wellbeing and fit with their daily lifeways (Wehbe-Alamah & McFarland, 2015a). As a result of conducting this study, the primary researcher is compelled to emphasize that, to discover truth, respect for the culture is paramount. Greater expressions of respect from the researcher elevate an exchange of respect and trust and result in authentic, credible data and study rigor. The researcher's respect for the informant and their culture and lifeways elevates the trust held by the study informant for the researcher (and vice versa, as trust from the informant elevates respect held by the researcher), and thus promotes study rigor. This relationship is depicted in Figure 20.1.

Care Constructs

As nurse researchers apply the Culture Care Theory using the Ethnonursing Method, new culture-specific meanings of care are discovered and extant meanings are re-confirmed. Care constructs are dominant care meanings and/or actions embedded in culture-specific values and/or practices. They are uncovered while using the CCT and facilitate the nurse researcher's understanding of the meaning of care. In the context of this

study, culturally competent research was conducted by seeking to understand the emic/Maasai view of care (McFarland & Wehbe-Alamah, 2015). The Maasai participants described specific meanings of care within their culture. Four care constructs found within the Maasai context were congruent with findings of other ethnonursing researchers who had also studied diverse cultures and are among those care/caring constructs listed in Chapter 3. The four constructs also identified among the Masaai were *respect for/about lifeways*; *acceptance*; *purging*; and *interest in/about* (McFarland & Wehbe-Alamah, 2015; Strang & Mixer, 2015). Three new care constructs were discovered from the Masaai in this study and build upon previous culture care knowledge: *Herbs as care*; *community as care*; and *praying to/for* (Refer to Table 20.3; C. W. Strang, 2014).

Both key and general informants spoke about the need for culturally congruent care that would demonstrate *respect for* and acknowledge the importance of their traditional and generic practices and *lifeways*. Informants consistently expressed an attitude of acceptance: *Acceptance* of malaria as an illness that was expected to occur in their contextual environment and *acceptance* that the malaria illness was an occurrence in need of care. *Purging*, through vomiting, diarrhea, or sweating, was shared as a necessary and accepted practice to dispel the malaria illness from the body. Key and general informants consistently verbalized their curiosity and *interest in/about* the malaria disease in order to learn about options for malaria care for their community (Strang & Mixer, 2015).

Although the current list of CCT care constructs includes use of folk foods/practices, *herbs as care* was a culture-specific and detailed generic care practice discovered during this study. Informants described the *first act of malaria care* as the use of herbs for purging the body. Herbs traditionally used for malaria care were collected near the village or in forests far away. Herbs were also used as additives to traditional foods such as soups during recovery from illness. The detailed process of using herbs as care was described by informants as the responsibility of the entire Maasai community. The consistent, passionate reference of herbs as the *first act of care* for persons ill with malaria qualifies it as a care construct that stands alone. While Moss (2010) did not specifically address this concept as a care construct, her ethnonursing research study among the Mestizo

TABLE 20.3. Care Constructs for Malaria Care Among Maasai.

Care Constructs	Definition within Maasai Context
Respect for/about lifeways	• Honoring the Maasai as a valued people group and appreciating similarities and differences among the Maasai and other people groups in Kenya • Respect for the use of traditional malaria care practices that stems from thousands of years of herbal care by traditional healers
Acceptance	• The malaria illness/symptoms are expected and perceived as a normal occurrence given certain environmental conditions (e.g., rainy seasons, green, evening, cool, standing water, mosquito presence) • Maasai take responsibility for malaria care
Purging	• Using an herb mixture to rid the body of malaria through vomiting and diarrhea • Usually the first care act for adults and children to treat symptoms recognized as active malaria illness
Interest in/about	• Interest in sharing their story with others through the research study process • Open to learning more about the science, prevention, and care of the malaria disease to benefit the community
Herbs as care	• A specific, detailed generic care practice to prevent and treat malaria • Used to sweat or purge to rid the body of the malaria disease • Used as base ingredient in recovery soups to regain strength
Community as care	• Responsibilities held by all members to care for those with malaria • Community referred to immediate family in the home village, close neighbors, and other Maasai, such as spiritual leaders or traditional caregivers
Praying to/for	• Caregivers prayed to God that the herbs/medicines would be effective and prayed for the sick person to fully heal • Prayers were often petitioned to *Enkai* [God] in song • Informants prayed to God for the researcher to be successful and return to offer malaria care in their communities

Reproduced, with permission from Strang, C. W. (2014). *Discovery of the meanings, expressions, and practices related to malaria care among the Maasai* [Doctoral dissertation]. Retrieved from http://trace.tennessee.edu/utk_graddiss/2734/

Ecuadorians also found that herbs were essential for culture care (Strang & Mixer, 2015).

Community as family has been previously identified as a culture care construct (Embler, 2012), but *community as care* was a unique care concept discovered in this study (Strang & Mixer, 2015). Whenever someone was ill with malaria, community members provided that person with physical and spiritual care and completed his/her daily tasks. The concept of *community* encompassed men, women, children, persons sick with malaria, family members, neighbors, and traditional herbalists—all of whom had responsibilities in the provision of malaria care. For example, a mother might need to sell the cow or borrow money from a neighbor to take a child for professional care or buy medicine to treat fever. If an adult was ill, community members cared for that person's children and did their chores such as collecting water and firewood or doing the laundry. The importance of each community member as an active participant in one another's daily lifeways was a phenomenon of care also found in the Amish culture where survival of the ill was dependent upon the fulfilled roles of each community member (Wenger, 2013). Within the Maasai lifeways, this pattern of care was offered by, within, and for the community toward the wellbeing of the entire community (C. W. Strang, 2014).

Praying to/for was also discovered as a new care construct, different from the previously reported construct *praying with* (McFarland & Wehbe-Alamah, 2015). Rather than describing *praying with* one another, Maasai informants universally described the practice of *praying to Enkai* [God] *for* healing of the sick. These prayers included praying for the traditional herbs and the clinic medicines to heal the patient. The informants also stated that they were praying to God for the researcher, that her work would prosper and she would return to improve the health of the Maasai (C. W. Strang, 2014).

Three Modes of Culture Care Decisions and Actions

Findings from this culturally congruent research study were further analyzed to formulate culture care decisions and actions related to the Maasai current and future malaria care preferences and needs. These decisions and actions are credible because the researcher took the time to enter into the emic culture, observe the overall and intricate patterns of daily living, and reflect on and confirm with participants any decisions and actions that displayed culturally congruent care.

Using the mode culture care preservation and/or maintenance, the researcher focused on assessing the research findings for discoveries of safe and beneficial malaria care practices that should be preserved and/or maintained. These community care actions included *physically caring for those who were sick and completing their daily chores*; *using herbs in illness-recovery soups*; and *acts of prayer*.

Culture care accommodation and/or negotiation for malaria care involved ensuring access to and availability of malaria preventive care measures in clinics. This included *respectful treatment when Maasai entered a professional care setting*; *the accessibility, affordability, and availability of rapid diagnostic testing and insecticide treated nets* (ITNs); and *culturally congruent health education for the Maasai and their professional caregivers.*

The primary researcher did identify potentially unsafe or harmful practices in malaria care that needed to be repatterned and/or restructured. One unsafe practice was the use of herbs as the first care action for children with malaria. Another was the nonuse of ITNs. The development of culturally competent educational approaches/materials and advocacy for local and national governmental policy changes are recommended to enable successful restructuring of harmful traditional care practices. In addition, the *Kenya World Malaria Report* (WHO, 2013) stated ITN and Artemisinin-based combination medication treatments for active malaria disease should be available and distributed free of charge to persons of all ages. However, this was not the practice discovered by the researcher. All key and general informants reported that everyone was required to pay for malaria medications and no

mass distribution of ITNs had taken place in this region for at least six years prior to the study period.

In Kenya, there are more than 42 people groups–each equally proud of their heritage. There is a great need to offer culturally competent and congruent care and respectful treatment within this cultural context. Pragmatic outcomes resulting from the discovery of malaria care among the Maasai encompassed multiple influences based on their worldview, cultural values, social structural dimensions, and environment. For example, the use of insecticide treated nets is an evidenced-based prevention measure for malaria (WHO, 2015). However, even if the economic factor is removed by offering ITNs at no cost, the current design of nets may never work given the structure of the traditional Maasai home. Evidenced-based research studies have stated that every child with a fever should go to a clinic to receive an accurate diagnosis using a rapid diagnostic test (RDT) and proper treatment (WHO, 2015). However, during the rainy, high-malaria season, roads are often impassable. In addition, RDTs or medications may not be available in rural care facilities. Professional caregivers, community health workers, and Maasai informants all requested education to help them differentiate malaria from other febrile-causing diseases that exhibit similar symptoms (D'Acremont et al., 2014; C. W. Strang, 2014).

■ SUMMARY

The authors reaffirm the need for nurse researchers who are culturally aware, sensitive, knowledgeable, and skilled in conducting culturally competent research. The Theory of Culture Care Diversity and Universality with the Ethnonursing Research Method provide an appropriate qualitative theoretical framework for such research.

Approaches for conducting culturally competent research have been threaded throughout this chapter by sharing the discovery process for malaria care among the Maasai. This study was the first use of the CCT and the Ethnonursing Method within the Maasai culture and in exploration about the topic of malaria care. The Maasai worldview and social structure dimensions, care constructs, and care decisions and actions shared in this chapter may be useful for nurses and other healthcare providers to further understand the Maasai cultural values, beliefs, and lifeways and enable them to provide culturally congruent professional malaria care. This information is also useful for other researchers who desire to conduct culturally competent research and then apply the data to healthcare decisions and actions, education, and policy that will fit with the daily lives of other indigenous, rural, or vulnerable cultural groups.

DEDICATION

This book chapter is dedicated to the beautiful Maasai people who shared their malaria stories.

ACKNOWLEDGEMENTS

The authors gratefully acknowledge the value of Leininger's Theory of Culture Care Diversity and Universality and the Ethnonursing Research Method and treasure the personal encouragement, mentoring, and friendship shown to us by Dr. Marilyn McFarland and Dr. Marilyn Ray.

DISCUSSION QUESTIONS

1. Describe how the ethnonursing research enablers facilitate authentic, credible qualitative research data.
2. When conducting a culturally competent research study and using a translator, discuss the various steps available to the researcher to ensure both linguistic accuracy and cultural sensitivity.
3. Compare and contrast the concepts of the emic and etic perspectives.
   - Discuss how characteristics of each are necessary to conduct a culturally competent research study.
4. Think of a vulnerable people group in your local community.
   - List four potential challenges you might face if you were to conduct culturally competent research within this culture's social and cultural dimensions.
   - Discuss how you would overcome these challenges.
5. Analyze how a transcultural nurse could help a community in a developing world respond to a disease such as malaria, Ebola, SARS, or influenza.

- Explore professional actions and decisions in the areas of education, research, and policy.

REFERENCES

Bussmann, R. W., Gilbreath, G. G., Solio, J., Lutura, M., Lutuluo, R. Kunguru, K., & Mathenge, S. G. (2006). Plant use of the Maasai of Sekenani Valley, Maasai Mara, Kenya. *Journal of Ethnobiology and Ethnomedicine, 2*(22), 1-11. doi: 10.1186/1746-4269-2-22

D'Acremont, V., Kilowoko, M., Kyungu, E., Philipina, S., Sangu, W., Kahama-Maro J., …Genton, B. (2014). Beyond malaria: Causes of fever in outpatient Tanzanian children. *New England Journal of Medicine, 370*(9), 809-817. doi: 10.0156/NEJMoa1214482

Embler, P. (2012). *End-of-life culture care expressions, meanings, patterns, and practices among Yup'ik Eskimo* [Unpublished doctoral dissertation]. University of Tennessee, Knoxville.

Haasnoot, P. J., Boeting, T. E., Kuney, M. O., & van Roosmalen, J. (2010). Knowledge, attitudes, and practice of tuberculosis among Maasai in Simanjiro district, Tanzania. *American Journal of Tropical Medicine and Hygiene, 83*(4), 902-905.

Hodgson, D. L. (2011). *Being Maasai, becoming indigenous: Postcolonial politics in a neoliberal world.* Bloomington, IN: Indiana University Press.

Homewood, K., Kristjanson, P., & Trench, P. C. (2009). Changing land use, livelihoods and wildlife conservation in Maasailand. In D. G. Bates (Ed.), *Staying Maasai? Livelihoods, conservation and development in East African rangelands* [Electronic resource]. New York, NY: Springer.

Kaiser Family Foundation. (2013, March 7). *Global malaria epidemic.* Retrieved from http://kff.org/global-health-policy/fact-sheet/the-global-malaria-epidemic-4/

Kenya National Bureau of Statistics. (2011). *Kenya malaria indicator survey 2010.* Retrieved from http://www.measuredhs.com/pubs/pdf/MIS7/MIS7.pdf

Koch, A., Tamez, P., Pezzuto, J., & Soejarto, D. (2005). Evaluation of plants used for antimalarial treatment by the Maasai of Kenya. *Journal of Ethnopharmacology, 101*(1-3), 95-99. doi: 10.1016/j.jep.2005.03.011

Malisa, A. L., & Ndukai, M. (2009). Knowledge and practices on malaria and its control among pastoralists in Simanjiro District, northern Tanzania. *Tanzania Journal of Health Research, 11*(4), 219-225.

Maneesriwongul, W., & Dixon, J. K. (2004). Instrument translation process: A methods review. *Journal of Advanced Nursing, 48*(2), 175-186.

McFarland, M. R. (2010). Culture care theory of diversity and universality. In M. R. Alligood and A. M. Tomey (Eds.), *Nursing theorists and their work* (7th ed., pp. 454-479). St. Louis, MO: Mosby.

McFarland, M. R., Mixer, S. J., Wehbe-Alamah, H. B., & Burk, R. (2012). Ethnonursing: A qualitative research method for studying culturally competent care across disciplines. *International Journal of Qualitative Methods*, *11*(3), 260-279.

McFarland, M. R., & Wehbe-Alamah, H. B. (2015). The theory of culture care diversity and universality. In M. R. McFarland and H. B Wehbe-Alamah (Eds.), *Leininger's culture care diversity and universality: A worldwide nursing theory* (3rd ed., pp. 1-34). Burlington, MA: Jones and Bartlett Learning.

Mol, F. (1996). *Maasai language and culture: Dictionary.* Lemek, Kenya: Maasai Centre.

Moss, J. A. (2010). *Discovering the healthcare beliefs and practices of rural Mestizo Ecuadorians: An ethnonursing study* [Unpublished doctoral dissertation]. Duquesne University, Pittsburgh, PA.

Polit, D. F., & Beck, C. T. (2012). *Nursing research: Generating and assessing evidence for nursing practice* (9th ed., pp. 371-372; 487-514). Philadelphia, PA: Lippincott Williams & Wilkins.

Papadopoulos, I. (2006). *Transcultural health and social care development of culturally competent practitioners.* Edinburgh: Churchill Livingstone, Elsevier.

Purnell, L. D. (2013). *Transcultural health care: A culturally competent approach* (4th ed.). Philadelphia, PA: FA Davis.

Rew, L., Becker, H., Cookston, J., Khosropour, S., & Martinez, S. (2003). Measuring cultural awareness in nursing students. *Journal of Nursing Education*, *42*(6), 249-257.

Saitoti, T., & Beckwith, C. (1980). *Maasai.* New York, NY: Harry N. Abrams.

Strang, C. W. (2014). *Discovery of the meanings, expressions, and practices related to malaria care among the Maasai* [Doctoral dissertation]. Retrieved from http://trace.tennessee.edu/utk_graddiss/2734/

Strang, C. W., & Mixer, S. J. (2015). Discovery of the meanings, expressions, and practices related to malaria care among the Maasai. *Journal of Transcultural Nursing*, 1-9. doi: 10.1177/1043659615573841

Strang, F. F. (2004). *Meisisi Enkai!: Claiming cultural identity in Maasai Christian worship in the Presbyterian Church of East Africa* [Unpublished doctoral dissertation]. University of Edinburgh, Scotland.

Thomson, J. (1885). *Through Masailand.* London, UK: Sampson Low, Marston, Searle and Rivington.

U. S. Department of Health and Human Services, Centers for Disease Control and Prevention. (2012). *U. S. President's malaria initiative* [Website]. Retrieved from http://www.cdc.gov/malaria/malaria_worldwide/cdc_activities/pmi.html

U. S. Department of Health and Human Services, Centers for Disease Control and Prevention. (2015). *Malaria* [Website]. Retrieved from http://www.cdc.gov/malaria/

U. S. Department of Health and Human Services, National Institutes of Health, National Institutes of Allergy and Infectious Diseases. (2008). *NIAID strategic plan for malaria research: Efforts to accelerate control and eradication of malaria through biomedical research.* Retrieved from http://www.niaid.nih.gov/topics/Malaria/Documents/strategic-plan.pdf

Wanzala, P., Hassanali, J., Kibet, P., & Dossajee, H. (2005). Perceptions of primary health care with regard to corresponding knowledge, attitude and practices amongst the Kenyan Maasai. *East African Medical Journal*, *82*(1), 24-27. doi: 10.4314/eamj.v82i1.9290

Wehbe-Alamah, H. B. (2011). The use of culture care theory with Syrian Muslims in the Midwestern United States. *Online Journal of Cultural Competence in Nursing and Healthcare*, *1*(3), 1-12.

Wehbe-Alamah, H. B., & McFarland, M. R. (2015a). The ethnonursing research method. In M. R. McFarland and H. B Wehbe-Alamah (Eds.), *Leininger's culture care diversity and universality: A worldwide nursing theory* (3rd ed., pp. 35-71). Burlington, MA: Jones and Bartlett Learning.

Wehbe-Alamah, H. B., & McFarland, M. R. (2015b). Leininger's enablers for use with the ethnonursing research method. In M. R. McFarland and H. B Wehbe-Alamah (Eds.), *Leininger's culture care diversity and universality: A worldwide nursing theory* (3rd ed., pp. 73-100). Burlington, MA: Jones and Bartlett Learning.

Wenger, A. F. (2013). The Amish. In L. D. Purnell (Ed.), *Transcultural health care: A culturally competent approach* (4th ed., pp. 115-136). Philadelphia, PA: F. A. Davis.

World Health Organization. (2013). *Kenya world malaria report.* Retrieved from http://www.who.int/malaria/publications/country-profiles/profile_ken_en.pdf?ua=1

World Health Organization. (2015). *Malaria.* Retrieved from http://www.who.int/mediacentre/factsheets/fs094/en/

Zurovac, D., Talisuna, A. O., & Snow, R. W. (2012). Mobile phone text messaging: Tool for malaria control in Africa. *PLoS Medicine*, *9*(2), 1-6.

CHAPTER 21

The Lived Experiences of African American Women Receiving Care from Nurse Practitioners in an Urban Nurse-Managed Clinic in the Midwestern United States[1]

Hiba B. Wehbe-Alamah, Marilyn R. McFarland, Janee F. Koc, and Nancy R. Riggs

> *I've learned that people will forget what you said, people will forget what you did, but people will never forget how you made them feel. Maya Angelou*

■ INTRODUCTION

Since 1965 when the first nurse practitioners were educated at the University of Colorado, the American Association of Nurse Practitioners (AANP, 2015) has grown to more than 205,000 members. A nurse practitioner may provide primary care in urban, rural, and suburban settings, and often functions singly or as a member of a small team in rural community settings (Barr, Johnston, & McConnell, 2000). As the number of nurse practitioners has continued to grow and the primary and specialty care roles have expanded, many African American women receive and actively seek primary and specialty health care from nurse practitioners. This has created the need to prepare and educate nurse practitioners to provide culturally congruent, sensitive, and meaningful care to African American women, which is predicted to improve their health and healthy lifeways. Nurse practitioners as primary care providers must have the knowledge to provide care to African American women while being sensitive to their cultural care values, beliefs, patterns, expressions, and practices.

A literature review revealed a dearth of knowledge regarding African American women and their insider (*emic*) care views and experiences about *health* and *healthy lifeways*. Previous research conducted with African American women was primarily done using quantitative research methods and focused mainly on health care from the provider's (*etic*) perspective rather than from the emic worldview of African American women about their experiences with the professional/etic healthcare system. This chapter presents the findings from a qualitative study that addresses this identified gap in the literature using Leininger's Theory of Culture Care Diversity and Universality as its *organizing framework* and Colaizzi's (1978) phenomenological research method.

[1] Revised reprint: Wehbe-Alamah, H., McFarland, M., Macklin, J., & Riggs, N. (2011). The lived experiences of women receiving care from nurse practitioners in an urban nurse- managed clinic. *The Online Journal in Cultural Competence in Nursing and Healthcare, 1*(1), 15-26.

RESEARCH PURPOSE AND GOAL

The purpose of this study was to discover the lived experiences of African American women receiving primary care from nurse practitioners in a nurse-managed clinic in an urban context. The goal of the research was to use findings from this study to guide nursing decisions and actions in providing culturally congruent care that could lead to improved health, wellbeing, and beneficial lifeways for African American women.

RESEARCH QUESTIONS

Research participants were encouraged to share their personal stories as well as life experiences related to care and health. The broad research questions that guided this study were:

1. What are the lived experiences related to care and health of African American women receiving primary care from nurse practitioners in a nurse-managed clinic?
2. In what ways do worldview and Leininger's culture and social structure dimensions influence the healthcare beliefs, practices, and expressions of African American women?
3. In what ways can Leininger's nursing decision and action modes be used by nurse practitioners to provide African American women with culturally congruent care?

THEORETICAL FRAMEWORK

Leininger's Theory of Culture Care Diversity and Universality (Culture Care Theory) was a perfect fit as the organizing framework for this study. The goal of the theory is the provision of culturally congruent and competent nursing care that results in health and wellbeing for people (Leininger, 2006b; McFarland, 2006; McFarland and Wehbe-Alamah, 2015). Leininger held that there were three modes of culture care decisions and actions designed to guide nurses and other healthcare professionals in the provision of culturally congruent care (Leininger, 1991, 2006a). The three modes are *cultural care preservation and/or maintenance, cultural care accommodation and/or negotiation,* and cultural care repatterning and/or restructuring (McFarland and Wehbe-Alamah, 2015). These culture care decisions and actions modes were predicted to assist people of different cultures retain, adapt to, and/or modify their lifeways to achieve beneficial health outcomes leading to health and wellbeing or to face death or disability (Leininger, 1991, 2006a).

The use of Leininger's Sunrise Enabler (Refer to Color Insert 1) guided the researchers in their discovery of the worldview; ethnohistory; religious (or spiritual) orientation; and folk and professional care practices as well as the kinship, political, economic, legal, educational, and technological factors affecting the health care received by urban African American women. Leininger developed 13 assumptive premises to support the tenets of the Culture Care Theory. Three of those were adapted as assumptive premises for this study:

1. Nurse practitioner care is essential for human growth, wellbeing, health, survival, and to face death as well as disabilities for African American women (adapted from Leininger, 1991, 2006a).
2. Leininger's three culture care modes offer new, creative, and different therapeutic ways to help African American women to promote [their own] health and wellness (adapted from Leininger, 1991, 2006a; McFarland & Wehbe-Alamah, 2015).
3. Qualitative research such as phenomenological methods offer important means to discover largely embedded, covert, epistemic, and ontological culture care knowledge as well as [the care] practices of African American women (adapted from Leininger, 1991, 2006a; Wehbe-Alamah & McFarland, 2015).

LITERATURE REVIEW

Studies with African American Women

African American women and their healthcare views, beliefs, and practices were the primary focus for this review of literature. As mentioned previously, the researchers found that a dearth of research existed about African Americans' insider or emic overall views regarding their health care and their satisfaction with the care provided to them. Exploring how African American women perceive their health care and the care provided by nurse practitioners in nurse-managed centers may help to address the gap discovered in the literature review and assist nurse practitioners and other healthcare providers to be able to better provide culturally congruent care to this cultural group.

African Americans have long reported racism and prejudice within the healthcare system (Cuevas, 2013). Literature review of published studies revealed that some African American women viewed the health care they received as substandard and often inadequate. These perceptions may be due in part to inadequate access to health care compared to their White counterparts (Kennedy, Mathis, & Woods, 2007). African Americans identified a strong correlation between experiencing racism and engaging in risky lifestyles and maladaptive coping behaviors (Shariff-Marco, Klassen, & Bowie, 2010). Nicolaidis et al. (2010) discovered that African American women mistrusted the healthcare system, which they viewed as a "White" system, and reported negative healthcare experiences that they attributed to racism. Benkert and Peters (2005) studied African American women's perceptions of prejudice in health care and looked at strategies for coping with those experiences. The study explored perceptions that African Americans received different care and experienced racial discrimination that could negatively affect healthcare outcomes (Benkert & Peters, 2005).

Johnson (2001) used a qualitative method to investigate the healthcare needs and perceived barriers to obtaining health care for children as well as urban and rural women in areas served by nurse practitioner (NP) and certified nurse midwife (CNM) clinics. The researcher discovered that it was important for patients to feel welcomed and valued when presenting themselves to a healthcare facility. He concluded that low-income minority women were more likely to experience discrimination during healthcare visits. Among the reasons cited for this were *Healthcare providers were unresponsive to their needs*; *patients received substandard care*; *practitioners lacked cultural sensitivity*; and *the women were treated with disrespect* (Johnson, 2001). All of these reasons thus contributed to the African American women's negative attitudes toward healthcare professionals.

Transcultural Studies Using the Culture Care Theory

Leininger's Theory of Culture Care Diversity and Universality affirms that people of different cultures are capable of informing and guiding professionals about the kind of care they desire or need to receive (Leininger, 2006a; McFarland & Wehbe-Alamah, 2015). Leininger (2006a) described the meaning of *culture* as the *patterned and valued lifeways of people that influence their decisions and actions*. Several studies using both the theory and the ethnonursing research method have been conducted with African Americans (Benkert & Peters, 2005; Ehrmin, 2005; McFarland, 1997; Plowden & Young, 2003). McFarland (1997) studied culture care with Anglo and African American elders in a long-term setting. Four major themes were discovered from this study: *Residents expressed and lived generic care to maintain their preadmission lifeways*; *nursing staff provided care to support satisfying lifeways*; *institutional care patterns were viewed as a continuing life experience*; and *culture of retirement home reflected unique lifeways*.

Plowden and Young (2003) used ethnographic methods to conduct in-depth individual interviews with urban African American men. They used the Stranger-to-Trusted Friend Enabler to develop trust with African Americans to gain access to their community and discover caring processes related to their culture. Ehrmin (2005) conducted an ethnonursing research study to discover meanings and expressions of care for substance-dependent African American women in an inner-city transitional home.

During a thorough review of the published literature, several common themes related to African American women and their overall care views, beliefs, and practices emerged. The literature review revealed that trusting the healthcare provider and perceiving a compassionate approach about their health care were important to African American women (Benkert & Peters, 2005). African American women described having more limited access to health care compared to their Caucasian counterparts and viewed the treatment provided by health care providers as substandard (Kennedy et al., 2007). Qualitative data was limited in regard to African American views about health care overall in the United States, and still fewer studies focused on their transcultural care. Specifically, no research addressed how African American women viewed health care when provided by nurse practitioners.

■ RESEARCH METHODOLOGY

This study was conceptualized using Leininger's (2006) Theory of Culture Care Diversity and Universality and followed Colaizzi's phenomenological approach (1978) for data analysis to allow the researchers to gain insight into the lived experiences of African American women receiving primary care from nurse practitioners. As both a philosophy and a research method, phenomenology enhances the discovery of the lived experiences of a phenomenon of interest and allows its essences to emerge (Colaizzi, 1978). The researchers chose the phenomenological method because it was the best fit for this study and its domain of inquiry. Phenomenological studies use data from prolonged conversations between researchers and study participants (Colaizzi, 1978). Researchers strive to discover the lived experiences of the participants without leading the interviews (Colaizzi, 1978). The researchers were careful to avoid allowing their preconceived beliefs or views to influence the research process. To further ensure this, they used bracketing, intuiting, and journaling while collecting, reviewing, and analyzing the data (Colaizzi, 1978).

Open-ended interview questions were designed to stimulate discussion and solicit the participants' stories during the interview process. Colaizzi's method of analysis is unique in that it requires researchers to return to participants to confirm findings as the study evolves (1978). Researchers used follow-up telephone interviews to confirm findings with participants. Approval for this study was obtained from the Institutional Review Board of the university with which the researchers were affiliated and all participants provided informed consent according to protocols.

Setting

An urban nurse-managed healthcare center was the setting selected for the study. One of the researchers for this study was a nurse practitioner who provided primary health care services at this clinic to university students and community adults (aged 18 to 64 years

and qualifying for a county-sponsored health plan). To qualify for service at the nurse-managed clinic, patients were required to have a limited income and no other health insurance coverage. All participants had been receiving their primary health care at the nurse-managed clinic during the time the study was conducted and had prior contact with the nurse managed clinic staff, stated that they were comfortable with the site, and verbalized eagerness to recall and discuss their healthcare experiences.

Sample

A convenience sample of 11 African American women (Please see Table 21.1) was selected from the patient panel at the nurse-managed urban clinic. Potential participants were approached by researchers in the waiting area of the clinic and given a flyer outlining the study. If interested in study participation, arrangements for an interview were made either during that visit or at another mutually agreed upon time. Eligibility criteria for participation in the study were: self-identification as an African American woman, being 18 to 64 years of age, being a current patient at the nurse-managed clinic, and willingness to participate in the study. To maintain confidentiality, the researchers assigned code names for all participants in the form of pseudo initials.

Data Analysis

Colaizzi's data analysis approach requires the researcher to abandon any desire to control the phenomenon in order to focus on the phenomenon itself. Colaizzi's (1978) seven steps of analysis were used to guide the analysis of the data collected during this study:

1. Reading transcripts of all the interviews to obtain a general sense of the whole content
2. Extracting significant statements related to the phenomenon under study
3. Deriving formulation of meanings from the significant statements
4. Organizing formulated meanings into categories, clusters of themes, and themes
5. Integrating findings into an exhaustive descriptions of the phenomena under study
6. Describing the fundamental structure of the investigated phenomena
7. Validating study findings with research participants and comparing with researchers' findings

TABLE 21.1. Demographics of Study Participants.

Participant	Age	Birth Place	Lives With	Religious Affiliation	Education	Occupation	Marital Status	Number of Children
BL	52	Flint	Alone	Baptist	12th grade	Unemployed	Single	1
HS	28	Flint	Husband and Children	Christian	1 yr. College	Employed	Married	2
JA	34	Mississippi	Children	Apostolic	11th Grade	Unemployed	Single	5
LK	42	Puerto Rico	Alone	Catholic	10th Grade	Unemployed	Single	2
LT	45	Virginia	Alone	Baptist	2 yrs. College	Unemployed	Single	4
ML	59	Arkansas	Husband	Christian	4 yrs. degree	Retired	Married	3
MX	28	Flint	Husband and Children	Christian	2 yrs. college	Employed	Married	1
NV	50	Flint	Alone	Baptist	1 yr. college	Unemployed	Single	2
OT	24	Oklahoma	Friend	Baptist	12th grade	Unemployed	Single	0
PD	55	Flint	2 Grown Children	SeventhDay Adventist	3.5 yrs. college	Unemployed	Widowed	5
RJ	49	Mississippi	Alone	Baptist	10thGrade	Unemployed	Single	1

Reproduced, with permission from Wehbe-Alamah, H., McFarland, M., Macklin, J., & Riggs, N. (2011). The lived experiences of African American women receiving care from nurse practitioners in an urban nurse- managed clinic. *The Online Journal in Cultural Competence in Nursing and Healthcare, 1*(1), 19.

The NVivo qualitative software package was used for management, classification, and coding of data, which was then analyzed under the supervision and guidance of two of the researchers who were qualitative research experts.

Each transcribed interview was reviewed and examined several times, allowing for discovery of recurring care patterns and themes which were coded using the Leininger-Templin-Thompson Ethnoscript Coding Enabler (Leininger, 1990). An example is shown in Table 21.2. The use of this enabler was extremely helpful to the researchers throughout the coding process, allowing for the processing and categorizing of large amounts of data. The analyzed narrative data was focused on participants' cultural values, beliefs, social structure, professional healthcare systems, environmental contexts, and worldviews.

■ RESEARCH FINDINGS

In keeping with Colaizzi's phenomenological approach, the study findings are presented using the format of listing categories **(bold)** first, then supporting themes (***bolded italics***), followed by their corresponding exhaustive descriptions (*italics*) with significant statements (participant quotations). Accordingly, the care

beliefs, practices, and expressions of African American women receiving primary care from nurse practitioners in a nurse managed clinic were compiled into the following three categories: *Professional Nurse Practitioner Care*; *Domains of Culture and Social Structural Dimensions*; and *Culture Care Modes for Health and Wellbeing.*

Category 1: Professional Nurse Practitioner Care

This category was supported by two themes, two exhaustive descriptions, and several significant statements.

Category 1, Theme 1: Nurse practitioners show more care than physicians

This theme was supported by the exhaustive description: *Nurse practitioners spend more time with patients and take more time to explain things better than physicians.* Participants in this study shared:

> "When she [nurse practitioner] explains stuff to me she is really down to earth. She doesn't talk over my head, you know. She even draws me pictures and stuff so I get it."

> "I just feel it was more personalized and not so rushed and harried and not so mechanical. I feel like a person instead of a number."

TABLE 21.2. Sample for the Leininger-Templin-Thompson Ethnoscript Coding Enabler used in this Study.

CATEGORIES AND DOMAINS OF INFORMATION
(includes observations, interviews, interpretive material, and nonmaterial data)

CATEGORY I: GENERAL CULTURAL DOMAINS OF INQUIRY DESCRIPTION CODE
1. Worldview
2. Cultural-social lifeways and activities (typical day/night)
3. Ethnohistorical (includes chrono-data, acculturation, cultural contracts, etc.)
4. Environmental contexts (i.e., physical, ecological, cultural, social)
5. Linguistic terms and meanings
6. Cultural foods related to care, health, illness and environment
7. Material and nonmaterial culture (includes symbols and meanings)
8. Ethnodemographics (numerical facts, dates, population size & other numerical data)
9. *Racism, prejudice, race**

CATEGORY II: DOMAIN OF CULTURAL AND SOCIAL STRUCTURAL DATA
(Includes normative values, patterns, function, and conflict)
10. Cultural values, beliefs, norms
11. Economic factors
12. Educational factors
13. Kinship (family ties, social network, social relationships, etc.)
14. Political and legal factors
15. Religious, philosophical, and ethical values and beliefs
16. Technological factors
17. Interpersonal relationships (individual groups or institutions)
18. *Recreation**

CATEGORY VIII: CULTURE CARE MODES
78. *Preservation and/or maintenance**
79. *Accommodation and/or negotiation**
80. *Re-patterning and/or restructuring**

*Italics indicate codes created specifically for this study
Reproduced, with permission from Wehbe-Alamah, H., McFarland, M., Macklin, J., & Riggs, N. (2011). The lived experiences of African American women receiving care from nurse practitioners in an urban nurse-managed clinic. *The Online Journal in Cultural Competence in Nursing and Healthcare, 1*(1), 21.

Category 1, Theme 2: Nurse practitioners develop strong relationships with patients to promote their health and wellbeing

The exhaustive description that supported this theme was: *Nurse practitioners develop strong and trusting relationships with their patients and provide nonjudgmental care to promote health and wellbeing.* Several participants in this research commented that:

"The nurse practitioner here, I say my doc 'cuz she is like a doc but better, she feels like a friend. I feel good around her, not worried what she thinks. She is so nice, she doesn't act like she is better or high up like my other doctors but she is smart. She knows how to help me."

"The doctor I went to before, he was not open to me. But here she [nurse practitioner] did not pass no [sic] judgment on me and she did not close her mind. That is what I respected the most. She still explored everything and didn't just blame my drugs. Sometimes my other doctor would make me feel so ashamed about my drug use that I just wouldn't go back when I needed to because it was a terrible experience for me mentally."

The African American women (participants) clearly conveyed that they felt the nurse practitioners showed respect, compassion, and concern while providing them with culturally congruent care. These participants expressed that the nurse practitioners gave holistic care and cared about them as a *whole person* and not just as a health problem. Many participants stated that the nurse practitioners cared for their other problems outside of the chief health concern and gave suggestions to help enrich and improve their overall quality of life. Trust was a repeated pattern discovered within the data that several of the participants verbalized. They perceived that the nurse practitioners cared about them as a person and therefore they felt safe and were able to trust the nurse practitioner's input in guiding their healthcare decisions.

Category 2: Domain of Cultural and Social Structural Dimensions: Religion, Family, and Economics

This category was supported by three themes, three exhaustive descriptions, and several significant statements:

Category 2, Theme 1: Religious care promotes health and wellbeing

This theme was supported by the exhaustive description: *Religion enhances spiritual health and wellbeing.* Participant statements included:

"It [religion] gives me some sense of inspiration…it kind of lifts me."

"I believe in God strongly and have a special relationship with Him. I think your life can go much better if you can just talk to Him. I believe He heals from all levels and helps me through the crisis in my life."

Category 2, Theme 2: Kinship and social factors influence care and health

The exhaustive description that supported this theme was: *Generic care from family and friends leads to health and wellbeing.* Several participants shared ways they had received social support from friends and family members that contributed to their overall wellbeing.

"Right now, with everything that I'm going through, not being very stable with my living situation and so forth, my family has been there for me. My kids and I are still real tight and we look after each other."

"My friends are busy but they show up and pay visits when they can. My best friend just moved to Ohio but she sends me cards and calls when she can."

Category 2, Theme 3: Local economic factors influence care and health

This theme was supported by the exhaustive description: *Patients are grateful for the affordable care provided at their local clinic because of their past experience of being uninsured and receiving poor and fragmented care.* Several participants shared their personal experiences:

"I was with a certain doctor you know, he talked down to me and I said, 'Don't do that just because you are a doctor and I'm poor…' They don't treat me like that here. I come here and they take good care of me and treat me with respect."

"It's nice coming here because they don't give me the run around … Here I can get everything at once and it is such a relief for me when I don't have to fuss with begging someone or paying people to get to around."

This study revealed that many African American women rely on religion and family to help guide their lifeways. Religion was a common theme noted throughout the interview process. The majority of the participants practiced spiritual care by attending church services, praying, or living with a strong belief in God. Many expressed the belief that these religious values, expressions, and practices influenced their health in a positive way.

The support of family and friends had a notable influence on the participants' healthcare decisions. Many participants revealed that the support of family and friends was invaluable during times of illness or stress. Family and friends also influenced self-care strategies that participants felt were essential for their health and wellbeing. Finally, participants valued the affordability of care they were able to receive at a healthcare setting that facilitated the delivery of comprehensive and respectful care.

Category 3: Culture Care Modes for Health and Wellbeing: Preservation and/ or Maintenance, Accommodation and/ or Negotiation, and Restructuring and/or Repatterning

This category was supported by three themes, three exhaustive descriptions, and numerous significant statements:

Category 3, Theme 1: Nurse practitioner care helps to assist and or preserve the state of health and wellbeing

The exhaustive descriptor that supported this theme was: *Nurse practitioners maintain holistic and culturally congruent care that helps to preserve and/or maintain the African American women's state of health and wellbeing.* Participants shared personal stories depicting their experiences with receiving comprehensive care and caring from nurse practitioners aimed at preserving and/or maintaining their overall wellbeing:

> "I was stressed and my blood pressure was elevated. She [nurse practitioner] took a holistic approach to find me the best treatment. Like she asked what was going on with me, my diet and stuff. She took time to figure out what was causing me stress. It was a temporary stress I was dealing with that was causing me the blood pressure problems and she helped me to alleviate that."

> "My nurse practitioner would say, just come on in when you're here for physical therapy to get a blood pressure check. It seems she was more concerned for my total health."

Category 3, Theme 2: Nurse practitioners accommodate and/or negotiate with participants to develop care strategies

This theme was supported by the exhaustive descriptor: *Culture care accommodation and/or negotiation with participants for culturally congruent professional nurse practitioner care.* Participants reported numerous concerns and shared how nurse practitioners worked with them to address such concerns in ways that were mutually satisfying:

> "She tells me that instead of going to the hospital when I'm not feeling well to just call her and let her know. She can help me or something so she is trying to keep me out of the hospital as much as possible."

In addition, the researchers observed nurse practitioners negotiating with participants to identify and prioritize their three most urgent health-related concerns. These negotiations often resulted in a mutually agreed upon plan to address remaining concerns at a future visit.

Category 3, Theme 3: Nurse practitioners and participants expressed the need for restructuring and/or repatterning the financial support of the clinic to continue providing culturally congruent care

This theme was supported by the following exhaustive descriptor: *Nurse practitioners and participants are concerned about the restructuring of community finances, which may impact the future viability of this clinic.* Participants shared their fear about losing future

health care access due to economic and financial constraints that affect the viability of their only source of professional healthcare:

> "If this clinic closes I don't know what I'll do. The insurance here isn't the best but if I didn't have this I'd have nothing."

One of the researchers noted in her observations: "Funding for the clinic is from grants and millages. With the high rate of unemployment in [this community], property tax values have decreased so less money comes to the clinic. There is now a disproportionate number of devalued housing. This clinic helps to combat the health disparities seen in this county."

The community where this study took place experienced severe economic losses in tandem with a significant decline in the automobile industry since the 1970s. The city's unemployment rate was and continues to be among the highest in the nation. The nurse-managed clinic was developed to provide healthcare coverage for low income, uninsured adults. Many participants reported that they previously had little or no access to care and would instead use local emergency departments or the only free medical clinic in the county. The nurse-managed clinic had reduced unnecessary and uncompensated emergency department use and likely reduced preventable and uncompensated hospital admissions. The researchers discovered that funding for this clinic was considered vulnerable and likely to be time-limited because large portions of the funds were generated through a property tax millage. As a results, restructuring efforts are needed to ensure viability of clinic.

■ SUMMARY

The researchers discovered that African American women valued the primary health care they received from nurse practitioners at an urban nurse-managed clinic in the Midwestern United States. These women appreciated the nonjudgmental, trusting relationships developed with nurse practitioners over time. Practicing spiritual and religious care, accepting generic care from family and friends, and receiving holistic and affordable health care from nurse practitioners at the clinic contributed to the participants' overall health and wellbeing. Discovering African American women's lived experiences with primary care may lead to a greater understanding of their unique cultural beliefs, expressions, and practices and assist nurse practitioners and other healthcare providers in providing culturally competent, beneficial, and satisfying care to African American women.

This phenomenological study conceptualized within Leininger's Theory of Culture Care Diversity and Universality provided an example of how the theory can be used with a nonethnonursing qualitative research methodology. The research findings from this study contributed to the body of nursing knowledge with evidence-based and best practices for nurse practitioners and may be applicable by other healthcare professionals as well. Leininger (1991, 2006a) predicted that knowledge gained from using the Culture Care Theory would constitute a substantive knowledge base to guide nursing care decisions and actions in the provision of care that is congruent with the patients' beliefs and practices. This study provides nurses, nurse practitioners, and other healthcare providers with holding knowledge about how African American women view the care they receive in a primary care setting.

The findings from this study contributed to the discipline of nursing by adding to the body of transcultural nursing knowledge and by providing insight into the patients' emic views of nurse practitioner care. Nurse practitioner students and practicing nurse practitioners may use such insights to mutually co-develop with their African American patients, culturally congruent care decisions and actions that may lead to improved health and wellbeing and enhanced quality of life.

■ ACKNOWLEDGEMENT

The authors would like to thank and acknowledge the contribution of the other researchers who participated in this study: Sherry Lenz and Jill Patterson.

■ DISCUSSION QUESTIONS

1. Discuss why nurse practitioners and other healthcare providers caring for African American patients should integrate cultural beliefs and practices in their professional practices.
2. Examine how the Culture Care Theory can be used as a theoretical framework for nonethnonursing qualitative research studies.
3. Discuss the study findings and implications to clinical practice.

■ REFERENCES

American Association of Nurse Practitioners. (2015). *NP facts* [Webpage document]. Retrieved from https://www.aanp.org/images/documents/about-nps/npfacts.pdf

Barr, M., Johnston, D. & McConnell, D. (2000). Patient satisfaction with a new nurse practitioner service. *Accident and Emergency Nursing, 8*(3), 144-147.

Benkert, R., & Peters, R. (2005). African American women's coping with health care prejudice. *Western Journal of Nursing Research, 27*(7), 863-889.

Colaizzi, P. (1978). Psychological research as the phenomenologist views it. In R. Valle and M. King (Eds.), *Existential-phenomenological alternatives for psychology* (pp. 48-71). New York, NY: Oxford University Press.

Cuevas, A. G. (2013). *Exploring four barriers experienced by African Americans in healthcare: Perceived discrimination, medical mistrust, race discordance, and poor communication* [Master's thesis]. Retrieved from http://pdxscholar.library.pdx.edu/cgi/viewcontent.cgi?article=1614&context=open_access_etds

Ehrmin, J. (2005). Dimensions of culture care for substance dependent African American women. *Journal of Transcultural Nursing, 16*(2), 117-125.

Johnson, M. (2001). Meeting health care needs of a vulnerable population: Perceived barriers. *Journal of Community Health Nursing, 18*(1), 35-52.

Kennedy, B. R., Mathis, C. C., & Woods, A. K. (2007). African Americans and their distrust of the healthcare system: Healthcare for diverse populations. *Journal of Cultural Diversity, 14*(2), 56-60.

Leininger, M. M. (1991). The theory of culture care diversity and universality. In M. Leininger (Ed.). *Culture care diversity and universality: A theory of nursing* (pp. 73-118). NY: National League for Nursing Press.

Leininger, M. M. (2006a). Culture care diversity and universality theory: Evolution of the ethonursing method. In M. M. Leininger and M. R. McFarland (Eds.), *Culture care diversity and universality: A worldwide nursing theory* (2nd ed., pp. 1-41). Sudbury, MA: Jones & Bartlett.

Leininger, M. M. (2006b). Ethnonursing: A research method with enablers to study the theory of culture care. In M. M. Leininger and M. R. McFarland (Eds.), *Culture care diversity and universality: A worldwide nursing theory* (2nd ed., pp. 43-81). Sudbury, MA: Jones & Bartlett.

McFarland, M. R. (1997). Use of culture care theory with Anglo and African American elders in a long-term care setting. *Nursing Science Quarterly, 10,* 186-192.

McFarland, M. R. (2006). Madeleine M. Leininger: Culture care theory of diversity and universality. In A. M. Tomey and M. R. Alligood (Eds.), *Nursing theorists and their work* (6th ed., pp. 472-496). St. Louis, MO: Mosby.

McFarland, M. R., & Wehbe-Alamah, H. B. (2015). The theory of culture care diversity and universality. In M. R. McFarland and H. B. Wehbe-Alamah (Eds.), *Leininger's culture care diversity and Universality: A worldwide nursing theory* (2nd ed., pp. 1-34). Burlington, MA: Jones & Bartlett Learning.

Nicolaidis, C., Timmons, V., Thomas, M., Waters, S., Wahab, S., Mejia, A., & Mitchell, R. (2010). "You don't go tell White people nothing:" African American women's perspectives on the influence of violence and race on depression and depression care. *American Journal of Public Health, 100*(8), 1470-1476.

Plowden, K., & Young, A. (2003). Socio-structural factors influencing health behaviors of urban African American men. *Journal of National Black Nurses Association, 14*(1), 45-51.

Shariff-Marco, S., Klassen, A., & Bowie, J. (2010). Racial/ethnic differences in self-reported racism and its association with cancer-related health behaviors. *American Journal of Public Health, 100*(2), 364-374.

Wehbe-Alamah, H. B., and McFarland, M. R. (2015). The ethnonursing research method. In M. McFarland and H. Wehbe-Alamah (Eds.), *Culture care diversity and universality: A worldwide nursing theory* (3rd ed., pp. 35-72). Burlington, MA: Jones & Bartlett Learning.

Wehbe-Alamah, H., McFarland, M., Macklin, J., & Riggs, N. (2011). The lived experiences of African American women receiving care from nurse practitioners in an urban nurse-managed clinic. *The Online Journal in Cultural Competence in Nursing and Healthcare, 1*(1), 15-26.

Yupiit: Alaska Native People of Southwest Alaska

Pamela J. Embler, Mary T. Weiss, and Sandra J. Mixer

> *"We call ourselves Yup'ik Eskimo or Yupiit (real people). In our language yuk means person or human being. Then we add pik (real or genuine). We are the real people"* (John, cited in Fienup-Riordan, 2007).

■ INTRODUCTION

In this chapter, the authors share their individual and collective experiences as nurse, nurse researcher, faculty member, and community member working with the Yupiit people. One author (Embler) has worked as a nurse in Alaska practicing exclusively in the intensive care unit. Living in Alaska and caring for Native Alaskan people has provided her with valued credibility among the Yupiit people who have allowed her to be accepted into the Yupiit culture in Bethel. Over a period of 14 years, she moved from being an observer to a participant in the end-of-life care practices of many Native Alaskan patients and their families. During this time, she witnessed many multifaceted end-of-life care interactions between non-Native care providers and Alaskan Native patients and their families and has come to recognize the complexity of healthcare delivery in Alaska, particularly at end-of-life.

Another author (Weiss) moved to Alaska in the early 1970s and has lived and worked in several urban and rural communities including Bethel. She is also an associate professor at the School of Nursing at the University of Alaska-Anchorage. Together, they collaborated in the writing of this chapter with a member of the nursing faculty (Mixer) from the University of Tennessee, Knoxville, who is recognized as a TCN

Scholar and leader, has published numerous studies using the Culture Care Theory and the Ethnonursing Research Method, and mentored Embler in her study of end-of-care among the Yupiit.

Findings from an ethnonursing research study that explored Yupiit end-of-life culture care expressions, meanings, patterns, and practices; the authors' cultural immersion experiences; and combined knowledge of and expertise in transcultural nursing theory have been synthesized to provide a rich discussion of the Yupiit culture.

■ RESEARCH STUDY

The end-of-life care needs of the Yupiit people were the focus of a qualitative Ethnonursing Research Study (Embler, 2012) that used the Theory of Culture Care Diversity and Universality (also known as the Culture Care Theory or the CCT) as its guiding framework. End-of-life care is multifaceted and its complexity increases when cultural perspectives are integrated into care decisions and actions (Embler, Mixer, & Gunther, 2015). This topic served as the domain of inquiry (DOI) for the study. The goal and purpose of this ethnonursing study was to discover culture care expressions, meanings, patterns, and practices at end-of-life among Yupiit people in community settings throughout the Yukon-Kuskokwim (Y-K) Delta and in Anchorage, Alaska using the CCT with the Ethnonursing Research Method. Key informants were Yupiit community members while general informants included healthcare providers, clergy, and non-Yupiit community members.

Research Questions

Four research questions guided the ethnonursing inquiry and served to generate new knowledge and address the limited extant information regarding Yupiit Eskimo end-of-life culture care.

- What are the culture care expressions, meanings, patterns, and practices related to end-of-life care among Yupiit Eskimo?
- In what ways do worldview and cultural and social structure factors, (religion [spiritual] & philosophical; kinship & social; political & legal; education; economics; technology; cultural values, beliefs and lifeways; ethnohistorical; and environmental) influence end-of-life culture care expressions, meanings, patterns, and practices for Yupiit Eskimo?
- In what ways do generic and professional care assist with or inhibit the end-of-life culture care expressions, meanings, patterns, and practices for Yupiit Eskimo?
- Based upon the discovery of Yupiit Eskimo end-of-life care, what nursing decision/action modes promote culturally congruent end of life care expressions, meanings, patterns, and practices for Yupiit Eskimo?

Three themes discovered in the study were supported by care patterns revealed from recurrent informant descriptors: Care is *uptete* (to get ready to go); care is *ilakellriit* (community and family); and professional care is *to do* (Embler, 2012). To provide culturally congruent end-of-life care to the Yupiit people, nurses need to know what they describe as important, fulfilling, useful, and meaningful within their unique cultural context.

■ THEORETICAL FRAMEWORK

The Theory of Culture Care Diversity and Universality is used as a guide to discover the relationships between *culture* and *health* phenomena (Leininger, 2006). The central concepts of the theory are *care*, *culture*, and *culture care* as the essence of nursing (Leininger,

2006). The theorist stated that care is embedded in culture, and culture care is necessary to promote health and facilitate meaningful nurse-patient interactions (Leininger, 2002). Research conducted using the CCT advances nursing knowledge about diverse and similar cultural groups.

Research studies conducted with the CCT guide nursing practice through application of the three modes of nursing actions and decisions: Culture care preservation and/or maintenance; culture care accommodation and/or negotiation; and culture care repatterning and/or restructuring (Leininger, 2006). The modes presented in a later section of this chapter were derived from the recurrent care findings discovered from the expressions, patterns, and practices of key and general informants. These discovered Yupiit end-of-life culture care practices will help nurses to coparticipatively make decisions and formulate actions that are culturally congruent for this cultural group.

Orientational Definitions

The purpose of orientational definitions is to maintain a qualitative participant/informant focus, not a researcher focus (Leininger, 2006, p. 12). The orientational definitions used for this study regarding end-of-life care were congruent with the National Institutes of Health/National Institute of Nursing Research (NIH/NINR) State of the Science Conference Statement on Improving End-of-Life Care (2004) and were adapted from the Theory of Culture Care Diversity and Universality and Leininger (2006), who held that there is cultural diversity inherent in words. Orientational definitions (as opposed to operational definitions) maintain fluidity and allow the researcher to discover culture care meanings (Leininger, 2006).

End-of-Life

There was no definitive or generally agreed upon definition of *end-of-life* in the nursing literature reviewed. The National Institutes of Nursing Research at the National Institutes of Health (NINR/NIH, 2004) proposed a definition based on attributes of chronic illness, symptoms, or impaired functional ability that are often irreversible, require formal assistance (professional care), or informal assistance (caregiver assistance), and can lead to death. For this study, end-of-life was defined broadly to include a sudden occurrence such as trauma or immediate pathophysiological event, and an expanded timeframe that includes the period during which an illness or disease that precipitates death occurs (Embler, 2012). Regardless of the brevity or the chronicity involved, end-of-life is a *process* (Baydala, Hampton, Kinunwa, Kinunwa, & Kinunwa, 2006; Bonura, Fender, Roesler, & Pacquiao, 2001; Gelfand, Balcazar, Parzuchowski, & Lenox, 2001; Kaufman & Morgan, 2005).

Emic

Folk or generic learned and shared knowledge of lifeways are the culturally-situated values, beliefs, meanings, and practices which explain health, nonhealth, and predict illness of individuals and groups (adapted from Leininger, 2006, p. 13).

Etic

Professional knowledge is formalized from cognitively and affectively learned knowledge from established educational institutions. Etic views are the outsider views (adapted from Leininger, 2006, p. 13).

Generic / Lay / Folk Care

Folk or generic care refers to "...learned and transmitted lay, indigenous, traditional, or local folk (emic) knowledge and practices to provide assistive, supportive, enabling, and facilitating acts for or towards others...to improve wellbeing or to help with dying" (Leininger, 2006, p. 14).

Professional Care

Care knowledge and practice that has been formally learned to prevent illness, improve wellbeing, or help with dying (Leininger, 2006, p. 14).

Assumptive Premises

The following study assumptions were derived from the assumptive premises of the CCT and guided the research discovery of culture care expressions, meanings, patterns, and practices related to end-of-life care among Yupiit Eskimo people:

- Care is essential to Yupiit Eskimo at end-of-life (adapted from Leininger, 2006, p.18);
- Culture care expressions, meanings, patterns, and practices for Yupiit Eskimo are influenced by and embedded in worldview and cultural and social structure factors, (i.e., religion [spiritual] & philosophical; kinship & social; political & legal;

education; economics; technology; cultural values, beliefs and lifeways; ethnohistorical; and environmental) (adapted from Leininger, 2006, p. 19);

- Every culture has generic (lay, folk, naturalistic; mainly *emic*) and usually some professional (*etic*) end-of-life care to be discovered and used for culturally congruent practices (adapted from Leininger, 2006, p. 19); and

- Leininger's three theoretical modes of care offer new, creative, and different therapeutic ways to help Yupiit Eskimo with end-of life care (adapted from Leininger, 2006, p. 19).

Ethnonhistory

The Yukon-Kuskokwim (Y-K) Delta in southwest Alaska was formed by the two largest rivers in Alaska, the Yukon and the Kuskokwim (refer Figure 22.1). The Y-K Delta was a lowland region roughly the size of Kansas (Barker, 2010). This region was home to a native Alaskan people known as the Yupiit. The Y-K Delta's subarctic tundra environment was a rich, giving, and sustaining environment for them and the seasonal variation in vegetation, fowl, fish, and mammals provided the Yupiit a relatively stable and settled life. Seasonal camps and winter settlements lined the rivers that connected villages and communities.

The Y-K Delta was situated 500 miles west of Anchorage, accessible only by aircraft. Two jets flew daily between Bethel and Anchorage. Many smaller planes flew in and out, but their numerous stops turned the normally one-hour trip into a multiple-hour journey. The weather had a huge effect on air travel. Fog, snow, or high winds could "weather planes *in* or *out*" meaning planes may or may not be able to take off or land. In the summer months, village-to-village travel was accomplished via boat on the Kuskokwim River, by three- or four-wheeled all-terrain vehicles, or on foot. In the winter months, the frozen Kuskokwim River "road" became a conduit for travel between villages by snow machine or automobile; the frozen tundra allowed for snow machine travel.

Study Setting

The village of Bethel, considered the economic hub for the Y-K Delta region, was a bush community which meant that no roads connected it to other major cities

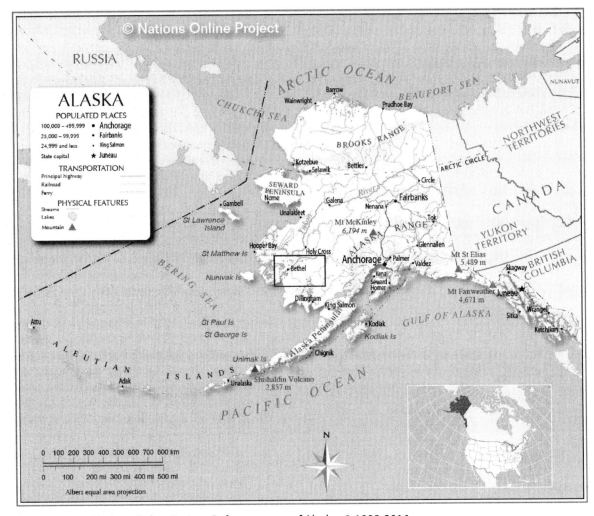

FIGURE 22.1 • Nations Online Project. Reference map of Alaska. © 1998-2016.
Retrieved from http://www.nationsonline.org/oneworld/map/USA/alaska_map.htm and used with permission.

(Refer to Figure 22.2). In rural off-road communities, Alaska Natives including the Yupiit of southwest Alaska, comprised the majority of the population (U. S. Department of Commerce/Census Bureau, 2012). The Yupiit people have been among the largest Native population in Alaska. Approximately 23,000 Yupiit lived scattered among the approximately 56 villages that ranged in population from 80 to 1,000 individuals (Fienup-Riordan, 2007). The population of Bethel was approximately 6,000 with the majority (65%) being Alaska Native/American Indian; the village was also home for a variety of other cultures, including Caucasians (23.3%); Asians (2.5%); Hispanics with Latinos (2.2%); African

Americans (0.9%); Native Hawaiian and Pacific Islanders (0.4%); and mixed heritage (7.3%; U. S. Department of Commerce/Census Bureau, 2012). Alaskan urban centers on the road system were populated predominately by Western, White, and non-Latino inhabitants (U. S. Department of Commerce/Census Bureau, 2012). However, Alaska Native cultural lifestyles—including food, dress, language, and behaviors—were commonly followed by Natives and non-Natives alike (Fienup-Riordan, 2007).

Several historical events have had devastating effects on the Yupiit people. The influenza epidemic of 1852-1853 wiped out entire villages when an estimated

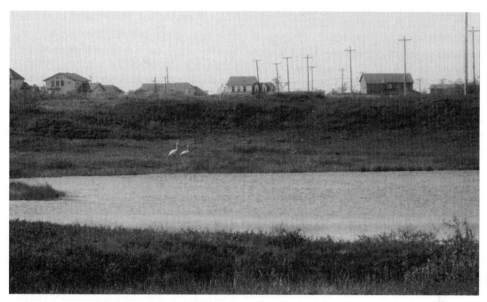

FIGURE 22.2. • Photograph of Bethel village. © P. Embler (2012).

60% of the Yupiit population died (Fienup-Riordan, 2007). In the early part of the 20th century, tuberculosis also caused a marked decline in the Yupiit population (Fortuine, 2005). Subsequently, as the Yupiit population declined, the region's non-native population grew exponentially (Fienup-Riordan, 2007).

Worldview

For the Yupiit, the world has existed on a continuum with no delineation between reality and dreams, life and death, or beginning and end (Burch, 1988; Fienup-Riordan, 1990, 2007; Kawagley, 2006). Cyclical energy exists in all things. All ceremonies and ceremonial practices were related. Family and community have been the foundation of Yupiit worldview: "...family is where our world begins."

Embler (2012) discovered that Yupiit culture care expressions, meanings, patterns, and practices generally focus on *what lies ahead*. Life has been viewed as cyclical and death not as final; spirits were believed to be born into future generations. The concept of human dominion over the natural environment, while part of the Eurocentric culture, has not been part of the Yupiit worldview that values balance and harmony among all things — time, places, and the living and nonliving (Embler). Everything has been viewed as connected and interrelated with each individual seen as a small part of the *web of life*, which must be respected. This belief "...extends to all creatures" as one general informant explained. This informant went on to describe the reverence that Yupiit give to the animals they hunt and eat: "....all parts are used or eaten and what isn't [sic] is carefully disposed of—the beaver is returned to the stream so it can live again and allow itself to be caught again." We have much to learn from this perspective.

Cultural and Social Structure Dimensions

Leininger's Sunrise Enabler (Refer to Color Insert 1) provided a cognitive map of the CCT that helped nurses to understand factors of the social structure dimensions that influence, describe, and give meaning to Yupiit cultural values, beliefs, expressions, and patterns. For the Yupiit Eskimo, the world has existed on a continuum with no demarcation or delineation between reality and dreams, life and death, or beginning and end (Burch, 1988; Fienup-Riordan, 1990, 2007; Kawagley, 2006). Cyclical energy has been viewed as existing in all things. Ceremonies and ceremonial practices connected everything, one to the other. Negotiated meanings between Yupiit Eskimo cosmology and Judeo-Christian worldview have forever transformed the lifeways and understandings of the Yupiik Eskimo (Fienup-Riordan, 1990, 2005, 2007).

Religious Factors

The Yupiit acknowledged and respected three major spirits. Contained in the wind and the weather, the *Spirit of the Air* was regarded as the most powerful, permeating the whole world, and influencing all things. The *Spirit of the Sea* controlled all the creatures of the ocean (Burch, 1988). The Bladder Festival was a ceremony central to honoring this spirit. The souls of seals were believed to be contained in their bladders; returning their bladders to the sea allowed the seals to be reborn (Fienup-Riordan, 1990, 2007). The *Spirit of the Moon* was believed to influence all land animals. Although the Yupiit revered these spirits, they did not worship them. However, when the spirits were being pleased, they directed caribou or whale so they could be taken by hunters (Burch, 1988).

The Yupiit acknowledged the universe has always been in flux but unified into one being. The cycle of death and rebirth was perhaps best exemplified by the ceremonial hooped mask. The mask was encircled by concentric rings called *ellanguat,* which meant "pretend or model cosmos" (Fienup-Riordan, 1990, p. 59). The central features of the mask were the *eyes of awareness.* More than a metaphor, the eyes allowed a view beyond this world and into another (Feinup-Riordan, 1990). Each mask was unique to the particular spirit or cyclical process it represented. The concentric rings and eyes of awareness allowed one to see *into* the spirit world and to be seen *by* the spirit world, thus making one capable of receiving spiritual knowledge and transformation (Fienup-Riordan, 1990, 2007).

The cyclical worldview of the Yupiit was also prominent in after-death rituals. The belief that birth and death are infinite was reflected in many Yupiit lifeways, such as child-naming practices, that showed reverence to all living things (Fienup-Riordan, 1990, 2007). The period of mourning after death was a blended practice of both Christian and traditional Yupiit observances. Embler (2012) discovered one common practice was *laying out* the body after death in the home of the deceased or a family member to allow loved ones the opportunity to pay their respects to the deceased person. For this observance, "…the person who died is in one room and an adjoining room is filled with persons who came to show respect." The period for laying out varied from one day to three weeks and visitors often stayed for weeks (Embler).

After death, there were periodic feasts or *potlatches* when the entire community was welcomed to come and remember the person who died (Embler, 2012). Practices used for feasts varied depending on the level of organized religious acculturation by and traditional orientation of the village members. In general, feasts took place after the funeral, on birthdays, and holidays. Specific patterns for feasting after a person's death occurred at 20 days, 40 days, and one year. A four-year feast marked a widow's formal availability to remarry (Embler).

Because the Y-K Delta had limited commercial value, missionaries were the first group of outsiders to settle in the region between 1840 and 1888 (Fienup-Riordan, 2007). Moravian missions were established in 1885 near the Yupiit village of Mumtrekhlogamute, which means "smokehouse people." Russian Orthodox and Roman Catholic missionaries also settled in the area (Fienup-Riordan, 2007). Much has been written about the atrocities inflicted upon the Yupiit by these missionaries (Napoleon, 1996). Language, traditional ceremonies, and subsistence practices were lost to subsequent generations as families were separated when children were sent to boarding schools (Napoleon, 1996). Fienup-Riordan (1990, 2005, 2007) noted that much of the Yupiit way was lost during the last 100 years when the *Kass'at* (White people), with their missionaries and schools, replaced the traditional teachings, the Yupiit language, and traditional ceremonies citing them as pagan rituals. In modern times, the Yupiit have again become the predominant inhabitants of the Y-K Delta as the elders have sought to renew cultural practices and diminish the traumatic outcomes (violence, substance abuse, and suicide) that resulted from years of oppression and threatened the health and vigor of future Yupiit generations (Fienup-Riordan, 2007). The Yupiit elders were uniting to revive these traditional ways, especially those in the Y-K Delta. However, the Yupiit cosmology and the beliefs, patterns, expressions, and practices of the Yupiit have been forever transformed by the imposition of the Judeo-Christian worldview (Fienup-Riordan, 1990, 2005, 2007).

Russian Orthodox, Roman Catholic, and Moravian were the predominant religions of the Yupiit of the Y-K Delta. As one informant explained, much care has been taken to "…bridge traditional practices and religious practices" and to "…sew back together traditions." Many religious ceremonies were conducted in Yupiit with hymnals continually being translated to Yupiit language. Blending traditional customs with Christianity was facilitated by both sides being open to the other. Religious services presented in both Yupiit and English created greater community cohesion. Christian religious beliefs and Yupiit traditional beliefs shared more commonalities than differences, such as the belief in life after death.

Embler (2012) observed a traditional Russian Orthodox Slavic celebration during which a Russian Orthodox congregation visited community-hosted homes during the first week of January. In the period leading up to this week-long Slavic celebration, curtains and blinds were kept open to allow the Holy Spirit to enter. In this celebration of Christ's birth, the congregation walked from home to home to give blessings for the coming year. The procession was led by the priest and two congregation members. One person carried a spinning Star of Christ and the other held a banner depicting the Holy Trinity.

Crowds of approximately 100 Slavic people—including men, women, and children of all ages—participated in this event on a cold January night in Bethel. Participants met early in the afternoon and the event lasted into the early morning hours of the following day. Each family hosting the event prepared food and provided gifts to all attendees. The size of a typical home in Bethel averaged about 1,250 square feet. Nevertheless, every effort was made to accommodate all of the approximately 100 Slavic participants. Furniture was removed from the main gathering rooms and every elder was given a place to sit while children sat on the laps of adults or older siblings.

At each home, the activities (prayers, hymns, feasting, and the passing of gifts) lasted approximately two hours. All prayers were said and hymns sung in the Yupiit language. The foods shared afterward consisted of nontraditional dishes as well as traditional Yupiit fish soup, dried fish, and *agutuk* (ice cream made from whale or seal fat, berries, and sugar). Children received candy and toys; the gifts were generally gloves and socks for men and sewing items and washcloths for women.

Kinship and Social Factors

Fienup-Riordan (1990, 2005, 2007) compiled the most comprehensive and detailed collection of *qanruyutet* (adages, words of wisdom, and oral instructions) known by the Yupiit elders of the Y-K Delta.

Throughout Yupiit history, the *qanruyutet* has served as the foundation for the relationships between men and women, parents and children, siblings, cousins, neighboring villages, and non-natives. "We talk because we love you" (John, 2000) has continued as the central ideology of historic Yupiit teachings. These teachings center on *humility, having compassion for all living things,* and *promoting tolerance* (Kawagley, 2006). Fienup-Riordan (2007) noted that Yupiit elders' beliefs about *love and guidance as discipline* have become lost to the modern-day Yupiit people.

A respectful greeting between Yupiit individuals establishes familiarity (Embler, 2012). The first questions asked were "…who is your family" or "….do you know …?" The researcher discovered it was considered important to remember names, because it showed respect to greet an individual by their name. When connections were thus made, conversations then easily unfolded from this common bond. This ritual was described most often in the context of relationships between Yupiit and non-Yupiit. When respectful common bonds were not established, relationships did not develop (Embler). The following quote from a Yupiit community member illustrates how Yupiit can feel disrespected by "….*kass'aq* [White people who] come out here [to name of village] [acting like] National Geographic taking pictures to post [on a website] without getting to know people or asking people first" (Embler).

Males

Early Yupiit seasonal settlements dictated village cohabitation (Feinup-Riordan, 2007). During the winter months, males and females lived together. During non-winter seasons, males and females lived separately. The *qasgi* (communal men's house) was a large, round, semi-subterranean log and sod structure where the men ate, slept, worked, entertained, and bathed (Feinup-Riordan, 2007). Most importantly, it was here that the men imparted *qanruyutet* to the boys. The qasgi was the school and the men were the teachers. Boys were considered men when they grew whiskers. Skills and responsibilities were taught according to individual capability and perceived receptivity, not age (Feinup-Riordan, 2007).

The *qasgi* served other important functions for the males of the village. All major village discussions, decisions, ceremonies, and celebrations took place there. The *angalkut* (shaman) tended to the sick and performed rituals there, asking for fair weather and successful hunts (Feinup-Riordan, 2005, 2007). Finally, all moral instruction for a properly-lived life was watched, listened to, and learned in this structure (Feinup-Riordan, 2005, 2007). Over decades of time, the *qasgi* gave way to single-family dwellings, churches, and traditional classrooms. According to Fienup-Riordan (1990, 2005, 2007), elders believed that the social problems plaguing the modern Yupiit people (domestic violence, suicide, substance abuse) resulted from losing the qasgi teachings.

Females
Fienup-Riordan (2005, 2007) noted that females received instruction by observing their mothers and other female village members. The *enet* (sod house) was the dwelling where females and children lived and worked. At five years of age, boys left their mother's dwelling to live in the *qasgi* with the men. Like their male counterparts, young females observed how adult women worked until they could function independently. Maturity was not defined by age but by the ability to complete tasks independently without constant instruction. For females, this stage usually coincided with the first menstruation (Fienup-Riordan, 2005, 2007).

On average, more than 350 babies were born in Bethel each year (Alaska Department of Health and Social Services, 2012). Childbirth education classes were not offered in Bethel because few babies were born to non-Yupiit families and Yupiit families managed the childbirth process within their own communities. When a Yupiit woman became pregnant, her extended family provided traditional antenatal teaching and support for all areas of her life, from morning until night, for the entire duration of her pregnancy. In Bethel, cesarean sections were done only in emergencies and epidurals were not given. There was still an aversion to the medicalization of the birth process. The Yupiit highly valued labor and delivery taking place in a manner congruent with their cultural belief of being in balance with nature (M. T. Weiss, personal communication, June 15, 2015).

Parents and Children
The Yupiit believed that the most essential of all human relationships was the one between parent and child (Fienup-Riordan, 2005, 2007). All responsibilities

and rules for living, surviving, functioning as a member of society, and living life properly were taught lovingly but firmly by a child's parents. While males and females received gender-specific instruction, the overriding goal of either parent was to impart obedience, compassion, and reverence for elders (Fienup-Riordan, 2005, 2007). The Yupiit believed that children were capable of learning before they can speak. Even in modern times, parenting has been held to be a reciprocal relationship. Children learned what they observed. Parents must embrace this responsibility, watch over them closely, and not ignore them (Fienup-Riordan, 2005, 2007). The Yupiit believed that a child's behavior reflected upon the parents.

In Yupiit culture, lessons were learned first through respectful observation and listening followed by replication. When individuals were asked to participate in community activities, it was culturally congruent for them to follow this pattern of respectful learning (Fienup-Riordan, 2005, 2007). By working alongside Yupiit adults and elders, younger observers were able to discover the experiences and practices inherent in these everyday activities. For example, during one encounter at a community fair, the researcher was invited by an informant to assist with meal preparation for a potluck gathering scheduled to take place later that evening (Embler, 2012). Several women (aged 40 to 60) were tearing meat from turkeys with their bare hands. The researcher was introduced to the other women who politely smiled. Following the informant's lead, the researcher began to assist with deboning the turkeys in similar fashion. Once this task was completed, one of the women invited the researcher to assist at another station. The researcher later learned from the informant that she must have made a favorable impression because otherwise she would not have been asked to continue helping with the preparations.

Embler (2012) also learned that the Yupiit believed that knowledge was in the sole possession of one individual; it must be earned. In other words, one did not find out because one asked; one was told when he or she was judged ready to hear, listen, and understand. Informants confided that, in the Yupiit worldview, persons who held a particular bit of knowledge— whether an elder or not—determined when to share it with others (Embler). This was communicated repeatedly in participant observations and in individual key and general informant interviews but in different ways. For example, one informant explained, "…it is about common bonds first.…much is not spoken, [and you] must be let in." Similarly, another informant shared, "…watch and the answer to a question will be revealed." Two favorite wisdoms, "…conversations turn to connections" and "…trust before revealing" represent the importance of respectful listening and learning (Embler).

Elders

Historically, elders were the central figures in educating Yupiit children and youth. Elders continued to be respected for their wisdom, which was passed down to children through stories and observational experiences as described by Fienup-Riordan (2005, 2007). The elders instructed by using carefully chosen words (Fienup-Riordan, 2005, 2007). It was understood that knowledge was not *property* to be owned by a chosen few, but rather it was to be a shared experience gained by engaging in the world and with others. Elders were cognizant of what young people needed to know and how they needed to learn (Fienup-Riordan, 2005, 2007). Being *upterralinarluta* or *ever prepared* was a common cautionary admonition spoken by Yupiit elders to young people. Implicit in this advice was the understanding that one must be wise in knowing what to prepare for and equally wise in being prepared for the unknowable (Fienup-Riordan, 2005, 2007).

Embler (2012) learned that the elders were considered "…the oak tree that holds the family together." When an elder spoke at a gathering, everyone listened respectfully. In addition, elders were greeted by everyone whenever they entered a room, seats were relinquished to them, and food was served to them. However, being *elderly* did not constitute being an *elder*. The Yupiit followed the premise that, "…a leader [is] identified by the wisdom of [their] actions, not by being the person who speaks first, speaks the loudest, or longest" (Embler). The Yupiit understood that elders held much of what was left of their traditional culture and language.

Childrearing and Moral Instruction

The elders who shared stories with Fienup-Riordan (2005, 2007) noted that *qanruyutet* guided their lives. The elders believed that ignoring *qanruyutet* invited disaster for people who followed their own minds and acted upon their own thoughts. In the past, children were taught all moral rules, guidelines, and standards

about how to behave as children, as adults, and as a spouse. Moral instruction provided all things needed to live a proper life. When the elders spoke, all worked stopped and everyone listened. Even in modern times, the Yupiit have believed that one should not speak more than needed. Their moral code was complicated and required a lifetime to learn and understand. Teaching and learning were regarded as lifelong pursuits as well as personal responsibilities (Fienup-Riordan, 2005, 2007).

By Yupiit tradition, childrearing was the responsibility of the family and community. However, Embler (2012) discovered that while "…discipline [is] everyone's business" many Yupiit expressed that "…technology is changing this" by re-creating their "social boundaries of action." Informants described a time when any parent could correct a child's action and not be questioned by that child's parent. More recently, some Yupiit observed that parents were less open to receiving this help and often requested that others not interfere.

Cultural identity and discipline, taught intergenerationally, served as strong, observable presences in the Yupiit culture. When they were born, children were bestowed the cultural Yupiit names of deceased family members. This act venerated and preserved the identity of the deceased person. The researcher observed many acts of respect for elders as well as the consequences of disrespect on more than one occasion. When disciplining a child, elders, adults, and parents alike did not make eye contact with the one being scolded; instead, their gaze was directed downward. Embler (2012) learned that this practice was a common "…scolding or ostracizing form of discipline." The reverence for elders, preservation of traditional names, and emphasis on discipline were prominent cultural practices in Yupiit culture.

Economic and Legal Factors

Health care was both the largest industry and largest employer in the greater Bethel area. There were 41 clinics in the Y-K Delta serving the approximately 56 villages (Embler, 2012). Clinics were staffed primarily by community health aides; the providers were either a nurse practitioner, physician assistant, or physician. Additional treatments and services were available at the regional healthcare facility in Bethel. Because there were no road systems, travel from outlying villages to

Bethel required air transport. For family or community members needing to travel with an ill person, the average round trip ticket between Bethel and the outlying villages would cost approximately $100 (Embler). For persons requiring medical care beyond the scope of services available in Bethel, the Yukon-Kuskokwim hospital provided free transportation only for the patient and one escort (Embler). Should more advanced medical treatment be required, air transport between Bethel and Anchorage with a round trip ticket would cost about $500. However, this fee did not include lodging in Anchorage or further travel for patients requiring out-of-state transport. Informants shared with the researcher that such costs were "… a *huge* hardship… family cannot afford to go to Anchorage for long term or often to visit… a person can end up dying alone, away from family, or away from the Delta."

The legal and economic factors affecting Alaska Natives, specifically the Yupiit people, were complex. Their subsistence rights (including fishing regulation), access to alcohol, and the jurisdiction of tribal courts reflected that they were subject to tribal, State of Alaska, and Federal policies. Many Yupiit people of the Y-K Delta depended on a subsistence lifestyle or a combination of subsistence and cash economies for their survival. *Subsistence* meant depending on the harvest of natural resources for food, clothing, and the necessities of life without cash or money (M. T. Weiss, personal communication, June 15, 2015).

The subsistence lifestyle consisted of hunting, fishing, and gathering food from the tundra. This lifestyle was congruent with the Yupiit values of being prepared for the unexpected (*upterrlainarluta*); seizing opportunities as they present themselves; embracing the uncertainty of the future; and staying in balance with nature. Seasonal variations in vegetation, fowl, fish, and mammals allowed the Yupiit a relatively stable and settled life (M. T. Weiss, personal communication, June 15, 2015). The Yupiit shared that they rarely made other plans "…if the fish are running" and harvest became a priority when "…the weather is ripe for berry picking" (Embler, 2012). While Alaska Natives historically practiced a subsistence lifestyle, Eurocentric culture and urbanization introduced a cash economy that threatened to erode this lifestyle (M. T. Weiss, personal communication, June 15, 2015).

A mainstay of the Yupiit diet was king salmon. Every spring and summer, king salmon returned from the sea and travel up Alaskan rivers to spawn. For centuries, Yupiit people survived because the salmon they caught and preserved each summer was the basis of their diet, providing their main source of protein for the following winter and spring. Over the past several years, the number of king salmon that traveled upstream in the Yukon and Kuskokwim rivers had steadily decreased, possibly due to several combined factors such as increased competition for fish by commercial interests on the rivers and high seas, sport fishing, and changing climate conditions. The State of Alaska managed the fisheries and developed management policies toward the goal of maintaining a sustainable fish yield while maintaining an equitable resource distribution among all Alaskans. These complex regulations also threatened traditional Yupiit lifeways (M. T. Weiss, personal communication, June 15, 2015).

Political and Legal Factors

The relationship between the Alaska state government and federally recognized tribal entities was variable and complex. There were approximately 300 federally recognized tribal entities in Alaska. However, recognition of tribal sovereignty by the state varied depending on the philosophy of the political leaders in power. Tribal traditions that emphasized restorative rather than punitive judgments conflicted with Alaska state sentencing requirements. Coordination between federal, state, and tribal systems required legal cooperation. The jurisdiction of tribal courts and their relationship with the state and federal court systems continued to be a work in progress (University of Alaska–Fairbanks, n. d.).

The Yupiit people experienced complex and confusing regulations from State and Federal agencies related to the buying, selling, and possession of alcohol. The Yupiit people desired tribal self-determination in regard to subsistence lifeways, fishing rights, and alcohol regulations rather than imposed state and federal mandates (M. T. Weiss, personal communication, June 15, 2015).

Educational Factors

Kawagley (2010) noted that historically, Eurocentric education was imposed upon the Yupiit people by religious missionaries and the federal government when it governed the Alaska territory. This educational system imposed a disjointed, segmented curriculum upon a culture that had a unified, holistic worldview. Kawagley emphasized that the system imposed a compulsory school attendance law that forced families to stay in one location during the school year which conflicted with the traditional Yupiit lifeway of responding to the cyclical animal migrations and timing of the tundra harvests needed to maintain their subsistence lifestyle. This Eurocentric education system taught English but not the Native languages. The teachers were not Yupiit and had no understanding of Yupiit culture. The educational system emphasized a philosophy that viewed the dominant culture as superior and the traditional Yupiit cultural values as inferior (Kawagley, 2010).

From the early 1800s, Alaskan children had been primarily educated in their local communities by Russian missionaries. Beginning in the 1920s, Yupiit children were separated from their communities and their families—often for years at a time—to attend boarding schools operated by the Federal Bureau of Indian Affairs in other Alaskan communities or even in other states (Kawagley, 2010) where the teaching emphasized assimilation into the dominant (White) culture. Native students were punished for speaking Yupiit or practicing traditional Yupiit traditions. Embler (2012) learned that when children returned home after being away for several years, they felt like a strangers among their people. Although they had learned the required reading, writing, and arithmetic at the boarding school, they had not learned how to perform the daily tasks of the traditional subsistence lifeway.

Legal attempts to reorganize the educational system regarding Alaska Natives (especially the issues of local control and access) included the Indian Reorganization Act of 1936; the Johnson-O'Malley Act of 1952; the Indian Education Act of 1972; the establishment of Alaska State Operated Schools in 1975; the Indian Self Determination and Educational Assistance Act of 1975; and the Establishment of Rural Educational Attendance Areas in 1975 (Barnhardt, 2001). Nevertheless, more than 204 Alaska Native students were sent to the boarding school in Chilocco, Oklahoma in 1976 because the boarding schools in Alaska and Oregon were already full and the other boarding schools in New Mexico, Colorado, and Kansas could not accept them (M. T. Weiss, personal communication, June 15, 2015).

Education for Alaska Natives continued to evolve. At the time of this study, Alaska Native students accounted for approximately 23% of students in grades 7 through 12 throughout the Alaska public school system (Alaska Department of Education and Early Development, 2010). Although the Native student dropout rate had decreased by approximately 3% during the 12-year period between 2001 and 2013 (Alaska Department of Education and Early Development, 2010), it nevertheless remained high (6.2%)—twice that of Caucasian students (3.0%)—in 2013.

Nursing Education

The School of Nursing at the University of Alaska-Anchorage (UAA) had been mandated to provide nursing education for the entire state of Alaska including Bethel and other remote areas. The rural communities differed from urban communities in two distinct ways: Each rural community had access to limited resources and each had its own unique cultural values. However, technology and the Internet had improved rural access to university-level educational services. The UAA used video conferences in combination with on-site local clinical experiences to provide nursing education in these rural Alaskan areas that was augmented by short-term intensive clinical experiences in the large urban centers of Anchorage and Fairbanks.

Yupiit students in the Bethel nursing program were frequently confronted with the differences between Yupiit and Western European cultures and lifestyles. Being successful in any nursing program involves reading, testing, individual achievement, active participation, and competition. The Yupiit culture has the tradition of a *collective* worldview. Yupiit students often reported that their reason for going to nursing school was to help their communities. The students valued being part of and contributing to the group over individual achievement and competition. Yupiit people valued observation as the main way of learning and stressed the importance of elders' wisdom. Yupiit students who were singled out for recognition invariably responded with expressions of embarrassment. For example, when an instructor asked a question during one of the video conference classes, the Yupiit students cast their eyes down and did not respond even though they all knew the answer. Meanwhile, non-Yupiit students from other teleconference class sites were competing to respond. When encouraged to answer questions, one Yupiit student respectfully shared that in her culture "…respect is earned by the observation of others [and in] the wisdom of one's actions, not [by] who speaks first, loudest, or longest." Volunteering to answer questions could be perceived as "bragging" or "being full of oneself." Humility was valued in the Yupiit culture but was contrary to the dominant Western cultural value of individual recognition. Furthermore, the Yupiit believed people should not take themselves too seriously. Some Yupiit have described this attribute as a sense of "lightness."

In order to be successful Yupiit people, these nursing students were expected to "…put themselves aside wherever they attend college." The Yupiit students must learn to balance the two cultures by "…hav[ing] one foot planted in each world." Yupiit students were extremely observant and easily discerned the nuances of non-verbal communication. During clinical skill demonstrations, Yupiit students became quite focused while they silently observed; they seldom asked questions but rarely need demonstrations repeated. After observing a demonstration, they usually could perform the skill and convey their understanding of the underlying concepts without need for additional instruction or further clarification. However, in order to succeed in the Western world of the university, these students needed to also learn to participate by reading and answering questions in class.

In many Yupiit homes, English was spoken as a second language. Although students were taught in English at school—some only after the third grade—most communicated in Yupiit at home and in their communities. Therefore, while Yupiit students could read and enunciate the words in their nursing textbooks, they often had limited comprehension of their meanings. Discussing textbook content in study groups has been an effective way of helping these students learn.

Yupiit students were closely connected to their families and communities. When introducing themselves, they stated to whom they were related. They did not share their job titles, interests, or plans as was commonly done in the dominant culture. The Yupiit students often struggled with separation from their families during the three-week intensive clinical session in Anchorage. For example, halfway through the first semester, one student who had left her village to attend school in Bethel planned to drop out because she missed her family so much. Another Yupiit woman who became aware of the situation helped the student to find an apartment for her family to occupy in Bethel. Having her family nearby enabled this student to complete the program.

Leaving Bethel for a nursing education in Anchorage or "outside" (outside of Alaska) was not possible for most Yupiit students. Cost, separation from family and community, and separation from the Yupiit lifestyle were major barriers. Many nursing students in the Yukon-Kuskokwim region, like much of rural Alaska, lived below the poverty level. Although their subsistence lifestyle made it possible for people to feed themselves without the benefit of cash, expenses such as tuition, books, and travel for clinical experiences made going to nursing school difficult. Two student trips outside of Bethel cost approximately $4,000—a significant part of a family's yearly income. Fortunately, the Yupiit community provided support for the students. The researcher (as faculty) was approached by community members with a contribution of nearly $5,000 to help defer education costs for Yupiit students. The hospital helped defray the cost of airline tickets and related transportation expenses so each student could travel to Anchorage for their clinical intensive experience. Employers worked closely with the students to accommodate their clinical schedules so they could continue to work as well.

A subsistence lifestyle is unpredictable and required constant work. Leaving the family to obtain an education meant there was one less person to help gather food. Some Yupiit nursing students shared that their parents encouraged them to become nurses while their grandparents discouraged them because going to school was perceived as a burden for the rest of the family. Several of the adolescent nursing students were single mothers who were embraced and supported by their nuclear and extended families without judgment. These students were able to pursue an education while their grandmothers and other relatives provided free childcare.

As the Yupiit continued to have more contact with Western lifeways, there was increasing motivation for them to seek an education. The temporary, short-term nurses working in Alaska (but whose permanent homes were elsewhere) were supportive of the Yupiit nursing students. They voiced their recognition of the need for a local nursing workforce and therefore provided consistent encouragement and mentorship to the Yupiit nursing students.

■ THREE MODES OF CULTURE CARE DECISIONS AND ACTIONS

Culture Care Theory research discoveries guide nursing practice using the three modes of nursing decisions and actions; they are *culture care preservation and/or maintenance*; *culture care accommodation and/or negotiation*; and *culture care repatterning and/or restructuring* (Leininger, 2006). The following culture-specific modes were abstracted from the Yupiit meanings, expressions, patterns, and practices described by the study informants to assist nurses and others in developing decisions and formulating actions to support the Yupiit people's health and wellbeing.

Culture Care Preservation and/or Maintenance

Culture care preservation and/or maintenance refers to those *supportive care decisions and actions that nurses and others can take to help Yupiit Alaskan Natives retain their beneficial cultural beliefs, values, and traditional lifeways, or face death* (Leininger, 2006). The Yupiit informants from the ethnonursing study emphasized that *community* and *family* were inseparable and that each had specific end-of-life care responsibilities. The end-of-life care practices that were regarded as important to be preserved or maintained were those that included the *community as family* perspective and acknowledged that *community has equal value to family* among the Yupiit. To preserve and maintain optimal Yupiit family and community involvement, the practices of *honoring* and *respecting* intergenerational connectedness extended beyond immediate and extended family members to include other community members.

Integrating the following four key recommendations into the education system could also help to preserve and maintain Alaska Native culture and traditional lifeways:

- Alaska Native children need an integrated education that includes the skills and values of both Alaska Native and dominant cultures.
- Education must involve the community and address the economic and societal issues of rural living, poverty, and inequality so that Native students can function with a clear understanding of both dominant culture and traditional heritage.

- Teachers and administrators need to respect, understand, and be able to integrate Native ways of learning.
- Alaska Native lifeways and values need to be fully integrated into school policy and decision-making (Kawagley, 2010).

Culture Care Accommodation and/or Negotiation

This mode refers to *decisions and actions that help professional caregivers negotiate for and accommodate Yupiit values and preferred care practices* (Leininger, 2006). To support the Yupiit cultural value that care is *uptete* (to get ready to go), nurses needed to accommodate and/or negotiate the integration of traditional end-of-life preparations, rituals, foods, and generic/folk care practices with professional care practices. Hosting large gatherings and serving traditional foods were important end-of-life traditions in the Yupiit culture (Embler, 2012). As long as consuming traditional foods is not contraindicated by the person's illness, condition, medications, or functional status, this practice should be accommodated. The aftercare ritual of *laying out* was especially important when death occurred away from the home and community. The laying out period after death provided time for the Yupiit to have loved ones come by and pay their respects. In the home and community contexts, this period could last days or weeks. Key and general informants also acknowledged the importance of using a traditional Yupiit healer during end-of-life care so that they could "…cure the soul" (Embler, 2012).

Culture Care Repatterning and/or Restructuring

This mode refers to *professional actions that help people "reorder, change, modify, or restructure lifeways for better health care patterns, practices, or outcomes"* (Leininger, 2006, p. 8). In this context, nurses were asked to modify actions that hindered the delivery of culturally meaningful care for Yupiit at end-of-life. Nurses often unconsciously carried personal emotions into the care setting that were perceived as culturally intrusive to the Yupiit during end-of-life care. In the Yupiit culture, *intention* was viewed as being as powerful as *action*.

The nurse-patient relationship was greatly affected by a nurse who was preoccupied and therefore not fully present with the Yupiit patient. Nurses need to be active in the development of hospital-based as well as community-based end-of-life care services that are culturally congruent. Nurses are encouraged to be fully present when providing end of life care. Finally, each nurse needs to be an active participant in social structure and policy measures to restructure professional end-of-life care so that it honors the preferences of the Yupiit Eskimos to remain in their home/community settings cared for by family and community. In this mode, the focus of nursing decisions and actions are to recognize, repattern, and restructure patterns of harmful professional care behaviors during Yupiit end-of-life and to restructure that professional end-of-life care so it honors the Yupiit desire to be in the home/community setting and cared for by family and community members.

SUMMARY

The Yupiit people lived in a sub-Arctic environment. Their worldview provided many lessons others can use to live in harmony with the environment. Sherry (2004) noted that the Alaska Native health system provided a model for sustainability and called for research about and with the Alaskan Natives to improve their health. The acute care services available in Alaska have already overcome major transportation, weather, and provider resource obstacles. The community healthcare needs for persons living in bush Alaska have been creatively addressed using community health aides, nurse practitioners, physician assistants, and telemedicine technologies.

DeCourtney, Jones, Merriman, Heavener, and Branch (2003) described the obstacles to successful palliative care programs for bush peoples. The Yupiit people preferred to remain in their community for health care, education, or end-of-life because they recognized the importance of strong people-to-people bonds. These Alaskan Native peoples had constrained educational, healthcare, and socioeconomic choices due to the limited availability of and access to assistive services. However, more work is needed to discover innovative ways to address logistic and geographic obstacles, and the lack of providers, that consistently plague the delivery of culturally congruent end-of-life care for rural/remote dwelling peoples. The findings from Embler's (2012) ethnonursing research study with the Yupiit has added substantively to the body of transcultural nursing knowledge related to end-of-life care for diverse cultural groups.

DEDICATION

This chapter is dedicated to Bing Santamour, a Yupiit healer and friend, who always teaches others to celebrate their time on earth.

ACKNOWLEDGEMENTS

We wish to acknowledge Yupiit community members Evelyn Pensgard, Elizabeth Lee, and Mary Pete for reviewing this chapter in regard to its cultural sensitivity. The Theory of Culture Care Diversity and Universality and the Ethnonursing Research Method were central in helping us to move from being strangers to trusted friends with the Yupiit people. We are especially grateful to the community of Bethel, the surrounding villages, and the gatekeepers, informants, and friends who shared their stories.

DISCUSSION QUESTIONS

1. Historically, the imposition of Eurocentric education on the Yupiit people was brought about by missionaries and the federal government as it governed over the Alaska territory. Cultural language, traditional ceremonies, and subsistence practices were lost to subsequent generations as families were separated when children were sent to boarding schools. How do you think these encounters affected their culture? What role has history played in the formation of Yupiit culture?
2. Discuss the various cultural roles of family members, especially parents and elders, for teaching children their Yupiit culture and compare them to your own culture. Compare them to another culture with which you have personal or professional experience.

REFERENCES

Alaska Department of Education and Early Development. (2010). *Statistics and Reports*. Retrieved from http://www.eed.state.ak.us/stats/

Alaska Department of Health and Social Services, Division of Public Health. (2012). *Hospital Reports*. Retrieved from http://dhss.alaska.gov/dph/VitalStats/Pages/data_quality/hospital_report.aspx

Barnhardt, C. (2001). A history of schooling for Alaska native people. *Journal of American Indian Education*, *20*(1), 1-30.

Baydala, A., Hampton, M., Kinunwa, L., Kinunwa, G., & Kinunwa, L., Sr. (2006). Death, dying, grieving, and end of life care: Understanding personal meanings of Aboriginal friends. *The Humanistic Psychologist, 34*(2), 159-176. doi: 10.1207/s15473333thp3402_4

Barker, J. H. (2010). Introduction. In J. H. Barker, A. Fienup-Riordan, and T. A. John (Eds.), *Yupiit yuraryarait: Yupiit Eskimo ways of dancing.* Fairbanks, AK: University of Alaska Press.

Bonura, D., Fender, M., Roesler, M., & Pacquiao, D. F. (2001). Culturally congruent end-of-life care for Jewish patients and their families. *Journal of Transcultural Nursing, 12*(3), 211-220.

Burch, E. S. (1988). *The Eskimos.* Norman, OK: University of Oklahoma Press.

DeCourtney, C. A., Jones, K., Merriman, M. P., Heavener, N., & Branch, P. K. (2003). Establishing a culturally sensitive palliative care program in rural Alaska Native American communities. *Journal of Palliative Medicine, 6*(3), 501-510. doi.org/10.1089/109662103322144871

Embler, P. J. (2012). *End-of-life culture care expressions, meanings, patterns, and practices among Yupiit Eskimo.* (Unpublished Doctoral Dissertation). University of Tennessee, Knoxville.

Embler, P. J., Mixer, S. J., & Gunther, M. (2015). End-of-life culture care practices among the Yup'ik Eskimo. *Online Journal of Cultural Competence in Nursing and Healthcare, 5*(1), 36-49. doi: 10.9730/ojccnh.org/v5n1a3

Fienup-Riordan, A. (1990). *Eskimo essays.* New Brunswick, NY: Rutgers University Press.

Fienup-Riordan, A. (2005). *Wise words of the Yupiit Eskimo people: We talk because we love you.* Lincoln, NE: University of Nebraska Press.

Fienup-Riordan, A. (2007). *Yuungnaqpiallerput: The way we genuinely live.* Seattle, WA: University of Washington Press.

Fortuine, R. (2005). *Must we all die?: Alaska's enduring struggle with tuberculosis.* Fairbanks, AK: University of Alaska Press.

Gelfand, D. E., Balcazar, H., Parzuchowski, J., & Lenox, S. (2001). Mexicans and care for the terminally ill: Family, hospice, and the church. *American Journal of Hospice and Palliative Care, 18*(6), 391-396.

John, P. (2000). Elders spoke and young people listened. In A. Fienup-Riordan (Ed.), *Wise words of the Yup'ik Eskimo people: We talk because we love you.* Lincoln, NE: University of Nebraska Press.

Kaufman, S. R., & Morgan, L. M. (2005). The anthropology of the beginnings and ends of life. *Annual Review of Anthropology, 34*, 317-314.

Kawagley, A. O. (2006). *A Yupiaq worldview: A pathway to ecology and spirit.* Long Grove, IL: Waveland.

Kawagley, A. O. (2010). *Alaska Native education: Views from within.* Fairbanks, AK: Alaska Native Knowledge Network Cross-Cultural Studies.

Leininger, M. M. (2002). Culture care assessments for congruent competency. In M. M. Leininger and M. R. McFarland (Eds.), *Transcultural nursing: Concepts, theories, research & practice* (3rd ed., pp. 117-145). New York, NY: McGraw-Hill.

Leininger, M. M. (2006). Culture care diversity and universality theory and evolution of the ethnonursing method. In M. M. Leininger and M. R. McFarland (Eds.), *Culture care diversity and universality: A worldwide theory of nursing* (2nd ed., pp. 1-39). Sudbury, MA: Jones and Bartlett.

Napoleon, H. (1996). *Yuuyaraq: The way of the human being.* Chicago, IL: University of Chicago Press.

Sherry, P. (2004). Health care delivery for Alaska Natives: A brief overview. *National Journal of Circumpolar Health, 63*(0, Suppl. 2), 54-62. doi: 10.3402/ijch.v63i0.17786

U. S. Department of Commerce, Economics and Statistics Administration, Census Bureau. (2012). State and County QuickFacts: Bethel (city), Alaska. Retrieved from http://quickfacts.census.gov/qfd/states/02/0206520.html

University of Alaska-Fairbanks. (n. d.). *Federal Indian law for Alaska tribes: TM112 course materials.* Retrieved from http://tm112.community.uaf.edu/

Understanding the Culture Care Needs of Appalachian Mothers Experiencing Homelessness

Rebecca C. Lee

> *We aren't homeless. We just don't have a house to put our home into. – Appalachian mother living in a family shelter*

■ INTRODUCTION

Family homelessness is an urgent public health issue. It is estimated that more than 600,000 American families, including more than 2.5 million children, will experience homelessness in any given year (National Center on Family Homelessness [NCFH], 2014). This historic high represents one in every 30 children living in the United States. From 2012 to 2013, child homelessness increased in 31 states and the District of Columbia representing an 8% increase nationally (U.S. Department of Housing and Urban Development [HUD], 2014). It is important to note that these numbers do not include the additional families precariously housed and living in doubled-up situations or in substandard housing.

Within many metropolitan areas of the United States, Appalachian families comprise one unique cultural group experiencing poverty and the extreme condition of homelessness. According to Leininger's Theory of Culture Care Diversity and Universality (also known as the Culture Care Theory or CCT), care is embedded in the worldview and social structure factors of cultural groups (McFarland & Wehbe-Alamah, 2015). The provision of culturally congruent nursing care, which supports the health and wellbeing

of Appalachian families experiencing homelessness, must be built upon an understanding of their unique experiences, values, beliefs, meanings, and practices within their cultural context. Based on a review of the literature; the author's research in the area of homelessness (Lee, 2012); her experience as a public health clinical nurse specialist working with homeless individuals, families, providers, and social service agencies; and first-person knowledge of Appalachian culture, this chapter provides the reader with holding knowledge regarding the culture care needs of urban Appalachian families experiencing homelessness in the Midwestern United States.

■ BACKGROUND ON FAMILY HOMELESSNESS

Among industrialized nations, the United States has the largest number of homeless women and children (NCFH, 2014). Families with children are now the fastest growing segment of the homeless population, accounting for 40% of the nation's homeless (HUD, 2014). Seventy-one percent of these families are headed by a single mother with two or more children under the age of six (NCFH, 2014; National Coalition for the Homeless, 2014). Many have lost jobs, become injured or ill, or are fleeing domestic violence and are on the edge of homelessness for several weeks or months prior to actually losing their housing (NCFH, 2014). These women are left alone to provide for the physical and emotional needs of their children while facing the daily challenges of the lifeways associated with homelessness.

There are several pathways to homelessness, including the context within which individuals and families live and the complex interactions that occur between personal, social, economic, and service system resources that impact wellbeing and housing security (Nooe & Patterson, 2010). Other factors contributing to the increase in family homelessness include scarcity of affordable housing, economic restructuring, poverty, and reductions in governmental financial assistance. The availability of housing for low-income persons has been greatly reduced through the gradual process of removing affordable housing units from circulation due to gentrification and urban renewal. As housing niches for the poor have been lost, those who were most vulnerable—including urban-dwelling minorities—have suffered greater losses. The availability of rental units affordable by low-income renters has consistently declined over recent decades (NCFH, 2014).

Economic restructuring to a low-wage, service economy has also contributed to the rise in family homelessness. Declining wages have put housing out of reach for many workers. In addition to the rising unemployment rates, current employment options offer low wages, less job security, and few if any benefits such as health care, leaving many families lacking the monetary resources necessary to secure and maintain housing (NCFH, 2014). According to the National Low Income Housing Coalition's 2014 figures, it takes approximately 2.6 full-time minimum wage jobs to afford a two bedroom apartment at the fair market housing rate. Homelessness and poverty are inextricably linked. Poor people are frequently unable to pay for housing, food, childcare, health care, and education. In 2013, 45.3 million individuals in this country lived in poverty. Furthermore, the 2013 poverty rate for children younger than 18 years was 19.9%—the highest rate for any age group (U.S. Department of Commerce, 2014).

Homelessness is a life experience that has a profound effect on the health and wellbeing of each member of a family. Research studies have demonstrated the influence of homelessness on the physical and mental health of all family members. Children who are homeless get sick twice as often as other children and have higher rates of asthma and ear infections. In addition, these children are twice as likely to experience hunger and four times as likely to have developmental delays (Herbers, Cutuli, Monn, Narayan, & Masten, 2014; NCFH, 2011; Park, Fertig, & Allison, 2011). Children who are homeless also experience more mental health problems such as anxiety, depression, and withdrawal. Nearly one in three children who are homeless have at least one major mental health disorder that interferes with daily activities compared to nearly one in five school-aged children who are not homeless (NCFH, 2014).

Mental health is a key component in a child's healthy development (Stagman & Cooper, 2010). Homeless children experience significantly more stress than housed children (NCFH, 2014). Over two-thirds of surveyed homeless mothers report that their children have experienced an *at-risk* number of stressful events during the last three months, including parents divorcing or permanently separating, changing schools, witnessing violence, and being hospitalized. Exposure to trauma and stress, coupled with the experience of homelessness, is strongly associated with emotional problems seen in these vulnerable children, both during the period in which they are homeless, and in the years following (Committee on Psychosocial Aspects of Child and Family Health, et al., 2012; NCFH, 2014).

Mothers suffer the ill effects of homelessness and poverty as well. Mothers who are homeless report increased major depressive symptoms as well as poorer physical health including chronic health conditions such as asthma, anemia, and ulcers (Hayes, Zonneville, & Bassuk, 2013). Mothers experiencing homelessness also report lifetime exposure to many of the same stressful events to which their children are exposed. These include their own childhood exposure to violence, recent divorce or separation from their spouse, and witnessing or being the adult survivor of violence (Hayes, et al., 2013). Some researchers have reported that up to 92% of homeless women have experienced severe physical and/or sexual assault at some point in their lives (Hayes et al., 2013). In addition, researchers working with homeless mothers find that one-third of the women surveyed reported having made at least one suicide attempt (Hayes, et al., 2013).

The lives of mothers and children experiencing homelessness often follow a tumultuous trajectory after loss of housing, resulting in families living "doubled-up" with extended family and friends, living on the streets, or living in abandoned cars or buildings (NCFH, 2011). Therefore, entry into a shelter can represent a stabilizing event in this cascade of uncertainty. However, despite this stabilization, congregate living within a shelter can also be a challenge and source of additional multiple stressors (Lee, 2012). Shared living space, congregate dining, and interaction with so many strangers, coupled with a lack of privacy, often create a sense of chaos and despair that can lead many mothers to feel overwhelmed. Within the "safe and secure" walls of the shelter, these women finally find themselves facing the realization of all they have lost during the process of becoming homeless–their own home, freedom, peace, and control over their lives and those of their children (Lee, 2012).

Despite the availability of previously cited descriptive and epidemiological studies of the effects of homelessness on mothers and children experiencing homelessness, a review of the literature revealed no articles describing the experience of family homelessness within a cultural framework prior to the author's own research. Such knowledge is vital to better address the health and wellbeing needs of Appalachian mothers struggling to survive and care for their children within the sociocultural context of homelessness. Thus the information presented in this chapter adds to the body of nursing knowledge; supports the assumptive premises of the theory; provides support for existing culturally congruent care practices; leads to the development of additional culturally relevant services; and enhances cultural competence among healthcare providers caring for homeless families.

■ THEORY AND RESEARCH METHOD TO DISCOVER CULTURE CARE FOR HOMELESS APPALACHIAN FAMILIES

Leininger's Theory of Culture Care Diversity and Universality (McFarland & Wehbe-Alamah, 2015) provides a theoretical framework within which to study holistic cultural lifeways to understand the worldview

of individuals and groups of people about health and care from within their cultural context. The author used Leininger's Ethnonursing Research Method to discover in-depth knowledge of the culture care meanings, experiences, and lifeways of Appalachian mothers who were caring for their children while living in an urban homeless shelter located within a recognized Appalachian community.

Leininger's (1991) Observation-Participation-Reflection Enabler (OPR) and the Stranger-to-Trusted Friend Enabler were used together to gain entry into the world of the Appalachian mothers. The Sunrise Enabler served as an overarching cognitive map for discovering meanings, patterns, and practices of care for these families embedded within the dimensions of ethnohistory, worldview, and social structure factors. Through observation, participant observation, and in-depth interviews, a group of 12 African-American and European-American Appalachian mothers shared with the author their first-person experiences of homelessness as well as the meaning of *home*. Reflections from these findings, along with the three modes of culture care decisions and actions, and an intensive review of the literature, serve as the basis for this chapter.

■ ETHNOHISTORICAL DIMENSIONS

The geographical area of the United States defined as Appalachia comprises a 205,000 square-mile region that extends from southern New York State to Mississippi (Appalachian Regional Commission [ARC], 2015). This region consists of 420 counties spread across all of West Virginia and parts of 12 other states: Alabama, Georgia, Kentucky, Maryland, Mississippi, New York, North Carolina, Ohio, Pennsylvania, South Carolina, Tennessee, and Virginia. Forty-two percent of the region's population is rural compared with 20% of the national population.

An outward migration away from the Appalachian region began in the last decade of the 19th century as Appalachian residents left the area in search of economic opportunities not found in the region (Obermiller, 1996). This migration, referred to as the *Great Migration*, spread Appalachians and their culture to many parts of the country including many of the cities of the Midwestern United States.

Both African-American and European-American Appalachians took part in the outward migration from Appalachia to urban centers in the North. In the 19th century, growing numbers of individuals living in Kentucky journeyed to work at the Champion Paper Company in Hamilton, Ohio (Obermiller, 1996). This was followed by waves of families who obtained seasonal employment harvesting vegetables in the fields of Indiana and Ohio. During this time, the rubber industry of Northeastern Ohio also attracted many migrants who filled the tire factories of Akron (Obermiller, 1996). The United States immigration restrictions following World War I led to a demand for a domestic labor force that brought Appalachians to cities such as Detroit, which ran bus lines from the county seats in eastern Kentucky directly to their factory gates (Obermiller, 1996). Similarly, following World War II, economic expansion and the demand for workers in industrial settings also sent millions of mountaineers into cities across the United States.

Throughout the Appalachian diaspora, much of its culture has remained relatively unchanged. Possessed with strong work ethic and armed with cultural values such as self-sufficiency, independence, and faith in God, Appalachians overcame the urban social, cultural, and economic barriers they encountered; passed down traditional Appalachian values to their children; and demonstrated that Appalachians are a people "… joined not by geography, or economics, but by a shared history" (Obermiller, 1996, p. 9).

■ WORLDVIEW OF APPALACHIAN CULTURE

Most cultures have a distinct way of looking out upon the surrounding world and understanding their place in that world. Leininger (1991) defined worldview as "…the way people tend to look out on the world or their universe to form a picture or a value stance about their life or world around them" (p. 47). Leininger further identified that cultural care values, beliefs, and practices are "…influenced by and tend to be embedded in the worldview" (p. 45).

Appalachians have forged a worldview influenced by geographical isolation as well as diverse backgrounds and values, including faith in God; self-reliance; and love of freedom, family, and independence. Experiences with those from outside the region who came

to pillage natural resources such as coal and timber, have left Appalachians—originally a very accepting people—more cautious with regard to those seen as outsiders (Blethen, 2004).

■ SOCIAL STRUCTURE DIMENSIONS OF APPALACHIAN CULTURE

Social structure factors were identified by Leininger (1991) as a rich and essential source of data to help nurses understand individuals for whom they provide care. In the Theory of Culture Care Diversity and Universality, Leininger (1991) conceptualized culturally congruent nursing care decisions and actions as being guided by the individual or group's social structure factors, including but not limited to cultural values, beliefs, and lifeways. An assumptive premise identified as an integral part of her Culture Care Theory is that culture care values, beliefs, and practices are influenced by and embedded in the worldview, social structure factors (e.g., religion, philosophy of life, kinship, politics, economics, education, technology, and cultural values) and the ethnohistorical and environmental contexts (McFarland & Wehbe-Alamah, 2015, p. 8).

Religious and Philosophical Factors

Religion is a strong force that shaped the early development of the Appalachian region and bound dispersed settlers together. Throughout this mountainous region, religious beliefs led to the formation of small sectarian groups rather than the large denominations found in other parts of the country (Blethan, 2004). Founded on the belief that salvation awaits all who seek the Lord, many Appalachians joined the more optimistic Methodist and Free-Will Baptist churches. Members depended on the grace of God to help them through a hard world and deliver them unto salvation in the end (Jones, 1994).

Jones (1994) notes that because Appalachian religious structures did not resemble more mainstream ideas of religiosity, home mission boards of mainline denominations outside the region usually looked upon Appalachians as unsaved masses awaiting redemption. The Appalachian people resented these implications. Life in the mountains did not allow for optimism. Hard work did not always bring a sure reward, so their religion supported a more fatalistic view. "The point is to get religion–get saved–and try to keep the faith and endure, hoping for a sure reward in the hereafter" (Jones, 1994, p. 46).

Faith in God transcends the concept of religiosity and permeates daily actions for many Appalachians. This faith and spirituality serves as a foundation for many societal values and perspectives. Spirituality for Appalachians encompasses a belief that God exists and participates in the daily lives of believers and that stronger connections to God occur in times of need (Diddle & Denham, 2011).

For Appalachian mothers living in the homeless shelter, spirituality provided the framework through which each mother viewed and derived meaning from the experience of homelessness (Lee, 2012). Rather than framing this event as a punishment, each mother instead spoke of this time in her life as being an important lesson from God to her, his child—an experience meant to teach her an important lesson that would leave her better for having lived it (Lee, 2012). Another unique facet of Appalachian culture— intergenerational transmission of knowledge—was also evident within this spiritual framework. Not only did every mother speak of God the Father teaching her (as His child) a lesson, but she also stated that by facing this challenge with dignity and hope, she was teaching her own children a valuable life lesson (Lee, 2012).

Spirituality also served as a source of strength and hope for Appalachian mothers experiencing home-lessness (Lee, 2012). Remaining strong during challenging lifeways and demonstrating resilience are two other cultural characteristics associated with Appalachian women in particular. Mothers shared stories of strong Appalachian women in their own lives who influenced their caring: Mothers, grandmothers, aunts, and sisters (Lee, 2012).

Kinship and Social Factors

Appalachians (Refer to Figure 23.1) place a strong value on family and kinship ties. This value influences many areas of their life. The influence of kinship can be traced back to the time of the early settlers. African American culture has always placed strong emphasis on extended *kinship patterns* while European immigrants to Appalachia brought with them a strong history of *clan ties* (Blethen, 2004).

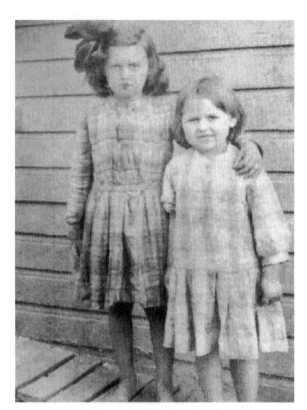

FIGURE 23.1 • Two Appalachian girls in Wytheville, VA in 1909. © Rebecca Lee (2015).

Appalachian people are family-centered. "Mountain people usually feel an obligation to family members and are more truly themselves when within the family circle" (Jones, 1994, p. 75). Appalachians eschew individualistic values and personal gain over the needs of their family. Appalachian families support each other during times of sickness, death, or a disaster, and these loyalties take precedence over all other obligations. When Appalachians migrated to northern industries in search of work, their ties to family and place led them to return home whenever possible (Refer to Figure 23.2).

This valuing of relationships extends beyond kin to other people with whom Appalachians come in contact. Appalachians relate to others "…on a personal basis rather than on how people dress or the credentials or accomplishments they claim" (Jones, 1994, p. 87). They tend to go to great lengths to extend respect to other persons and to keep from offending them. This cultural value of personalism speaks to the importance of getting along with one another rather than pushing

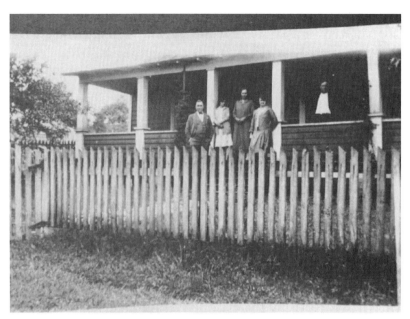

FIGURE 23.2 • Appalachian homeplace, Wytheville, VA. © Rebecca Lee (2015).

one's own views. Therefore, Appalachians tend to be reluctant to confront and alienate someone if it can be avoided. While respecting the rights of other people to be themselves, Appalachians expect those same rights to be afforded to them (Jones, 1994).

Kinship and social factors greatly influence Appalachian family homelessness. A lack of supportive relationships is one risk factor contributing to a family becoming homeless. Due to geographic boundaries, interpersonal conflict, or economic limitations, some Appalachian families are not able to provide needed support. Because of the expectation of familial care, this lack of support during a time of crisis can be even more painful for Appalachian mothers (Lee, 2012). Once mothers enter the shelter, many seek to create a sense of family and community with other people living there to meet this cultural care need for human connectedness (Lee, 2012).

Cultural Values, Beliefs, and Lifeways

According to Jones (1994), the values held in esteem by Appalachian people are spirituality, independence, self-reliance, pride, neighborliness, familism, personalism, humility and modesty, love of place, patriotism, sense of beauty, and humor. Many of these cultural values can be seen embedded in relationships—with God, self, others, and place. Forged from the strong themes of kin and clan found within the African-American and European-American cultures of early settlers and the geography of the region, Appalachians learned to value the importance of relationships from those who came before (Jones, 1994).

Pride, independence, and self-reliance are also characteristics valued in Appalachian culture. Appalachians are inclined to try to do things for themselves, resisting asking others for help. "Pride is mostly a feeling of not wanting to be beholding to other people … The value of independence and self-reliance, and our pride, is often stronger than desire or need" (Jones, 1994, p. 68).

While Appalachians take great pride in self-reliance, they also place great value on neighborliness— welcoming, assisting, and supporting others in need (Jones, 1994). This value was seen as vitally important to facilitate survival during the migration experiences of Appalachians moving from the region to urban communities in other parts of the country (Helton & Keller, 2010). Neighborliness was seen as creating a sense of community based on respect and a deep sense of caring for one another (Helton & Keller, 2010). Similarly, dominant cultural values among Appalachian mothers living in a family shelter were observed to include pride, independence, self-reliance, spirituality, familism,—and personalism (Lee, 2012).

For some Appalachian mothers, entering the shelter required them to "swallow their pride" (Lee, 2012). This event was seen as shameful, resulting in a lack of independence and inability to be self-reliant. These mothers were often especially distraught during the intake process to the program (Lee, 2012). However, for another group of Appalachian mothers, entry into the shelter was seen as a source of pride and a demonstration of their independence from the support of family and friends, and was viewed as an act of self-reliance (Lee, 2012). These mothers saw the homeless shelters as a necessary community resource in times of need as well as an opportunity to connect with programs designed to support their return to self-sufficiency. During intake, these mothers were much more at ease with themselves and their decision (Lee, 2012).

The values of spirituality, familism, and personalism were evident in Appalachian mothers' sustaining connections (Lee, 2012). The dominant connection that all mothers spoke about was their connection to a loving God as previously discussed. Beyond this all-important relationship with God, Appalachian mothers struggled to sustain relationships with self and others including their children, other families living in the shelter, shelter staff, and family and friends outside of the shelter (Lee, 2012).

Political and Legal Factors

Early settlers to the Appalachian region came to America seeking changes in their lives for economic and political reasons such as relief from heavy taxation and punitive inheritance laws (Blethen, 2004). Therefore, these individuals were less likely to become involved in political activities other than at the family and sometimes community levels.

Access to land was the primary means to the formation of social stratification in preindustrial Appalachia (Blethen, 2004). Latecomers to the region and the poor, frequently found the more desirable land already taken and therefore moved on to the remaining land located higher in the mountains (Blethen, 2004). Owning land gave Appalachians power and this power was passed down to their children through gifts or inheritances of land. Those Appalachians who did not own their own land had less incentive to remain in the area. Therefore, during periods of outmigration from the region, those individuals lacking access to land—and thereby, political power—often chose to leave (Obermiller, 1996).

Early Appalachian settlers found that having a place to call one's own equated with power. Lacking such a place to "be" in the world left some Appalachian families feeling especially vulnerable and lacking a voice (Lee, 2012). For Appalachian mothers living in a shelter for the homeless, lack of power and societal marginalization were an all too familiar source of stress (Lee, 2012).

Economic Factors

The early economy of Appalachia between the Revolutionary War and the Civil War was based on a shared core of skills—farming, herding, and hunting—held by the three main groups settling the area: Native Americans, Africans, and Europeans. Native Americans had long-established patterns of sustainable agriculture. Africans and Europeans adopted skills such as slashing and burning to fertilize fields and grow crops of corn, beans, squash, and tobacco; grains such as wheat, rye, barley, oats, and millet; and watermelons, okra, peas, peanuts, and yams, as well as medicinal herbs (Blethen, 2004). Europeans introduced the herding of cattle, sheep, and hogs to the Appalachian region, a new tradition for Native Americans, who in turn shared with both the Europeans and Africans skills needed to dress, track, and hunt wild game (Blethen, 2004). A distinct mountain culture based on self-sufficiency and independence flourished.

Salt mines and iron forges were among the first industries to develop in the mountains of Appalachia (Blethen, 2004). Later the coal industry was developed in central section of the region (Blethen, 2004). With the arrival of the railroad in the 1850s, Appalachia became connected to eastern factories and outside industrialists eager to capitalize on the natural resources of the area—coal and timber (Eller, 2004). Regional speculators, similarly eager to profit, purchased land and mineral rights from local residents for small amounts of money and then sold them to outside corporations at a higher price (Eller, 2004). With economic interests of the area controlled by outside investors, the Appalachian people had little power over their own resources. Discrimination in awarding jobs was also commonly practiced, with African Americans and newly arriving immigrants being assigned the harder, more dangerous tasks. Thus, Appalachian resources, both environmental and human, were seen as the means by which to advance the financial wellbeing of outside interests who did not invest in nor respect the area and its residents.

In the 1960s, President Kennedy and President Johnson spearheaded efforts to battle persistent poverty in the nation, focusing attention on the Appalachian region, which at that time had an overall poverty rate of 31% (ARC, 2015). In his first State of the Union address in January 1964, President Johnson brought the attention of the rest of the country to the Appalachian region and people when he declared a "War on Poverty" (Eller, 2004). While this effort resulted in some funding for Appalachian infrastructure and those in need, it also resulted in an influx of missionaries, teachers, welfare workers, and writers into the region, all determined to save the people of this part of the country who were described by the President as being "...located in America, but not a part of America" (Obermiller, 1996, p.). More recently, some progress has been made in growing the Appalachian economy through economic diversification. From 2008 to 2012, the overall poverty rate for the Appalachian region was 16.6%. During this same time period, the number of high-poverty counties in the Appalachian region (defined as those with poverty rates more than 1.5 times the U.S. average) declined from 295 in 1960 to 107 in 2012 (ARC, 2015).

Homelessness represents an extreme result from a lack of economic resources. Appalachian mothers entering a shelter for homeless families often reported job loss as one of the major factors contributing to their becoming homeless (Lee, 2012). Unemployment typically resulted from family illness—either that of a child or the mother. As these women typically had been employed in low-wage jobs without benefits such as sick leave, an illness represented much more than just a threat to physical wellbeing, it was a risk to their ability to maintain housing (Lee, 2012). Once families entered the shelter, it was challenging to arrange child care and schedules to seek employment and affordable housing. In addition, Appalachian mothers saw a lack of money as a significant barrier to providing care to their children. The inability to provide shelter, food, clothes, and health care was viewed as an ongoing threat to each mother's sense of identity and self-respect (Lee, 2012).

Educational Factors

Although many of the early immigrants to the Appalachian region were literate, subsequent generations left formal schooling behind, focusing instead on making a life in the harsh terrain (Jones, 1994). During the period of migration, urban Appalachian children often started preschool with positive self-images, were verbal, and playful. However, by junior high those same students had negative self-images, were shy and withdrawn, and eventually dropped out—at rates in some urban Appalachian neighborhoods approaching 70% (Timm, 1996). Children frequently missed school to care for sick relatives or other family responsibilities (Timm, 1996). When forced to choose between school and family, Appalachian children made a culturally appropriate, if harmful, choice by caring for and placing family first (Timm, 1996). Appalachian mothers believed education was the key to family stability and future success, yet they found the schools to be an unwelcoming, alienating environment, which led them to allow their children to drop out in order to avoid feelings of discomfort (Timm, 1996).

In the ethnonursing research conducted with Appalachian mothers in a shelter for homeless families, most of the Appalachian mothers had high school diplomas or general educational development (GED) equivalents; one African-American Appalachian mother had earned her associates degree (Lee, 2012). Because the mothers placed a high value on their children's education, children living in the shelter were either enrolled in the neighborhood school or were provided transportation to their former school whenever possible. Shelter living took a toll on the children's school success due to their chaotic schedules and lack of private space in which to complete homework (Lee, 2012).

Generic (Folk) and Professional Care Beliefs and Practices

During the early settlement of Appalachia, medical practice combined the best available science with an intimate knowledge of the healing properties of native plants and homemade potions (Obermiller, 1996). Gathering of medicinal plants and herbs was a natural part of the culture. The plant materials used for making folk medicines included roots, bark, wood, sap, and leaves. Roots came from blackberry, ginger, ginseng, goldenseal, ironweed, jimsonweed, and sassafras (Cavender, 2003). Bark from the dogwood, hickory, red oak, sweetgum, willow, and wild cherry trees was also used (Cavender, 2003). Some of the more common treatments included drinking tea made from blackberry plants and red oak bark to treat diarrhea; applying a poultice of cottonseed to the neck for a sore throat; drinking tea brewed with wild ginger root and peppermint leaves to relieve colic in infants; smoking the leaves of jimsonweed to treat asthma and other respiratory ailments; using a mixture of castor oil, Epsom salts, and water to treat constipation; and drinking teas of sassafras root bark or wild cherry bark or a half cup of vinegar to treat hypertension (also known as *high blood*) (Cavender, 2003).

Many Appalachians made their own medicinal brushes for oral care, using willow, sassafras, birch, and blackgum twigs to scrape teeth and gums (Cavender, 2003). Treatments for ailments were focused on contravening the suspected cause of the health problem. For example, it was believed that earaches were caused by cold air blowing into the ear; folk treatment consisted of blowing of warm air or instilling of warm liquids into the affected ear (Cavender, 2003). The author's grandfather would smoke his pipe and blow warm air into her own ear, followed by a plug of cotton, to treat her childhood earaches.

Denham (1999) conducted ethnographic research with families living in an Appalachian area of southeast Ohio and discovered that home is the central focus of health for Appalachian families with mothers serving as a primary healthcare resource for the family, acting as gatekeepers as well as care providers. Health was seen as a holistic combination of physical, emotional, social, spiritual, and ecological dimensions, with an emphasis placed on family rather than individual health (Denham, 1999), a finding that also reflected the cultural value of familism. Other cultural norms associated with the Appalachian worldview can have a negative influence on health practices. These include a fatalistic outlook, distrust of outsiders, and distrust of formalized medical systems (McGarvey, MaGuadalupe, Killos, Guterbock, & Cohn, 2011).

For Appalachian mothers living in a homeless shelter, health was seen as a multidimensional construct comprising physical, emotional, and spiritual factors (Lee, 2012). However, the priority for each mother was ensuring the health of her children, sometimes at the expense of her own health. These women spoke of the importance of her role in providing "mother care" to their children. From the perspective of Appalachian culture, *mother care* promotes health and wellbeing and consists of love, nurturance, discipline, and instilling hope for the future (Lee, 2012). Self-care was often based on treatments passed down from previous generations. One Appalachian mother reported that since running out of her hypertensive medications, she had been drinking vinegar several times a day—a home remedy she had learned from her grandmother (Lee, 2012).

Each of the Appalachian mothers shared stories of noncaring experiences with healthcare providers who were quick to judge them based on their economic or social status or physical characteristics (Lee, 2012). These experiences served to reinforce existing cultural distrust of healthcare systems and the professionals who work there. Appalachian mothers living in the homeless shelter stated that professional caring needs to be based on treating patients "…the same way they would treat their own family members" (Lee, 2012).

Review of the ethnohistory, worldview, social structure dimensions, and generic (folk) and professional care beliefs and practices has enabled a deeper understanding of the Appalachian culture and its influence on the experience of family homelessness. Nurses must consider these historical and cultural factors to provide culturally congruent care. Lessons from Appalachia show us that partnering with the people, the true "knowers" of their experiences and needs is the best way to provide care that respects, honors, and builds upon the strengths found within their cultural values, beliefs, and practices.

■ THREE MODES OF CULTURE CARE DECISIONS AND ACTIONS

The goal of the Theory of Culture Care Diversity and Universality is the provision of culturally congruent care (Leininger, 1991). Transcultural nursing advocates for the provision of nursing care that is congruent with the expressed care needs of diverse people in ways that are meaningful and beneficial to them (Leininger, 1991). Within the Culture Care Theory, there are three care modes that guide nursing decisions and actions. By examining care within the theory framework, the clinician can provide care that is congruent with the client's culture and would benefit and hold meaning for the client. The three modes of culture care are: Culture care preservation and/or maintenance; culture care accommodation and/or negotiation; and culture care repatterning and/or restructuring (McFarland & Wehbe-Alamah, 2015). The modes facilitate the nurse's decisions and actions toward helping clients to meet their healthcare goals in a culturally congruent and acceptable manner (Leininger, 1991) as explained in greater detail in Chapters 3 and 4 of this text.

Based on the holding knowledge presented, as derived from a review of the literature and the ethnonursing research study discussed, the author formulated the following culturally congruent nursing care decisions and actions. These nursing decisions are based on the experiences, values, beliefs, meanings, and practices of Appalachian mothers providing care for themselves and their children with the context of homelessness and while living in an urban homeless shelter.

Culture Care Preservation and/or Maintenance

To preserve and/or maintain the culture care of Appalachian mothers experiencing homelessness, nurses and other healthcare providers may engage in the following actions:

- **Recognize, appreciate, and acknowledge the personal strength, courage, and resiliency of each Appalachian mother entering a homeless shelter**

Pride, independence, and self-reliance are core values within Appalachian culture (Jones, 1994). A mother's decision to enter a homeless shelter and struggle through those harsh lifeways in the days that follow is not a decision that is made lightly, but is done to promote the health and wellbeing of her children. Recognition, appreciation, and acknowledgement of these qualities by nurses can help re-establish feelings of self-worth in mothers struggling with shelter entry, while also reaffirming [preserving] the decision by those for whom shelter entry was seen as a statement of pride and independence.

- **Respect and support the Appalachian mother's role in the life of her child**

Maintaining family relationships and connections is at the core of Appalachian culture. Further, the mother is seen as the keeper of family health. Nurses and other healthcare providers and shelter staff need to respect a mother's desire to continue providing *mother care* for her children through expressions of love, nurturance, and discipline (Lee, 2012). Health education activities can be planned in which mothers spend time with children coloring and reading pages from health promotion booklets, or reinforcing content learned in classes about hand-washing and safety. Partnering with mothers and supporting them as they provide health education to their children allows mothers to feel in control and respected in their role as competent caregivers.

Culture Care Accommodation and/or Negotiation

To accommodate and/or negotiate the culture care of Appalachian mothers experiencing homelessness, nurses and other healthcare providers may engage in the following actions:

- **Assist families as they accommodate and negotiate losses**

Appalachian mothers and children experience a series of traumatic events leading up to their entry into a shelter. New lifeway experiences such as doubling-up can often result in conflict with families and friends, thus eroding these fragile caring connections (Lee, 2012). Kinship connections are crucial for promoting the health and wellbeing of mothers and children, not only during the period in which they are experiencing homelessness, but also when lifeways are threatened in the period following placement in permanent or transitional housing (Lee, 2012). For Appalachian families, whose cultural heritage is steeped in the importance of kinship ties, the effects from damaged or severed family ties cannot be underestimated. Healthcare providers need to accommodate or negotiate culture care practices as indicated and appropriate in order to provide the necessary support for Appalachian mothers and children (Lee, 2012). Examples of culturally sensitive accommodations include expansion of supportive networks and referrals to community and healthcare agencies.

- **Provide anticipatory guidance to empower Appalachian mothers to better support their children during the chaotic period of shelter-living**

As previously stated, recognition of the important role of mothers in an Appalachian family is the foundation of providing them with culturally congruent care (Lee, 2012). Because of the lifeways associated with becoming and being homeless, children staying in a shelter often express their needs in ways that are different than before coming to the shelter. Despite recognizing their own stress, many of the mothers in shelters failed to appreciate the potential negative effects that altered lifeways had on their children (Lee, 2012). Nurses need to provide mothers with anticipatory guidance to raise their awareness about some of the typical expressions displayed by children at various ages when faced with stressful shelter lifeways. Prepared with this knowledge, mothers can explore with nurses ways of supporting their children and can negotiate care practices that accommodate their children's changing needs, thus assisting them in adapting to this period of uncertainty and instability.

- **Facilitate healthy communication patterns and greater understanding between shelter staff and Appalachian mothers**

The nurse is in a unique position to enhance understanding between shelter staff and families, providing guidance to shelter staff on how to accommodate Appalachian mothers and their families and how to negotiate shelter rules and expectations of programming to foster an atmosphere that is conducive to health and wellbeing and so that mothers feel respected in their role as head of their family. Nurses can also work with shelter staff to provide education that promotes a greater understanding of the health and wellbeing of mothers and children who are homeless so that their needs can be accommodated whenever possible within the framework of the shelter programming and therefore reduce the stress level of Appalachian families within the homeless shelter environment.

Culture Care Repatterning and/or Restructuring

To repattern and/or restructure the culture care of Appalachian mothers experiencing homelessness, nurses and other healthcare providers may engage in the following actions:

- **Assist mothers in repatterning and restructuring culture care practices that are in violation of shelter rules**

For some Appalachian mothers caring for their children in a shelter, rules barring corporal punishment can be seen as noncaring and as interfering with parental authority (Lee, 2013). However, shelter rules supporting nonviolent expressions have been instituted in order to foster/promote an atmosphere of respect and safety for all shelter residents. To restructure care patterns that do not fit within these guidelines, nurses can provide mothers with health education related to child development and alternative forms of discipline.

- **Engage in process of self-examination in order to identify potential biases and stereotypes related to homelessness**

Pride and respect are fundamental values of Appalachian culture (Lee, 2012). Treating mothers in a disrespectful manner by making assumptions about their situation is viewed as a noncaring expression which diminishes their sense of self-worth and human dignity; therefore, such actions will not have the desired outcome of promoting their health and wellbeing. Nurses who work with families experiencing homelessness must examine and repattern their own practices to reflect an understanding that these individuals are not defined by their shelter or homelessness experiences. Homelessness is not a simple phenomenon and those experiencing it do not represent a homogenous population (Lee, 2012). Rather than categorizing based solely on this common lifeway experience, the differing needs of individuals and families experiencing homelessness must be discovered and supported through culturally congruent programming (Lee, 2012).

- **Advocate on behalf of all individuals and families experiencing homelessness**

Nurses have a social mandate to provide care and respect for all persons (ANA, 2010) and an ethical duty to speak up when they see others devaluing personhood for any reason (ANA, 2015). While nurses and other healthcare providers need to continue delivering healthcare services to families and individuals who are homeless, they also must move their advocacy efforts beyond the traditional scope of service provision and into the arena of public policy advocacy related to housing and employment reform. From this perspective, culture care for Appalachian mothers means having access to: Safe, affordable housing;

employment opportunities that provide a living wage; and affordable, quality childcare for working families (Bassuk, Volk, & Olivet, 2010).

SUMMARY

Appalachian mothers face a multitude of challenges when attempting to provide care for their children within the context of family homelessness. Threatening lifeways experienced during the period before entering a shelter can have lasting negative effects on the health and wellbeing of all family members. Supporting families during this vulnerable transition period by providing respectful care that recognizes the inherent dignity of each mother and child is vital.

Culturally congruent care provided to homeless families must be based on an understanding of their unique situation and the contextual factors that contribute to their experience. Women who are guiding their families as they navigate homelessness need to be respected and supported in their roles as mothers and valued for the strength, dignity, and resilience they have shown while enduring traumatic life experiences.

The reader has been presented with holding knowledge of Appalachian culture in general, as well as family homelessness, as viewed through this cultural lens. The knowledge gained can provide the foundation for culture care preservation and/or maintenance; accommodation and/or negotiation; and repatterning and/or restructuring for culturally congruent care practices by mothers and children navigating the lifeways of homelessness. Ultimately, the health and wellbeing of these women and their children can be improved by the application of culture-specific knowledge in designing programs that meet the needs of Appalachian mothers in a holistic manner. Services provided for families who are experiencing homelessness must be based on an understanding of their unique situation and the contextual factors that contribute to their experience. These mothers and children cannot simply be treated as if they have the same needs as individuals who are homeless. African-American and European-American Appalachian mothers who are experiencing homelessness need programs that build upon their cultural strengths, not those that identify and highlight their deficits. These women need to be respected and supported in their roles as mothers and valued for the strength they have shown in facing challenging lifeways.

DEDICATION

I would like to dedicate this work to the Appalachian mothers who walked with me on a wonderful journey of exploration. I would also like to dedicate this work to the Appalachian women in my own family who have taught me lessons in caring, strength, hope, and faith, and nurtured in me a love of God and family that has been my foundation. To each of these Appalachian women who have been a part of my life, especially my beloved grandmother Eva Mae Hutchins, the lessons you have taught and the wisdom you have shared will always be a part of who I am. Finally, I would like to dedicate this chapter to the memory of my dear father, Rev. Samuel William Crews—my first and greatest teacher of lessons in human caring.

ACKNOWLEDGEMENTS

I wish to acknowledge the support of those who made this research possible. My sincere appreciation goes to Dr. Edith Morris, who originally opened my eyes to the wonders of transcultural nursing. In addition, gratitude is extended to the International Association for Human Caring whose awarding of the Leininger Research Award provided financial support for the ethnonursing study that contributed many of the findings included in this chapter.

DISCUSSION QUESTIONS

1. How are the ethnonursing research method and accompanying enablers useful for conducting research with vulnerable populations such as families experiencing homelessness?
2. Discuss how your nursing care practices will be influenced by the holding knowledge provided in this chapter when you are caring for members of the Appalachian culture.
3. Discuss the impact of migration on the health and wellbeing of Appalachians.
4. Discuss strategies for providing families living in a homeless shelter with culturally congruent care to support their health and wellbeing.

■ REFERENCES

Appalachian Regional Commission. (2015). *The Appalachian region.* Retrieved from http://www.arc.gov/appalachian_region/TheAppalachianRegion.asp.

American Nurses Association. (2015). *Code of Ethics for Nurses: With interpretive Statements.* Silver Spring, MD: American Nurses Association.

American Nurses Association. (2010). *Nursing's Social Policy Statement.* Silver Spring, MD: American Nurses Association.

Bassuk, E. L., Volk, K. T., & Olivet, J. (2010). A framework for developing supports and services for families experiencing homelessness. *The Open Health Services and Policy Journal,* S3, 34-40. doi: 10.2174/1874924001003010034

Blethen, H. T. (2004). Pioneer settlement. In R. A. Straw and H. T. Blethen (Eds.), *High mountains rising: Appalachia in time and place* (pp. 17-29). Urbana, IL: University of Illinois Press.

Cavender, A. (2003). *Folk medicine in southern Appalachia.* Chapel Hill, NC: The University of North Carolina Press.

Committee on Psychosocial Aspects of Child and Family Health, Committee on Early Childhood, Adoption, and Dependent Care, Section on Developmental and Behavioral Pediatrics Shonkoff, J. P., Garner, A. S.,...Wood, D. L. (2012). [Policy Statement] Early childhood adversity, toxic stress, and the role of the pediatrician: Translating developmental science into lifelong health. *Pediatrics, 129*(1), e224-e231. doi: 10.1542/peds.2011-2662

Denham, S. A. (1999). The definition and practice of family health. *Journal of Family Nursing, 5*(2), 133-159.

Diddle, G., & Denham, S. A. (2010). Spirituality and its relationships with the health and illness of Appalachian people. *Journal of Transcultural Nursing, 21*(2), 175-182.

Eller, R. (2004). Modernization. In R. A. Straw and H. T. Blethen (Eds.), *High mountains rising: Appalachia in time and place* (pp. 197-219). Urbana, IL: University of Illinois Press.

Hayes, M., Zonneville, M., & Bassuk, E. (2013). The SHIFT study final report: Service and housing interventions for families in transition. Newton, MA: National Center on Family Homelessness.

Helton, L. R., & Keller, S. M. (2010). Appalachian women: A study of resiliency assets and cultural values. *Journal of Social Service Research, 36*(2), 151-161.

Herbers, J. E., Cutuli, J. J., Monn, A. R., Narayan, A. J., & Masten, A. S. (2014). Trauma, adversity, and parent-child relationships among young children experiencing homelessness. *Journal of Abnormal Child Psychology, 42*(7), 1167-1174. doi: 10.1007/s10802-014-9868-7

Jones, L. (1994). *Appalachian values.* Ashland, KY: Jesse Stuart Foundation.

Lee, R. C. (2012). Family homelessness viewed through the lens of health and human rights. *Advances in Nursing Science. 35*(2), e47-e59.

Leininger, M. (1991). *Culture care diversity and universality: A theory for nursing.* New York: National League for Nursing Press.

McFarland, M. R., & Wehbe-Alamah, H. B. (2015). The theory of culture care diversity and universality. In M. R. McFarland and H. B. Wehbe-Alamah (Eds.), *Culture care diversity and universality: A worldwide nursing theory.* (3rd ed., pp. 1-31). Burlington, MA: Jones and Bartlett Learning.

McGarvey, E. L., MaGuadalupe, L., Killos, L. F., Guterbock, T., & Cohn, W. (2011). Health disparities between Appalachian and non-Appalachian counties in Virginia USA. *Journal of Community Health, 36*(3), 348-356. doi: 10.1007/s10900-010-9315-9

National Center on Family Homelessness. (2011). *The characteristics and needs of families experiencing homelessness.* Retrieved from http://www.familyhomelessness.org/media/278.pdf

National Center on Family Homelessness. (2014). *America's youngest outcasts: A report card on child homelessness.* Retrieved from http://www.homelesschildrenamerica.org/

National Coalition for the Homeless. (2014). Homeless families with children. Retrieved from http://nationalhomeless.org/wp-content/uploads/2014/06/families_children-Fact-Sheet.pdf

National Low Income Housing Coalition. (2014). *Housing wage calculator.* Retrieved from http://nlihc.org/library/wagecalc

Nooe, R. M., & Patterson, D. A. (2010). The ecology of homelessness. *Journal of Human Behavior in the Social Environment, 20*(2), 105-152.

Obermiller, P. J. (1996). Introduction. In P. J. Obermiller (Ed.), *Down home, downtown: Urban Appalachians today* (pp. 1-10). Dubuque, IA: Kendall/Hunt Publishing.

Park, J. M., Fertig, A. R., & Allison, P. D. (2010). Physical and mental health, cognitive development, and healthcare use by housing status of low-income young children in 20 American cities: A prospective cohort study. *American Journal of Public Health, 101*(S1), S255-S261.

Stagman, S. M., & Cooper, J. L. (2010). *Children's mental health: What every policymaker should know.* New York, NY: National Center for Children in Poverty.

Timm, P. Z. (1996). Pushed out the door: An intergenerational study of early school leaving among Appalachians. In P. J. Obermiller (Ed.), *Down home, downtown: Urban Appalachians today,* (pp. 107-114). Dubuque, IA: Kendall/Hunt Publishing.

U.S. Department of Commerce, Economics and Statistics Administration, Census Bureau. (2014). *Income and poverty in the United States: 2013*. Washington, D. C.: Author. Retrieved from https://www.census.gov/content/dam/Census/library/publications/2014/demo/p60-249.pdf

U.S. Department of Housing and Urban Development, Office of Community Planning and Development. (2014, October). *Part 1: The 2014 point-in-time estimates of homelessness: The 2014 Annual Homeless Assessment Report to Congress*. Washington, DC: Author.

CHAPTER 24

Culture Expressions, Meanings, Beliefs, and Practices of Mexican American Women During the Postpartum Period: An Ethnonursing Study

Valera A. Hascup

> *"If we are to have a richer culture, rich in contrasting values, we must recognize the whole gamut of human potentialities, and so weave a less arbitrary social fabric, one in which each diverse human gift will find a fitting place"* (Margaret Mead, 1935, p. 300).

■ INTRODUCTION

The need for nurses to be knowledgeable about the culture care beliefs and practices of Mexican American women for whom they provide care is an imperative within the profession. Learning about the cultural values, beliefs, practices, and expressions of Mexican American women is essential to the development of cultural competency skills. The ability to provide culturally competent care will help ensure client safety and optimal maternal-child health outcomes during the puerperium (Boyle, 2011).

Background and Significance

Nursing has a long history of being concerned for the basic rights of people to live with dignity regardless of their socioeconomic status or ethnicity. Zoucha (2001) urged that "…we put aside deep-seated feelings of ethnocentrism and accept that every health worldview is equally valid" (p.157). Nursing research studies have indicated that compared to Caucasian or African American women, Hispanic women in the United States (U. S.) do not effectively utilize healthcare services due to cultural, socioeconomic, and linguistic barriers that may

pose critical challenges for pregnancy and postpartum outcomes (Cristancho, Garces, Peters, & Mueller, 2008). It is imperative that nurses develop an understanding of the postpartum period as experienced by Mexican American women in order to be able to provide culturally congruent and competent care for this rapidly growing Hispanic subgroup.

Mexican American Demographics

Projections estimate that by the year 2060, the number of Hispanic people in the U. S. will be over 128 million, constituting 30% of the nation's population (Brown & Patten, 2015). According to the U. S. Census Bureau, *Hispanic or Latino* refers to "…a person of Cuban, Mexican, Puerto Rican, South or Central American, or other Spanish culture or origin, regardless of race" (Humes, Jones, & Ramirez, 2011, p. 1). Of the Hispanic subgroups, Mexican Americans number more than 31 million people, representing approximately 64% of the overall Hispanic population in the U. S. (Humes, Jones, & Ramirez, 2011).

Gonzalez-Barrera and Lopez (2013) projected that more than 10 million Mexican American women will be living in the U. S. by the year 2050. The birth rate among Mexican Americans in the U. S. accounted for 63% of the 11.2 million increase in national population between the years 2000 to 2010, a rate approximately 50% higher than among non-Hispanics (Gonzalez-Barrera & Lopez, 2013). This has tremendous significance for the healthcare system and especially for maternal-child nurses in terms of providing quality care and the associated economic expenditures.

THEORETICAL FRAMEWORK

Culture care values, beliefs, practices, and expressions are unique to each culture and have meanings that influence health, wellness, and illness (Berry, 2002; Leininger, 2006a). The theorist (Leininger, 2006b, p. 55) explicated cultural context as a construct of the Theory of Culture Care Diversity and Universality (also known as the Culture Care Theory or CCT), stating that the "…ethnonursing method requires that the researcher focus on the cultural context of whatever phenomena are being studied." Leininger further explained that the cultural context referred to the comprehensiveness of the present lifeway.

The Culture Care Theory and the Sunrise Enabler* (Refer to Color Insert 1), a visual representation of Leininger's theory, were used as the guiding framework for this study along with the Ethnonursing Research Method. Other enablers used to enhance this discovery of emic, or insider, data included the Observation-Participation-Reflection (OPR) Enabler and the Stranger-to-Trusted Friend Enabler. The Domain of Inquiry (DOI) Enabler developed by the researcher, the ethnodemographic data sheet, and Leininger's Semi-Structured Inquiry Guide Enabler to Assess Culture Care and Health* (Wehbe-Alamah & McFarland, 2015, p. 81-84) were used to explicate culture care phenomena from the emic perspective of Mexican American women during their childbirth experience.

DOMAIN OF INQUIRY (DOI)

This chapter discusses the findings from the doctoral research study and professional nursing experiences of the author in labor and delivery/maternal-child health. The DOI for the ethnonursing study was *to discover, understand, describe, explicate, and analyze the cultural expressions, meanings, beliefs, practices, and experiences of postpartum Mexican American women living a county in New Jersey* (USA).

RESEARCH QUESTIONS

The open discovery process with focused research questions was used by the author to elicit in-depth data regarding the cultural expressions, meanings, practices, beliefs, and experiences of Mexican American women during the postpartum period. The findings were inductively derived from the data using Ethnonursing Research Method (Leininger, 2006a, 2006b) and Leininger's Four Phases of Data Analysis Enabler for Qualitative Data* (Wehbe-Alamah & McFarland, 2015, p. 89). The research questions that guided this study were as follows:

- How do Mexican American women describe the postpartum experience?
- What are the generic cultural expressions, meanings, beliefs, health and self-care practices, and experiences of Mexican American women during the postpartum period?
- In what ways do worldview, cultural and social structure [dimensions], and ethnohistory influence the care expressions, meanings, beliefs, practices, and experiences in the home and community contexts for Mexican American postpartum women?

ASSUMPTIVE PREMISES OF THE STUDY

The assumptive premises of the study discussed in this chapter were based on the assumptive premises of culture care theory. They are as follows:

- Care meanings and experiences within the cultural context of care contribute to understanding of health, illness, and wellbeing and add to the body of nursing knowledge.
- Care meanings and experiences are embedded in the Mexican American worldview and social structure and can be identified within a naturalistic environmental context.
- Culture care concepts, expressions, meanings, practices, beliefs, practices, experiences, possess diversities and universalities among all cultures, including that of Mexican Americans.
- The Mexican American culture has specific attitudes toward the postpartum experience.

* The titles for Leininger's enablers have been updated and reflect current designations.

ETHNONURSING INQUIRY GUIDE FOR DISCOVERING CARE MEANINGS AND EXPERIENCES WITHIN THE CULTURAL CONTEXT

NUMBER:

NAME:

I. Introduction

As a maternal child nurse, I am interested in learning about your culture and way of life in order to assist healthcare providers in providing culturally appropriate care for Mexican American women, particularly new mothers after the birth of a baby.

II. Cultural Values, Beliefs, Lifeways

As a nurse, I am interested in your cultural values and beliefs in order to be able to plan appropriate care for you.

1. What values or beliefs do you possess that are important to you?

III. Kinship and Gender Roles

I am interested in knowing more about your ideas on family.

1. Tell me about your family. Who do you consider to be part of your family?
2. Who is important in your life?
3. Can you tell me what the women do in your family? What do the men in the family do? Can you tell me what the children do?
4. Tell me what it means for you to have children.
5. Can you describe for me some of the family beliefs and values that are important to you to pass on to your children?

IV. Political Factors

I would like to know more about your community.

1. Can you tell me who the important leaders are in your community?
2. Can you tell me if you feel they are helpful to you?
3. Is your routine similar or different from other Mexican Americans that you know in your community?

V. Religious and Spiritual Factors

I am interested in knowing about church and religion in your life.

1. Would you tell me what religion means in your everyday life?
2. During pregnancy and childbirth? After delivery?
3. Can you tell me your thoughts on religion and health?

VI. Meanings and Experiences of Care

I would like to know more about how you care for yourself and keep healthy.

1. What does good health and being healthy mean to you?
2. Can you explain for me what care means to you?
3. How do people show care?
4. Can you describe for me what you would consider to be non-caring?

VII. Prenatal, Childbirth and Postpartum Practices and Beliefs

I would like to learn about your practices and beliefs about pregnancy, childbirth and after delivery.

1. Can you share with me your thoughts about pregnancy? Childbirth? After delivery?
2. Who is a good person to provide advice for either a pregnant woman or new mother?
3. What might some of the older women in your family or community tell you about pregnancy? Childbirth? After delivery?
4. Describe for me what a healthy pregnancy means to you?
5. Who would you like to be with you in labor? What would they do for you?
6. How does a person show care for a new mother?
7. Would you tell me how you recover and gain strength after delivery?
8. What does it mean for you to have a healthy baby?

VIII. Meanings and Experiences of Care After Delivery

I would like to talk with you about who gives you care after delivery when you come home.

1. What happened after your baby was born? Your feelings? Thoughts?
2. After delivery, how do you express how you feel? What words do you use? Feelings? Who would you share your feelings with?
3. How would people react when you told them how you felt (after delivery)?
4. What would care be like for a Mexican American woman at home after delivery?
5. How would you like to be cared for after delivery? By family? By friends?
6. Is there something you would have liked them to do for you that they didn't do?
7. Is there anything else you would like to tell me about what it was like for you at home during the first few weeks and months after delivery?
8. How is care different or similar to what would happen in Mexico or with relatives/friends in Mexico?
9. Is there anything else you would like to share with me about what we talked about?

FIGURE 24.1 • Ethnonursing Inquiry Guide for Discovering Care Meanings and Experiences Within the Cultural Context. © V. Hascup (2011).

Adapted, with permission, from *The cultural context of culture care practices of Mexican American women.*

- The Mexican American culture has generic (e.g., lay, folk, and indigenous) care knowledge and practices as well as professional care knowledge and practices that may differ from the Anglo American culture. These may change over time in women distanced from their homeland and culture.

ORIENTATIONAL DEFINITIONS

Leininger (2006a) described orientational definitions as "...not operational to encourage the researcher to discover new qualitative knowledge and to avoid being focused solely on the researcher's quantitative definitions or Western ideas" (p. 12). The orientational definitions used in this chapter include the following:

- *Culture*: Those learned and shared beliefs, values, and lifeways of Mexican American women that are generally transmitted intergenerationally and influence their thinking and action modes (as adapted by Berry, 2002, p. 28).
- *Care*: Those assistive, supportive, enabling, and facilitative culturally based ways to help Mexican American women in a compassionate, respectful, and appropriate way to improve a human condition or lifeway (as adapted by Berry, 2002, p. 28).
- *Culture-specific care (culturally congruent care)*: Care that is tailored to fit with specific cultures in appropriate ways (as adapted by Berry, 2002, p. 29).
- Mexican American *Woman (Women)*: Woman (Women) living in the United States who self-identified as a Mexican American.
- *Postpartum; Postpartum period; Puerperium; Fourth trimester*: A 6-week interval that begins after the birth of the newborn and ends upon the return of the reproductive organs to their normal, nonpregnant state. The physiologic changes that occur during this time, while distinctive, are normal (Bobak, Perry, & Lowdermilk, 2000).
- *Generic (Emic) care*: "...Refers to the local, indigenous, or insiders' cultural knowledge and view of specific phenomena" (Leininger, 2006a, p. 14).
- *Etic care*: "...Refers to the outsider's or stranger's views and often health professionals views and institutional knowledge of phenomena" (Leininger, 2006a, p. 14).

- *Cultural context*: "...the totality of the situation or lifeway at hand (Leininger, 2006a, p. 10).
- *Generic postpartum care*: Refers to culturally learned and transmitted lay, traditional, or folk caring behaviors or concerns by family, friends, or healthcare professionals who assist, support, or enable Mexican American women during the postpartum period (as adapted by Berry, 2002, p. 29 from Leininger, 2002).
- *Ethnocentrism*: "....Refers to the belief that one's own ways are the best, most superior, or preferred ways to act, believe, or behave (Leininger, 2002b, p. 50).

LITERATURE REVIEW

The review of the literature revealed a paucity of extant nursing research specific to Mexican American women's cultural beliefs, practices, and experiences related to the postpartum period (Hartweg & Isabelli-Garcia, 2007; Ramirez & Suarez, 2007). Research has focused on Mexican immigrant women during the antepartum (Berry, 1996, 1999, 2002) and intrapartum periods (Gallo, 2003) but has excluded the postpartum period. It has been hypothesized that the longer these women remain in the U. S. it is less likely they will adhere to traditional cultural beliefs and practices that they had perceived as offering protection. The literature review affirmed that care issues exist among Mexican American women that may threaten maternal-child wellbeing during the postpartum period.

Access to Healthcare

Johnson (2005) discussed the *Latina paradox*, revealing that Mexican immigrant women have better pregnancy outcomes than Mexican American women born in the United States (McGlade, Somnath, & Dahlstrom, 2004). What is striking about the *Latina paradox* is that favorable birth outcomes are not associated with socioeconomic status, given that Latinos are among the most disadvantaged ethnic populations in the U. S. (McGlade, Somnath, & Dahlstrom, 2004). Because they have lower levels of education than White females, almost 50% of Mexican American females live below the poverty level, and they are the least likely to have a regular healthcare provider or source of health care (Callister, 2005; Ramirez & Suarez, 2007). At the same time, Mexican American women have the strongest advantages in birth outcomes due to cultural protective factors and social support (McGlade et al., 2004).

Mexican American Women: Perceptions of Health and Wellbeing

Divine will, Folk Systems, and Health

Worldview is an encompassing perspective that guides one's thinking and decisions about all aspects of life, including care decisions and actions (Leininger, 2006a). The Mexican American worldview was tightly woven with [in] the concept of 'divine will' that [had] "...ultimate control over their lives" (Madsen, 1964, p. 16 as cited by Berry, 1996, p. 52) and although they prayed asking God to intercede, the view persisted that "God's will takes care of me" (Berry, 1996). As a manifestation of Mexican American women's faith and spirituality (Berry, 1996; Mendelson, 2002; Mendelson-Klauss, 2000; Rojas, 1991) prayer was a part of their daily routine and served as a conduit through which to give thanks, develop strength, make decisions, seek protection for one's children, and maintain emotional support, balance, and harmony (Mendelson, 2002).

Combined with the emphasis on divine will are indigenous and Spanish folk traditions, resulting in *curanderismo*, "...a synergetic, eclectic, and holistic ... mixture of beliefs derived from Aztec, Spanish, spiritualistic, homeopathic, and modern 'scientific' medicine" (Rojas, 1991, pp. 2-3). The mind, body, and spirit are inseparable and any disruption in balance and harmony may produce illness (Zoucha & Zamarripa, 2008). Mexican American women have achieved harmony by participating in interrelated health practices drawn from folk healers with no medical expertise (Refer to Table 24.1) as well as from professional healthcare sectors (Sanchez, 1997). Although reliance upon traditional healers in acculturated Hispanic women has decreased, their persistent use of self-care and home-based remedies point to the continued need for of low-cost care and cultural empathy in care, which are often missing in the Western biomedical healthcare system (Berry, 2002; Lopez, 2005).

Prenatal Health Behaviors, Beliefs, and Practices

Historically and to the present, the folk beliefs and practices surrounding pregnancy in Mexican American culture (Berry, 1996; dePacheco & Hutti, 1998; Kay, 1980;

Zoucha, 1998) have been handed down intergenerationally through the elder women in the family. Depending on degree of acculturation to U. S. lifeways, prenatal care–while valued–may not be sought until late in the pregnancy after family advice has been sought (Purnell & Paulanka, 2003). Mexican American women are modest and the pelvic exam is distressing for them. Gender-congruent care is provided by the midwife who is culturally perceived as able to conduct pelvic exams without violating cultural taboos that prohibit men from viewing intimate female body parts (Galanti, 2004; Zoucha, 1998).

Childbirth Practices and *Matrescence*

In Mexican American culture, attending a woman during delivery is a woman's role, ideally the midwife and the woman's mother (Galanti, 2004). Healthcare providers should respect the practice of not allowing any men in the delivery room including the child's father (Zoucha & Zamarripa, 2003, p. 272) and should encourage gender-congruent supportive care by mothers, sisters, relatives, or friends in the labor and delivery setting. At the same time, some childbearing practices changed abruptly when Mexican American wives of servicemen began to deliver in hospitals during World War II (Kay, 1980) creating an acute alienation from the traditional practices. There was no need for her mother's knowledge and support in this biomedical environment dominated by male physicians and technology (Kay, 1980).

Motherhood, or *matrescence,* in Mexican American culture is considered the fulfillment of the ultimate role of womanhood (Gonzalez-Swafford & Gutierrez, 1983; Melville, 1980). Motherhood establishes a degree of status and respect that is unrivaled in any other role, male or female. However, a mother's power extends only to her children, within her household (Melville, 1980). This aspect of Mexican American culture has also been altered by Anglo American culture and societal values including economic productivity. While Mexican American mothers are expected to be mothers first, they are also expected to contribute to the economic wellbeing of their family.

The Postpartum Period for Mexican-American Women

In contrast to mainstream U. S. culture, where pregnancy is viewed as the vulnerable period, the postpartum period is considered a time of vulnerability

TABLE 24.1. Cultural Beliefs and Healthcare Practices of Childbearing Puerto Rican Women and Mexican American Women.

Cultural Affiliation	Hispanic Term	English Term	Associated Belief
Puerto Rican (PR) and Mexican American (MA)	*Curandera*	Folk Healer Spiritualist	Chosen by God and highly respected; cures or breaks hexes, illnesses, and ailments.
PR and MA	*Yerbero*	Herbalist	An expert in herbal medicine; intervenes to help cure ailments of natural or supernatural origin.
PR	*Santera*	Sainterist	Prescribes prayers, teas, and herbal mixtures.
PR and MA	*Espiritista*	Psychic	Has divine power to analyze dreams, foresee the future, and explain the present situation related to hidden experiences or in another life.
PR and MA	*Brujeria Bruja*	Witchcraft	Has supernatural power to place hexes and curses and cause bad luck or despair; believed to be capable of "healing" through potions, verses, and magic.
PR	Intermediator	Medium	Has supernatural power to serve as a spiritual receiver or channel communication from the dead, similar to someone who conducts a séance.
MA	Intermediator	Medium	Treats emotional problems and physical illness by transporting the spiritual self of the victim; treats the spirit, body, and mind; prescribes teas, medicinal baths, and prayers.

Reproduced with permission from dePacheco, M. R., & Hutti, M. H. (1998). Cultural beliefs and healthcare practices of childbearing Puerto Rican women and Mexican American women: A review of the literature. *Mother Baby Journal, 3*(1), 16-17.

for mother and baby in Mexican American culture. *La cuarenta/la cuarentena* (a postpartum 40-day rest period) includes protective seclusion, restriction from bathing or washing hair, and adherence to the hot-cold theory to restore balance in the mother's body after delivery, because childbirth is considered to be a *cold* state due to the heat lost during pregnancy, which is considered a *hot* state (dePacheco & Hutti, 1998). Social support from family and friends, proscription from household chores, and education and assistance from female relatives are perceived to prevent future uterine problems, breastfeeding difficulties, or arthritis (dePacheco & Hutti, 1998; Zoucha & Zamarripa, 2003).

The extent to which practices of *la curantena* are followed depends on the availability of female relatives and friends to provide needed assistance. Epidemiologists have noted that such support may shelter pregnant women from adverse health issues including postpartum depression. According to Stern and Kruckman (1983), postpartum depression in the U. S. is a culture-bound syndrome resulting from the *lack of social structuring of the postpartum period; social recognition of the new role of mother; and social support for the new mother* (p. 1027). Although this study dates back to 1983, it still has merit in view of the high rate of postpartum depression in the U. S., which may be due in part to the fact that there is no sociocultural structuring of the postpartum period unlike that found in Mexican American culture (Beck, 2002; Beck, Froman, & Bernal, 2005; Beck & Gable, 2000, 2003). In non-Western cultures, birth involves moral and social values and the environment as well as the body, whereas with Western births, the focus is on the biomedical aspects of the birth process (Kim-Godwin, 2003). Postpartum rituals of enforced rest, seclusion, and adherence to the hot-cold theory mitigate the development of postpartum depression among Mexican American women.

■ DATA COLLECTION

The Ethnonursing Research Method

Leininger's Ethnonursing Research Method is an inductive, naturalistic, and emic-focused open inquiry mode that was ideal for this study due to its congruence with the DOI, purpose, and goal of the study discussed in this chapter (Leininger, 2006a, 2006b). Discovering the similarities and differences between generic care and professional care enables nurses to provide meaningful, beneficial, and culturally congruent care in alignment with CCT (Leininger, 2006a). Using Leininger's three modes of culture care decisions and actions (maintenance and/or preservation; accommodation and/or negotiation; and repatterning and/or restructuring) to provide clients with culturally congruent, beneficial, and meaningful care is crucial for nurses' understanding of Mexican American women's naturalistic forms of cultural expressions, meanings, beliefs, and practices during the postpartum period.

Setting: Entry into the Community

A county in an Eastern seaboard state of the U. S. was selected as the location for this study because it had a large Mexican American population. The county saw a large influx of immigrants from Central America, South America, and Mexico after World War II, who settled in the eastern section of the city, an aging urban center near the business and transportation districts that had been the former home of European immigrants. The downtown business district has since become dominated by small family-style businesses catering to the Latino community.

To help the researcher gain entry into the community, her Latino university colleagues facilitated an introduction to the Director of the Hispanic Information Center. This community gatekeeper (someone in a position of authority to grant or refuse entry into the community [Luna, 1989]) expressed verbal approval of the study and promised support with informant recruitment. Because the researcher did not speak fluent Spanish, a Mexican American Registered Nurse (RN) who was known in the community was selected by the community gatekeeper to serve as interpreter/gatekeeper and facilitate the introductions of participants to the researcher. The researcher's status as a maternal child RN who was interested in helping Mexican American women by understanding their culture also facilitated entry and helped to establish rapport. Combined with the gatekeeper's assistance, knowing about the researcher's skills helped to alleviate informants' feelings of apprehension, prevent cultural misunderstandings, and encourage participation in the study.

The Community Context

Leininger stated that the ethnonursing researcher does not have subjects, samples, or populations but rather, works with key and general informants. Key informants "… are held to reflect the norms, values, beliefs, and general lifeways of the culture." Eight key and 15 general informants were chosen based on the following selection criteria as adapted from Leininger: Self-identification as Mexican American; age 18 years or older; ability to read, write, and speak English and/or Spanish; and willingness to share information about the domain of inquiry. Key informants were those who personally experienced the postpartum period and were willing to be interviewed by the researcher one to three times for approximately two hours. General informants were not as knowledgeable about the domain of inquiry but were willing to participate (Leininger, 2002c, 2006b) and may have personally experienced or had knowledge of the postpartum period. Most general informants were willing to be interviewed one time for approximately one hour to reflect on how similar or different their ideas were from those expressed by the key informants.

After receiving approval by the university Institutional Review Board and the community gatekeeper, informants were recruited with the assistance of the interpreter/gatekeeper using the Snowball method, "… an effective strategy for identifying participants who know other potential participants who can provide the greatest insight and information…" (Grove, Burns & Gray, 2013, p. 366). Interviews were conducted in Spanish or English, based on informant preference. To protect informants' rights, a written informed consent, provided in English and Spanish, was obtained. Permission to tape record the interviews and take notes during the interview process was requested. The purpose and use of the notes and recordings were explained, and the interpreter was present for all interviews. Given that the Ethnonursing Research Method provides for the study to take place in a naturalistic setting, interviews were conducted at the informants' homes, the Hispanic Information Center, the Catholic Church annex, or another place of their choosing. In collaboration with the interpreter and researcher, informants chose the time and place, to assure privacy and keep distractions to a minimum.

Research Enablers

Interviews were conducted using Leininger's Semi-Structured Inquiry Guide Enabler to Assess Culture Care and Health* (Wehbe-Alamah & McFarland, 2015, p. 81-84) as adapted for the study (Refer to Figure 24.1) as well as an ethnodemographic data sheet (Refer to Figure 24.2) developed by the researcher based on the CCT. Leininger's (2002a) Stranger-to-Trusted Friend Enabler and Observation-Participation-Reflection Enabler* were also used to aid the researcher in establishing trust between the researcher and informants. Throughout the data collection process with informants, the researcher was careful with protected cultural data or potentially sensitive topics. Data collection was regarded as complete when no new data was discovered or saturation was reached (Leininger, 2006b).

■ DATA ANALYSIS

All gathered information was reviewed and rigorously analyzed using Leininger's Four Phases of Data Analysis Enabler for Qualitative Data* (Wehbe-Alamah & McFarland, 2015, p. 89) and were evaluated to ensure that the six major qualitative criteria were met (Leininger, 2002a, 2006b). These criteria are credibility; confirmability; meaning-in-context; recurrent patterning;

saturation; and transferability (Leininger, 2002c, p. 88) and were used throughout the data collection and analysis process (Hascup, 2011).

■ RESULTS AND FINDINGS

Culture Care Worldview According to the Culture Care Theory

Seventeen categories, six patterns, and three themes emerged from the data analysis (Refer to Figure 24.3) and correlated with the cultural and social structure dimensions of Leininger's CCT as depicted in the Sunrise Enabler*. These categories, patterns, and themes were supported by data from the researcher's observations and field journal and provide a contextual perspective into the culture care worldview of Mexican American women.

Categories

During the process of data collection and concurrent analysis, 17 identified categories emerged from the data (Refer to Figure 24.3): *La familia (family); religion and God; everyday life*; valores *(values); traditions; caring and non-caring behavior; folk beliefs; prenatal beliefs; intrapartum beliefs; postpartum beliefs; differences in living*; machismo; *motherhood; circle of violence; gender roles; health*; and melancolía de bebé *(baby blues)* and depresion postparto *(postpartum depression*; Hascup, 2011, p. 91).

FAMILY. *Familism* was one of the most important cultural values held by Mexicans and Mexican Americans identified in the study. The traditional family, *la familia,* was the core of their society and came before all else (except for God)–including work. Individuals derived personal strength from family ties and relationships. One informant stated:

> One of the most important values is family, *la familia*. Family is God. I think that it's willing to support a lot of our decisions in our daily life. I would include our extended family, not only our nuclear like we used to … you know the most important is family; to always keep your family together. That the distance doesn't have to matter or the time, anything else doesn't matter, but if you have your family, that's the important thing.

All informants viewed the family as being of primary importance; for the informants, family consisted

---

* The titles for Leininger's enablers have been updated and reflect current designations.

Ethnodemographic Data Sheet
Number: _____
Name: _____
Age: _____ Marital Status: ☐ Single ☐ Married ☐ Divorced ☐ Separated ☐ Widowed ☐ Partnered Ethnicity: ☐ Mexican American Occupation: You _____ Your Spouse/Partner _____ Religion: _____ Birthplace: _____ How many years lived in U. S. (you) _____ Highest Education: ☐ Elementary ☐ Middle School ☐ High School ☐ College ☐ Graduate School Number of Pregnancies: _____ Experience with:

*The titles for Leininger's enablers have been updated and reflect current designations.

FIGURE 24.2 • Ethnodemographic Data Sheet. © V. Hascup (2011).

Adapted from *The cultural context of culture care practices of Mexican American women.*

of not only husband and children but also parents, aunts, uncles, cousins, grandparents, and friends, which also confirmed findings found in the literature.

RELIGION AND GOD. Mexican American women were found to be deeply spiritual and depended on God as part of their spiritual worldview. It was noteworthy that the women in this study did not necessarily attend church on a regular basis yet still considered themselves to be devout Catholics. Many of the women displayed statues and other religious symbols in their homes. Their religion influenced every action in their daily lives

Miscarriage:	☐Yes ☐No	
Stillbirth:	☐Yes ☐No	
Ectopic Pregnancy:	☐Yes ☐No	
Pregnancy Planned:	☐Yes ☐No	

Number of Living Children: _____

Number: _____

Age of youngest child: ☐Girl   ☐Boy

Age of oldest child: ☐Girl   ☐Boy

Primary Language Spoken: _____

Fluency in other Languages (speaking, reading, writing) _____

Household composition (who lives with you at home?) _____

Where do you live? (Private home, apartment?) _____

*The titles for Leininger's enablers have been updated and reflect current designations.

FIGURE 24.2 • (*Continued*)

including their health-seeking behaviors. Another informant stated, "I have a lot of faith, faith moves mountains, and God will cure anything. God also has the medicine, which would be the doctors, so I know to take Tylenol for a headache or Advil for headache or pain."

EVERYDAY LIFE. Everyday life for the informants involved children, family, and work but especially God and prayer. The first informant stated that religion gave her a sense of security:

You see from the time I wake up in the morning, even from the time we get out of the house, I just say "God protect me and be with me," and so it's from the time you wake up until the time you go to sleep and you thank him with prayers.

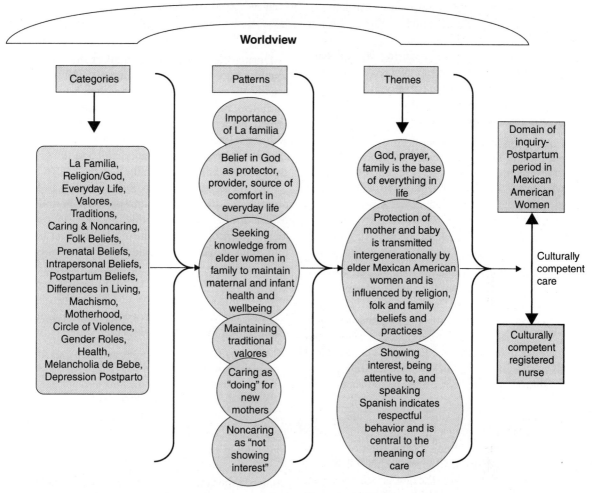

FIGURE 24.3 • Culture Care Practices of Mexican American Women. © V. Hascup (2011).
Adapted from *The cultural context of culture care practices of Mexican American women.*

VALORES (VALUES). *Respeto* (respect), honesty, belief in God, hard work, family unity, and education were highly valued among Mexican American informants. Yet another informant stated that "…The most important thing that I have is *mi familia* [my family]. I would like to be able to help my family in the difficult moments. Also, it's important to respect those around me. It's important to be honest."

TRADITIONS. Traditional beliefs and customs have persisted in spite of acculturation into U. S. lifeways. Mexican Americans had re-created a piece of Mexico for themselves in the U. S. county where the study was conducted that reflected a strong attachment to their homeland. One informant spoke again, sharing about cultural and religious traditional values that were important not only for her but also for her to teach her children:

In Christmas, I teach my children the nativity scene. We also put up the tree. We also put up the tree that is a tradition from here. We celebrate the 16th of September, which is important day for us. My youngest argues with me because she's an American, but I tell her that I respect her flag, so that she has to respect ours so we also celebrate the Fourth of July. Another traditional difference is Halloween and Day of Saints. They are celebrated the same day in two types of ways and we celebrate both.

Folk beliefs. The study informants revealed that Mexican American women used a variety of folk medicine practices. Herbs used for the treatment of headache or stomach ache and during *la cuarentena* included arnica; *Mexicana* (camphor weed); *ruda* (rue); *pirul* (pepper tree); *manzanilla* (chamomile); mint; and *romero* (rosemary). Another informant gave the following description of herbal usage during *la cuarentena*:

> Drink the teas for at least three days, arnica, romero, peru, ruba, boil the herbs in water—take a little bit of that drink that to clean yourself and you also have to bathe yourself with that. This takes out all of the air you had in your stomach. Then you bind yourself [with the *faja*] and you have to cover your head as well.

Informants also acknowledged the use of folk healers (*curanderos*). The informant continued by stating, "In my family and my husband's family too… we go to the *curandero* first and then the doctor." However, this informant preferred to see the doctor first: "Personally, for me I always use the doctor first. Not the *curandero* first. I am not accustomed to seeing a *curandero*, but the majority of Mexicans are." Regardless of individual family practices, reliance on folk medicine reflected an inner cultural harmony: One must be in balance with God, family, and spirit.

Informants also described specific folk beliefs and practices, such as avoiding starchy foods to prevent *empacho* (constipation) during the postpartum period. Informants also held several other folk beliefs, such as *mal de ojo* (evil eye). The first informant stated, "Baby wears a bracelet with red bead on it to ward off evil eye." Another informant shared, "*Mal de ojo*. It's when the baby starts crying and their forehead gets warm, not a fever, just heat. Suppression in both eyes. [So far] nothing has happened to my children; I have always dressed them in red."

Prenatal beliefs. The study informants also stated that they believed in obtaining prenatal care in the U. S., although it was not always an option in Mexico or may not have been seen as necessary because pregnancy is viewed in Mexican culture as a natural event. In addition, among Mexicans the prenatal period has many "old wives tales" and folk beliefs, such as those held by the grandmother of the first informant:

> She said cravings must be satisfied, if not it might "mark the baby." No early baby shower, it brings bad luck. Baby wears a bracelet with red bead on it to ward

off evil eye. Mother follows diet—stay away from spicy foods, hot foods. Mother is to "eat for two." Herbal bath to be done following delivery.

During the prenatal period, all of the informants sought advice first from a respected family member, usually their mother or grandmother, and then the *curandero* or a physician. Another informant confirmed this with her perspective: "I think your mother is the best [person] to provide advice. She has experience and knows about the good and bad things to do since she has been through [life]."

The presence of God in these women's lives was prominent during the intrapartum period and reflected the fatalistic worldview with an external locus of control, including during delivery. Yet another informant stated, "You would just entrust yourself to the Virgin to make sure all goes well." This informant further stated that the doctor told her that her baby might be born with Down Syndrome and because she was very frightened, she turned to prayer, to God, and to the Virgin for support:

> I was scared, but well, I got him, and then I asked the Virgin of Guadalupe for her health, and the baby was fine … I kept prayer all of the time during labor and delivery about that, for religion to give me support.

Postpartum beliefs. The major belief and practice surrounding the postpartum period among Mexican American women was *la cuarentena*. Friends and older women in the family cared for the new mother and baby by providing meals; caring for other children; and helping with routine household tasks. The custom of following some, if not all, of the practices of *la cuarentena* was common among the study informants. Comments by the first informant reflected the magicoreligious paradigm found in *la cuarentena* as well as the limitations of living in the U. S. away from family:

> We have, oh my God, you know we … we are not only religious but superstitious [laughing]. You know, it used to be years ago, I honestly don't follow it, but my Grandmother will tell me, "You are not supposed to wash your hair after you have a baby, because, God forbid, the coldness is gonna get into your body and then years from now you are gonna be in severe pain, from muscles because you are not supposed to do anything." …actually just [the new mother is] supposed to be on bed rest, not do anything. God forbid you touch a broom. …But you see, in Mexico, that's possible. You

can afford to do those things because your family is close to you. In Mexico, you tell family, they take care of you. But here, you know, if my mom is not here, then I am by myself, so I wasn't really able to do what my grandmother wanted me to do.

Differences in living. Informants painted a revealing contrast between life and healthcare in the U. S. and in Mexico. One informant revealed that, in Mexico, all three of her babies were delivered by a doctor from a rural area who came to her home:

Yes, he would go to my house and just come for the delivery. I never got any other care. For my second delivery, he came to my in-laws' home; he told me to go upstairs and I had the baby right then. Where we live, only those with money and insurance go to the hospital.

Another informant also confirmed that lifestyle differences made it difficult to follow *la cuarentena* in the U. S., although it was strictly followed in Mexico:

Yes in Mexico, they stay in bed, are taken care of by the other women in the family, because the women don't work, but here everybody works so it's hard to follow the *cuarentena*. We have an herbal bath after delivery, sometime during the first seven days. I don't remember what herbs they put in, but it's like a sauna and feels so good. Then they wrap you in a blanket. Your hair is also washed in the herbal water, and you are also given some of the same water to drink to cleanse you inside and out.

Machismo. *Machismo* is defined as overly assertive or exaggerated masculine behavior reflected by male behaviors of superiority, dominance, sexual infidelity, aggression, and alcohol consumption. *Machismo* is legitimized by a patriarchal social system that promotes and condones this behavior (Gilmore & Gilmore, 1979; Mayo & Resnick, 1996; Stevens, 1973). While acculturation has changed some aspects of gender roles, informants confirmed the continued presence of *machismo* in Mexican American culture. The first informant discussed how her grandmother cared for her grandfather:

She did everything for him, everything. Even when my grandfather, by the end of his illness, he was still able to do a lot of things for himself …the women of the house took care of him completely. My grandmother, you know I wouldn't do it for my husband, but she would dress

him, and you know, I'm talking about when you are 50 years old, and completely healthy. She would help him shower, she would dress him, don't ask me why …she never did mention it …that's the way she was.

Motherhood. All of the informants believed that to be a mother and care for their children was their sole purpose in life. One informant shared that, "…Having children is something beautiful, something sacred." For most, their children were more important to them than their husbands. The first informant confirmed this value:

They are the reason that I live for. My children are the most important and valuable things that I have; I would do anything for them … I never imagined myself without children, like I wouldn't have children.

Circle of violence. Domestic violence is rarely spoken about within the Mexican American culture, although one-in-three Latinas report experiencing it (Breiding, Chen, & Black, 2014; Clark, Galano, Grogan-Kaylor, Motalvo-Liendo, & Graham-Bermann, 2014). The trust developed among the informants, the interpreter, and the researcher enabled the informants to reveal verbal and physical abuse as a pervasive cultural problem (Hascup, 2011). For some, domestic violence appeared following the birth of a baby. When one informant came home from the hospital and was resting in bed after having their baby, her husband made her get up out of bed and cook for him and threatened physical abuse if she did not. The informants believed that the *circle of violence* was created and perpetuated by the mother, a concept supported by the research findings of some psychologically-oriented anthropologists (Gilmore & Gilmore, 1979). Another informant stated, "Mothers perpetuate it because they treat the boys differently. It is that way in Mexico. Men are treated differently, they are treated better."

Gender roles. Gender roles were clearly defined within Mexican American culture of the informants. Children were expected to respect to their elders; be honest, obedient, and polite–not "talk back" to adults. The male was the decision maker and financial provider for the family. The female was wife, mother, and caretaker of the home, children, and family. Although gender roles were undergoing some transformation within the U. S. population (Knapp, Muller, & Quiros,

2009), one informant stated that in Mexico the men preferred to have the women stay at home:

> [The men] don't give [the women] much money to dress, to eat, and they don't like them to go out, and for the woman to obey the husband. The men always bring just enough to eat, but they love to drink in Mexico. Very few women actually go out to work in my country. Back in Mexico, the men want to keep the women at home.

HEALTH. *General health* as defined by the informants focused on their ability to be active in daily activities, regardless of how they actually felt physically or emotionally, and included thinking positive thoughts, relying on God, eating healthy, and exercising. One informant stated, "Good health is just being able to do your everyday chores, being able to get out and take a walk if you'd like." Another informant shared that she asks God for help in terms of health: "…I think it's up to God to whether I am healthy or not, and that if I get sick it's in God's hands."

MELANCOLÍA DE BEBÉ (BABY BLUES) AND DEPRESION POSTPARTO (POSTPARTUM DEPRESSION). Almost half of the informants self-reported experiencing *melancolía de bebé* (baby blues) and felt depression in the postpartum period. None received medical treatment for their symptoms.

One informant described her feelings:

> I think that I felt… alone…I felt sad, um…not helpless, because I kind of at the same time thought that I had my son and he was the one that was giving me happiness, but…I felt like in the sense I didn't have anyone to share it with.

CARING AND NONCARING BEHAVIORS. The informants' perspective of caring and noncaring behaviors also emerged from the data. The first informant stated, "Caring—care means support, people show care by calling you to see how you are, what can they do for you, do you need anything." For another informant, caring was "…others being there for you, asking how you are, calling you—just being interested." Noncaring for this informant was not being interested; she provided an example of her sister not taking the time to pick up the phone to see if she needed anything, to see if she wanted to talk, or to ask how she felt.

> …I think with my sister, she is so busy with her job, she has so much on her mind with my grandfather, my

mother being there, worrying about how my mother is doing … coming home to her family, she doesn't have enough time to …maybe …I know she thinks of me but it's not how I want it …I don't think it takes much time …

This informant also shared the following regarding noncaring behavior:

> …before they let the baby's father in, they started [the cesarean section], and I was scared, and one of the nurses came in and held my hand and [said], "Oh, don't do it too hard, you are going to break my hand." …It wasn't a caring remark and it wasn't professional…No, they were not interested in me! I was shaking, I was trembling, and I remember perfectly well the shakes. When it was time that my daughter was coming, I didn't have the attention from the nurses or the doctor. I feel they just let me suffer. They gave me no pain medication, nothing.

Patterns

Six patterns of care were synthesized from the descriptors in the raw data following the guidelines for the second and third phases of Leininger's Data Analysis Enabler (Wehbe-Alamah & McFarland, 2015, p. 89): The importance of the family; belief in God as protector, provider, and source of comfort and strength in everyday life; seeking knowledge from the elder women in the family to maintain maternal and infant health and wellbeing; maintaining traditional values; caring as "doing" for new mothers; and non-caring as "not showing interest" (Hascup, 2011, p. 116).

PATTERN 1: THE IMPORTANCE OF THE FAMILY. Categories supporting this pattern are family; religion and God; and everyday life (Hascup, 2011, p. 116). For the study informants, the family, or *la familia,* was the foundation of Mexican American culture, as every aspect of life revolves around it. One informant stated, "I think in the Mexican culture and I see it in my family… family, it's everything. The family provides for every–and any--support you need, emotionally and financially."

PATTERN 2: BELIEF IN GOD AS PROTECTOR, PROVIDER, AND SOURCE OF COMFORT AND STRENGTH IN EVERYDAY LIFE. This pattern is supported by the categories of family; religion and God; everyday life; values; traditions; prenatal beliefs; intrapartum beliefs; and health (Hascup, 2011, p. 117). All of the informants believed that God was in full control of every aspect their lives, but they also stated that they have to do their part. Another informant shared, "The most important thing is to believe in God. If you believe in God, everything will go well."

PATTERN 3: SEEKING KNOWLEDGE FROM THE ELDER WOMEN IN THE FAMILY TO MAINTAIN MATERNAL AND INFANT HEALTH AND WELLBEING. This pattern is supported by the categories of family; religion and God; traditions; folk beliefs; prenatal beliefs; intrapartum beliefs; postpartum beliefs; gender roles; values; caring and non-caring behavior; and differences in living (Hascup, 2011, p. 118). Informants revealed a strong respect for elder women, both family and friends, and relied on them during the childbirth continuum. Their advice and support provided a cloak of protection for mother and baby. Yet another informant conveyed her family's beliefs about pregnancy and the postpartum period:

> Mother would tell me to not get upset. There's also a belief to not eat everything you crave because then the child is born with its mouth always open. We have a Mexican believe that after birth we take a bath in herbs.

PATTERN 4: MAINTAINING TRADITIONAL VALUES. This pattern was supported by the categories of family; religion and God; valores (values); folk beliefs; traditions; differences in living; everyday life; gender roles; health; motherhood; prenatal beliefs; intrapartum beliefs; postpartum beliefs; melancholia de bebé (baby blues); and *despresion postparto* (postpartum depression; Hascup, 2011). For the informants, traditional values included not only the intrinsic personal, moral, and societal *valores* (values) such as respect and honesty, but also included traditional values and practices related to the entire childbirth continuum. *La cuarentena* was the most significant postpartum practice discussed by informants, who indicated that it was disturbing for them to be unable to adhere to *la cuarentena* practices as described by their mothers and grandmothers. The first informant stated:

> …when you have a baby, there are family and friends that will help you and you can follow the traditional practices. This is not possible here. Everyone works, many do not have their moms or grandmothers here, so it is difficult.

PATTERN 5: CARING AS "DOING" FOR NEW MOTHERS. This pattern was supported by the categories of family; traditions; caring and noncaring behaviors; folk beliefs; prenatal beliefs; intrapartum beliefs; postpartum beliefs; machismo; gender roles; and health (Hascup,

2011, p 120). The concept of care for the informants was action-oriented. The act of doing included "showing interest," which was perceived as caring. One informant stated that for a new mother, caring is "giving actions, not material [things]." Confirming this, another informant described what she believed caring to be:

> When my husband sees that I'm sick during pregnancy or after delivery he takes care of me carefully; he would go to the pharmacy and get my medicine. My sisters through the phone or coming to visit me–they take care of me. When I lost my baby, my sister came to cook. When my babies were born, my sisters come over to help with the children. They do things for me.

PATTERN 6: NONCARING AS "NOT SHOWING INTEREST." This pattern was supported by the categories of family and caring and noncaring behaviors (Hascup, 2011, p 121). Lack of interest was typically interpreted as noncaring. One informant stated, "…It feels bad if a person doesn't care for you, then they don't call you or doesn't show any interest." Informants also shared their perception that healthcare providers who did not speak Spanish demonstrated noncaring behavior by not attempting to communicate with them in their own language. Another informant revealed that she perceived healthcare providers to be noncaring because they did not speak Spanish to her; she did not speak English and a translator was not provided during these interactions.

Themes
From these patterns were derived three major themes, as follows:

THEME 1: GOD, PRAYER, AND FAMILY ARE THE BASE OF EVERYTHING IN LIFE AND PROVIDED SUPPORT, STRENGTH, AND PROTECTION FOR DEALING WITH THE TRIALS AND TRIBULATIONS OF EVERYDAY LIFE, WHICH WERE DISCOVERED AS BEING INTENSIFIED DURING THE POSTPARTUM PERIOD. This universal theme is supported by the patterns of *the importance of* la familia; belief in God as protector and provider; seeking knowledge from elder women in the family; and maintaining traditional values (Hascup, 2011). The informants' deep spirituality was revealed by their constant prayer, especially during postpartum. The informants in this study identified that God, prayer, and family were interwoven and provided support for dealing with the trials and tribulations of everyday life, which were intensified during the postpartum period. Their deep faith and spirituality was revealed by constant prayer, especially during postpartum (p. 122). One informant shared, "...Every day I would pray, but after the first [delivery], I had complications and I would pray more because I became very sick."

Another Informant stated that her mother and significant other were not supportive of her, and she prayed constantly after delivery to *La Virgen* and God, "Now is the time where I will go to church often, I would ask the Virgen and God to help me through this, I would pray her and God ... ." A third informant confirmed the importance of *La Virgen de Guadalupe* and prayer: "In Mexico, we believe a lot in the Virgin of Guadalupe and you can see when we all get together to pray to her during her day." This woman also shared that she prayed more after delivery not simply for herself but because of her concerns for her baby.

It is noteworthy that, for the majority of the informants, religion and God were separate. The informants connected religion with attending formal church services. All informants except one were Roman Catholic, but none attended church services on a regular basis. Informants expressed that in Mexico, they were more likely to attend church on a regular basis, as one woman stated: "In Mexico, I would go to church every day, but here I have gotten away a little a bit from it, I don't know why, I still have faith." Regardless of church attendance, God offered a sense of security in daily life for the informants, many of whom prayed daily for protection, faith, and strength (p. 123). This belief was repeated throughout the interviews by all informants.

THEME 2: PROTECTION OF THE MOTHER WAS TRANSMITTED INTERGENERATIONALLY BY THE ELDER MEXICAN AMERICAN WOMEN AND INFLUENCED BY RELIGION, FOLK AND FAMILY BELIEFS AND PRACTICES. This theme is supported by the following patterns of la familia; belief in God as protector and provider; seeking knowledge from elder women in the family; maintaining traditional values; and caring as "doing" (Hascup, 2011, p 123). The informants relied completely on the wisdom and advice of the elder women in the family or among female friends (both in Mexico and the U. S.) during all phases of the childbirth continuum but more so during the postpartum.

Informants shared their feelings of vulnerability as first-time mothers and felt comforted and protected by the elder women and by traditional postpartum beliefs and rituals such as *la cuarentena*. The informants did attempt to adhere to these traditional rituals and practices but acculturation into the lifeways of the U. S. often limited them from doing so. The first informant stated, "Without my mom or grandmother after delivery made it impossible for me to follow grandmother's traditions." Religion and folk practices were also influential during the postpartum period as confirmed by another informant:

> I prayed every day for a safe delivery and a quick recovery. [My mother and grandmother] took me to shower when I had my first daughter. My mom took me a shower with weeds, not with a lot of them, but I don't remember the name of them. I felt good when they took me a shower with water and that I was able to recuperate very quickly. It felt good that they took me a shower.

Many of the study informants did not have mothers, grandmothers, or aunts present in the United States and relied on either friends or sisters-in-law during the postpartum period, revealing a "family of women" who provided support (p. 124). One informant stated that she came to the United States while she was pregnant, "...but since I did not have the support of my grandmother, mother, and aunts, I returned to Mexico to have the baby, and then I returned to the United States after *La Cuarentena*." Another informant stated that she also had no grandmother or mother here, so she relied on her sister-in-law for help: "She helps me with my children a lot, and after I had the babies and any problems I may have with the family or if I need advice, I go to my sister-in-law."

The influence of religion and folk practices were also present during the postpartum period.

One informant described her reliance on religion and family practices for protection:

> I am constantly asking God to help me with the pregnancy, the delivery ... hopefully all will go well during labor, and the baby, and that everything will be ok. Once the baby is born, after a month, I go to church, and I feel that definitely take that baby to God and thank him for allowing the child to be ok and for having him. That's my custom and my mother's and my sister's as well.

Many informants also confirmed the folk practice of herbal baths after delivery, as one woman shared:

> You can do one or the other, either sauna with alcohol and Sulphur, or herbal bath. The herbal bath is more effective, but some people prefer the other. You go to a steam bath; they bathe us there with the herbs. That helps get us clean. They say that when you are having a baby your bones are separated, so the steam bath helps the bones with the warm air. We also believe that woman that can't get pregnant should take those baths to help them have a baby. Those are beliefs we have; we don't know if they work or not, but we still do them.

Another informant described a *temescal* bath, which is a very hot vapor bath using the earth:

> They give us an herbal bath. They add rosemary and a holy herb to boiling water. They cover us so that we sweat it in. It is believed that this helps with the cooking the milk for the baby. Otherwise, the baby will get sick and get diarrhea.

Another described the bath she received:

> It's like a steam bath. They usually recommend to do it during the 40 days, I recently did it and you feel the difference. You sweat a lot cause it's a steam bath with all of those herbs that's melting, and it relaxes your body, and they wrap you around with blankets with a lot of heavy blankets after you get out of the bath…they wrap you as soon as you get out. You don't even dry yourself; you only dry your face. And you'd be wrapped from head to toe.

A third informant stated she helped her daughters after their delivery, although they did not believe in the traditional practices:

> I didn't feel sad; they think differently and I have to respect that. I cannot force my beliefs on them. I did help them for 3 weeks. I would feed them, Help them with the baby, and take care of them. …My mom would say the bath was to help your body get strong. They didn't believe in that, so maybe their body is not strong now.

Regarding superstitions, protection of the baby from "evil eye" or *mal de ojo* is very important, as one informant shared:

> Evil eye—*mal de ojo*—I believe in that, when the baby is born I use a red bracelet (hand or foot) or under the T-shirt, or use the T-shirt backward, break an egg in water to see if the baby had a problem. Then, you give the baby an egg bath.

THEME 3: SHOWING INTEREST, BEING ATTENTIVE, CARRYING OUT "ACTS OF DOING" AND SPEAKING SPANISH INDICATE RESPECTFUL BEHAVIOR AND ARE CENTRAL TO THE MEANING OF CARE. This theme is supported by the following patterns of la familia; maintaining traditional values; caring as "doing;" and noncaring as not showing interest (Hascup, 2011, p 126). Theme 3 speaks to relational aspects of caring for postpartum Mexican American women. Mexican American informants described showing respect; being attentive to; carrying out acts of "doing;" and speaking Spanish as the best way to express care to an individual. The Spanish verb *attender* translates "to care for or look after," which was the verb informants most commonly used to describe caring behavior. Caring acts by family and friends during the postpartum period included helping with the new mother and baby; helping with household tasks; cooking, and caring for other children (p. 127). *Caring* for these women was taking action, and the action of doing something for the new mother would assist her during the postpartum period as well as show interest in her [as a person]. Telephone calls, visits, keeping in touch, and asking how they were doing were all perceived as indications of caring and interest. One informant defined caring acts as being: "…to take care of me and be considerate. I would like for them to help me and cook and help me with the baby so that I can sleep." Another woman stated, "Right now, since I had the baby, my mom always shows she cares for me, and she always calls. She has seen me through all of my pregnancies when the babies were born." A third informant added: "…My family who would me call ask me how I am doing, and my friends – just one friend who is religious who always calls me, the nurse that takes care of my daughter."

Healthcare providers who spoke to the women while maintaining eye contact; answered their questions; showed an interest in their lives; and spoke Spanish were perceived to be caring individuals. One informant described an act of caring by a nurse at the hospital who was caring for her after delivery: "…A nurse that worked in St. Joseph's, her name was Ana. She gave me a stamp of the Divine Child of Jesus; it's very miraculous. Most children could die, but my daughter is healthy."

Healthcare providers who spoke Spanish were very important to the informants. One informant perceived caring behavior from her healthcare providers to be as she described:

> Yes, the doctors will sit down next to me and start talking to me. They would ask me where did I work and what I do. They gave me trust, and I trusted them too. They would tell me everything was going to be okay, and …They would tell me since it was my first time not to be scared. I had good support, and that was important. By sitting next to me and talking to me not like a doctor but as a friend and speaking to me in Spanish.

The informants believed respectful behavior to be listening to them; allowing them to ask questions; explaining information to them; and acknowledging and addressing their individual needs and concerns (p. 127). Another informant stated:

> The majority of the doctors, they treat me very well. They are not Hispanic, one is Filipino, the other is Dominican, both speak Spanish. If they don't speak Spanish, the nurse will translate for me, but I am not sure she is saying everything the doctor is saying. It is much better if I can communicate directly with the doctor. Then, I can be sure of what he is saying.

Noncaring behavior for all of the informants was "not doing" such as not calling; not visiting; not asking if the new mother needed anything at all; and not showing interest in the new mother. One informant described noncaring behavior as follows:

> Not to call me, I don't receive any mail [from Mexico], and if there is something they know I like to eat … if none of those things are happening, then I know that people don't care, I am not important to them.

Leininger's Three Modes of Culture Care Decisions and Actions

The three modes of culture care decisions and actions are used by the researcher with cultural informants or clinicians during assessment care practices to discuss and discover how to provide culturally congruent, beneficial, and meaningful care to clients (Leininger, 2002c, p. 78). According to the theorist (Leininger, 2002c, p. 78), the modes may be used singly, in pairs, or all three together with clients in a coparticipative manner to identify appropriate care that fits with their cultural values, beliefs, and lifeways (p. 78). These three care modes are culture care preservation and/or maintenance; culture care accommodation and/or negotiation; and culture care repatterning and/or restructuring. A major

care difference with Leininger's theory compared to other theories was that the use of the three theoretically based decision and action modes enabled nurses to provide culturally congruent care in a creative way to Mexican and Mexican American women during the postpartum period.

Culture care preservation and/or maintenance refers "…to those assistive, supportive, facilitative, or enabling professional acts or decisions that help cultures to retain, preserve, or maintain beneficial care beliefs and values or to face handicaps and death" (Leininger & McFarland, 2006a, p. 8). Nurses and other healthcare providers must recognize the key values that are important in the Mexican American culture. Nurses must also understand the importance of family religion, faith, and God within this culture for maintaining health and wellbeing as well as their very strong adherence to folk beliefs and practices, particularly during the postpartum phase of delivery. Culturally knowledgeable nurses will be able to provide culturally competent, congruent, sensitive, and safe postpartum care in the hospital or community settings and ensure both patient satisfaction and positive clinical outcomes.

Culture care accommodation and/or negotiation are "…those assistive, accommodating, facilitative, or enabling creative provider actions or decisions that help cultures adapt to or negotiate with others for culturally congruent, safe, and effective care for their health, wellbeing, or to deal with illness or dying" (Leininger & McFarland, 2006a, p. 8). Within the current maternal-child hospital setting, nurses still adhere to many outdated "sacred cows" such as rigidly restricted visiting hours. Informants shared experiences of having to labor and deliver alone, and about how frightening it was for them to not have anyone explaining procedures in Spanish. Nurses need to proactively seek ways to negotiate and accommodate family into the plan of care because family support is what comprises caring and security for Mexican American women. Similarly, many less acculturated Mexican American men do not want to be present during labor or delivery because of their cultural perspective that this is "women's domain." Nurses need to recognize this belief, avoid passing judgment, and maintain open communication with expectant fathers while they are waiting for their wives to deliver. Understanding the importance of adhering to the "hot-cold" theory particularly during the postpartum period is an imperative–not doing so undermines a key cultural value of maintaining balance and harmony in health to promote recovery.

Culture care repatterning and/or restructuring refers to "...those assistive, supportive, facilitative, or enabling professional actions and mutual decisions that would help reorder, change, modify, or restructure the patient's lifeway or the healthcare institution for better healthcare patterns, practices, or outcomes" (Leininger & McFarland, 2006a, p. 8). Repatterning and/or restructuring harmful generic care practices of Mexican American postpartum women required having an established trusting relationship between patient and nurse. Nurses must take the time to show interest in and gain knowledge about Mexican American women's postpartum beliefs and practices. For example, some herbal remedies used by Mexican American women may be harmful, especially if combined with prescribed medications. Nurses need to gain knowledge of such remedies in order to be able to accurately and sensitively repattern or restructure their use of contraindicated herbal or generic care remedies to prevent harmful outcomes by providing information to the patient and her family.

■ DISCUSSION

The interconnectedness of categories, patterns, themes, and descriptors reflected the overarching components of worldview present within the Mexican American culture that directly influenced the postpartum experiences of the informants (Refer to Figure 24.3). The three themes discussed above represented the worldview of Mexican American women interviewed during this study. Nurses need to improve their cultural competency by understanding this worldview because it influences the postpartum experience for Mexican American women. In addition, cultural competence enables nurses to better provide their patients with professional care knowledge about the antepartum and intrapartum periods. Most importantly, by understanding how worldview influences all three periods of the delivery process the nurse can provide culturally congruent, sensitive, and competent care that is holistic, meaningful, and beneficial to Mexican American women.

Theoretical Implications of the Study

The Theory of Culture Care Diversity and Universality with the Ethnonursing Research Method served as the philosophical, theoretical, and analytical foundations for this study. Both the theory and the method provided the researcher with the means to discover rich, detailed, and covert emic data vitally important to gaining an understanding of the specific folk beliefs and practices of Mexican American women during the postpartum period. Serendipitous findings included the discovery of additional in-depth cultural data about the beliefs and practices of informants during the antepartum and intrapartum periods. This study supported the importance of understanding the worldview and social structure dimensions of Mexican American women from within a naturalistic environmental context. The Mexican American culture has both generic care and professional care knowledge that differ from Anglo American cultural practices. Mexican American beliefs have similarities and differences with Mexican that have changed over time and yet continue to influence postpartum generic care beliefs, values, expressions, and practices. The findings from this study have contributed to the body of transcultural nursing knowledge about the care meanings and experiences of Mexican American women during the postpartum period and the cultural context of their care regarding health, illness, and wellbeing.

Implications for Nursing Practice, Research, and Education

This research study highlighted the fact that there was no extant nursing research pertinent to the stated Domain of Inquiry. Without such cultural knowledge about the postpartum period, nurses cannot effectively provide culturally congruent, and sensitive, and competent care that is meaningful and beneficial to postpartum Mexican American women. The study supported the importance of combining generic care with professional care to promote health among postpartum Mexican American Mexican American women.

However, simply adding to the body of nursing knowledge in this domain of inquiry is not sufficient. All nurse researchers have an ethical and moral responsibility to disseminate their research findings in a clear and understandable way to illustrate their relevance in clinical practice to nurses who care for people from diverse cultures–in this case, postpartum Mexican American women and the findings of the study discussed in this chapter. Most importantly, nurses must be educated about transcultural nursing, the conduct of transcultural nursing research, and the application of the Theory of Cultural Diversity and Universality across the spectrum of nursing practice, education, administration, and research.

■ SUMMARY

In Mexican American culture, meanings and expressions of postpartum culture care are embedded in their worldview, language, social structure, and environmental context. To provide holistic care that is culturally congruent, sensitive, and competent for this population, it is important for nurses to understand the perspectives of Mexican American women regarding care and caring (and noncaring) behaviors during all three phases of the childbirth continuum, but especially during the postpartum when cultural beliefs and practices are heightened.

■ DEDICATION

This chapter is dedicated to my late husband, William, who died just as I entered the dissertation phase of my research study. William so hoped he would see me finish my PhD, but it was not meant to be. My love, my confidante, my closest friend, my everything—this is for you. You earned it as much as I did.

■ ACKNOWLEDGEMENTS

I am especially indebted to Dr. Rick Zoucha who worked tirelessly in helping me understand Leininger's theory and the ethnonursing research method. An ancient metaphysical proverb states, "When the student is ready, the teacher will appear." I was ready to learn, and Rick encouraged me to reach beyond anything I ever thought possible. Rick epitomizes for me what a professor should be.

I would also like to acknowledge the Transcultural Nursing Society, Epsilon Phi, and Duquesne University's Carmella Zoucha Research Award for their partial funding of my dissertation.

■ DISCUSSION QUESTIONS

1. Discuss how Leininger's three care decision and action modes can be used in providing care to postpartum Mexican American women in clinical practice. Give specific examples for each one of the decision and action modes.
2. Discuss how *your* understanding of the lifeways, cultural beliefs, and practices of Mexican American women can lead to providing culturally sensitive, appropriate, and congruent care.
3. Discuss the importance of family in the Mexican American culture and how it influences care delivery to childbearing Mexican American women. Give specific examples.
4. Using critical thinking skills, discuss how providing culturally congruent care can lead to patient satisfaction and positive patient outcomes in prenatal, intrapartum, and postpartum Mexican American women. Be specific.
5. Describe and discuss the differences between the postpartum period in Mexican American women and Anglo American women.

■ REFERENCES

Beck, C. (2002). Revision of the postpartum depression predictors inventory. *Journal of Obstetric, Gynecological, and Neonatal Nursing, 31*(4), 394-402.

Beck, C., Froman, R. D., & Bernal, H. (2005). Acculturation level and postpartum depression in Hispanic mothers. *American Journal of Maternal Child Nursing, 30*(5), 299-304.

Beck, C., & Gable, R. K. (2000). Postpartum depression screening scale: Development and psychometric testing. *Nursing Research, 49*(5), 272-282.

Beck, C., & Gable, R. K. (2003). Postpartum depression screening scale: Spanish version. *Nursing Research, 52*(5), 296-306.

Berry, A. (1996). *Culture care expressions, meanings and experiences of pregnant Mexican American women within Leininger's culture care theory* (Unpublished doctoral dissertation). Wayne State University, Detroit, MI.

Berry, A. (1999). Mexican American women's expressions of the meaning of culturally congruent prenatal care. *Journal of Transcultural Nursing, 10*(3), 203-212. doi: 10.1177/104365969901000311

Berry, A. (2002). Culture care of the Mexican American family. In M. M. Leininger and M. R. McFarland (Eds.), *Transcultural nursing: Concepts, theories, research and practice* (3rd ed., pp. 363-373). New York: McGraw Hill.

Bobak, I. M., Perry, S. E., & Lowdermilk, D. L. (2000). *Maternity and women's health care* (7th ed.). St. Louis, MO: Mosby.

Boyle, J. S. (2011). *Transcultural concepts in nursing care* (6th ed.). New York, NY: Wolters Kluwer|Lippincott Williams & Wilkins.

Breiding, M., Chen, J., & Black, M. (2014). *Intimate partner violence in the United States – 2010*. Atlanta, GA: National Center for Injury Prevention and Control, Centers for Disease Control and Prevention.

Brown, A., & Patten, E. (2015). *Statistical portrait of Hispanics living in the United States, 2012*. Washington, DC: Pew Research Center. Retrieved from http://www.pewhispanic.org/2014/04/29/hispanic-nativity-shift/

Callister, L. C. (2005). What has the literature taught us about culturally competent care of women and children? *American Journal of Child Nursing, 30*(6), 380-388.

Clark, H., Galano, M., Grogan-Kaylor, A., Montalvo-Leindo, N., & Graham-Bermann, S. (2014, November 11). Ethnoracial variation in women's exposure to intimate partner violence. [Published online ahead of print]. *Journal of Interpersonal Violence, 33*(3), 531-552. doi: 10.1177/0886260514555871

Grove, S., Burns, N., & Gray. J. (2013). *Practice of nursing research: Appraisal, synthesis and generation of evidence* (7th ed.). New York, NY: Elsevier.

Cristancho, S., Garces, M., Peters, K., & Mueller, B. (2008). Listening to rural Hispanic Immigrants in the Midwest: A community-based participatory assessment of major barriers to healthcare access and use. *Qualitative Health Research, 18*(5), 633-46. doi: 10.1177/1049732308316669

dePacheco, M. R., & Hutti, M. H. (1998). Cultural beliefs and health care practices of childbearing Puerto Rican Women and Mexican American women: A review of the literature. *Mother Baby Journal, 3*(1), 14-23.

Galanti, G. (2004). *Caring for patients from different cultures* (3rd ed.). Philadelphia, PA: University of Pennsylvania Press.

Gallo, A. (2003). *The lived experience of Latina women giving birth in the United States*. (Doctoral dissertation). Available from ProQuest Dissertations and Theses database. (UMI No. 3088659)

Gilmore, M., & Gilmore, D. (1979). "Machismo": A psychodynamic approach. *Journal of Psychological Anthropology, 2*(3), 281-299.

Gonzalez-Barrera, A., & Lopez, M. H. (2013). *Pew research Hispanic trends project: Appendix A: Geographic distribution of Mexican immigrants in the U. S.* Washington, DC: Pew Research Center.

Gonzalez-Swafford, M. J., & Gutierrez, M. G. (1983). Ethnomedical beliefs and practices of Mexican Americans. *The Nurse Practitioner Journal, 8*(10), 29-38.

Hartweg, D., & Isabelli-Garcia, C. (2007). Health perceptions of low-income, immigrant Spanish-speaking Latinas in the United States. *Hispanic Health Care International, 5*(2), 53-63. doi: 10.1891/154041507780978914

Hascup, V. A. (2011). *Cultural expressions, meanings, beliefs, and practices of Mexican American women during the postpartum period: An ethnonursing study*. (Doctoral dissertation). Available from ProQuest Dissertations and Theses database. (UMI No. 863965498)

Johnson, C. A. (2005). *Understanding the culture care practices of rural immigrant Mexican American women*. (Doctoral dissertation). Available from ProQuest Dissertations and Theses database. (UMI No. 317585)

Humes, K. R., Jones, N. A., & Ramirez, R. R. (2011, March). *Overview of race and Hispanic origin: 2010* [2010 Census Brief]. Washington, DC: U. S. Department of Commerce, Economics and Statistics Administration, Census Bureau.

Kay, M. (1980). Mexican, Mexican American, and Chicana childbirth as seen in eHRAF Collection of Ethnography on the Web, Document Number 51, 2002 computer file. In M. B. Melville (Ed.), *Twice a minority: Mexican American women* (pp. 52-65). St. Louis: Mosby.

Kim-Godwin, Y. S. (2003). Beliefs and practices among non-Western cultures. *The American Journal of Maternal Child Nursing, 28*, 74-80.

Knapp, J., Muller, B., & Quiros, A. (2009). Men, women, and the changing role of gender in immigration. *Institute for Latino Studies, University of Notre Dame, 3*(3), 1-14. Retrieved from https://latinostudies.nd.edu/assets/95245/original/3.3_gender_migration.pdf

Leininger, M. M. (2002a). Culture care assessments for congruent competency practices. In M. M. Leininger and M. R. McFarland (Eds.), *Transcultural nursing: Concepts, theories, research & practice* (3rd ed., pp. 117-143). New York, NY: McGraw-Hill.

Leininger, M. M. (2002b). Essential transcultural nursing care concepts, principles, examples, and policy statements. In M. M. Leininger and M. R. McFarland (Eds.), *Transcultural nursing: Concepts, theories, research & practice* (3rd ed., pp. 45-69). New York, NY: McGraw-Hill.

Leininger, M. M. (2002c). Part I. The theory of culture care and the ethnonursing research method. In M. M. Leininger and M. R. McFarland (Eds.), *Transcultural nursing: Concepts, theories, research & practice* (3rd ed., pp. 71-98). New York, NY: McGraw-Hill.

Leininger, M. M. (2006a). Culture Care Diversity and Universality and evolution of the ethnonursing method. In M. M. Leininger and M. R. McFarland (Eds.), *Culture care diversity and universality: A worldwide nursing theory* (3rd ed., pp. 1-41). Sudbury, MA: Jones & Bartlett.

Leininger, M. M. (2006b). Ethnonursing research method and enablers [Revised reprint]. In M. M. Leininger and M. R. McFarland (Eds.), *Culture care diversity and universality: A worldwide nursing theory* (3rd ed., pp. 43-81). Sudbury, MA: Jones & Bartlett.

Lopez, R. A. (2005). Use of alternative folk medicine by Mexican American women. *Journal of Immigrant Health, 7*(1), 23-31. doi: 10.1007/s10903-005-1387-8

Luna, J. L. (1989). *Care and cultural context of Lebanese Muslims in an urban U. S. community: An ethnographic and ethnonursing study conceptualized within Leininger's theory* (Unpublished doctoral dissertation). Wayne State University, Detroit, MI.

Mayo, Y. Q., & Resnick, R. P. (1996). The impact of machismo on Hispanic women. *AFFILIA: Journal of Women and Social Work, 11*(3), 257-277. doi: 10.77/088610999601100301

McGlade, M. S., Somnath, S., & Dahlstrom, M. (2004). The Latina paradox: An opportunity for restructuring prenatal care delivery. *American Journal of Public Health, 94*(12), 2062-2065. doi: 10.2105/AJPH.94.12.2062

Mead, M. (1935). *Sex and temperament in three primitive societies.* New York, NY: Harper Collins.

Melville, M. B. (1980). *Twice a minority: Mexican American women* (pp. 11-16). St. Louis, MO: Mosby. Retrieved from eHRAF Collection of Ethnography, Document No. 48, Kean University eHRAF database.

Mendelson-Klauss, C. (2000). *Mexican American women's struggle to create health.* (Doctoral dissertation). Available from ProQuest Dissertations and Theses database. (UMI No. 9992091)

Mendelson, C. (2002). Health perceptions of Mexican American women. *Journal of Transcultural Nursing, 13*(3), 210-217. doi: 10.1177/10459602013003010

Purnell, L., & Paulanka, B. (2003). *Transcultural health care: A culturally competent approach* (2nd ed.). Philadelphia, PA: Davis.

Ramirez, A. G., & Suarez, L. (2007). Cancer in Mexican American women: Key points (2007). In National Cancer Institute Cancer Control and Populations Sciences (Ed): National Cancer Institutes of the U. S. National Institutes of Health. Bethesda: Maryland. Retrieved from http://cancercontrol.cancer.gov/womenofcolor/pdfs/mexican-chapter.pdf

Rojas, D. Z. (1991). *Perceived health status, spiritual well-being, and selected health practices among Mexican-American women.* (Unpublished doctoral dissertation, Texas Woman's University, Denton.) Retrieved from Photocopy, Ann Arbor, MI: University Microfilms International, 1992, 135 p.; 22 cm.

Sanchez, M. S. (1997). *Pathways to health: A naturalistic study of Mexican-American women's lay health behaviors.* (Doctoral dissertation). Available from ProQuest Dissertations and Theses database. (UMI No. 9822698)

Stern, G., & Kruckman, L. (1983). Multi-disciplinary perspectives on post-partum depression: An anthropological critique. *Social Science and Medicine, 17*(15), 1027-1041. doi: 10.1016/0277-9536(83)90408-2

Stevens, E. (1973). Machismo and marianismo. *Society, 10*(6), 57-63. doi: 10.1007/BF02695282

Wehbe-Alamah, H. B., & McFarland, M. R. (2015). Leininger's enablers for use with the ethnonursing research method. In M. R. McFarland and H. B. Wehbe-Alamah (Eds.)., *Leininger's theory of culture care diversity and universality: A worldwide nursing theory* (3rd ed., pp. 75-97). Burlington, MA: Jones and Bartlett Learning.

Zoucha, R. (1998). The experiences of Mexican Americans receiving professional care: An ethnonursing study. *Journal of Transcultural Nursing, 9*(2), 34-44.

Zoucha, R. (2001). President's message. *Journal of Transcultural Nursing, 12*(2), 157.

Zoucha, R., & Zamarripa, C. (2003). People of Mexican heritage. In L. Purnell and B. Paulanka (Eds.), *Transcultural health care: A culturally competent approach* (2nd ed.). Philadelphia, PA: FA Davis.

Zoucha, R., & Zamarripa, C. (2008). People of Mexican heritage. In L. Purnell and B. Paulanka (Eds.), *Transcultural health care: A culturally competent approach* (3rd ed., pp. 374-390). Philadelphia, PA: FA Davis.

CHAPTER 25

Culture Care of Syrian Muslims in the Midwestern United States: An Ethnonursing Research Study

Hiba B. Wehbe-Alamah

> *Your Lord has commanded that you worship none but Him, and that you be kind to your parents. If one or both of them reach old age with you, do not say to them a word of disrespect, or scold them, but say a generous word to them. And act humbly to them in mercy, and say, 'My Lord, have mercy on them, since they cared for me when I was small (The Holy Qur'an- 17: 23-24).*

Revised reprint from Wehbe-Alamah, H. (2011). The use of Culture Care Theory with Syrian Muslims in the Midwestern United States. *Online Journal of Cultural Competence in Nursing and Healthcare, 1*(3), 1-12.

■ INTRODUCTION

Leininger (2002b) predicted that by the year 2020, healthcare worldwide would be based on transcultural principles in order to appropriately care for the needs of diverse people (Leininger, 2002b). The initial impetus for Syrian immigration was the lure of economic opportunity; by 1940, 350,000 persons of Syrian/Lebanese birth were living in the United States (U.S.; Bennett, 2000). According to the U.S. Census Bureau (Asi & Beaulieu, 2013), 147,426 people self-identified their ethnic origin as "Syrian" on the 2006-2010 American Community Survey. However, it is important to keep in mind that the U.S. Census count does not accurately reflect the number of Syrians living in the U.S. as it does not take reflect those Syrians identifying themselves as either White or Asian. In addition, the 2010 Census data do not include the number of Syrian immigrants or refugees who have sought refuge in the U.S. since the beginning of the Syrian Arab Spring Uprising on January 6, 2011.

On that date, a series of small peaceful protests remonstrating the torture of students who had publicly written anti-government graffiti in the city of Daraa escalated into a nationwide Syrian revolution and civil war (Cornell University Library, 2015). Since the beginning of the Syrian war in 2011, 1 in 10 Syrians or 1.88 million have been wounded; more than 20,000 individuals have been detained in regime prisons; about 470,000 Syrians were confirmed as dead (Boghani, 2016) and more than 50% of the Syrian population has been displaced as of the autumn of 2015 (Amnesty International, 2016). About 11 million Syrians have left their homes since the outbreak of the Syrian revolution in 2011, seeking refuge in neighboring and other countries and/or other regions within Syria (Migration Policy Center, 2016). Of these, 2.5 million have immigrated to/sought asylum in Turkey; 1.1 million in Lebanon causing a 25% increase in the country's population; 635,324 in Jordan; 245,022 in Iraq; 117,658 in Egypt; 98,700 in Germany; 64,700 in Sweden; 18,800 in Hungary; 11,300 in Denmark; 7,000 in the United Kingdom; 6,700 in France, and 1,500 in the United States (Amnesty International, 2016; Martinez, 2015). Ten thousand additional Syrians were to be granted refuge in the U.S. in 2016 (Martinez, 2015). Learning about the generic (lay, folk, or indigenous) and professional care meanings, beliefs, and practices related to health and illness of traditional Syrian Muslims living in the U.S. will assist nurses and other healthcare professionals to provide them with culturally congruent and sensitive care.

■ ETHNOHISTORY

The Syrian Arab Republic lies at the Eastern end of the Mediterranean Sea and is bordered to the North by Turkey, to the East by Iraq, to the West by Lebanon and the Mediterranean Sea, to the South by Jordan (Bateman, 2002), and to the Southwest by Palestine/Israel. Present day Syria was once part of a land called Greater Syria, which encompassed Jordan, Lebanon, and Israel in addition to modern Syria (South, 2006). After receiving their independence from the French mandate, people from the regions of Syria and Lebanon immigrating to the U.S. continued to identify themselves as "Syrians" until the 1950s.

It has been estimated that more than 80% of Syrians are Muslim; Christians accounted for 10% of the population and included mainly Syrian Orthodox, Greek Orthodox, Armenian Orthodox but also some Roman Catholic, Protestant, and Russian Orthodox believers (South, 2006). An offshoot group of Islam known as the Druze accounts for approximately 3% of the population (South, 2006). There were also small groups of Jews as well as Yazidis, a sect that combines aspects of Judaism, Christianity, and Islam (South, 2006).

■ PURPOSE, GOAL, AND DOMAIN OF INQUIRY

The domain of inquiry for this ethnonursing research study was the generic and professional care meanings, beliefs, and practices related to the health and illness of Syrian Muslims living in several urban communities in the Midwestern United States. The purpose of this study was to discover, describe, and analyze the influences of worldview, cultural context, technological, religious, political, educational, and economic factors on traditional Syrian Muslims' generic and professional care meanings, beliefs, and practices. The goal of this study was to provide the nurses with holding knowledge for use in the development of care decisions and actions in the provision of culturally congruent care for diverse Syrian Muslims living in urban communities in the Midwestern United States. The major findings from this study are presented in the form of themes, patterns, and descriptors. The generic care practices discovered in this study have been described in another publication (Wehbe-Alamah, 2015).

■ THEORETICAL FRAMEWORK

The theoretical framework for this study was Leininger's Theory of Culture Care Diversity and Universality (also known as the Culture Care Theory or CCT) which holds *care as the essence and unifying focus of nursing* (Leininger, 1991). According to the Culture Care Theory, care is embedded in people's social structure, worldview, language, and environmental context (Leininger, 2006; McFarland & Wehbe-Alamah, 2015). Cultural diversities and universalities about human care exist among and within all cultures worldwide, and discovering culture-specific care knowledge can be used to guide nursing care decisions and actions beneficial to clients' health (Leininger, 2002a). When the cultural care values, beliefs, expressions, and practices for people of diverse or similar cultures are discovered and used in appropriate, sensitive, and meaningful ways, culturally congruent and therapeutic care occurs (Leininger, 2006; McFarland & Wehbe-Alamah, 2015).

■ ETHNONURSING RESEARCH METHOD

Leininger's qualitative ethnonursing research method along with the Culture Care Theory fit well with the goal and purpose of this study. Ethnonursing research is an open discovery and naturalistic people-centered research method developed by Leininger with the goal of teasing out complex and largely unknown people's emic (local) viewpoints about nursing dimensions such as human care, wellbeing, health, and environmental influencers (Leininger, 2006; Wehbe-Alamah & McFarland, 2015). According to Leininger (1991) a major reason for establishing this method was her interest in discovering the differences and similarities of generic care and professional nursing care among diverse cultures.

The study was conducted in several urban Midwestern communities over the period of two years with informant interviews held in locations such as homes, mosques, offices, Middle-Eastern restaurants, and other places of the informants' choosing. Ten key informants (see Table 25.1) and 20 general informants (see Table 25.2) were interviewed for this study. Informants were recruited using the Snowball method as long as they met the following recruitment criteria: 18 years of age or older; born to Syrian parents in any country in the world but later relocated to the U.S. *or* born in the U.S. to Syrian parents; currently living in the U.S.; stated cultural identity as Syrian Muslim; knowledgeable about the domain of inquiry; and willing to participate in the study.

Key informants were considered to be more knowledgeable than general informants about the domain under study and were interviewed on two separate occasions. The interviews lasted anywhere from 45 minutes to 1.5 hours and consisted of asking semi-structured questions derived from Leininger's Semi-Structured Inquiry Guide to Assess Culture Care and Health (Wehbe-Alamah & McFarland, 2015). Consent from the Institutional Review Board was secured and a written consent to participate in the study and audio record interviews was obtained from each of the informants. The use of Leininger's Stranger-to-Trusted-Friend Enabler and the Observation-Participation-Reflection Enabler helped the researcher in establishing with informants; developing sensitivity to the informants' verbal and visual clues; and maintaining the researcher's objectivity during data collection and analysis.

For the purposes of this study, data saturation was reached after interviewing 10 key and 20 general Syrian Muslim informants who ranged between the ages of 18 to 79 years and were knowledgeable about the domain of inquiry. The majority of the informants identified themselves as traditional Syrian Muslims. A written explanation of the study and consent form was read, explained, and given to all informants to sign in either the English or their Arabic language depending upon each informant's stated preference. Informants were given the option of signing their names or leaving a mark on the consent form that was meaningful to them (such as an X) to further preserve the confidentiality of their identity.

TABLE 25.1. Demographic Characteristics of Key Informants.

Informant Codename	Age	Gender	Place of Birth	Years in the U. S.
K01	46	Male	Syria	23
K02	46	Female	Syria	30
K03	46	Male	Syria	13
K04	36	Female	Syria	13
K05	65	Male	Syria	35
K06	38	Female	Saudi Arabia	16
K07	48	Female	Syria	31
K08	42	Female	Syria	15
K09	27	Male	Syria	6
K10	28	Female	Syria	9

Reproduced with permission from Wehbe-Alamah, H. (2011). The use of Culture Care Theory with Syrian Muslims in the Midwestern United States. *Online Journal of Cultural Competence in Nursing and Healthcare, 1*(3), 3.

TABLE 25.2. Demographic Characteristics of General Informants.

Informant Codename	Age	Gender	Place of Birth	Years in the U.S.
G01	32	Female	Syria	15
G02	38	Female	Syria	22
G03	49	Female	Syria	29
G04	42	Female	Syria	12
G05	30	Male	Midwestern U.S.	30
G06	29	Female	Syria	9
G07	33	Female	Syria	10
G08	25	Female	Syria	7
G09	32	Female	Syria	13
G10	64	Female	Syria	1
G11	35	Female	Midwestern U.S.	29
G12	47	Female	Syria	13
G13	23	Male	Midwestern U.S.	18
G14	35	Female	Syria	15
G15	79	Female	Syria	3
G16	44	Female	Syria	28
G17	23	Female	Syria	6
G18	35	Female	Syria	13
G19	29	Female	Syria	10
G20	36	Female	Syria	17

Reproduced with permission from Wehbe-Alamah, H. (2011). The use of Culture Care Theory with Syrian Muslims in the Midwestern United States. *Online Journal of Cultural Competence in Nursing and Healthcare, 1*(3), 4.

Data was collected through field notes, observations, daily journal notes, photographs of material objects, and videotaping informant interviews (while preserving anonymity). All audiotapes were returned to informants following data transcription as is congruent with the Syrian Muslim culture and religion. Rigorous data analysis was conducted through the use of Leininger's Phases of Ethnonursing Analysis for Qualitative Data and the QSR NUD*IST 4 software program for qualitative data analysis. Leininger's (2006) ethnonursing research evaluation criteria of credibility, confirmability, meaning-in-context, recurrent patterning, saturation, and transferability were also used throughout the data analysis.

■ MAJOR RESEARCH FINDINGS AND DISCUSSION

Three major themes (see Table 25.3) were discovered from the data analysis. In the following sections, these themes will be presented with selected patterns and descriptors.

Theme I. Traditional Syrian Muslim Men and Women Share Caregiving Responsibilities and Practices to Promote Healthy Family and Community Lifeways

This universal theme was derived from the informants' worldview and religious and cultural beliefs, values, and practices and was supported by four care patterns and numerous descriptors. One example of a descriptor that supported the care pattern of *deriving pride and satisfaction from caring for others* included an informant statement that "…When you care for your family and friends and neighbors, like cooking for them or giving them medications, Allah is pleased with you, and you are pleased with yourself because you pleased God." Generic care practice exemplars of this pattern were *outstanding hospitality; personally caring for elderly relatives at home versus admitting them to nursing homes; extending confidential financial assistance to the needy; offering sick persons chocolates or flowers when visiting them; delivering home-cooked meals; and caring for the children of sick community members.*

TABLE 25-3. Themes and Related Patterns.

Themes	Related Patterns
I. Traditional Syrian Muslim men and women share caregiving responsibilities and practices to promote healthy family and community lifeways	1. Deriving pride and satisfaction from caring for others 2. Shared care decision-making and practices 3. Caring as being honest, respectful, tolerant, and accommodating of others 4. Caring as worrying about others
II. Traditional Syrian Muslims view caring for family members, friends, all living creatures, and oneself as embedded in religion	1. Caring as an act of worship 2. Caring as family and community unity 3. Caring as being honest, respectful, tolerant, and accommodating of others 4. Caring as worrying about others
III. Traditional Syrian Muslims rely on Islamic spiritual care to promote health and prevent illness	1. Abstaining from noncaring actions according to Islam as preventing illnesses 2. Engaging in caring actions according to Islam to promote physical and psychological health 3. Illness as a caring practice from God 4. Language as a religious protective caring practice

Source: Wehbe-Alamah, H. (2011). The use of Culture Care Theory with Syrian Muslims in the Midwestern United States. *Online Journal of Cultural Competence in Nursing and Healthcare, 1*(3), 5-9.

The care pattern of *shared care decision-making and practices* reflected some commonalities as well as diversities. While both Syrian Muslim men and women similarly engaged in the provision of emotional and physical care, the men tended to express their care through actions whereas the women tended to be more emotional and verbal in their care expressions. In addition, while both Syrian Muslim men and women engaged in the delivery of physical care, men took pride in being able to provide financial care for their families and community. Examples of these generic care practices were such activities as *taking time off from work to care for a sick spouse* and *hiring maids to assist the wife in housework*. One informant proudly stated that:

> My husband shows his caring for me when I am sick by buying food so I don't have to cook. He also pays for me to have a cleaning lady so I don't get tired from doing the housework. This is how he demonstrates his caring.

The care pattern of *caring as being honest, respectful, tolerant, and accommodating* was derived from the Syrian Muslims' worldview that arises from the teachings of Islam. Generic care practices related to this pattern include *kissing the right hand of parents and grandparents*; *refraining from raising the voice when addressing them*; *accommodating the religious beliefs of others*, and *being friendly to people of different faiths*.

The care pattern of *caring as worrying about others* was expressed through the generic care practices of *calling or visiting to check on sick people; bringing home-made healthy meals; offering rides to physicians' offices; developing empathy towards the plight of others; the provision of spiritual care;* and *checking the background of future husbands and wives for family members*. One informant explained that "…We have a system in our community, we check on each other and cook or babysit for each other when we are sick."

Interestingly, many key and general informants reported sharing personal left-over medications or providing professional medication samples to individuals who cannot afford these professional services as *caring actions*. An example of this is the informant statement that:

> We never bought health insurance because we can always get samples from doctor friends and we can be checked by them for free. We can also call a friend who has the same illness and take leftover medications. The only problem is if we need surgery!

These caring actions were viewed as ways of accommodating the healthcare needs of others.

In her 1989 study conducted with Lebanese Muslims in a Midwestern community, Luna discovered that *care encompassed equal but different gender role responsibilities* and also that *care reflected individual and collective meanings of honor* which were later supported by the findings of a separate study with Luna's study also identified *care as a source of pride and satisfaction*. However, the findings of the Syrian Muslim study demonstrated that reflected more universal gender-based caring roles and responsibilities. The discovery that Syrian Muslim men and women engage in similar caring roles and responsibilities were different from the findings in the earlier studies conducted with Lebanese Muslims (Luna, 1998; Wehbe-Alamah, 2006).

Theme II. Traditional Syrian Muslims View Caring for Family Members, Friends, All Living Creatures, and Oneself as Embedded in Religion

There were four care patterns derived from the informants' worldview; religious and cultural beliefs, values, and practices; and kinship dimensions that supported this theme. The universal pattern of *care as an act of worship* was derived from the worldview and religious beliefs and practices of Syrian Muslims. The majority of informants identified care as an act of worship and maintained that Islam mandates caring for Muslim and non-Muslim family and community members, animals, and oneself, as one informant confirmed: "Caring for family members such as parents, grandparents, siblings, aunts, uncles, as well as unrelated people is a religious obligation." These Syrian Muslims believed that the human body and mind are gifts entrusted to them by God; therefore they are required to care for and preserve this trust, as described by another informant: "Sleeping is believed to be an act of worship because it rests and regenerates the body and mind, which are two gifts trusted to human beings by God."

Informants shared stories about how the Prophet cared for animals and recited verses from the *Qur'an* that supported their belief that caring for all of God's creatures is a religious duty. Generic care practices that supported this care pattern included *feeding and being kind to animals*; *eating healthy foods*; *going to bed and waking up early*; *abstaining from actions that are known to be harmful to the body such as smoking*; and *organizing a schedule for community members to take turns cooking and caring for sick people requiring assistance*. Two

informant descriptors that provided credibility and confirmability to the researcher's observations and supported this care pattern included: "When you care for others, you do your Muslim duty" and "… you are caring when you respect people who are or are not Muslim."

The care pattern of *care as family and community unity* was derived from the worldview, cultural, religious, and kinship dimensions of Syrian Muslims. *Caring for family members, friends, and neighbors* fosters unity and cohesion. The social structure of the Syrian Muslim informants was characterized by a close kinship system continuously reinforced through caring actions. Syrian Muslims maintained family and community unity through *social visitations, phone calls, and caring network systems* devised at the local community level; *caring for elderly parents in their own homes* rather than sending them to nursing homes; and *traveling to visit family members in Syria during the summer* to maintain and nurture kinship bonds. One informant shared: "My husband traveled three times to Syria this year to check on his sick mother. He also calls on an almost daily basis. If he doesn't, he would not be considered caring."

Another pattern that supported Theme II was that *care is being honest, respectful, tolerant, and accommodating of others*. This pattern was embedded in the worldview and religious beliefs and practices of Syrian Muslims as previously discussed. The pattern of *care as worrying about others* described under Theme I was also reflected in the findings for Theme II. Caring expressed through worrying about others was found to be embedded throughout the teachings of Islam. Islam's emphasis on fostering family and community unity and on caring for relatives and strangers promotes a feeling of solidarity and responsibility toward others in need, as exemplified by the following informant statement that "…by caring for community members and neighbors the way we do, we become family, a big family."

The theme of *caring for family members, friends, all living creatures, and oneself as embedded in Islam* was also found in a previous study conducted with Lebanese Muslims in the Midwestern U.S. wherein Lebanese Muslims in general considered *caring as a religious duty* (Wehbe-Alamah, 1999). Luna (1989) also discovered that Lebanese Muslims' family obligations to provide care were embedded in the religious worldview of Islam.

Theme III. Traditional Syrian Muslims Rely on Islamic Spiritual Care to Promote Health and Prevent Illness

This theme was supported by four care patterns derived from the worldview and cultural and religious dimensions of Syrian Muslims. The care pattern of *abstaining from noncaring actions according to Islam as preventing illnesses* was supported by the Syrian Muslims' belief that *religion prohibits noncaring actions that are harmful to health* such as *eating in excess; smoking cigarettes or using water pipes; consuming pork products (including gelatin); drinking alcohol or consuming blood; taking illicit drugs;* and *engaging in sexual activities outside of the marriage bond.* Abstaining from all of these activities prevents illness. Additional *noncaring actions* according to traditional Syrian Muslims included *going to bed late* and *shaking hands, hugging, kissing, and intermingling in intimate ways with members of the opposite sex*, as one informant substantiated: "When you stay up and go to bed late, you ruin your health. The Prophet, *peace be upon him*, told us that we should eat in moderation, go to bed early, and wake up early; this is good for our health."

Applying Islamic teachings yields protective care effects such as preventing sexually transmitted diseases, drug addictions, and alcohol problems, as another informant elaborated:

> Islam shields people from several problems that are common in other cultures such as the high divorce rate, broken families, and drug and alcohol abuse. Of course, this does not mean that other cultures are bad. Many young Syrians are now smoking *Argeeleh* (please see Color Insert 5), they think it's cool, they don't understand how harmful it is. If they followed their religion, they would not smoke and they would be healthier.

The care pattern of *engaging in caring actions according to Islam to promote physical and psychological health* was supported by the belief that Islam fosters care actions that positively influence physical and psychological health. These Syrian Muslims believed that the teachings of Islam and having faith in them provided a sense of peace that promoted spiritual health. Generic care practices such as *reading the holy book* and *engaging in prayer* were credited for enhancing spiritual, emotional, physical, mental, and psychological health. Informants maintained that *drifting away from religion* is believed to be detrimental to their wellbeing whereas getting close to it lifts their spirits and improves emotional and psychological health, as one informant clearly stated: "...Trusting in my religion makes me feel safe, stable, happy, and stress-free."

Health promotion was valued by the Syrian Muslim informants who believed that they had to *maintain good health* to be able to practice and meet the requirements of their faith. The belief that Muslims should care for their bodies and health was also supported by Abdal Ati (1998) who affirmed that Muslims believe that they are *trustees of the gifts bestowed upon them by God* and should therefore handle this trust to the best of their abilities. Caring actions that promoted health according to Islam included *exercising; sleeping early; waking up early; fasting; praying; eating in moderation;* and *following the examples of the Prophet.* The Syrian Muslim generic care practice of cleanliness was maintained by *performing ablution; brushing the teeth* with a toothbrush or a small tree stick (called a *Miswak*); *showering; cleaning the genitalia after using the toilet* by using watering cans; and *trimming nails.*

The care practices of fasting and praying, reported by informants as benefiting health, were supported by the findings of several other authors. According to the findings of Hamid (1996), *fasting fine tunes the body* and *sheds it of obesity.* In addition, it *ensures the body and the soul against all the harm* that results from overburdening the stomach (Abdal Ati, 1998). Ramadan fasting was identified as the ideal care practice for the treatment of obesity, essential hypertension, and mild to moderate stable Type II diabetes as it was found to lower blood sugar and systolic blood pressure (Athar, 2008). Furthermore, along with the benefits of exercise, the care practice of prayer was found to help Muslims in maintaining a *sense of health and wellbeing; intellectual meditation; spiritual devotion;* and *moral elevation* (Abdal Ati, 1998; Luna, 1989; Wehbe-Alamah, 1999, 2015).

Illness as a caring practice from God was the third pattern identified in support of Theme III. Syrian Muslim informants viewed *illness as a sign of love from God.* They believed that illnesses erased their sins in this lifetime and took away from their punishment in the afterlife, as noted in the informant description that "...illness is a blessing in disguise and as a sign of mercy and loving care from God." In addition, illness was viewed by these Syrian Muslims as *a physiologic and spiritual wakeup call* because it alerted them to the *need to pay attention* and *provide better care* to their body. It also reminded them of the *need and duty to remember and worship God*, as detailed by one informant that "…When I get sick, it's God's way of telling me wake up! I have strayed away from Him, and I need to try to be closer to Him through prayer. It also means I have to be patient because God is erasing my sins when I suffer from illness, even when I get a paper cut." *Illness as a care practice to erase one's sins* was similarly discovered in two separate studies conducted with Lebanese Muslims (Wehbe-Alamah, 1999, 2006).

Syrian Muslim informants used their *language as a religious protective caring practice*, revealing that they use Arabic religious expressions such as *Inshaallah* (God willing); *MashaAllah* (what God wills); and *Subhanallah* (Glory be to God) to praise God and His prophets, protect people from the evil eye, and preserve or bless material possessions. All informants stated that

language is used to recite specific chapters from the Qur'an known as *Al-Muawwathat* or The Exorcists, a practice which is believed to ward off and treat the evil eye. This protective care practice was described by one informant: "When women go into labor or someone is having surgery, we meet and read a chapter from the Qur'an called *Surat Yasseen* to help the woman in labor and to protect the person having surgery." Also, reading *Surat Al Baqarah* (see Figure 25.1) every three days is believed to prevent the devil from entering the house and causing trouble between the husband and wife.

In addition, Syrian Muslim informants used language to *recite supplications to God* known as *Dua'* before performing simple daily activities such as eating, sleeping, and making love to their spouses in an effort to protect themselves from harm, as one informant shared: "…When I married my husband and before

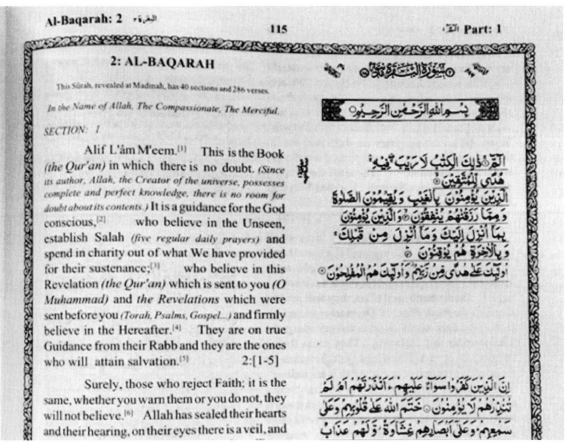

FIGURE 25.1 • Opening of Surat Al Baqarah.

Photo © Hiba Wehbe-Alamah (2018). From Malik, M. F. A. (1997). English translation of the meaning of Al-Qur'an: The guidance for mankind. (p. 115). Houston, TX: The Institute of Islamic Knowledge. With permission from Muhammad Farooq-i-Azam Malik.

we made love for the first time, we said a special prayer so God would bless our union and so we would have a blessed child if I was to get pregnant." Language as protective care was also discovered in another Middle Eastern Arab culture. Lebanese Muslims were also found to consider *language as protective care* in two other studies (Luna, 1989; Wehbe-Alamah, 1999 & 2006).

Theme III was also supported by an earlier study. Abdal Ati (1998) found that the beliefs that *God's prescriptions were in the best interest of mankind* and *His prohibitions were aimed to protect mankind* were commonly shared by the majority of Muslims. The review of the literature also revealed that religious people tended to have healthier lifestyles and fewer physical and mental disorders (Athar, 2008; Koenig, 2001). In addition, religion was seen to have a direct preventive health effect by *promoting the avoidance of unhealthy habits* and the *promotion of a strong social support network* (Koenig, 2001).

■ CULTURE CARE MODES WITHIN THE SYRIAN MUSLIM CULTURE

Leininger (2006) proposed that the discovery of universalities and diversities in human care in a specific culture enables nurses to plan and provide culturally congruent care for members belonging to that culture. The holding knowledge of culture care meanings, beliefs, and practices of Syrian Muslims discovered in this study could enable nurses to make culturally congruent care decisions and initiate care actions that fit with the lifeways of traditional Syrian Muslims living in the Midwestern U.S. and possibly elsewhere, as well as with other traditional Arab Muslims.

Culture Care Preservation and/or Maintenance

To preserve and/or maintain the culture care of the Syrian/Arab Muslim patients, nurses and other healthcare providers are encouraged to abstain from initiating shaking hands with patients of the opposite gender and to assign same sex healthcare providers whenever possible, especially for female patients in radiology, operating and recovery rooms, and obstetrics. Most (not all) Syrian and other Arab Muslims only shake hands with, hug, or kiss people from the same sex and believe this practice to be congruent with their religion. Congruent with the findings of this

study, Connelly, Hammad, Hassoun, Kysia, and Rabah (1999) maintained that handshakes between non-related men and women were against Islamic norms and that same-sex care providers should generally be made available to Arab Muslim patients with the exception of life-threatening circumstances.

Hospitals are encouraged to provide alcohol-free and pork-free meals and medications to Syrian Muslim and other Muslim patients. Foods containing lard or gelatin such as Jell-O; pork based insulin; elixirs and mouthwashes containing alcohol; gelatin encapsulated medications; and vitamins and drugs that contain gelatin as an ingredient are not acceptable to the majority of Muslim patients. Reading the contents in medicine and food labels to rule out the presence of gelatin and/or alcohol can preserve this cultural and religious belief and practice. Connelly et al. (1999) maintained that lard, gelatin (unless specified as beef gelatin), and some forms of nonsoy lecithin are pork products that are widely used in processed foods and frequently added to prepared foods, which justifies the wariness felt by Arab Muslim patients toward unfamiliar food offerings, especially hospital meals. Finally, because Syrian Muslims consider their bodies to be a gift from God and deem themselves to be the trustees of this gift, nurses are encouraged to avoid pressuring relatives of a deceased Muslim patient to give consent for autopsy or organ donation.

Culture Care Accommodation and/or Negotiation

To accommodate for and/or negotiate culture care with Syrian/Arab Muslims, nurses and other healthcare providers are encouraged to accommodate or negotiate the number of visitors in an inpatient setting as well as the duration of the hospital visit. The presence of a supportive network of family members and friends is extremely important for Syrian Muslims, especially because this is considered a sign of caring as well as a social, religious, and cultural obligation and expectation. The literature supported the finding that it is common for Muslim community members who are not related to the patient to visit the sick (Luna, 1989, 1998; Wehbe-Alamah, 1999 & 2006). Healthcare professionals need to understand that the extensive social support received by the hospitalized Arab patient is an important part of recovery, and does not impede recovery (Connelly et al., 1999). Nurses need to negotiate with the patient, family, and friends to ensure the patient receives privacy for nursing care and necessary rest as well as social support.

Other ways of providing culture care accommodation for Syrian Arab Muslim patients included requesting hospitals to provide *Halal* (lawful) or seafood meals or allowing patients to have homemade foods brought into the hospital. Nurses can also negotiate with hospital officials to provide Muslim patients with culturally congruent hospital gowns that reach all the way down to the ankles and cover the arms in order to accommodate the modesty needs of Muslim patients. Finally, nurses working in labor and delivery, surgery, and radiology are encouraged to accommodate their patients by keeping their body covered and exposing only the areas required during care or procedures.

Culture Care Repatterning and/or Restructuring

To repattern and/or restructure some of the potentially harmful health practices of Syrian Muslims, nurses are encouraged to educate clients about the risks of medication sharing and taking medications without receiving proper diagnosis by a primary healthcare provider. Similarly, nurses can encourage clients to consult with a primary care provider such as a physician, a nurse practitioner, or a physician assistant before consumption of any lay or self-prescribed medications. In addition, nurses are encouraged to educate new Syrian Muslim immigrants who smoke cigarettes or use a water pipe about the health dangers associated with smoking as well as the effects of secondhand smoke inhalation (passive smoking) on nonsmokers to promote smoking cessation. Finally, nurses should explain the potential dangers from relying solely on a social network for healthcare delivery, and provide Syrian Muslim clients with information about appropriate resources that can assist them in purchasing or locating affordable health care.

■ IMPLICATIONS FOR THE DISCIPLINE AND PRACTICE OF NURSING

Findings from this study contribute to the body of knowledge for discipline of nursing and supports Leininger's Theory of Culture Care Diversity and Universality by adding to the evolving body of transcultural nursing care knowledge related to the care of Syrian Muslims. These discoveries will expand the awareness of the importance of generic and professional care in the promotion of the health and wellbeing of Syrian Muslims in the U.S. Findings from this study may be used by U.S. healthcare providers such as registered nurses, nurse practitioners, and others to provide Syrian Muslims with culturally congruent and holistic care using Leininger's three care modes of culture care decisions and actions within hospital and community contexts. Syrian Muslim patients are diverse in their generic care beliefs and practices. Nurses and other professional healthcare providers cannot assume that all Syrian Muslim patients share the traditional generic care beliefs and practices discovered in this study. A cultural assessment of each patient is crucial to discovering their cultural beliefs and practices and in providing culturally congruent care that is tailored to the individual client. The knowledge gained from this study may be integrated into nursing curricula when addressing culture-specific care practices and may lay the foundation for future research with other cultural groups.

■ SUMMARY

Nurses are caring for greater numbers of patients from cultures other than their own due to increased immigration and expanding diversity within the U.S. Findings from this study may be used by U.S. healthcare providers such as registered nurses, nurse practitioners, and others to provide traditional Syrian Muslims with culturally congruent, and holistic care. Providing culturally congruent care is a goal all nurses share or should share. Learning about the generic (lay, folk, or indigenous) care beliefs, expressions, and practices related to health and illness of Syrian Muslims will assist U.S. nurses and other healthcare professionals to provide this group with culturally meaningful care and lessen the potential for cultural pain, clashes, imposition, and conflicts. Although this study discovered important cultural values, beliefs, and lifeways of traditional Syrian Muslims living in the Midwestern United States, it is important to remain vigilant to the fact that diversities and similarities exist within and among all cultures. Nurses and other healthcare providers may use information in this chapter as holding knowledge to guide them as they engage in individual cultural assessments and as they plan culturally congruent decisions and actions. With the influx of Syrian and other refugees and immigrants from around the world, it is imperative that nurses be prepared with the knowledge needed to provide culturally sensitive care to diverse individuals, families, and groups.

■ DEDICATION

This chapter is dedicated to Syrian immigrants and refugees worldwide, and especially those who contributed to the findings of this study.

■ DISCUSSION QUESTIONS

1. Discuss the sociopolitical factors that have historically prompted Syrian immigration to the United States and other nations worldwide and the implications for nursing practice.
2. What are some of the important cultural beliefs, practices, and lifeways of traditional Syrian Muslims? How are they significant for the provision of culturally congruent care?
3. What are ways nurses and other healthcare providers can provide culturally sensitive and meaningful care to traditional Syrian Muslims using the three modes of culture care decisions and actions?

■ REFERENCES

Abdal Ati, H. (1998). *Islam in focus*. Beltsville, MD: Amana Publications.

Amnesty International. (2016, February 3). *Syria's refugee crisis in numbers*. Retrieved from https://www.amnesty.org/en/latest/news/2016/02/syrias-refugee-crisis-in-numbers/

Asi, M., & Beaulieu, D. (2013). *Arab households in the United States: 2006-2010 American Community Survey Briefs*. Washington, DC: U.S. Department of Commerce, Economics and Statistics Administration, U.S. Census Bureau. Retrieved from https://www.census.gov/prod/2013pubs/acsbr10-20.pdf

Athar, S. (2008). *The spiritual and health benefits of Ramadan fasting*. Retrieved from: http://www.islam-usa.com/index.php?option=com_content&view=article&id=168:the-spiritual-and-health-benefits-of-ramadan-fasting&catid=68:health--medicine&Itemid=137

Bateman, G. (2002). *The Encyclopedia of World Geography*. England, UK: Andromeda Oxford Ltd.

Bennett, S. H. (2000). Lebanese or Syrian ancestry. *Genealogy Today*. Retrieved from http://www.genealogytoday.com/family/syrian/

Boghani, P. (2016). A staggering New Death Toll for Syria's War-470,000. Retrieved from: http://www.pbs.org/wgbh/frontline/article/a-staggering-new-death-toll-for-syrias-war-470000/

Connelly, M., Hammad, A., Hassoun, R., Kysia, R., & Rabah, R. (1999). *Guide to Arab culture: Health care delivery to the Arab American community*. Dearborn, MI: Access Community Health Center.

Cornell University Library (LibGuides/Near Eastern Studies). (2015, July 13). *Arab Spring: A research and study guide:_Syria*. Retrieved from http://guides.library.cornell.edu/c.php?g=31688&p=200753

Hamid, A. W. (1996). *Islam Natural Way*. Chicago, IL: Kazi Publications, Inc.

Koenig, G. H. (2001). *The healing power of faith: Science explores medicine's last great frontier*. New York, NY: Simon & Schuster.

Leininger, M. M. (1991). *Ethnonursing: A research method with enablers to study the theory of Culture Care*. New York, NY: NLN Publications.

Leininger, M. M. (2002a). Part I. The theory of culture care and the ethnonursing research method. In M. M Leininger and M. R. McFarland (Eds.), *Transcultural nursing: Concepts, theories, research, and practice* (3rd ed., pp 71-98). New York, NY: McGraw-Hill.

Leininger, M. M. (2002b). Transcultural nursing and globalization of health care: Importance, focus, and historical aspects. In M. M. Leininger and M. R. McFarland (Eds.), *Transcultural nursing: Concepts, theories, research, and practice* (3rd ed., pp 3-43). New York, NY: McGraw-Hill.

Leininger, M. M. (2006). Culture care diversity and universality theory and evolution of the ethnonursing research method. In M. M. Leininger and M. R. McFarland (Eds.), *Culture care diversity and universality: A worldwide nursing theory* (2nd ed., pp. 1-41). Sudbury, MA: Jones & Bartlett.

Luna, L. J. (1989). *Care and cultural context of Lebanese Muslims in an urban U.S. community: An ethnographic and ethnonursing study conceptualized within Leininger's theory*. (Unpublished doctoral dissertation). Wayne State University, Detroit, MI.

Luna, L. J. (1998). Culturally competent health care: A challenge for nurses in Saudi Arabia. *Journal of Transcultural Nursing, 9*(2), 8-14.

Martinez, M. (2015). *Syrian refugees: Which countries welcome them, which ones don't*. Retrieved from http://www.cnn.com/2015/09/09/world/welcome-syrian-refugees-countries/

McFarland, M. R., & Wehbe-Alamah, H. B. (2015). The Theory of Culture Care Diversity and Universality. In M. R. McFarland and H. B. Wehbe-Alamah (Eds.), *Leininger's culture care diversity and Universality: A worldwide nursing theory* (3rd ed., pp. 1-34). Burlington, MA: Jones and Bartlett Learning.

Migration Policy Center. (2016, September). Syrian refugees: A snapshot of the crisis—in the Middle East and Europe. Retrieved from http://syrianrefugees.eu/

South, C. (2006). *Syria (Cultures of the World)*. New York, NY: Benchmark Books.

Syrian Observatory for Human Rights. (2015, October). *310,000 people killed since the beginning of the Syrian revolution.* Retrieved from http://www.syriahr.com/en/2015/04/310000-people-killed-since-the-beginning-of-the-syrian-revolution/

Wehbe-Alamah, H. (1999). *Generic health care beliefs, expressions, and practices, of Lebanese Muslims in two Urban U.S. communities: A mini ethnonursing study conceptualized within Leininger's theory.* (Unpublished master's thesis). Saginaw Valley State University, University Center, MI.

Wehbe-Alamah, H. (2006). *Generic care of Lebanese Muslim women in the Midwestern USA.* In M. M. Leininger and M. R. McFarland (Eds.), *Culture care diversity and universality: A worldwide nursing theory* (2nd ed., pp. 307-325). Sudbury, MA: Jones and Bartlett.

Wehbe-Alamah, H. (2011). The use of Culture Care Theory with Syrian Muslims in the Midwestern United States. *Online Journal of Cultural Competence in Nursing and Healthcare, 1*(3), 1-12.

Wehbe-Alamah, H. B. (2015). Folk Care Beliefs and Practices of Traditional Lebanese and Syrian Muslims in the Midwestern United States. In M. R. McFarland and H. B. Wehbe-Alamah (Eds.), *Leininger's culture care diversity and universality: A worldwide nursing theory* (3rd ed., pp. 137-182). Burlington, MA: Jones and Bartlett Learning.

Wehbe-Alamah, H. B., & McFarland, M. R. (2015). The Ethnonursing Research Method. In M. R. McFarland and H.B. Wehbe-Alamah (Eds.), *Leininger's culture care diversity and universality: A worldwide nursing theory* (3rd ed., pp. 35-72). Burlington, MA: Jones and Bartlett Learning.

Appendix: Studies conceptualized within Leininger's Culture Care Theory and/or Ethnonursing Research Method [1966-2017]

	Name	Title	Year of Publication
1	Leininger, Madeleine M.	Convergence and divergence of human behavior: An ethnopsychological comparative study of two Gadsup villages in the eastern highlands of New Guinea	1966
2	Adair, S. A.	An ethnoscientific approach to identify the perceptions and experiences as perceived by an urban Mexican-American group in relation to medical and nursing care	1974
3	Horn, B. M.	An ethnoscientific study to determine social and cultural factors affecting Native American Indian women during pregnancy	1975
4	Glittenberg, J. K.	A comparative study of fertility in highland Guatemala: A Ladino and an Indian town	1976
5	Ray, Marilyn Anne	An applied anthropological study of role behavior within the profession of nursing within the complex institution of the hospital	1978
6	Wison, J.	An ethnoscientific study to determine the perception, description, causation, resolution, and categorization of the illness domain for Mexican Americans	1979
7	Ray, Marilyn Anne	A study of caring within an institutional culture	1981
8	Bradford, Dorothy M. Ellington	Health survey of international students at Kent State University (Cultural, transcultural, self-Care, foreign)	1985
9	Kinney, Genevieve Lehuan Aniokilauea	Caring values and caring practices of native Hawaiians in a Hawaiian Home Lands Community (Transcultural)	1985
10	Al-Darazi, Fariba Abdulwahab	Assessment of Women's health and illness cognitions and practices	1987
11	Poznanski, Cynthia Anne	Types and meanings of caring behaviors among elderly nursing home residents	1987
12	Telford, Lorraine Aline	Adolescent health an emic perspective	1987

	Name	Title	Year of Publication
13	Welch, Alice Z.	Concepts of health, illness, caring, aging and problems of adjustment among elderly Filipinas residing in Hampton Road, Virginia	1987
14	Birk, Hasana Ann	Initiating outreach home visits PHN approaches	1988
15	Bottorff, Joan Lorraine	Breastmilk the emic perspective of mothers	1988
16	Gates, Marie Frances Gutowski	Care and cure meanings, experiences and orientations of persons who are dying in hospital and hospice settings	1988
17	Wenger, Anna Frances Z.	The phenomenon of care in a high context culture: The old order Amish	1988
18	Ingram, Mary Regina	Ethnohealth and ethnocaring practices among the Lakota	1989
19	Jambunathan, Jayalakshmi	An exploratory study of the sociocultural factors in depression among women in southeast India	1989
20	Luna, Linda Jacqueline	Care and cultural context of Lebanese Muslims in an urban U.S. community: An ethnographic and ethnonursing study conceptualized within Leininger's theory	1989
21	Beauchamp, Charles James	The structure of the lived experience of struggling with making a decision in a critical life situation, for a group of individuals with HIV	1990
22	Cameron, Cynthia Frederika	An ethnonursing study of the influence of extended caregiving on the health status of elderly Anglo-Canadian wives caring for physically disabled husbands	1990
23	Parnicza, Diana Rose	Analysis of rural Appalachian caregivers' use of social support	1990
24	Rosenbaum, Janet Nancy	Cultural care, cultural health, and grief phenomena related to older Greek Canadian widows within Leininger's Theory of Culture Care	1990
25	Thompson, Teresa Louise Cervantez	A qualitative investigation of rehabilitation nursing care in an inpatient rehabilitation unit using Leininger's theory	1990
26	Weaver, Rosella A.	A phenomenological study of caring in the nurse-patient relationship: The patient's perspective	1990
27	Cameron, Cynthia	An ethnonursing study of health status of elderly Anglo-Canadian wives providing extended care giving to their disabled husbands	1991
28	Kearney, Carol Lynne	The patient perspective of caring expressed by nurses through patient explaining (teaching)	1991
29	Pask, Eleanor G.	Caring [microform]: The changing essence of nursing	1991

	Name	Title	Year of Publication
30	Paul, Donna Marie	Description of the health experience of Athabascans living in Galena: A modified ethnographic approach	1991
31	Spangler, Zenaida de los Santos Soriano	Nursing care values and caregiving practices of Anglo-American and Philippine-American nurses conceptualized within Leininger's theory	1991
32	Bunting, Sheila M.	Negotiating the journey: A grounded theory study of family/friend caregiving in the context of AIDS	1992
33	Davis, Anne Walendy	Discovering Comanche health beliefs using ethnographic techniques	1992
34	Edmunds, Kathryn	Ethnonursing Study of Mennonites with Leininger's Culture Care Theory	1992
35	Holliger, Victor Harry	Retirement housing preferences of the homosexual elderly	1992
36	Pereira, Rosane Carrion Jacinto	Untold stories: The lived experience of Brazilian novice nurses	1992
37	Ruppert, Susan D.	Wives' perceptions of situational experiences during critical care hospitalization: A phenomenological study	1992
38	Scott, Shari Hughes	Experiences of battered women: The impact of childhood sexual abuse on adult relationship choices	1992
39	Williams, Charles Wayne	The confidence of general duty nurses in caring for ethnically diverse inpatient populations within a general hospital setting	1992
40	Basuray, Joanna Shakila	Meaning of caring in the academic culture of nurse educators: An ethnography	1993
41	Chiara, Maria	"Making a difference": An ethnography of women's career motivations, values, and work satisfaction in nursing (Volumes I and II)	1993
42	Ethier, Marlene	Patients' perceptions of caring in the rural culture	1993
43	Finn, Julianna M.	Professional nurse and generic care of childbirthing women conceptualized within Leininger's Culture Care Theory and using Colaizzi's phenomenological method	1993
44	Fischer, Dorothy Konowitz	Stories, styles, and perceptions of practice constructs among intensive care nursery nurses	1993
45	Villarruel, Antonia Maria	Mexican-American cultural meanings, expressions, self-care and dependent-care actions associated with experiences of pain	1993
46	Williams, Myra Dee	Epistemological perspectives and education experiences of female registered nurse baccalaureate students	1993

	Name	Title	Year of Publication
47	Zwane, Thembi Isabel	Developing a curriculum for professional nursing education in Swaziland: Views from Ministry of Health officials and nursing leaders	1993
48	Cohen, Judith Ann	A tapestry of caring: The lived experience and meaning of caring within nurse student/faculty relationship	1994
49	Foley, Sandra Joy	Parental care practices of the Hmong refugees	1994
50	Ford, Donna-Mae	The viability of the Primary Health Care model for women's health: An ethnographic study of women's health beliefs, values, and practices in rural Vanuatu	1994
51	Gelazis, Rauda	Humor, care, and well-being of Lithuanian Americans: An ethnonursing study using Leininger's Theory of Culture Care Diversity and Universality	1994
52	Gichia, Jannie E. Underwood	Mothers and others: Afro-American women's descriptions of motherhood	1994
53	MacNeil, Joan Mary	Culture care [microform]: Meanings, patterns and expressions for Baganda women as AIDS caregivers within Leininger's theory	1994
54	Morgan, Marjorie Anne	Prenatal care of African-American women in selected USA urban and rural cultural contexts conceptualized within Leininger's Cultural Care Theory	1994
55	Strodtman, Linda Kay Tanner	Becoming a "real woman": Historical analysis of the characteristics, ethos and professional socialization of diploma nursing students in two midwestern schools of nursing from 1941 to 1980	1994
56	Drury, Lin Joan	Lifeways of homeless chronically mentally ill individuals in a community housing program	1995
57	Ekstrom, David N.	Gender and perceived nurse caring in nurse-patient dyads	1995
58	Garteig, Jennie Laureen	Health meanings and dynamics among urban residing Native women	1995
59	Goddard, Nancy Carol	The fourth dimension: Conceptualization of spirituality	1995
60	Higgins, Barbara Joan	Puerto Rican cultural beliefs: Influence on infant feeding practices in western New York	1995
61	Hunnibell, Laura S.	The experience of caring by nurses who work in the intensive care unit	1995
62	McFarland, Marilyn	Culture Care Theory and Ethnonursing Mini-study of care experiences in residential nursing homes and Mexican-American communities	1995

	Name	**Title**	**Year of Publication**
63	McFarland, Marilyn Ruth	Cultural care of Anglo- and African-American elderly residents within the environmental context of a long-term care institution	1995
64	Wuest, Judith Anne	Precarious ordering: A theory of women's caring	1995
65	Alexander, Barbara Harris	Self-perceived cultural competence of Delaware nurses	1996
66	Berry, Anita B.	Culture care expression, meanings, and experiences of pregnant Mexican-American women within Leininger's Culture Care Theory	1996
67	Chiu, Lyren	Spirituality of women living with breast cancer in Taiwan: A phenomenological study	1996
68	Curtis, Marguerite	Advanced practitioners in nursing as a subculture	1996
69	Frese, Carlyn	Parents' and adolescents' experiences in family therapy: A qualitative study	1996
70	Herp, Cheryl Ann	Meanings of folk and professional health care experienced by Guatemalan Mayans in southeast Florida	1996
71	Hummel, Faye Colglazier	The role of nursing in the Vietnam health care system	1996
72	Miller, June	Politics and care: A study of Czech-Americans within Leininger's Theory of Culture Care Diversity and Universality	1996
73	Omeri, Akram	An ethnonursing study conceptualized within Leininger's Culture Care Theory focused on "the Care Meanings, Experiences, and Expressions of Mexican-American Women During Pregnancy"	1996
74	Racine, Louise	Étude des perceptions culturelles d'un groupe d'aînées et d'aînés de la communauté juive et d'un groupe d'infirmières sur les soins infirmiers de maintien à domicile du CLSC	1996
75	Selzler, Bonnie Kay	The health experiences of Dakota Sioux and their perceptions of culturally congruent nursing care	1996
76	White, Patrice Michele	Crossing the river: A study of Khmer women's beliefs and practices during pregnancy, birth and postpartum	1996
77	Ark, Pamela Dale	Health risk behaviors and coping strategies of African-American sixth graders	1997
78	Banfield, Barbara E.	A philosophical inquiry of Orem's self-care deficit nursing theory	1997
79	Berardinelli, Candace Gearing	The health care experiences and health-seeking patterns of native Americans in an urban environment	1997

	Name	Title	Year of Publication
80	Curtis, Marguerite Robertson	Cultural care by private practice APRNs in community contexts	1997
81	Deevey, Sharon	Bereavement experiences in lesbian kinship networks in Ohio	1997
82	Garcia, Lillian Denise	Intergenerational analysis of dietary practices and health perceptions of Hispanic women and their adult daughters	1997
83	Garland, Hettie Lou	Reactions of native southern Appalachian children and youths to sudden death	1997
84	Perry, Tonya Evette	The lived experiences of Ghanaian women with HIV/AIDS: A phenomenological study	1997
85	Sanchez, Mabel Sandra	Pathways to health: A naturalistic study of Mexican-American women's lay health behaviors	1997
86	Sonninen, A. L.	Testing reliability and validity of the Finnish version of the Appraisal of Self-Care Agency (ASA) scale with elderly Finns	1997
87	Suttharangsee, Wandee	Concepts and protective factors related to positive mental health from Thai adolescents' perspectives: An ethnonursing study	1997
88	Vlasses, Frances Rita	Too familiar for words: An analysis of "invisible" nursing work	1997
89	Woodland, Darlene Dostiee	Perceptions of professional nurses toward the delivery of health care to culturally diverse populations in a suburban San Antonio hospital	1997
90	Zoucha, Richard Dennis	The experience of Mexican-Americans receiving professional nursing care: An ethnonursing study	1997
91	Chase-Ziolek, M. A.	Health ministry in the life of a congregation with a parish nurse: Caring and connecting through Christ	1998
92	Claus, Inga Bryde	Helseopplevelse på landsbygda i Gambia: hvordan opplever gambiske kvinner nytten av et dagsenter for helsetjenester?	1998
93	Cornelius, Ilana S.	Folk beliefs about health promotion and disease prevention behaviors among Hispanic women in southeastern New Mexico	1998
94	Ehrmin, Joanne Therese Hirscher	Culture care: Meanings and expressions of African-American women residing in an inner-city transitional home for substance abuse	1998
95	Gagnon, Linda	Signification pour les aînées inuites du soin offert par leurs proches	1998
96	George, Tamara Bloom	Meanings, expressions, and experiences of care of chronically mentally ill in a day treatment center using Leininger's Culture Care Theory	1998

	Name	Title	Year of Publication
97	Horton, Betty J.	Nurse anesthesia as a subculture of nursing in the United States	1998
98	Kawulich, Barbara Bussell	Muscogee (Creek) women's perceptions of work	1998
99	Lamp, Judith Kilmer	Generic and professional culture care meanings and practices of Finnish women in birth within Leininger's Theory of Culture Care Diversity and Universality	1998
100	Taylor, Janette Yvette	Resilience and recovering among African-American women survivors of domestic violence	1998
101	Baluyot, Cynthia M. A	Primary nursing health care services and ethnic minority elderly patients: Are nurses able to give this group of patients the nursing care they want and need?	1999
102	Cooksey-James, Tawna Jean	Utilization of prenatal care by women of St. Thomas, United States Virgin Islands: A descriptive study	1999
103	Duran, Graciela S.	A cultural analysis of Hispanic Canadian young adult males' lived experiences with addictions	1999
104	Edwards, Nicki Ellen	Registered nurses "in the middle" in clinical practice	1999
105	Fox-Hill, Emily Jean	The experiences of persons with AIDS living-dying in a nursing home	1999
106	Hólmfríður S. Kristjánsdóttir	What is the theoretical and practical framework which shapes the nurse - patient relationship?	1999
107	Kidner, Molly A.	The lived experiences of persons dependent on hemodialysis	1999
108	Kim-Godwin, Yeoun Soo	Sensitivity, knowledge, and skills prerequisites of provision of culturally competent care to Mexican migrant farmworkers: A Delphi study	1999
109	Martin-Paruta, Helenann	Homeless women and hope: An exploratory study	1999
110	Pharris, Margaret Louise Dexheime	The process of pattern recognition as a nursing intervention with adolescent males convicted of murder	1999
111	Rogers, Willetta Howell	Psychological well-being of family caregivers of dementia patients in nursing homes	1999
112	Tretton, Jacquelyn Lois	Caring behaviors of nurses as perceived by patients and nurses	1999
113	Wehbe-Alamah, H.	Generic and health care beliefs, expressions, and practices of Lebanese Muslims living in the Midwestern United States - A Mini-study	1999
114	Wekselman, Kathryn	The culture of natural childbirth	1999

	Name	Title	Year of Publication
115	Castro, Maria Clara Dias da Costa Correia de	Para um cuidado cultural congruente com a cultura familiar	2000
116	Grotbo, Anna Christine	Recognizing and responding to spiritual need in clinical settings: A nursing study	2000
117	Kioke, Sandra Jean	...Revisiting the past...: Discovering traditional care and the cultural meaning of pregnancy and birth in a Cree community	2000
118	Kuhns-Hastings, Judy Jane	Middle-aged daughters' transitions from non-caregiver to caregiver for elderly dependent parents	2000
119	Lazure, Ginette	Le soin générique et le soin professionnel à la période prénatale [microforme]: l'expérience de femmes de la région du sud de la Tunisie	2000
120	Levin, Julie T.	A descriptive study of adult Jewish women's perceptions of the influence of a significant other's addiction on the health and harmony in their life	2000
121	Penny, Jane Therese	The influence of a supportive network on the journey to motherhood of primiparous white women living in rural communities in eastern Nova Scotia	2000
122	Rink, Doris Gail	Health beliefs and practices of Russian immigrant families	2000
123	Sagar, Priscilla Limbo	The lived experience of Vietnamese nurses: A case study	2000
124	Sanders, Nancy Lee Williamson	The relationship of spirituality and health among the Yup'ik of southwestern Alaska: An exploratory study	2000
125	Smith, Brenda Hanson	The balancing act: How working mothers manage home, work, and family	2000
126	Benavente, Gladys Susan	Si Dios Quiere: Cultural beliefs of the Mexican-American impacting secondary prevention	2001
127	Farrell, Linda Schofield	Cultural care: Meanings and expressions of caring and noncaring of the Potawatomi who have experienced family violence	2001
128	Hagman, Lynda Wilson	Cultural self-efficacy of licensed Registered Nurses in New Mexico	2001
129	Hsueh, Kuei-Hsiang	Family caregiving experience and health status among Chinese in the United States	2001
130	Liang, Hwey-Fang	Understanding culture care practices of caregivers of children with cancer in Taiwan: An ethnonursing study	2001

	Name	Title	Year of Publication
131	Lin, Pay-Fan	Development and psychometric evaluation of the Caring Behaviors Scale of baccalaureate nursing student in Taiwan	2001
132	Lowe-Nurse, Doris D.	Assessment of nurses' confidence levels when caring for culturally diverse patients	2001
133	Moffitt, Pertice Marie	The spirit of the drum	2001
134	Nelson, Jean	Factors influencing care expressions, patterns and practices in adult day care	2001
135	Padilla, Rosalia Aquino	Cultural influences in Southeast Asian nurses' perceptions of caring	2001
136	Rosa, Ninon Girardon da	Dilemas éticos no mundo do cuidar de um serviço de emergência	2001
137	Schaaf, Sharon M.	The relationship between acculturation level and patient satisfaction among adult Mexican American emergency department patients	2001
138	Thomas, Patricia A.	Managed to care: Transcultural encounters and business as usual in nurses' work narratives	2001
139	Adepoju, Joseph Adetunji	An exploratory study of health beliefs and practices of the Yoruba living in the Philadelphia-Wilmington metropolitan area (United States of America)	2002
140	Clark, Elizabeth-Ellen Hills	Quality of life: Psychiatric nurses hearing the voices of individuals with severe mental illness	2002
141	Debs-Ivall, Salma	The meaning of social support: The perspective of Arab Canadians with congestive heart failure	2002
142	Dhaliwal, Sukhwarsha	Dietary practices of older Punjabi women living in Canada	2002
143	Enns, Carol L.	Expressions of caring by contemporary surgical nurses: A phenomenological study	2002
144	French, Melody Weaver	El corazon de la cebolla: A mini-ethnographic study of Mexicana/o symptom interpretation and management	2002
145	Genung, Vanessa Marie	Health perspectives of world religions: An exploratory investigation	2002
146	Gustafson, Diana Lynn	Cultural sensitivity as a problematic in Ontario nursing policy and education: An integrated feminist con/textual analysis	2002
147	Kelley, Lisa Skemp	Expectations and elder care networks in a Saint Lucian village	2002

	Name	Title	Year of Publication
148	Schwartz, Karon Stitt	Breast cancer and health care beliefs, values, and practices of Amish women	2002
149	Silva, Iolanda Giordano	A Promoção da saúde e a prevenção da doença na prática curativa da enfermagem na comunidade : Perspectivas do enfermeiro	2002
150	Smith, Mary Ellen	Bone marrow donation: Factors influencing intention in African-Americans	2002
151	Thyli, Bente	A qualitative study of male nurse educators' and male students' perceptions of caring: A gender perspective	2002
152	Voigtman, Janet Louise	Learning to suffer: Pain response in a community of Saudi Arab children with sickle cell disease	2002
153	Weissheimer, Anne Marie	O parto na cultura teuto-gaúcha	2002
154	Wilson, Tina Marie	Onion Lake First Nations women: Knowledge, attitudes and health beliefs of cervical cancer and cervical cancer screening	2002
155	Yu, Boas Judy	The caregiving practices of Korean-American families: A descriptive study using an ethnographic approach	2002
156	Zaidi, Saira M.	Gift of Allah: An ethnographic study of mothers who care for children with disabilities	2002
157	Aitken, J. A.	The psychosocial impact of epilepsy in later life: An ethnonursing study	2003
158	Campesino-Flenniken, Maureen	Voces de Las Madres: Traumatic bereavement after gang-related homicide	2003
159	Fliszar, Rosemary Schleicher	Culture care of Puerto Rican elderly in a community setting	2003
160	Florczak, Kristine Louise	The lived experience of sacrificing something important	2003
161	HoSang, Margaret R.	Perceptions of community health nurses of their preparedness to care for culturally diverse clients	2003
162	Lapasaran, Alex Santa Ana	Learning the ethnonursing research methodology within the domain of Filipino elders residing in a nursing home in northern Nevada	2003
163	Le Balch, Deborah Lynn	Examining the role of ethnonursing research enablers	2003
164	Missal, Bernita Eileen	The Gulf Arab woman's transition to motherhood	2003
165	Ott, Renee Anne	Euro-American women substance abusers in an Alcoholics Anonymous program, their culture care needs	2003

	Name	Title	Year of Publication
166	Pasco, Alberta Catherine Ybalan	The experiences of Filipino-Canadian patients: "One of us" (hindi ibang tao) and "not one of us" (ibang tao)	2003
167	Schulling, Sharon Kay	Differences and similarities between Yup'ik generic care and professional nursing care: Implications for nursing education	2003
168	de Vera, Noemi Zabala	Saving women's lives by spacing births: A qualitative study	2004
169	Hunter, Linda M.	Traditional Aboriginal healing practices: An ethnographic approach	2004
170	Kagan, Paula Nadine	Feeling listened to: A lived experience of human becoming	2004
171	Kardong-Edgren, Suzan	Cultural competency of nursing and health education faculty	2004
172	Lenir Maria Baruffi	O cuidado cultural à mulher durante a gestação: uma contribuição para a humanização	2004
173	Morris, Edith J.	An ethnonursing culture care study of the meanings, expressions, and lifeways experiences of selected urban African American adolescent gang members	2004
174	Nailon, Regina Eileen Ruskamp	Expertise in the care of Latinos: An interpretive study of culturally congruent nursing practices in the emergency department	2004
175	Nolan, Pearline C.	Recently immigrated young adult Hispanic males' lived experience with drug addiction	2004
176	Sobralske, Mary C.	Health care seeking beliefs and behaviors of Mexican American men living in south central Washington	2004
177	Stinson, Lori Guenthner	An exploration of native nurse leadership: Stories "of the people"	2004
178	St-Onge, Maude	La difference culturelle du point de vue d'usagers participant a une demarche ergotherapique de maintien a domicile: Etude exploratoire	2004
179	Andress, Peggy B.	Culture care and the Northwestern Native Alaskan within their rural environmental context of Alaska	2005
180	Butler, Georgene A.	Protective factors associated with delayed sexual activity among urban African American females	2005
181	Gallagher, Martina	Child health promotion and health protection practices used by mothers of Mexican descent	2005
182	Gillespie, Marjorie May	HIV/AIDS-preventive behavior in recent-immigrant Jamaican women	2005
183	Johnson, Catherine Archibald	Understanding the culture care practices of rural immigrant Mexican women	2005

	Name	Title	Year of Publication
184	Kelsey, Beth Marie	Culture care values, beliefs, and practices of Mexican American migrant farm workers related to health promoting behaviors	2005
185	Lange, Bernadette M.	The Clarity-Parity Community Nursing Practice framework: A critical ethnonursing study of women in recovery from chemical dependence and their return to the community	2005
186	Marrone, Stephen Richard	Attitudes, subjective norms, and perceived behavioral control: Critical care nurses' intentions to provide culturally congruent care to Arab Muslims	2005
187	Mooney, Sharon Fish	Worldviews in conflict: A historical and sociological analysis of the controversy surrounding therapeutic touch in nursing	2005
188	Noble, Anita	Cultural competence and ethnic attitudes of Israeli midwives concerning Orthodox Jewish couples in labor and delivery	2005
189	Parucha, Grace Victoria G.	Barriers preventing registered nurses from accommodating the culture-specific health beliefs and practices of hospital patients	2005
190	Prince, Lola Mari	Culture care and resilience in minority women residing in a transitional home recovering from prostitution	2005
191	Robles, Melanie M.	Factors influencing treatment expectations for an upper respiratory infection in employed adults	2005
192	Schlickau, Jane M.	Prenatal breastfeeding education: An intervention for pregnant immigrant Hispanic women	2005
193	Smith, Shirley Ann Powe	Promoting the health needs of homeless women residing in a shelter in an urban community: A participatory action research study	2005
194	Vallee, Marie-Noelle	Etude sur les dimensions des competences culturelles des infirmieres qui interviennent dans la rencontre de soin avec des femmes immigrantes victimes de violence	2005
195	Wehbe-Alamah, Hiba	Generic and Professional Health Care Beliefs, Expressions and Practices of Syrian Muslims Living in the Midwestern United States	2005
196	Whitten, LaDonna Jean	Factors that influence the decisions of at-risk African American men to seek HIV testing	2005
197	Cantu, Adelita G.	Sociocultural context of physical activity in older Mexican American women: A life history approach	2006
198	Coleman, Jennifer Jeames	Culture care meanings, beliefs, lifeways, and care experiences of African American parents related to infant mortality and sleep positioning	2006

	Name	Title	Year of Publication
199	Pollard, Joy A.	Cognitive maps of women with coronary heart disease: Describing the content	2006
200	Pollard, Myrtle Denise	Meaning of maternal care giving and health perceptions in Ghana, West Africa: A visual ethnography	2006
201	Reif, Lu Ann Mary	Perceptions of health and health promotion behaviors and their meaning of Mexican-born men living in the United States	2006
202	Rife, Jill M.	Understanding heart disease in women: A focused ethnographic approach	2006
203	Schumacher, Gretchen	Culture care meanings, beliefs and practices of rural dominicans in a rural village of the Dominican Republic: An ethnonursing study conceptualized within the Culture Care Theory	2006
204	Pereira de Almeida, Shirley	A vivência no grupo: a experiência para as pessoas diabéticas	2006
205	Simmons, Bonnie J.	Understanding teen pregnancy through the younger sister's voice: A focused ethnography	2006
206	Witt, Diane	Growing old on the farm: An Ethnonursing examination of aging and health within the Agrarian rural subculture	2006
207	Yosef, Abdel-Raheem O.	Male Arab-Muslims health and health promotion perceptions and practices	2006
208	Yount, Susan Marie	Use of manzanilla tea during the childbearing period among women of Mexican origin who reside in the United States-Mexico border region	2006
209	Zammata, Pauline	Kulturella värden, tro, levnadssätt och livsstil	2006
210	Acharya, Manju Prava	Constructing cultural diversity: A study of framing clients and culture in a community health centre	2007
211	Alvarez, Emilia	Palliative care in multicultural communities: A phenomenological study exploring the lived experiences of nursing staff	2007
212	Camila Augusta dos Santos	Gravidez e Soropositividade para o HIV: vivências de mulheres atendidas em um centro de referência em HIV/AIDS	2007
213	Carlson, Sonja Birgitta	Children's voices about HIV/AIDS-related stigma in Uganda: A descriptive study of adolescents experiencing stigma	2007
214	Chuang, Yeu-Hui	Exploration of elderly residents' care needs in a Taiwanese nursing home: An ethnographic study	2007
215	Godbout, Pierre	Habilitation a l'autoprise en charge de sa sante, representations des infirmieres des soins a domicile	2007

	Name	Title	Year of Publication
216	Gunn, Jennie Ann Nause	Beliefs, meanings, and practices of healing with botanicals recalled by elder African American women in the Mississippi Delta	2007
217	Jasmine, Tayray	The elderly client's perception of caring behaviors	2007
218	Oliveira Fernandes, Maria Teresinha de	Trabalho com grupos na Saúde da Família: concepções, estrutura e estratégias para o cuidado transcultural	2007
219	Tyree, Elizabeth Maly	Culture care values, beliefs and practices observed in empowerment of American Indian community health representatives	2007
220	Aitken, R. L.	Internationalizing nursing education in Central Java, Indonesia: A postcolonial ethnography	2008
221	Brandao, Sandra Maria Oliveira Caixeiro	Vivência do acolhimento da mulher encaminhada da Casa de Parto David Capistrano Filho à unidade de referência	2008
222	Cataldi Flores, Gisela	Eu Cuido Dela E Ela Me Cuida: Um Estudo Qualitativo Sobre O Cuidado Intergeracional Com O Idoso	2008
223	deRuyter, Lana Marie	Culture care education and experiences of African American students in predominantly Euro American Associate Degree Nursing Programs	2008
224	Fabiane do Amaral Gubert	Report on dialogue of mothers about sexual and reproductive health with their adolescent daughters	2008
225	Feitoza, Aline Rodrigues	Elderly culture and its influence to HIV/Aids risk	2008
226	Fox-Kuhner, Susan	Cultural factors influencing prenatal care in the Amish	2008
227	Gagnon, Lissa	An exploration of nurse autonomy in cancer care	2008
228	Gonzalez-Guarda, Rosa Maria	Substance abuse, intimate partner violence and risk for HIV among a community sample of Hispanic women	2008
229	Harper, Mary G.	Evaluation of the antecedents of cultural competence	2008
230	Hartford, Lori Ann	Cultural perceptions of American Indian women in southcentral Montana regarding pre-diabetic education	2008
231	Johnson, Debra A.	Job satisfaction in the operating room: An analysis of the cultural competence of nurses	2008
232	Johnston, Mary Suzanne	Northern British Columbian mothers: Raising adolescents with Fetal Alcohol Spectrum Disorder	2008
233	Jovanovic, Maja	Cultural competency in hospice care: A case study of hospice Toronto	2008

	Name	Title	Year of Publication
234	KlÃvia Regina de Oliveira Saraiva	Obesidade infantil: a famãlia como unidade promotora da saãde	2008
235	Kokko, Raija	Aiming at culture conscious and tailored nursing	2008
236	Lee, Rebecca Crews	Culture care meanings, expressions, and lifeways of African American Appalachian and European American Appalachian mothers caring for their children in an urban homeless shelter	2008
237	Lima, Tatiane Cardoso de	Revelando o processo de recriação do banho no leito no cenário da terapia intensiva: produto da sustentabilidade da enfermagem em incorporar o conhecimento êmico a sua práxis	2008
238	Martin-Plank, Lorraine	A study of health care practices and health beliefs of Puerto Rican women in southeastern Pennsylvania	2008
239	Mixer, Sandra Jean	Nursing faculty care expressions, patterns, and practices related to teaching culture care	2008
240	Ribeiro Farias, Doris Helena	Vivências de cuidado da mulher: a voz das puérperas	2008
241	Srivastava, Rani H.	Influence of organizational factors on clinical cultural competence	2008
242	Bodin, Ida	Stödfaktorer av betydelse för flyktingar med psykisk ohälsa	2009
243	Bourbonnais, Anne	Les sens des cris de personnes âgées vivant avec une démence en centre d'hébergement et de soins de longue durée	2009
244	Bowles, Margaret	Culture care beliefs, meanings and practices related to health and well-being of South Sudanese "Lost Boy and Lost Girl" refugees	2009
245	Brito, Maria Eliane Maciel de	The influence of the familiar culture in the care of a child victim of burn	2009
246	Chao, Ying-Hua	A comparative study of the effects of a health care package on knowledge, attitudes and self-care behaviours in older Taiwanese aboriginal and non-aboriginal adults with type 2 diabetes in Taiwan	2009
247	Kgwatalala, Gomotsang	Health seeking behaviour among the people of the Africa Gospel Church in Francistown	2009
248	Knowles, Amy	"I am a Living History": A qualitative descriptive study of atomic bomb survivors	2009
249	Mdondolo, Nosipho	Cultural factors associated with management of a breast lump amongst Xhosa women	2009
250	Moulder, Maureen	Senior nursing student level of preparation, attitudes, awareness, and competence in ethnocare	2009

	Name	Title	Year of Publication
251	Santos, Alessandro Marques dos	Práticas de cuidado no cotidiano das famílias de mulheres que vivenciam o alcoolismo	2009
252	Souza, Adalbi C.	O itinerário terapêutico das famílias de crianças com diarréia	2009
253	Tegano, Sylvia	Configurations of site-based financial leadership practice within school contexts	2009
254	Addington, Andrea	Caring for refugees: Measuring cultural competence in nursing students	2010
255	Ahvenainen, Leena	Providing a good death: The importance of culturally sensitive end of life care in the acute ward setting	2010
256	Bell, Annalita Shireen	Exploring understandings and/or knowledge of maternity nurses in caring for immigrant/refugee women of African origin	2010
257	Böhmig, C.	Ghanaian nurses at a crossroads: Managing expectations on a medical ward	2010
258	Budd, Linda-Jennifer	Den röda tråden: en empirisk studie om barnmorskors kulturella kompetens i samband med vården av födande kvinnor från andra kulturer	2010
259	Gillum, Deborah R.	Cardiovascular knowledge, beliefs and healthcare practices of the Amish in Northern Indiana	2010
260	Höglund, Ida	Kulturella faktorer som påverkar sjuksköterskans omvårdnad av patienter med smärta	2010
261	Jackson, Everlyne Cosey	The influence of cultural beliefs and attitudes on the perceptions of health, body size, and health behaviors among over-weight and obese African American women	2010
262	McGee, Michèle	L'expérience de vieillir au quotidien de femmes âgées montré-alaises vivant seules à domicile dans un contexte de précarité économique	2010
263	Moss, Julie A.	Discovering the healthcare beliefs and practices of rural Mestizo Ecuadorians: An ethnonursing study	2010
264	Ntsaba, Mohlomi Jafta	The delivery of cultural care by health professionals among the hospitalized AmaXhosa male initiates of traditional circumcision in the Eastern Cape	2010
265	Ortiz-Morales, Hilda	A cultural analysis of Hispanic registered nurses' career selection: A quantitative descriptive study	2010
266	Pennafort, Viviane Peixoto dos Santos	Crianças E Adolescentes Em Tratamento Dialítico: Aproximações Com O Cuidado Cultural Da Enfermagem	2010

Name	Title	Year of Publication
267 Porrett, Theresa	Coping and help seeking behaviour in women with Pelvic Floor Dysfunction: The emic perspective	2010
268 Savage, Angela Ruth	Child vulnerability in the Iraqw and Datoga of Haydom village, northern Tanzania	2010
269 Schroeder, Amy	The health beliefs and practices of the Amish	2010
270 Scott, Korto L.	The development of cultural competence among community college nurses from the classroom to the work setting	2010
271 Scott, Shari Hughes	The impact of the father-daughter relationship on eating disorder treatment: A qualitative study	2010
272 Soyring, Jenikka	Barriers for Latinas in prevention and screening of cervical cancer: A literature review	2010
273 Wright, Pauline Rita	Care, culture, and education nursing students' perceptions of care and culture: Implications for practice	2010
274 Zajac, Lynne K.	The culture care meaning of comfort for ethnically diverse pre-licensure baccalaureate nursing students in the educational setting	2010
275 Alzoubi, Fatmeh Ahmad	Motherhood and childbirth experiences among newcomer women in Canada: A critical ethnographic study	2011
276 Amirehsani, Karen A.	Self-care expressions, patterns, and practices of Latinos/Hispanics for the management of type 2 diabetes	2011
277 Burke, Patricia M.	Cultural competency of associate degree nursing faculty	2011
278 Gaudreau, Sylvie	Facteurs culturels liés au maintien des comportements de santé chez des femmes algonquines ayant souffert de diabète gestationnel	2011
279 Gonçalves, Isménia de Fátima	A criança e a família em contexto muticultural	2011
280 Goonetilleke, Habaragamuwe Radalalage Ajith	Growing old amongst strangers and staying healthy, as experienced by elderly Sri Lankan immigrants living in Norway	2011
281 Hardy, Linda K.	Cultural competence and racist attitudes of direct patient care registered nurses in a Midwestern state	2011
282 Hascup, Valera A.	Cultural expressions, meanings, beliefs, and practices of Mexican American women during the postpartum period: An ethnonursing study	2011
283 Hemgren, Mia	Kulturmöten i vården	2011

	Name	Title	Year of Publication
284	Herranen, Juuli	Burmalaisten maahanmuuttajien kotoutumisen edistäminen	2011
285	Holland, Ann Elizabeth	The place of race in cultural nursing education: The experience of White BSN Nursing Faculty	2011
286	Howell, Mary Ellen	From darkness turning to light: A study of spirituality in homeless African American women	2011
287	Lizama, Tricia A.	How are traditional Chamoru healing practices being perpetuated and preserved in modern Guam: A phenomenological study	2011
288	Namora, Anabela Oliveira	Cuidar a criança / família oriunda dos Palop: a diferença na igualdade...	2011
289	Oliveira, Ana Sofia Matos Rodrigues de	Um olhar sobre a comunidade na perspectiva do centro de saúde e hospital	2011
290	Ramos Lafont, Claudia Patricia	Prácticas culturales de cuidado de gestantes indígenas que viven en el Resguardo Zenú ubicado en la Sabana de Córdoba	2011
291	Reneau, Margaret	Teaching nurses sight unseen: Comparing the cultural competency among on-campus and online baccalaureate degree nursing faculty	2011
292	Ruskeeniemi, Anna	Perheen hoitotyö Suomessa: Esite vuorovaikuksen tueksi	2011
293	Shviraga, Bonita Ann	A critical ethnographic study of the cultural values, beliefs, and practices of recently immigrated Mexican primiparas regarding infant feeding with a focus on exclusive breastfeeding	2011
294	Street, Darlene J.	Infant feeding attitudes, feeding method choice, and breastfeeding initiation among African American and Caucasian women	2011
295	Wünsch, Simone	Cuidado Em Saúde Nas Famílias Em Assentamento Rural: Um Olhar Da Enfermagem	2011
296	Adams, Theresa Mary Ann	The evaluation of service-learning as an innovative strategy to enhance BSN students' transcultural self-efficacy	2012
297	Bloch, Carol	Hispanic nurses' perception of pain assessment and management	2012
298	Bloch, Carolyn	Cultural competency intervention program for healthcare workers	2012
299	Chávez Alvarez, Rocío Elizabeth	O cuidado das crianças no processo saúde-doença: crenças, valores e práticas nas famílias da cultura kabano da amazônia peruana ; The care of children in the health-illness process: Beliefs, values and practices in the families of kabanos culture from the peruvian amazon	2012

	Name	Title	Year of Publication
300	Cregg, Wendy	Adult children's perceptions of critical caregiving conversations with their aging parents: A pilot study	2012
301	Embler, Pamela J.	End-of-life culture care expressions, meanings, patterns, and practices among Yup'ik Eskimo	2012
302	Furuhagen, Hanna	Att famla i blindo; Flying blind	2012
303	Gilmon, Margaret E.	Cultural diversity and the experiences of Alaska Native nursing students	2012
304	Gonçalves, Luís Miguel da Cunha	A pessoa em situação crítica e o cuidado de enfermagem transcultural	2012
305	Jones, Sharon M.	The development of trust in the nurse-patient relationship with hospitalized Mexican American patients	2012
306	MacDonald, Carla J.	Faculty leadership in baccalaureate study abroad programs: The relationship between faculty preparedness and intercultural competence	2012
307	Moreira da Silva, Marciele	Experiência Com O Diabetes Mellitus Tipo Ii Em Uma Comunidade Rural: Contribuições Para A Enfermagem	2012
308	Montufar, Raul	Rectal examinations and the Hispanic male	2012
309	Ribar, Alicia Kay	The Meaning and Experiences of Healthy Eating in Mexican American children: A focused ethnography	2012
310	Sullivan, Katherine L.	An ethnonursing study of the culture care values, beliefs and practices of new baccalaureate-prepared registered nurses regarding the primacy of an ethical commitment to the patient within a Magnet hospital	2012
311	Suomela, Melina	Kulttuurilähtöinen hoitotyö asiakkaan kohtaamisessa: Aikuisen somalipotilaan kipukäyttäytyminen	2012
312	Veräjänkorva, Irene	Women's health and health promotion in the Luo community of Omboga area in Kenya	2012
313	Wanchai, Ausanee	Care practices in complementary and alternative medicine in Thai breast cancer survivors	2012
314	Allen, Susan Roth	An ethnonursing study of the cultural meanings and practices of Clinical Nurse Council Leaders in Shared Governance	2013
315	Asakura, Yuki	Perceptions of future and advance care planning for Japanese women with early stage gynecological and breast cancer	2013

	Name	Title	Year of Publication
316	Brinkman, Mary Adams	A focused ethnography: Experiences of registered nurses transitioning to the operating room	2013
317	Burkett, Karen W.	Culture care meanings, expressions, and cultural lifeways of urban African American family members caring for their child with autism	2013
318	Caruth, Roger	Staying connected to home: The use of social media by the Howard University English-Speaking Caribbean Student Diaspora	2013
319	Castelblanco, Frank	Cultural bias education of Nursing Faculty	2013
320	Coleman, Jami-Sue	The lived experiences of acute-care bedside registered nurses caring for patients and their families with limited English proficiency	2013
321	Cortese-Peske, Marisa A.	Improving cultural competency and disease awareness among oncology nurses caring for adult T-cell leukemia and lymphoma patients	2013
322	Daly-Gordon, Edris	The effects of a cultural immersion on the cultural competence of student nurses	2013
323	Davy, Gloria Margaurita	Cultural understanding and interpretation of postpartum depression in a Caribbean immigrant community in the United States	2013
324	Edward, Jean S.	Understanding social determinants of healthcare access from the perspective of Hispanic Latino immigrants in Louisville, KY	2013
325	Ferranto, Mary Lou Gemma	An interpretive qualitative study of baccalaureate nursing students following an eight-day international cultural experience in Tanzania	2013
326	Gottlieb, Jeanne Chatham	Suffering in the midst of technology: The lived experience of an abnormal prenatal ultrasound	2013
327	Helin, Janine	Faktorer som inverkar på handhygienbeteenden i Etiopien	2013
328	Hernandez, Jesus A.	The struggle for balance: Culture care worldview of Mexican Americans about diabetes mellitus	2013
329	Huang, Liang-Guei	The patient and caregiver interaction of Vietnamese pregnancy women in Taiwan	2013
330	Imes, Helen Susan Berry	Discovering the culture care meanings and care expressions of men with a spinal cord injury from the Appalachian region of west Virginia: An ethnonursing study	2013
331	Jenkins, Olivia	Does use of culturally focused literature enhance cultural competence of nursing students?	2013

	Name	Title	Year of Publication
332	Muñoz Henríquez, Maribel	Significado de las prácticas de cuidado cultural de sí y de su hijo por nacer, de un grupo de gestantes adolescentes de Barranquilla	2013
333	Rogers, Laura M.	Opening the Black Box: Understanding adult inpatient falls	2013
334	Wolf, Kimberly M.	Somali immigrant perceptions of mental health and illness: An ethnonursing study	2013
335	Abdulrehman, Munib S.	Exploring cultural influences of self-management of diabetes in coastal Kenya	2014
336	Chiatti, Beth Desaretz	Culture care beliefs and practices of an Ethiopian immigrant community: An ethnonursing study	2014
337	Guerrero Camacho, Deysi Melissa	Caracteristicas de la consejería nutricional que brinda la enfermera a las amdres de niños entre 6 y 12 meses, desde la perspectiva transcultural en la microed los olivos 2013	2014
338	Nelson, Monica Marie	NICU culture of care for infants with Neonatal Abstinence Syndrome: A focused ethnography	2014
339	O'Harra, Pamela S.	Nursing students' lived experiences in learning communication skills in a theater class taught by theater faculty	2014
340	Okegbile, Elizabeth Oladayo	South Sudanese refugee women's healthcare access and use	2014
341	Olaivar, Oliver Kampitan	Transcultural self-efficacy perceptions of nurse practitioners in Fresno, California	2014
342	Rogers-Walker, Monique M.	Examining the relationship between participation in service-learning and the levels of transcultural self-efficacy reported by associate of science in nursing students	2014
343	Smith, Mikal	The experience of refugee women in a perinatal nutrition education program	2014
344	Strang, Cecily Weller	Discovery of the meanings, expressions, and practices related to malaria care among the Maasai	2014
345	Vandenberg, Helen	Concepts of culture, diversity and cultural care among undergraduate nursing students: A nursing education perspective	2014
346	Wolf, Sherry L.	Homeless young adults caring for their health	2014
347	Gerszbejn, Sharon	Kommunikation vid omvårdnad hos patienter med annan kultur	2015
348	Hussein, Abdul-Kadir	An examination of the care provided to Arab Muslim clients with type 2 diabetes receiving health care in Australia in order to expand our understanding of culturally congruent care	2015

	Name	Title	Year of Publication
349	Rousseau, Karen S.	An exploration of the culture care experiences of Puerto Rican families with a child with special health care needs as perceived by the family caregiver	2015
350	Grant, Ernest J.	Self-reported reasons for acting or not acting on safety recommendations taken by older black and white men who reside in North Carolina	2015
351	Sobon Sensor, Constance	Health-related beliefs, practices and experiences of migrant Dominicans in the northeastern United States	2015
352	Darden, Shavon	How are the dimensions of technology, culture, kinship, and economics and the experience of stress described by African American students who gained weight during their freshman year in college?	2015
353	Rakes, Valerie N.	Interprofessional Education: Implementation into curriculum	2016
354	Kalinowski, Maria	Nursing faculty's feelings of teaching cultural competence in the nursing education curriculum	2016
355	Sowicz, Timothy Joseph	Exploring sexual history taking in one health center: A focused ethnography	2016
356	Rodriguez, Luana	A Curriculum on culturally competent practices to prevent retraumatization in diverse survivors	2016
357	Fang, Dao Moua	Social-cultural, religious, and health system barriers to hepatitis B screening among Hmong: A case study	2016
358	Rahemi, Zahra	Iranian-American older adults' attitudes and proactive actions toward planning ahead for end-of-life care	2017
359	Nwamu, Anita	Barriers to healthcare: A phenomenological study of Nigerian immigrants	2017
360	Clarey-Sanford, Catherine M.	Unavoidable pressure ulcers: An ethnonursing study	2017
361	Scott, Thecly Hines	Perceptions of care during the prenatal period: An ethnonursing study of African American childbearing women in the Military Health System	2017

INDEX

Note: Page numbers followed by *f* or *t* refer to the page location of figures or tables, respectively.